Library of
Davidson College

VOID

Diseases of Amphibians and Reptiles

Diseases of Amphibians and Reptiles

Edited by
Gerald L. Hoff
Kansas City Health Department
Kansas City, Missouri

Frederic L. Frye
Veterinary Consultant
Davis, California

and

Elliott R. Jacobson
College of Veterinary Medicine
Gainesville, Florida

Plenum Press · New York and London

Library of Congress Cataloging in Publication Data

Main entry under title:

Diseases of amphibians and reptiles.

Includes bibliographical references and index.
1. Amphibians—Diseases. 2. Reptiles—Diseases. I. Hoff, Gerald L. (Gerald Lawrence), 1945-   . II. Frye, Frederic L. III. Jacobson, Elliott R., 1945-
SF997.5.A45D57   1984   639.3′760423   84-8385
ISBN 0-306-41711-1

©1984 Plenum Press, New York
A Division of Plenum Publishing Corporation
233 Spring Street, New York, N.Y. 10013

All rights reserved

No part of this book may be reproduced, stored in a retrieval system, or transmitted, in any form or by any means, electronic, mechanical, photocopying, microfilming, recording, or otherwise, without written permission from the Publisher

Printed in the United States of America

PREFACE

While diseases of free-ranging and captive mammalian and avian wildlife species have received considerable interest in the past 25 years, those of amphibians and reptiles (collectively, the herptiles) generally have been assigned lesser importance. The literature concerning disease in herptiles is widely scattered, consisting chiefly of case reports and prevalence surveys, and with heavy emphasis on captive reptiles. The dynamics of the host-agent-environment relationship have been studied for only a few diseases. This diverse data base is primarily a function of the paucity of investigators whose chief interest is in diseases of herptiles.

This first edition represents an effort to bring together some of the diffuse knowledge on infectious and non-infectious diseases of free-ranging and captive herptiles. Issue may be taken with the choice of topics; however, predominant diseases, as well as some diseases of lesser prominence, are presented. The editors were forced to accept certain omissions, particularly with amphibian diseases, simply for lack of contributors. The resulting text, however, we hope will be of value to veterinarians, herpetologists, wildlife disease investigators, wildlife managers, zoo curators, and university students.

G.L. Hoff
F.L. Frye
E.R. Jacobson

CONTENTS

Mycobacteriosis 1
    D.G. Brownstein

Pasteurella in Reptiles 25
    K.P. Snipes

Pseudomonas 37
    E.R. Jacobson

Areomonas 49
    E.B. Shotts, Jr.

Serratia 59
    G.L. Hoff

Salmonella and Arizona 69
    G.L Hoff and D.M. Hoff

Edwardsiella tarda 83
    F.H. White

Leptospirosis 93
    G.L. Hoff and F.H. White

Q Fever 101
    G.L. Hoff

Arboviruses 107
   K.F. Shortridge and A. Oya

Reptilian Rhabdoviruses 149
   C.B. Cropp

Herpesviruses of Reptiles 159
   G.L. Hoff and D.M. Hoff

Amphibian Chromomycosis 169
   R.E. Schmidt

Fungal Diseases in Reptiles 183
   G. Migaki, E.R. Jacobson, and
     H.W. Casey

Pentasomiasis 205
   G.E. Cosgrove, D.E. Deakins, and
     J.T. Self

Lungworms 213
   R.E. Brannian

Ascaridoid Nematodes 219
   J.F.A. Sprent

Platyhelminths 247
   D.R. Brooks

Non-hemoparasitic Protozoans 259
   W. Frank

Haemoparasites of Reptiles 385
   S.R. Telford, Jr.

Neoplasia in Reptiles 519
   S.V. Machotka, II

CONTENTS

Lucke Tumor of Frogs 581
    R.G. McKinnell

Physical Influences 607
    J.E. Cooper

Aging and Degenerative Diseases 625
    G.E. Cosgrove and M.P. Anderson

Nutritional Disorders in Reptiles 633
    F.L. Frye

Immunologic Aspects of Infectious Disease 661
    G.V. Kollias, Jr.

Resistance of Reptiles to Venoms 693
    V.P. Philpot, Jr. and R.L. Stjernholm

Euthanasia, Necropsy Techniques and
        Comparative Histology of Reptiles 703
    F.L. Frye

Contributors 757

Index 761

MYCOBACTERIOSIS

David G. Brownstein

School of Medicine

Yale University

INTRODUCTION

Mycobacteriosis of amphibians and reptiles is a group of infectious diseases caused by bacteria of the genus Mycobacterium. While insidious chronicity is the rule, peracute and acute cases occur; reflecting the heterogeneous biological behavior of the various mycobacterial species as well as the heterogeneity of host responses.

Mycobacteriosis is the oldest known infectious disease of amphibians and reptiles with a history dating back to the latter part of the nineteenth century. Seven years after Robert Koch isolated Mycobacterium tuberculosis in 1882, Sibley reported the first case of spontaneous mycobacteriosis in a poikilotherm (Sibley, 1889). The distinction went to a snake, Natrix natrix, necropsied at the London Zoological Society Gardens several months after its capture in Italy. It was not until 1905 that amphibian mycobacteriosis emerged with a report on hepatic mycobacteriosis in three frogs (Kuster, 1905). Until 1953, these sporadic reports were regarded as interesting novelties. However, with the recognition of human susceptibility to some of the mycobacteria isolated from poikilotherms and subsequent confirmation of their importance as human pathogens came a broader interest in mycobacteriosis of amphibians and reptiles (Marks and Schwabacher, 1965; Moore and Frerichs, 1953). Several recent reports have proposed herpeteofauna as reservoirs for mycobacteria of public health significance based on experimental evidence (Kazda and Hoyte, 1972; Marcus et al., 1975,1976). However, there has been no subsequent confirmation that reptiles or amphibians are true reservoirs for those mycobacteria of public health concern.

Mycobacteriosis has been most frequently reported among exhibited reptiles and amphibians as well as laboratory maintained amphibians utilized for research purposes. This reflects more diligent observation of confined specimens rather than a lack of spontaneous mycobacteriosis among free-living populations. When attention has been directed towards these free-living animals, mycobacteriosis has been identified as an enzootic disease, at least in amphibians. Such enzootics may be important modulators of population densities through the culling of debilitated individuals since some form of host impairment appears to be important in predisposing individuals to mycobacteriosis. Incidences as high as 20% have been reported for mycobacteriosis among South American anurans (Machicao and LaPlaca, 1954). In well managed captive populations of amphibians and reptiles, incidences of 0.1 to 0.5% have been reported (Brownstein, 1978; Griffith, 1939).

ETIOLOGY

Mycobacteriosis is caused by a ubiquitous and versatile group of bacteria belonging to the order Actinomycetales, gram-positive aerobic or facultatively anaerobic bacilli that tend to form filaments in culture. The members of the family Mycobacteriaceae are distinguished from other families within the order by a cell wall rich in lipids, arabinose, and galactose. The cell wall is resistant to decolorization by acidified organic solvents once stained by basic dyes.

Mycobacteria are ubiquitous within the environment and may be divided into obligate vertebrate parasites, obligate or accidental vertebrate commensals, and saprophytes. The parasitic forms include the agents of the classical mycobacterioses; tuberculosis (human, avian, bovine and vole), leprosy (human, armadillo and murine), and bovine paratuberculosis. In recent years, attention has been directed towards the commensal and saprophytic mycobacteria with the recognition that they are occasionally capable of initiating disease among vertebrates. It is these commensal and saprophytic mycobacteria that account for the majority of cases of mycobacteriosis in amphibians and reptiles. These usually innocuous mycobacteria generally have optimum growth at temperatures below those encountered within the bodies of higher vertebrates. It is, therefore, among the poikilotherms that they most frequently emerge as pathogens.

There are currently 26 mycobacterial species of accepted taxonomic status (Runyon et al., 1974b). As previously mentioned, seven of these species are primary pathogens of homeothermic vertebrates. The remaining 19 species include 6 species isolated from amphibians and reptiles with spontaneous mycobacteriosis. Several other mycobacteria are capable of inducing mycobacteriosis in amphibians and reptiles under experimental conditions, although their status as spontaneous pathogens is unknown. Mycobacterial pathogens of amphibians and reptiless are listed in Table 1.1.

Due to the low incidence of mycobacteriosis among captive populations of amphibians and reptiles, few investigations have encompassed sufficient cases to draw conclusions about the relative frequencey of mycobacterial isolates. The largest series of cases was reported by Griffith at the London Zoological Park (Griffith, 1939). Twenty of the 28 cases of mycobacteriosis of reptiles included in the report were caused by M. marinum with the remainder caused by M. chelonei and M. thamnopheos. However, among anurans, M. fortuitum (ranae, giae) has been most frequently reported (Darzins, 1952; Gonzales, 1938; Kuster, 1905).

The mycobacteria recovered from spontaneously diseased amphibians and reptiles represent 3 of the 4 Runyon groups used to characterize atypical mycobacteria (Runyon, 1970). The criteria used include growth rate and pigment production in culture. M. marinum, a group I slow growing photochromogen, is a ubiquitous inhabitant of fresh and salt water (Aronson, 1926; Linell and Norden, 1954). Epizootics among humans have been associated with aqueous environments from which M. marinum was isolated (Linell and Norden, 1954).

In contrast to M. marinum, M. xenopi, usually classified as a group III slow growing non-chromogen (actually a delayed scotochromogen), appears to have limited environmental distribution other than as a vertebrate commensal (Marks and Schwabacher, 1965; Runyon et al., 1974b). However, the presence of saprophytic sources is suggested by a report of M. xenopi isolated from water taps (Bullin et al., 1970). A second group III non-chromogen, M. avium, was recently isolated from a turtle and represents the first confirmed case of spontaneous mycobacteriosis

Table 1.1. Mycobacterium Species Reported to Produce Disease in Amphibians and Reptiles.

Mycobacterium Species	Category[a]	Reference
Amphibians		
M. fortuitum	1	Gonzales, 1938; Kuster, 1905
M. fortuitum	2	Darzins, 1952
M. fortuitum	3	Gonzales, 1938
M. marinum	1	Aronson, 1957; Shively et al., 1981
M. marinum	3	Clark and Shepard, 1963
M. thamnopheos	3	Aronson, 1929a
M. xenopi	1	Schwabacher, 1959
Reptiles		
M. avium	1	Thoen et al., 1977
M. avium	3	Griffith, 1941
M. chelonei	1	Friedmann, 1903; Griffith, 1939
M. fortuitum	3	Darzins, 1952; Gonzales, 1938
M. intracellulare	1	Friend and Russell, 1979
M. marinum	1	Griffith, 1919, 1939
M. marinum	3	Clark and Shepard, 1963
M. thamnopheos	1	Aronson, 1929a,b
M. thamnopheos	3	Aronson, 1929a
M. tuberculosis	3	Bertarelli, 1905; Sibley, 1892
M. ulcerans	3	Marcus et al., 1975; 1976

[a] 1=spontaneous disease among captive animals; 2=spontaneous disease among free-living animals; 3=experimentally induced disease

in a poikilotherm caused by the avian organism (Thoen et al., 1977). Oophidian susceptibility to experimental M. avium infection has been known since 1941 (Griffith, 1941). Early investigators had implicated avian sources for spontaneous mycobacteriosis among exhibited snakes, but cultural confirmation was lacking (Aronson, 1929b; Gibbes and Shurley, 1890).

M. fortuitum, M. chelonei (abscessus) and M. thamnopheos are rapid growers of Runyon group IV. Both M. fortuitum and M. chelonei have wide environmental distribution, being found in soil, dust and water and as vertebrate commensals and opportunistic pathogens (Darzins, 1952; Runyon et al., 1974; Smith, 1972). M. thamnopheos has only been recovered from reptiles with mycobacteriosis (Aronson, 1929a,b; Griffith, 1939). The status of M. thamnopheos as a legitimate member of the genus has been questioned on the basis of the small carbon skeleton of the cell wall mycolic acids which more closely resemble those of Nocardia (Lechevalier and Gerber, 1971). Indeed, M. thamnopheos is the least acid-fast of all the mycobacteria.

Several mycobacteria isolated from spontaneous cases in reptiles have not been given species status in the eighth edition of Bergey's Manual of Determinative Bacteriology. M. schlangen, a non-chromogen, caused disseminated mycobacteriosis in several snakes at the Berlin Aquarium (Rabinowitsch-Kempner, 1938). M. tropidonotus was recovered from several cases of oophidian mycobacteriosis at the London Zoological Park (Griffith, 1970).

PATHOGENESIS

The ubiquity of saprophytic and commensal mycobacteria and the generally low incidence of mycobacteriosis in amphibians and reptiles attests to the high degree of innate resistance possessed by these two classes of vertebrates. This is in contrast to the classical mycobacteriosis of higher vertebrates where pathological changes are the rule when host and bacterium interact. Disease production in amphibians and reptiles not only requires contact with these potential pathogens but also some form of host defense impairment to augment the infectious process (Reichenbach-Klinke and Elkan, 1965; Schwabacher, 1959).

Host impairment may include acid-fast bacillary access to tissues through breaches in surface epithelium and failure of specific and non-specific defense mechanisms to contain acid-fast bacilli in tissues. Disruption of epithelial barriers such as skin or respiratory or alimentary mucosa by physical, chemical, microbiological or nutritional injury may create a conduit for mycobacterial invasion. Cutaneous trauma is believed to be important in certain cases of atypical mycobacteriosis of man (Linell and Norden, 1954).

There is some evidence that surface epithelium may not be an effective mycobacterial barrier in normal hosts. In an experiment involving intragastric inoculation of Anolis carolinensis with M. ulcerans, 3 of 17 lizards became chronic hepatic carriers. Two of these lizards had identifiable acid-fast bacilli within the wall of intrahepatic bile ducts unaccompanied by pathological alterations. The authors concluded that ascending biliary infection accounted for the presence of acid-fast bacilli in the liver since M. ulcerans reaching the liver embolically produces a granulomatous response (Marcus et al., 1976). It therefore appears that, in certain apparently healthy individuals, some degree of host invasion does occur and that latent mycobacterial infections of the liver may not be uncommon. Alimentary (biliary) epithelium is not a barrier and bacterial progression is inhibited by other host factors. Other investigators have found a high incidence of chronic hepatic carriers among frogs, Rana temporarin, in an environment contaminated with M. intracellulare serotype Davis (Kazda and Hoyte, 1972).

Arguing against the activation of latent hepatic infections in the pathogenesis of mycobacteriosis are two observations: 1) acid-fast bacilli in the liver of cases of hepatic mycobacteriosis are not demonstrable outside granulomas, including intrahepatic bile ducts, and 2) a diligent search of the gastrointestinal tract in cases of hepatic mycobacteriosis will usually confirm the presence of micro- or macrotubercles, supporting hepatic portal embolization rather than ascending biliary infection as the source of acid-fast bacilli in the liver (Fig. 1.1). Such tubercles characteristically occur within the lamina propria of the small intestine beneath intact epithelium. Whether this represents invasion of intact epithelium or regenerated, previously disrupted epithelium is not known.

The skin and respiratory tract may also serve as portals of mycobacterial entry in amphibians and reptiles. Both of these portals have been implicated in chelonian mycobacteriosis (Friedmann, 1903; Rhodin and Anver, 1977). Cutaneous mycobacteriosis has been reported in Xenopus laevis infected with M. xenopi (Schwabacher, 1959).

There is no evidence that species susceptibility to mycobacteriosis exists among amphibians and reptiles although individual susceptibility certainly does occur. Current information based on experimentally produced mycobacteriosis suggests a broad host range for those mycobacteria isolated from spontaneously diseased amphibians and reptiles.

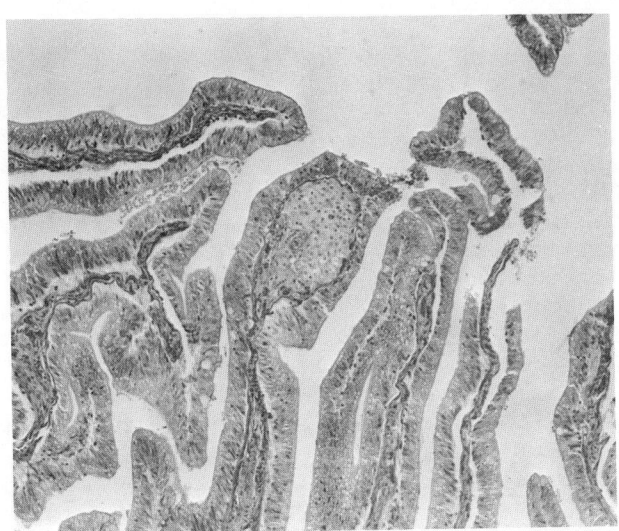

Fig. 1.1. Microtubercle in the lamina propria of a small intestinal villus from a snake with hepatic mycobacteriosis. H&E X100

TRANSMISSION

As a complex of diseases, poikilothermic mycobacteriosis exhibits a variety of transmission patterns. Contagion has not been a feature of reported cases in amphibians and reptiles, although it appears likely in certain epizootics among fish (Baker and Hagan, 1942; Besse, 1949; Winsor, 1946). More likely modes of transmission among amphibians and reptiles are contact with environmental sources. Infected insects have been implicated in alimentary mycobacteriosis of anurans (Machicao and LaPlaca, 1954). The importance of dietary sources of poikilothermic mycobacteriosis has been confirmed in salmon under intensive aquaculture (Wood and Ordal, 1958). When young fry and fingerlings are fed uncooked carcasses of adult salmon the incidence of mycobacteriosis approaches 100%.

The simultaneous isolation of mycobacteria from aquatic environments inhabited by amphibians and reptiles with spontaneous mycobacteriosis has been reported on several occasions (Darzins, 1952; Reichenbach-Klinke and Elkan, 1965; Schwabacher, 1959). The majority of cases of mycobacteriosis probably originate from contaminated water.

SIGNS AND PATHOLOGY

Mycobacteriosis of amphibians and reptiles may present as peracute, acute or chronic diseases. Peracute mycobacteriosis is strictly an experimental disease caused by parenterally administered rapidly growing mycobacteria of Runyon group IV (Aronson, 1929; Clark and Shepard, 1963; Gonzales, 1938). The disease is characterized by high acute mortality associated with massive intravascular proliferation of acid-fast bacilli and minimal host inflammatory response.

Acute mycobacteriosis is an uncommon disease in which bacterial proliferation is largely extracellular. The resulting inflammatory response is suppurative and therefore mimics both clinically and pathologically infections by more frequently encountered bacteria. This type of reaction is usually encountered in primary pulmonary infections of reptiles and nasopharyngeal infections of anurans (Machicao and LaPlaca, 1954). Reptiles with acute respiratory mycobacteriosis present with anorexia, depression, dyspnea and occasional rales. Gross necropsy findings include diffuse, edematous thickening of respiratory membranes and irregular, raised cream to yellow flocculent accumulations of exudate within the air sacs. Microscopically, the exudate is composed of heterophils infiltrating regions of caseous necrosis. Macrophages and fibroplasia are minimal. Within the inflammatory exudate are large numbers of extracellular acid-fast bacilli, measuring 1 to 10 microns, best demonstrated by Fite-Faraco method of acid-fast staining (Luna, 1968). Because this form of mycobacteriosis presents clinically and morphologically as an acute disease, the diagnosis is likely to be missed unless acid-fast stains are routinely performed on tissues with acute inflammatory reactions, especially lungs.

A variant of this acute type of inflammatory response was encountered by the author in the oviduct of a coachwhip snake, _Masticophis flagellum_, with chronic disseminated mycobacteriosis. There was an acute, diffuse necrotizing inflammation of the oviduct characterized by widespread inflammatory destruction of arteries and veins (Fig. 1.2). The vascular walls were edematous, indistinct and infiltrated with heterophils. Unlike the predominantly intracellular acid-fast bacilli that characterized the infection in other organs, those within the oviduct were extracellular. The association of acid-fast bacilli with necrotizing inflammation of arteries and veins has been described in erythema nodosum leprosum in leprosy patients

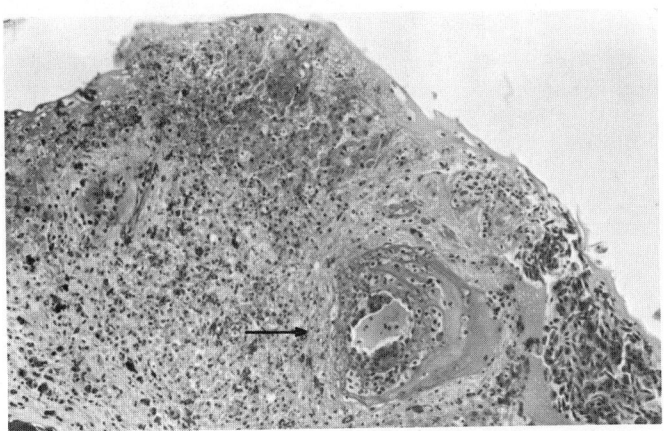

Fig. 1.2. Oviduct from a snake, Masticophis flagellum, with disseminated mycobacteriosis. Unlike the more typical granulomatous response, this acute response is characterized by vasculitis (arrow) and widespread tissue necrosis accompanied by massive extracellular proliferation of acid-fast bacilli. H&E X100

treated with sulfones (Wemambu et al., 1969). This side effect of leprosy therapy is believed to represent an Arthus reaction to mycobacterial antigens.

Anurans with acute nasopharyngeal mycobacteriosis usually have a cararrhal or suppurative nasal discharge with large numbers of extracellular acid-fast bacilli (Machicao and LaPlaca, 1954).

Chronic mycobacteriosis is the most frequent form of mycobacteriosis in amphibians and reptiles. The hallmark of this form of infection is granulamatous inflammation with tubercle formation. Like mammalian and avian tubercles, the tubercles of amphibians and reptiles undergo sequential changes as the tubercles age. However, there are a number of differences between tubercles of poikilotherms and those of mammals and birds.

The earliest event in spontaneous amphibian and reptilian tubercle formation is the accumulation of a compact nest of macrophages in various states of activation (Fig. 1.3 upper left). The macrophages are plump, polyhedral with distinct plasma membranes and abundant pink, often foamy cytoplasm. The vesicular nuclei are oval or indented and nucleoli are indistinct. Acid-fast bacilli are intracellular at this stage and have a slightly beaded appearance (Fig. 1.3 upper right).

These small nests of macrophages begin to expand to form a more complex tubercle in which the central area of activated macrophages becomes surrounded by a zone of spindle-shaped histiocytes and reticulin producing spindle cells (Fig. 1.3 lower left). Within this marginal zone are numerous heterophils with globular eosinophilic granules (Fig. 1.3 lower right). These granules are moderately acid-fast when stained with Fite-Faraco or Ziehl-Neelsen stains. Many of the activated macrophages are epithelioid at this stage having large vesicular oval nuclei with prominent nucleoli. Mycobacteria are still intracellular at this stage.

Central caseation marks the third stage of tubercle development (Fig. 1.4 left). There is some fibroplasia and a mild lymphoid infiltrate within the marginal zone. A feature of the central caseation that distinguishes it from mammalian and avian caseation is its acid-fastness. While acid-fast caseation is a nuisance when attempting to identify acid-fast bacilli within these foci, it may also be an important clue to the pathogenesis of caseation in amphibians and reptiles. Heterophil granules, as previously mentioned, are acid-fast and these cells are conspicuous in tubercles. They are often numerous at the margins of areas undergoing caseation and can be found in various stages of disruption within caseous foci (Fig. 1.4 left, insert). The presence of acid-fast heterophil granules within these acid-fast caseous centers suggests a role for heterophils as mediators of caseation in . amphiibians and reptiles. This is in contrast to caseation in mammalian and possibly avian tuberculosis where delayed type hypersensitivity is believed to initiate caseation through cytotoxic effects of sensitized thymus derived lymphocytes or the release of enzymes from macrophages stimulated by sensitized lymphocytes. Different mechanisms for caseation may explain the relative dearth of lymphocytes in the marginal zones of amphibian and reptilian tubercles when compared to the profusion of lymphocytes that usually infiltrate mammalian and avian tubercles.

The final stage of tubercle formation is characterized by expansion of the caseous region to involve the entire tubercle with obliteration of the tubercle architecture and often confluence with adjacent tubercles (Fig. 1.4 right). With the progression of caseation large numbers of extracellular acid-fast bacilli appear (Fig.

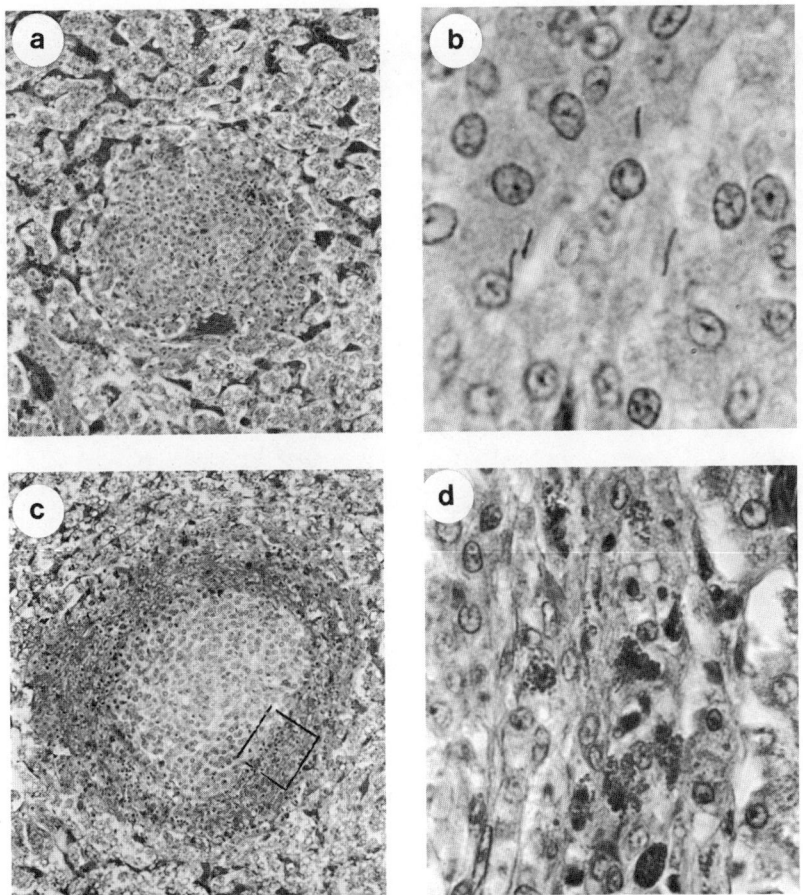

Fig. 1.3. Pre-caseous stages of reptilian tubercle formation.
Upper left. Compact nest of activated macrophages. H&E X100
Upper right. Intracellular acid-fast bacilli. Ziehl-Neelsen X1024
Lower left. Expanding tubercule with margin of spindle shaped histiocytes, reticulum cells and heterophils. Square denotes field covered in photo on lower right. H&E X100
Lower right. Marginal zone showing spindle cells and heterophils with globular eosinophilic granules. H&E X512

1.4 right, insert). These bacilli are usually more beaded than those located intracellularly. Whether this irregular carbol-fuchsin staining represents reduced

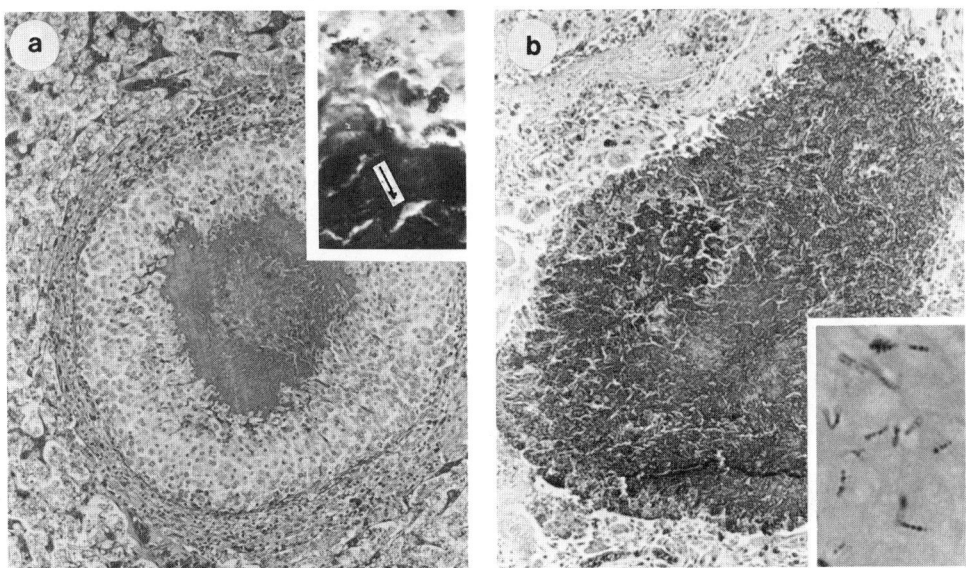

Fig. 1.4. Caseous stages of reptilian tubercle formation. Left. Central caseation. H&E X100 Insert-- Caseous margin demonstrating acid-fast staining of central caseation and incorporation of acid-fast heterophil granules at the margin and in the center (arrow). Ziehl-Neelsen X512 Right. Predominately caseous lesion. Tubercle architecture has been obliterated. H&E X40 Insert--Extracellular acid-fast bacilli in caseous tubercle. The organisms are more beaded-appearing than the intracellular bacilli. Ziehl-Neelsen X1024

viability, as has been proposed for the leprosy bacillus (McFadzean and Valentine, 1960), or other differences produced by extracellular versus intracellular growth is not known.

The gross morbid appearance of chronic mycobacteriosis is that of disseminated granulaomatosis with varying of caseation. The most frequently encountered form in amphibians and reptiles is hepatosplenic mycobacteriosis of alimentary origin. Affected individuals generally present with non-specific signs that include anorexia and cachexia. Occasional individuals die with no premonitory signs. The normal liver architecture is effaced by multiple, discrete cream to yellow nodules measuring up to one

centimeter in diameter. These nodules bulge above the
capsular surface and are easily enucleated. On sectioning,
these nodules may be homogeneous or have varying degrees
of central caseation. Tubercles are found throughout the
hepatic parenchyma (Fig. 1.5). Livers which are heavily
pigmented with melanin will often release significant
quantities in severe cases of mycobacteriosis
(Reichenbach-Klinke and Elkan, 1965). The released
melanin is subsequently taken up by the proximal uriniferous tubules. A second hepatic pigment, hemosiderin,
also may be released in cases of mycobacteriosis and
Accumulate in the kidneys. Hemosiderin, unlike melanin,
is deposited along the glomerular basal lamina.

The spleen is generally enlarged and contains superficial and deep tubercles similar to those described for
the liver. Although grossly visible gastrointestinal
tubercles are uncommon in reptiles with hepatosplenic
mycobacteriosis of alimentary origin, they are a common
finding in amphibians. The serosal surface of the
intestines and the mesentery of amphibian cases is often
studded with discrete tubercles. There is generally less
tendency for caseation in amphibian mycobacteriosis than
in reptiles and the formation of massive sarcomatous
masses composed of epithelioid cells is not uncommon.

Most cases of alimentary mycobacteriosis are not confined to hepatosplenic tubercles produced by bacillary
embolization from the portal vein. Attainment of the
systemic circulation also occurs relatively early in the

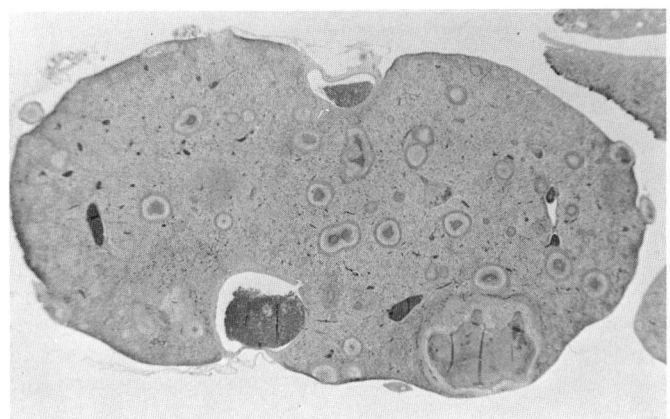

Fig. 1.5. Hepatic mycobacteriosis in a snake, having
tubercles in all stages of development. H&E X6

course of the disease, resulting in tubercles in a variety of organs. Generally these secondary tubercles are not as exuberant as those of the liver and spleen. Kidneys, fat bodies, gonads, heart and mediastinum are commonly affected in amphibians. Lung, bone and central nervous system are usually spared. Secondary sites of mycobacteriosis in reptiles frequently include bone, lungs and subcutis. Osseous localization in reptiles is often dramatic due to the destructive nature of the lesion (Fig. 1.6). Extensive osteolysis results from an expanding mass of fibrovascular tissue, rich in mycobacteria-laden macrophages. Concurrently, there is usually periosteal new bone formation. These foci of osteomyelitis most frequently occur within vertebrae by expansion of areas of mycobacterial disconspondylitis. Such lesions may dominate the clinical signs by producing pathological fractures resulting in central or peripheral nerve dysfunction. These osseous lesions are frequent enough in reptilian cases to warrant survey radiographs of suspected cases even in the absence of neurologic disorders. Mycobacterial osteomyelitis in chelonians frequently develops in the plastron or carapace (Besse, 1949; Scott, 1930) and should be easily recognized radiographically.

Secondary pulmonary tubercles of reptiles tend to be much more caseating than tubercles of parenchymous organs. Like osseous mycobacteriosis, mycobacterial pneumonia may dominate the clinical signs by producing severe dyspnea.

Secondary subcutaneous localization frequently occurs in snakes. These generally present as firm, well circumscribed swellings of the neck over which the skin is freely movable. These swellings may approach the size of a hen's egg although most are less than 5 cm. Subcutaneous tubercles must be distinguished from swellings produced by parasites, neoplasms and bacterial infection.

Primary chronic cutaneous mycobacteriosis is frequent in anurans and has been reported in turtles (Rhodin and Anver, 1977). This form is characterized by well circumscribed dermal indurations which gradually expand to form fungating lesions. Cutaneous mycobacteriosis rarely disseminates in amphibians, in part, due to the the relatively early death resulting from loss of cutaneous osmoregulation. Dissemination of primary cutaneous mycobacteriosis has been reported in a terrapin, _Phrynops hilari_, which developed secondary hepatosplenic tubercles (Rhodin and Anver, 1977). A tendency for mycobacteria to invade dermal nerve fibers has been reported in some

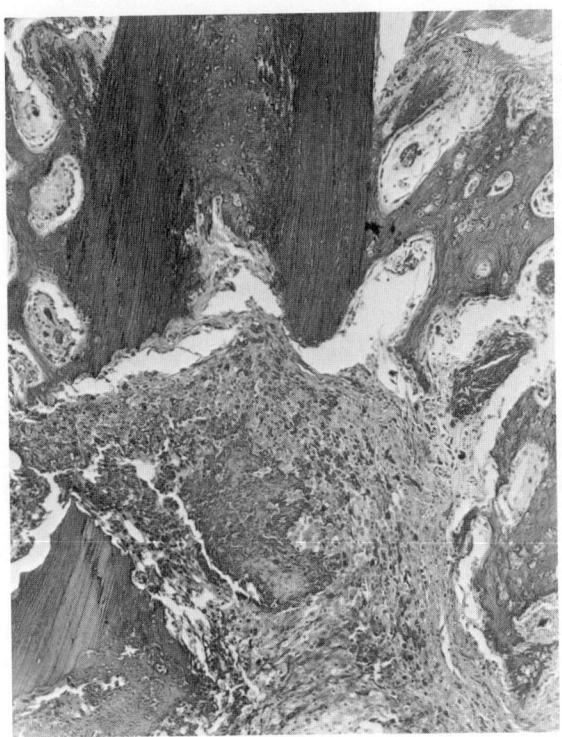

Fig. 1.6. Mycobacterial spondylitis in a snake. Both osteolysis and reactive new bone formation are occurring. H&E X40

cases of cutaneous mycobacteriosis (Machicao and LaPlaca, 1954).

Primary chronic respiratory mycobacteriosis is uncommon but has been described in turtles (Friedmann, 1903) and anurans (Darzins, 1952; Reichenbach-Klinke and Elkan, 1965). Restlessness, dyspnea and anorexia were described in the chelonian cases, caused by severe caseating, cavitating pulmonary lesions. Anuran cases are much less caseating than reptilian cases and usually consist of homogeneous gray to white nodules scattered throughout the air spaces, usually near the carina. Because of the anuran capacity for cutaneous respiration, pulmonary tubercles may be extensive before signs appear.

DIAGNOSIS

A definitive antemortem diagnosis of mycobacteriosis is currently practical only when there is cutaneous, subcutaneous or nasopharyngeal involvement. However, a high degree of suspicion should be generated by the combination of a chronic, debilitative disease accompanied by radiographic evidence of focal osteolytic lesions in reptiles.

The gross necropsy findings in disseminated mycobacteriosis are usually characteristic, but must be distinguished from other causes of disseminated granulomatosis. Due to the relatively primitive nature of the poikilotherm inflammatory response a broader spectrum of agents are capable of eliciting a granulomatous response when compared with higher vertebrates. Therefore, the differential diagnosis must include mycoses, distomiasis, larval cestodiasis, larval helminthiasis and botryomycotic reactions to a variety of gram-positive and gram-negative bacteria. Chronic infections with Escherichia coli (coligranuloma) and Pseudomonas aeruginosa commonly produce granulomatous responses in amphibians and reptiles.

Histopathologically, mycobacterial granulomas can be distinguished from parasitic, non-acid-fast bacterial and mycotic granulomas. Unlike tubercles, parasitic granulomas tend to be large and asymmetrical. Instead of having homogeneous caseous centers, the centers of parasitic granulomas usually consist of concentric lamellae which often calcify. The centers of mycobacterial granulomas rarely calcify. There is also a prominent connective tissue capsule surrounding parasitic granulomas. Mycotic granulomas can usually be distinguished from mycobacterial granulomas by the presence of giant cells. Botryomycotic reactions are usually most difficult to distinguish since the granuloma may closely resemble that of mycobacteriosis. The acid-fast stain is often the only way to make the diagnosis morphologically, but care must be exercised that over decolorization of mycobacteria does not occur. Generally, more heterophils infiltrate botryomycotic than mycobacterial granulomas. Because acid-fastness is not confined to bacteria of the genus Mycobacterium bacterial isolation is essential to confirm a diagnosis.

The isolation of mycobacteria from tissues or exudates of amphibians and reptiles requires careful control of contaminating organisms. Decontaminating agents are useful in this respect but care must be used to optimize their effectiveness. These agents are bacteriacidal and excessive treatment of tissues exudates can adversely affect mycobacterial viability as well as that of contaminating microorganisms. The concentration and duration of treatment will depend on the site of infection, whether the material is ante- or post-mortem and, in the latter case, the postmortem interval. Generally, fresh necropsy material from parenchymous organs, such as liver and spleen, does not require decontamination. Ulcerated cutaneous lesions from animals dead for several hours should be decontaminated.

Decontaminating agents are divided into alkalies and surface-active agents. The latter are more effective in maintaining mycobacterial viability. Specifics on decontaminating techniques can be found in most clinical microbiology texts (Runyon et al., 1974).

Tubed or bottle egg media, such as Lowenstein-Jensen, are preferable for primary mycobacterial isolation. Cultures obtained from amphibian or reptilian sources should be sealed and incubated at several temperatures (24, 32, 37 and 45 C). Runyon group IV rapid growers will appear within one week while groups I, II and III require at least a week and as long as six weeks to be visible.

The classification of mycobacteria is based on growth rate, temperature requirements, colony morphology, pigment production and specific biochemical reactions. These characteristics are briefly listed in Table 1.2.

TREATMENT AND CONTROL

Mycobacteriosis occurs when two prerequisites are met, host contact with potentially pathogenic mycobacteria and host debility. Control, therefore, must be directed at reducing environmental sources and maintaining colony health. Most captive amphibians and reptiles are exposed to mycobacteria through water. Slime within water dishes or other aquatic media is especially high in saprophytic mycobacteria. Spigots are also potentially rich sources of mycobacteria. Mechanical removal of organic films is the single most effective means of reducing mycobacterial populations.

Mycobacteria are resistant to most commonly used disinfectants. They resist chlorine at concentrations of 0.7 micrograms free chlorine per milliliter (Carson et al., 1978). Concentrations of aqueous formaldehyde

Table 1.2. Characteristics of *Mycobacterium* Producing Disease in Amphibians and Reptiles.

	avium	xenopi	marinum	chelonei	fortuitum	thamnopheos
Growth rate	Slow	Slow	Slow	Rapid	Rapid	Rapid
Growth temp. (C)	25-45	40-45	25-35	22-40	22-40	25-32
Pigment	P[a]-late	S[b]-late	P	-	-	-
Urease	-	-	+	+	-	-
Catalase	-	-	-	+	+	+
Tween 80 hydrolysis (5 day)	-	-	+	-	-	+
Arylsulfatase	-	+	+/-	+	+/-	-
Tellurite	+/-	-	-	+/-	+/-	-
Iron uptake	-	-	-	-	+/-	+
Growth on MacConkey agar	-	-	-	+	+	-

[a]photochromogen
[b]scotochromogen

that readily inactivate gram-negative bacteria are not effective in eliminating saprophytic mycobacteria (Katz et al., 1976). Several investigators have reported on the effectiveness of 2% alkaline glutaraldehyde in disinfecting hospital equipment contaminated with saprophytic mycobacteria (Collins and Montalbine, 1976; Miner et al., 1977).

Attention also should be directed at dietary sources of mycobacteria. Almost any invertebrate or lower vertebrate food source may be heavily contaminated or infected with mycobacteria. Several zoological parks routinely sample poikilotherms used as food animals to reduce the incidence of distomiasis and larval cestodiasis among valuable reptiles. Such sampling could include a search for evidence of mycobacteriosis.

There are no reports on the treatment of amphibians or reptiles with mycobacteriosis. Antibiotic sensitivity of the atypical mycobacteria varies widely. The group IV rapid growers tend to be highly resistant to most antituberculous drugs. M. xenopi, on the other hand, is usually sensitive to the antituberculous drugs including: rifampin, streptomycin, ethambutol, isoniazid, cycloserine and para-aminosalicylic acid (Beck and Stanford, 1968). M. marinum is resistant to isoniazid and para-aminosalicylic acid but sensitive to rifampin, ethambutol, ethionamide, cycloserine and kanamycin (Banerjee and Holmes, 1976; Leach and Fenner, 1954; Rynearson et al., 1971; Silcox and David, 1971). The toxicity of the various antituberculous drugs has not been evaluated in amphibians or reptiles.

REFERENCES

Aronson, J.D., 1926, Spontaneous tuberculosis in salt water fish, J. Infect. Dis., 39:315-320.
Aronson, J.D., 1929a, Spontaneous tuberculosis in snakes. Arch. Pathol., 8:159.
Aronson, J.D., 1929b, Spontaneous tuberculosis in snakes; n. sp. Mycobacterium, J. Infect. Dis., 44:215-223.
Aronson, J.D., 1957, Tuberculosis of cold blooded animals, Leprosy Briefs, 8:21-24.
Baker, J.A., and Hagan, W.A., 1942, Tuberculosis of the Mexican platyfish, J. Infect. Dis., 70:248-252.
Banerjee, D.K., and Holmes, I.B., 1976, In vitro and in vivo studies of the action of rifampicin, clofazimine and B1912 on Mycobacterium marinum, Chemotherapy, 22:242-247.

Beck, A., and Stanford, J.L., 1968, Mycobacterium xenopei: A study of sixteen strains, Tubercle, 49:226-321.

Berarelli, E., 1905, Einige untersuchungen uber die tuberkulose der reptilien, Zentralbl. Bakteriol. Parasitenkd., 38:403-408.

Besse, P., 1949, Epizootic a bacilles acid-resitants chez des poissons exotiques, Bull. Acad. Vet. Fr., 22:151-154.

Brownstein, D.G., 1978, Reptilian mycobacteriosis, in: "Mycobacterial infections of zoo animals," R.J. Montali, ed., Smithsonian Institution Press, Washington.

Bullin, C.H., Tanner, E.I., and Collins, C.H., 1970, Isolation of Mycobacterium xenopei from water taps, J. Hyg., 68:97-100.

Carson, L.A., Petersen, N.J., Favero, M.S., and Aguero, S.M., 1978. Growth characteristics of atypical mycobacteria in water and their comparative resistance to disinfectants. Appl. Environ. Microbiol., 36:839-846.

Clark, H.F., and Shepard, C.C., 1963, Effect of environmental temperature on infection with Mycobacterium marinum (balnei) of mice and a number of poikilothermic species, J. Bacteriol., 86:1057-1069.

Collins, F.M., and Montalbine, V., 1976, Mycobacteriacidal activity of glutaraldehyde solutions, J. Clin. Microbiol., 4:408-412.

Darzins, E., 1952, The epizootic of tuberculosis among the Gias bahia, Acta Tuberc. Scandinav., 26:170-174.

Friedmann, F.F., 1903, Spontaner lungentuberkulose bei schildkroten und die stellung des tuberkelbazilus in system, Zeitschr. f. Tuberk, u. Heilstattenw., 4:439-457.

Friend, S.C.E., and Russell, E.G., 1979, Mycobacterium intracellulare infection in a water monitor, J. Wildlife Dis., 15:229-233.

Gibbes, H., and Shurly, E.L., 1890, An investigation into the etiology of phthisis. V. Tubercle peritonitis, Amer. J. Med. Sci., 100:145-158.

Gonzales, L.M., 1938, Tuberculosis in a frog, Puerto Rico J. Public Health Trop. Med., 13:399-412.

Griffith, A.S., 1928, Tuberculosis in captive wild animal, J. Hyg., 28:198-218.

Griffith, A.S., 1939, Infections of wild animals with tubercle bacilli and other acid-fast bacilli, Proc. Royal Soc. Med., 32:1405-1412.

Griffith, A.S., 1941, The susceptibility of the water (or grass) snake (Tropidonotus natrix) to the avian tubercle bacillus and to reptilian strains of acid-fast bacilli, J. Hyg., 41:284-288.
Griffith, A.S., 1970, Tuberculosis in cold-blooded animals, A System of Bacteriology in Relation to Medicine, 5:326-332.
Katz, D., Laney, H., Linquist, J.A., and Persike, E.C., 1976, Formaldehyde disinfection to eliminate bacterial contamination of deionizers, Dialy. Transplant, 5:42-44.
Kazda, J., and Hoyte, R., 1972, Zur okologie von Mycobacterium intracellulare serotype Davis. Zentralbl. Bakteriol. Hyg., I. Abt. Orig. A, 222:506-509.
Kuster, E., 1905, Uber kaltblutertuberculose, Munchen med. Wchnschr., 52:57-59.
Leach, R.H., and Fenner, F., 1954, Studies of Mycobacterium ulcerans and Mycobacterium balnei. III. Growth in the semi-synthetic media of Dubos and drug sensitivity in vitro and in vivo. Australian J. Exp. Biol., 32:835-841.
Lechevalier, H.A., and Gerber, N.N., 1971, Chemical composition as a criterion in the classification of Actinomycetes, Adv. Appl. Microbiol., 14:47-72.
Linell, L., and Norden, A., 1954, Mycobacterium balnei: A new acid-fast bacillus occurring in swimming pools and capable of producing skin lesions in humans, Acta Tuberc. Pneumol. Scand. Suppl., 33:1-84.
Luna, L.G., 1968, "Manual of histologic staining methods of the Armed Forces Institute of Pathology," McGraw-Hill, New York.
Machicao, N., and LaPlaca, E., 1954, Lepra-like granulomas in frogs, Lab. Invest., 3:219-227.
Marcus, L.C., Stottmeier, K.D., and Morrow, R.H., 1975, Experimental infection of anole lizards (Anolis carolinensis) with Mycobacterium ulcerans by the subcutaneous route, Amer. J. Trop. Med. Hyg., 24:649-651.
Marcus, L.C., Stottmeier, K.D., and Morrow, R.H., 1976, Experimental alimentary infection of the anole lizard (Anolis carolinensis) with Mycobacterium ulcerans, Amer. J. Trop. Med. Hyg., 25:630-632.
Marks, J., and Schwabacher, H., 1965, Infection due to Mycobacterium xenopei, British Med. J. 1:32-33.
McFadzean, J.A., and Valentine, R.C., 1960, The examination and determination of the viability of Mycobacterium leprae by electron microscopy, Leprosy Rev., 31:6-14.

Miner, N.A, McDowell, J.W., Willcockson, G.W., Bruckner, N.I., Stark, R.L., and Whitmore, E.J., 1977, Antimicrobial and other properties of a new stabilized alkaline glutaraldehyde disinfectant sterilizer, Amer. J. Hosp. Pharm., 34:376-382.

Moore, M., and Frerichs, J.B., An unusual acid-fast infection of the knee with subcutaneous, abscess-like lesions of the gluteal region, J. Invest. Dermatol., 20:133-169.

Rabinowitsch-Kempner, L., 1938, Tuberculosis of cold-blooded animals, in: "The mycobacterial diseases," F.R. Moulton, ed., Amer. Ass. Adv. Sci., Washington.

Reichenbach-Klinke, H., and Elkan, E., 1965, "The principle diseases of lower vertebrates," Academic Press, New York.

Rhodin, A.G., and Anver, M.R., 1977, Mycobacteriosis in turtles: Cutaneous and hepatosplenic involvement in a Phrynops hilari, J. Wildlife Dis., 13:180-183.

Runyon, E.H., 1970, Identification of mycobacterial pathogens utilizing colony characteristics, Amer. J. Clin. Pathol., 54:578:586.

Runyon, E.H., Karlson, A.G., Kubica, G.P., and Wayne, L.G., 1974a, Mycobacterium, in: "Manual of clinical microbiology," 2nd ed., E.H. Lennette, E.H. Spaulding and J.P. Truant, eds., Amer. Soc. Microbiol., Washington.

Runyon, E.H., Wayne, L.G., and Kubica, G.P., 1974b, Mycobacteriaceae, in: "Bergey's manual of determinative bacteriology," 8th ed., B.E. Buchanan and N.E. Gibbons, eds., William and Wilkins Co., Baltimore.

Rynearson, T.K., Shronts, J.S., and Wolinsky, E., 1971, Rifampin: In vitro effect on atypical mycobacteria, Amer. Rev. Respir. Dis., 104:272-278.

Schwabacher, H., 1959, A strain of Mycobacterium isolated from skin lesions of a cold-blooded animal, Xenopus laevis, and its relation to atypical acid-fast bacilli occurring in man, J. Hyg., 57:57-67.

Scott, H.H., 1930, "Tuberculosis in man and lower animals," Med. Res. Council Sp. Report, His Majesty's Stationary Office, London.

Shevely, J.N., Songer, J.G., Prchal, S., Keasey, M.S., and Thoen, C.O., 1981, Mycobacterium marinum infection in Bufonidae, J. Wildlife Dis., 17:3-7.

Sibley, W.K., 1889, Uber tuberkulose bei wirbelthieren, Arch. f. Pathol. Anat., 116:104-115.

Sibley, W.K., 1892, Inoculated tuberculosis in snakes, Trans. Pathol. Soc. London, 53:430-436.
Smith, D.T., 1972, Other species of mycobacteria, in: "Zinsser microbiology," W.K. Joklik and D.T. Smith, eds., Meredith Corp., New York.
Thoen, C.O., Richards, W.D., and Jarnagin, J.L., 1977, Mycobacteria isolated from exotic animals, J. Amer. Vet. Med. Ass., 170:987-990.
Wemambu, S.N., Turk, J.L., Waters, M.F., and Rees, R.J., 1969, Erythema nodosum leprosum: A clinical manifestation of the Arthus phenomenon, Lancet, 2:933.
Winsor, H., 1946, Cold-blooded tuberculosis from the Fairmount Park Aquarium, Proc. Pennsylvania Acad. Sci., 20:43-46.
Wood, J.W., and Ordal, E.J., 1958, Tuberculosis in Pacific salmon and steelhead trout, Oregon Fish Comm., 25:1-38.

PASTEURELLA IN REPTILES

        Kurt P. Snipes

        School of Veterinary Medicine

        University of California

INTRODUCTION

    For many years pasteurellosis has been recognized as a significant infectious disease in domestic ruminants and fowl, as well as free-flying fowl. The two species of this bacterium most frequently associated with disease are Pasteurella multocida and P. haemolytica. Clinical signs in mammals and birds have included those characteristic of pneumonia, hemorrhagic septicemia and mastitis.

    This chapter will focus primarily on P. testudinis, a recently described species isolated from desert tortoises, Gopherus agassizi. Information in the literature concerning the recovery of other species of Pasteurella from reptiles has consisted primarily of isolated case reports which have not entered into great detail regarding the nature of the infection or the particular species involved.

    Reports of Pasteurella isolations from reptiles are relatively recent, but evidence is accumulating that implicates bacteria of this genus as potential pathogens of poikilotherms. Reichenbach-Klinke (1966) noted that Newsom and Cross recovered P. haemolytica from cases of ulcerative stomatitis in reptile collections. Unfortunately, a detailed account of the biochemical identification and the pathology pertaining to these isolations was not provided. Pneumonia in reptiles due to Pasteurella has been postulated to occur afer aspiration of exudate into the respiratory system resulting from similar cases of stomatititis (Frye, 1977).

Pasteurella spp. are included in a list compiled by Wallach (1969), listing gram-negative bacteria which are found in specific infections (non-mixed) in reptiles. Henricksen and Graham (1972) reported Pseudomonas spp. and Proteus spp. to be the most common bacterial disease agents in turtles and tortoises, followed by other less common offenders, including Pasteurella spp., Escherichia coli and Erysipelothrix insidiosa. These bacteria are stated to cause similar disease syndromes, which may manifest themselves as gastroenteritis, diarrhea, constipation, anorexia or pneumonia. Terminal septicemic forms of these syndromes may arise, leading to depression and death. Wallach (1971) felt that certain non-specific infections in captive reptiles may be due to opportunistic organisms, e.g., Pseudomonas or Proteus, attacking stressed or debilitated animals. As will be discussed later, this may very well be true of more specific infections due to Pasteurella.

A case of P. multocida associated pneumonia was reported in Alligator mississippiensis in the "Alligator Gardens" in San Antonio, Texas (Mainster et al., 1973). P. multocida was cultured from a pneumonic lung noted upon necropsy of an alligator that died following foreign body penetration of the stomach which resulted in peritonitis. Many of the other alligators in the enclosure had begun to cough and sneeze, with some demonstrating mucopurulent discharge from their nares. Results of nasal cultures from these animals were not given.

Pasteurella, among many other genera of bacteria, has been isolated from reptilian and amphibian abscesses (Frye, 1977). It has been recovered from a middle ear abscess in a tortoise and from multiple abscesses of another tortoise (Mayer and Frank, 1974). P. testudinis and P. haemolytica were cultured from axillary abscesses in a desert tortoise, G. agassizi (Snipes, 1978).

P. testudinis has been reported to be associated with apparently stress-induced pneumonia in captive desert tortoises (Fowler, 1977; Snipes, 1978). This bacterium was found in various clinical samples, i.e., oral swabs, cloacal swabs and respiratory cultures, obtained from healthy as well as clinically ill tortoises. It has been isolated from the mouth and trachea of free-ranging tortoises in the Mojave Desert in California. Tracheal washes and lung culture of moribund captive tortoises demonstrating respiratory pathology consistently yielded P. testudinis as well as a variety of other bacteria. Experimental exposure of healthy tortoises to this particular bacterium produced equivocal results. One case of ulcerative stomatitis in a non-experimentally exposed animal progressed to osteomyelitis with necrotizing tracts extending to the brain. P. testudinis, Proteus and other bacteria were isolated from the tracts, pneumonic lung and trachea.

DISTRIBUTION

The genus Pasteurella is worldwide in geographic distribution. P. multocida and P. haemolytica have been reported from all parts of the world while P. ureae has been found in Europe, Africa and North America (Biberstein, 1978). P. testudinis, a newly described species, thus far has been reported only from tortoises in California. Many of the previous reports from Europe and the United States of Pasteurella infections in reptiles have not discussed the particular species encountered. Pasteurellosis has been noted in reptile collections and in general reptilian bacterial surveys. Specific reports to date have been limited to turtles, tortoises and alligators.

ETIOLOGY

Members of the genus Pasteurella are gram-negative pleomorphic bacteria which are non-motile, fermentative, and catalase and oxidase positive. The basic biochemical tests used to differentiate species of Pasteurella are indole production, urease activity, beta-galactosidase activity, growth on MacConkey agar and hemolysis on beef or sheep blood agar. Pasteurella spp. utilize carbohydrates by fermentation. In general, there is variability between strains of the different species of Pasteurella regarding their ability to ferment various carbohydrates tested. The bacteria are readily isolated on sheep blood agar incubated aerobically for 24 to 48 hours. Pasteurella spp. appear to possess capsule-like suface layers as evidenced by colony appearance, serologic reactivity and stained impression smears of the bacterium in tissues.

P. testudinis, P. multocida and P. haemolytica are highly virulent when inoculated intraperitoneally into mice. The LD_{50} of P. testudinis roughly approximates that of P. haemolytica when inoculated intraperitoneally. P. testudinis also is virulent when inoculated intranasally into laboratory mice.

TRANSMISSION

Pasteurella spp. are found principally on the mucous membranes of the cranial ends of the respiratory and alimentary tracts of their hosts. Colonization of mucus membranes of new hosts occurs mainly via inhalation or ingestion (Biberstein, 1978). *P. testudinis* in desert tortoises is similary disseminated. Additionally, in tortoises, isolation of *P. testudinis* is not uncommon from the cloaca. Deposit of nasal or stomatitic exudate containing *P. testudinis* in the environment could certainly provide a focus for exposure.

Indirect transmission via formites or animal products is a theoretical possibility, but in reptiles these methods probably do not play a major role in disease transmission. Pasteurellas are not particularly adept at surviving in the external environment for extended periods of time, probably not enduring over three weeks. It has been noted that survival times in nature for *P. multocida* can be extended when the organisms are supported by animal carcasses or excretions (Titche and Snipes, 1978).

In desert tortoises, *P. testudinis* appears to be part of the normal flora. In experiments exposing healthy tortoises to clinically ill tortoises shedding *P. testudinis* in nasal exudate, transmission of clinical disease did not occur. At this time it is believed that respiratory disease in captive desert tortoises is primarily stress-related, possibly involving the *Pasteurella* found in many tortoises. The possibility of predisposing or concomitant viral infection contributing to the respiratory disease observed also must be considered. Viral isolation in conjunction with the bacterial surveys has not been attempted, nor have any electron microscopic studies of the respiratory epithelium of clinically ill tortoises been carried out. It appears unlikely that epizootics in the wild involving *P. testudinis* and desert tortoises would occur. However there is the possibility of a particular strain increasing in virulence in a debilitated host and then somehow being transmitted to other tortoises. This phenomenon could possibly occur in winter dens where the tortoises might occasionally gather to hibernate and while their immune systems are depressed. As yet, respiratory epizootics have not been reported in free-ranging desert tortoises, nor have any tortoises from the wild been reported displaying clinical signs of respiratory disease.

PATHOGENESIS

It has been postulated that respiratory problems arising in desert tortoises are not solely due to an infectious agent, e.g., Pasteurella, but rather that decreased resistance of the tortoise due to stress predisposes the animal to infection by normal bacterial flora (Fowler, 1977). A desert tortoise when removed from its natural habitat and placed in captivity is subjected to a variety of potentially detrimental conditions. Among these conditions are: temperature extremes, improper humidity, inability to burrow, photoperiod discrepancies and malnutrition. Malnutrition is a definite problem in many captive tortoises and is probably the chief offender in the extrinsic stress category. Intrinsic stress related changes occur when an animal is prevented from responding to stress in its natural behavioral manner over an extended period of time. Excessive adrenal steroid hormones that are secreted in response to the stress can actually have deleterious effects. This is known to occur in mammals (Fowler, 1978) and it would no doubt also be true in reptiles. Some deleterious changes assumed to be the result of stress as noted by Fowler (1977) are:

1. changes in blood leukocyte cell counts which decrease the host's ability to combat infection;
2. interference with and dampening of the immune response;
3. poor wound healing; and
4. behavioral changes, e.g., refusal of food, increased aggression and failure to exhibit normal reproductive response.

Conclusive documentation of these changes has not been reported in tortoises given corticosteroids, however the above alterations certainly could apply to the problems seen in tortoises with chronic respiratory infection. Once the lungs become inflamed, removal of exudate and drainage of debris through the narrow and tortuous respiratory tract is difficult (Fowler, 1977; Frye, 1977). The tortoise's respiratory tract is composed of a series of small sacs connected by narrow "bronchioles" easily occluded by inflammatory debris. As the accumulation of debris progresses, a chronic situation is established.

It is apparent that captivity may impose many deleterious changes in the life of a captive desert tortoise. These changes may lower the resistance of the tortoise, possibly allowing a normal bacterial inhabitant of that tortoise to become opportunistic, resulting in respiratory disease.

SIGNS AND PATHOLOGY

Clinical signs of respiratory disease in reptiles consist of listlessness and anorexia, purulent nasal discharge and dyspnea. The eyes and their adnexae may become inflammed. These signs are consistent with those observed in tortoises suffering from respiratory disease which harbor P. testudinis. Alligators suffering from P. multocida associated pneumonia demonstrated similar signs (Mainster et al., 1973).

P. haemolytica and Pasteurella spp. have been reported to be associated with ulcerative stomatitis in reptiles (Reichenbach-Klinke, 1966; Wallach, 1971). Signs of stomatitis in reptiles include anorexia, oral mucosal ulcerations, gingeval edema and cloudy oral mucus containing clumps of caseous material (Burke, 1978). P. testudinis has been isolated from a desert tortoise demonstrating severe ulcerative stomatitis with extensive fistulous tracts extending into the hard palate.

P. haemolytica, P. testudinis and Pasteurella spp. have been recovered from abscesses from a variety of locations in reptiles, including subcutaneously in the axillary region and the middle ear.

Naturally infected captive desert tortoises which displayed clinical signs of respiratory disease and harbored P. testudinis in nasal exudates usually revealed evidence of chronic pneumonia upon necropsy. Bronchial involvement was inconsistent. The pneumonia observed was characterized as pyogranulomatous, multifocal and moderate to severe. Gross pulmonary pathology consisted of areas of dark red, patchy, pneumonic-like parenchyma. Histopathologically, lung sections displayed multiple focal to diffuse inflammatory lesions consisting of heterophil leukocytic and mixed mononuclear cell infiltrates subjacent to the respiratory epithelium. Exudate was usually observed within pulmonary air spaces. Gram stained smears of lung tissue revealed gram-negative bacterial rods. However, recovery of P. testudinis did not always occur when specimens of lung tissue were submitted to culture.

A suppurative or pyogranulomatous, multifocal, severe hepatitis sometimes has been observed in tortoises with pulmonary pathology but no correlation can be inferred at this point. On histopathology, these lesions resemble those observed in the lungs. Evidence of chronic starvation, i.e., serous atrophy of fat, often was revealed in some of these naturally infected pneumonic tortoises. Occasionally the spleen was enlarged two to three times its normal size.

In desert tortoises experimentally exposed to P. testudinis via intratracheal inoculations, granulomatous, multifocal, severe broncho-pneumonia was observed. Gross pathologic findings included grossly inflamed, firm, consolidated lungs. Histopathologically, pulmonary tissues contained multiple pyogranulomatous inflammatory lesions and mixed leukocytic infiltration throughout the submucosal connective tissue, particularly adjacent to mainstem bronchi and larger bronchioles. Well developed granulomata with multinucleated giant cells were seen. Direct smears of lung tissue revealed gram-negative rods, but culture failed to retrieve these bacteria.

In some of the experimental tortoises, a pale, mottled, yellow-grey liver was seen upon necropsy. Histopathologic examination revealed a suppurative, focal and generally mild hepatitis. Also occasionally observed upon histopathologic examination of various tissues was multifocal, suppurative interstital and/or glomerular nephritis. In some cases small gram-negative rods were observed from impression smears of liver but culture was negative.

Captive desert tortoises experimentally inoculated with P. testudinis intratracheally and receiving adrenal corticosteroid hormone, revealed lungs with patchy red fields, some consolidation and occasionally caseous debris in the hilar portions. Stained impression smears of lung tissue usually demonstrated short gram-negative rods. Cultures were negative. Quite often the liver was pale pink-grey with accentuated lobular pattern and quite friable. Histopathologically, these experimental tortoises revealed multifocal suppurative inflammatory lesions (heterophilic and mixed mononuclear leukocytic infliltrations) in the liver, pancreas, kidney, myocardium and lung. This would appear to reflect septicemia during the recent past history of the tortoises, and possibly may reflect the markedly reduced immune response due to administration of the potent adrenal corticosteroids. Respiratory lesions observed in the group receiving bacteria plus steroids were essentially the same as those in tortoises exposed only to bacteria.

DIAGNOSIS

In tortoises dying of apparently stress-related respiratory disease, P. testudinis has been cultured from affected lung tissue and trachea. This is true also of Pasteurella associated pneumonias in other reptiles. In cases of Pasteurella associated ulcerative stomatitis, the organism may be recovered from swabs of the inflamed lesions. Isolation of Pasteurella from these clinical samples can be made by simply streaking the material on conventional sheep blood agar plates and incubating at either 37 C or room temperature. Increased CO_2 tension (10%) may enhance growth in some cases. Biochemical and other criteria used for identification of the bacterium as P. testudinis have been mentioned previously.

PROGNOSIS AND TREATMENT

If the aforementioned stressors, presumably allowing a commensal P. testudinis to become pathogenic and predisposing a desert tortoise to respiratory disease, are eliminated early in the course of the pneumonia while clinical signs are mild, the prognosis is favorable. On the other hand, if the condition is allowed to smolder over an extended period of time and become chronic, the tortoise will have great difficulty in overcoming the problem. This will be aggravated by the anatomy of the respiratory tract and the passiveness of expiration.

As with general prognosis, a direct correlation exists between the extent and chronicity of pneumonia on one hand, and the efficacy of treatment on the other. Treatment of pneumonia in tortoises, other than stressor elimination, aimed at P. testudinis should consist of systemic bactericidal antibiotics, vitamin B-complex, vitamin A and perhaps aerosolized gentamicin or similar bactericidal antibiotic. Potential renal toxicity must be considered when aminoglycoside antibiotics are used. Aerosol therapy with antibiotic diluted in normal saline or a wetting agent appears to be an important part of this treatment, if for no reason other than to induce drainage of respiratory debris. Moistening of inspissated inflammatory debris lodged in the narrow passageways of the tortoise's lower respiratory tract might allow it to be broken up and transported to the exterior for elimination. This increased drainage will hypothetically expel infectious agents along with other debris once the pathway is clear for the normal defense mechanisms of the animal to become operative. Dosages for respiratory therapeutics in tortoises for P. testudinis are given in Table 2.1.

Table 2.1. Respiratory Theraputics for _Pasteurella testudinis_ in Tortoises.

Theraputic Agent	Dosage	Duration
Ampicillin (injectable)	20 mg/kg b.i.d. intra-coelomically	7 to 9 days
Gentamicin	10 mg/kg every 48 hours intramuscularly (I.M.) (Frye, 1981)	Up to 8 days, then abstain 1 week before resumption if necessary
Gentamicin	10 to 20 mg/15 cc normal saline b.i.d. nebulized for 30 minutes	Persistence of clinical signs
Vitamin A	50,000 I.U. every 2 weeks I.M.	Persistence of clinical signs
Vitamin D_3	7,500 I.U. every 2 weeks I.M.	Persistence of clinical signs
Vitamin B-complex	Pyridonxine hydrochloride 2 mg Thiamine hydrochloride 1 mg Ribovlavin 2 mg Panthenol 5 mg Nicotinamide 10 mg every 2 weeks I.M.	

IMMUNITY AND CONTROL

In domestic mammals, effective immunizing procedures exist for the prevention of hemorrhagic septicemia due to Pasteurella utilizing a bacterin containing critical surface antigens (Biberstein, 1978). Bacterins are currently avavailable for use in domestic fowl which have been reported to provide immunity against the homologous P. multocida (Biberstein, 1978). However, attempts at immunizing against other forms of pasteurellosis have met with much less success. For example, no effective immunizing agent has been developed yet for the various pneumonic pasteurelloses in domestic livestock.

The state of the art of immunizing against Pasteurella is not complete in domestic mammals and birds, much less in captive reptiles. If pneumonia in desert tortoises is indeed due to P. testudinis, much more work is required on the antigenic structure of the bacterium before attempts at bacterin production could be conducted. Since many zoos and private reptile collections possess tortoises and other reptiles prone to succumbing to chronic respiratory disease, such a bacterin might provide useful in preventing this problem in the future. Reptiles are capable of producing immune responses against complex antigenic components associated with infectious agents (See chapter 26).

Regarding endangered free-ranging desert tortoises, immunization against pneumonia would be valuable in situations where large numbers of them were brought together and confined, and therefore stressed for the purpose of relocation to other areas of desert not at carrying capacity. Currently, a reptilian version of shipping fever erupts when this is attempted.

Control of potentially P. testudinis related pneumonia is best effected by avoiding the stressors which apparently precipitate the problem. Providing the reptile with its native habitat and climate or a reasonable approximation will usually prevent this commensal bacterium from exhibiting it potential pathogenicity. If the pneumonia does arise, antibiotics will partially assist in resolution.

REFERENCES

Biberstein, E.L., 1978, The pasteurelloses, in: "Handbook of zoonoses," J. Steele, ed., CRC Press, Boca Raton.

Burke, T.J., 1978, Infectious diseases of reptiles, in: "Zoo and wild animal medicine," M.E. Fowler, ed., W.B. Saunders Co., Philadelphia.

Fowler, M.E., 1977, Respiratory disease in desert tortoises, Amer. Ass. Zoo Vet. Ann. Proc., 1977:79-99.

Fowler, M.E., 1978, "Wild and domestic animal restraint," Iowa State University Press, Ames.

Frye, F.L., 1977, Bacterial and fungal diseases of captive reptiles, in: "Current veterinary therapy VI," R.W. Kirk, ed., W.B. Saunders Co., Philadelphia.

Frye, F.L., 1981, "Biomedical and surgical aspects of captive reptile husbandry," V.M. Publ. Co., Bonner Springs.

Henriksen, P., and Graham, D.L., 1972, Diagnosis and treatment of disease in the turtle, Iowa State Univ. Vet., 34:29-32.

Holt, P.E., and Cooper, J.E., 1976, Stomatitis in the Greek tortoise (Testudo graeca), Vet. Rec., 98:156.

Mainster, M.E., Lund, F.T., Cragg, P.C., and Karger, J., 1973, Treatment of multiple cases of P. multocida and staphlococcal pneumonia in Alligator mississippiensis on a herd basis, Amer. Ass. Zoo Vet. Ann. Proc., 1973:33-36.

Mayer, H., and Frank, W., 1974, Bacteriological investigations on reptiles and amphibians, Zentralbl. Bakteriol. Hyg. Abt. I Orig. A, 229:470-481.

Reichenbach-Klinke, H., and Elkan, E., 1966, "The principle diseases of lower vertebrates," Academic Press, New York.

Snipes, K.P., 1978, Respiratory disease in captive desert tortoises (Gopherus agassizi): Investigation of bacterial role and characterization of possible agent involved, M.S. Thesis, Univ. California, Davis.

Titche, A., and Snipes, K.P., 1978, Unpublished data, Dept. Med., School of Vet. Med., Univ. California, Davis.

Wallach, J.D., 1969, Medical care of reptiles, J. Amer. Vet. Med. Ass., 155:1017-1034.

Wallach, J.D., 1971, Diseases of reptiles and their clinical management, in: "Current veterinary therapy IV," R.W. Kirk, ed., W.B. Saunders Co., Philadelphia.

PSEUDOMONAS

Elliott R. Jacobson

College of Veterinary Medicine

University of Florida, Gainsville

INTRODUCTION

Organisms of the genus Pseudomonas are mostly free-living bacteria which are widely distributed in the soil and water. At least four species are considered potential pathogens and are associated with diseases in man and animals: P. aeruginosa, P. maltophila, P. pseudomallei and P. mallei (Carter, 1973). Additional species have been associated with reptilian diseases. Since there is a strong feeling that a normally functioning immune system protects against colonization with Pseudomonas it is not surprising that these microorganisms are important pathogens for the immunocompromised reptile. Captive squamates are more commonly affected than other reptilian orders with the oral cavity, respiratory system and integumentary system most often involved.

ETIOLOGY

Organisms of the genus Pseudomonas are aerobic (except for those species which can use denitrification as a means of anaerobic respiration), non-spore forming, gram-negative rods. Pseudomonads exhibit respiratory metabolism, never fermentative metabolism. They are catalase positive, oxidase positive (except P. maltophila) and split sugars by oxidation. Some strains produce water soluble yellow-green fluorescent pigments, whereas others, in addition, can synthesize a variety of type specific phenazine pigments; still others are non-pigmented (Davis et al., 1973).

With the exception of P. mallei, all species are motile by means of one or more polar flagella (Buxton and Frazer, 1977).

HISTORY AND DISTRIBUTION

Squamata

Patrick and Werkman (1930) isolated P. jaegeri, P. smaragdina, P. viscosa and P. puris from snakes suffering from a condition which resembled typhoid. Subsequently P. fluorescens liquefaciens was described by Burtscher (1931) as being the causative agent of an ulcerative stomatitis in snakes that he called "Mouth Rot" or "Mundfaule". Caldwell and Ryerson (1940) isolated a new pseudomonad species, P. reptilovorus, which was considered pathogenic for horned lizards, Phrynosoma solare, Gila monsters, Heloderma suspectum, and chuckawallas, Sauromalus obesus. All of nine horned lizards inoculated intraperitoneally with a suspension of organisms died within 48 hours. Autopsy findings included hemorrhagic areas in the serosa of the stomach, congested and hemorrhagic lungs and hemorrhage at the site of inoculation. Although Page (1961; 1966) isolated P. aeruginosa from several cases of ophidian ulcerative stomatitis, Aeromonas hydrophila was considered the most significant pathogen in his study. Pseudomonas spp. have been commonly isolated from the oral cavity of a variety of clinically healthy snakes (Ledbetter and Kutscher, 1969; Parrish et al., 1956).

Gray et al. (1966) found that one of the two major causes of death among reptiles at the National Zoological Park was a necrotizing enteritis from which P. aeruginosa was consistently cultured. Keydar et al. (1971) found that Palestine vipers, Vipera xanthina palestinae, suffered 80% mortality from infection with P. aeruginosa. Cooper (1973) cultured Pseudomonas, Aeromonas and Proteus from African snakes suffering from ulcerative stomatitis. A Pseudomonas respiratory disease was described from a rainbow boa, Epicrates cenchris (Levy, 1974). Pseudomonas spp. were isolated from 23 of 127 snakes which died of a septicemic disease in an East African snake farm (Cooper and Leakey, 1976). The lung and liver were the organs most severely affected. Although Pseudomonas was suspected of being the causative agent of a fatal endemic infection of fer-de-lances, Bothrops atrox, in a serpentarium in Switzerland, lung suspensions of affected snakes injected into embryonic eggs resulted in the isolation and identification of a paramyxovirus as the etiologic agent (Folsch and Leloup, 1976). Murphy and Armstrong (1978) reported isolation of P. aeruginosa, in addition to other microorganisms, from swellings on the heads of four crotalid species at the Dallas zoo. The same authors reported the isolation of P. aeruginosa as well as Corynebacterium xerosis, Staphylococcus spp., Streptococcus spp. and Citrobacter freundii from a necrotizing dermatitis in a Crotalus mitchelli pyrrhus. Additional cases of Pseudomonas spp. isolated from reptiles submitted to the Veterinary Medical Teaching Hospital, University of Florida, are presented in Table 3.1.

Chelonia

The only reports of Pseudomonas spp. associated with chelonian disease are the data of Dieterich (1967) collected from necropsy specimens and that of Jacobson (1978) who identified Pseudomonas spp. in lung washings of a box turtle, Terrapene carolina, that was suffering from a respiratory disease. Pseudomonas was isolated also from a lung washing of a gopher tortoise, Gopherus polyphemus, suffering from respiratory disease; from pericardial fluid aspirated from a gopher tortoise with a severe pericarditis; and, from the oral cavity of a chicken turtle, Deirochelys reticularia, with ulcerative stomatitis (Jacobson, unpublished data).

TRANSMISSION, SIGNS AND PATHOLOGY

As stated above, the genus Pseudomonas is ubiquitous in nature being found in soil and water. Captive reptiles would be expected to be challenged constantly with these microorganisms, especially in natural exhibits where bacteria would tend to accumulate in the substrate. In addition, Pseudomonas spp. are commonly isolated from the oral cavity (Ledbetter and Kutscher, 1969; Parrish et al., 1956) and intestinal tract (Jacobson, unpublished data) of healthy squamates and thus can be considered part of the normal flora. Disease results from an interplay of factors that tend to simultaneously increase the virulence of the microorganism and immunosuppress the host.

Environmental conditions, nutritional status of the host and traumatic injury to tissues are all important factors which may influence the initiation of a lesion and the course of disease. Each reptile species tends to have a preferred temperature range that in the wild is maintained by behavioral and physiological mechanisms (Benedict and Dawson, 1979). Below optimum environmental

Table 3.1. Pseudomonas spp. Isolated from Reptiles, University of Florida, College of Veterinary Medicine, 1977-1980.

Species	Pseudomonas sp.	Lesion: Localization/Characterization
Anolis carolinensis	aeruginosa	Palpebrae, orbital adnexal structures
Dipsosaurus dorsalis	aeruginosa	Periconjunctival abscess
Tiliqua gigas	aeruginosa	Dermatitis, coelomic mass
Eublepharis macularis	undetermined	Ulcerative stomatitis
Elaphe subocularis	aeruginosa	Ulcerative stomatitis
Constrictor constrictor	maltophila	Respiratory disease: tracheal wash cultured
	cepacia fluorescens	Ulcerative stomatitis
Python m. molurus	aeruginosa	Ulcerative stomatitis
Python m. bivittatus	fluorescens cepacia	Respiratory disease: tracheal wash cultured
	fluorescens cepacia	Dermatitis
Python regius	fluorescens aeruginosa	Dermatitis
Python reticulatus	aeruginosa	Systemic infection: lung, kidney and small intestine
Terrapene carolina	undetermined	Respiratory disease: tracheal wash cultured
Gopherus polyphemus	cepacia	Respiratory disease: tracheal wash cultured
	fluorescens aeruginosa	Pericarditis: pericardial fluid cultured
Deirochelys reticularia	cepacia fluorescens	Ulcerative stomatitis

conditions in captivity may lead to a depressed humoral immune system (Evans, 1963) which may predispose to invasion by opportunistic pathogens. Thus it would not be surprising to find an increased incidence of Pseudomonas oral disease and respiratory disease in reptiles maintained at suboptimum environmental temperatures. Trauma to oral mucous membranes also predisposes to infection. Cooper

and Leakey (1976) found a higher incidence of infection
in mambas, Dendroaspis angusticeps, D. jamesoni and
D. polylepis, that were milked for venom compared to those
not milked. The stress of venom extraction was considered
to be a contributing factor. Recently imported reptiles
suffering from a combination of problems including oral
and skin abrasions resulting from attempts at escaping
confinement, poor nutritional status and dehydration,
are all excellent candidates for a bacterial stomatitis
and subsequent systemic disease. It is only logical to
expect that the immune status of these animals would be
at a suboptimum level, allowing invasion by opportunistic
pathogens. Thus, a high incidence of Pseudomonas stomatitis and septicemias would be expected and indeed is found
in recently imported reptiles.

P. aeruginosa colonizes 60% of human burn patients
by the fifth day after the burn (Dogget, 1979). The
clinical syndrome is referred to as invasive burn wound
sepsis and two cases including sepsis in a Burmese python,
Python molurus bivittatus, and a boa constrictor,
Constrictor constrictor, followed burning of the integument
by improper use of electrical heating pads within the
cages of these snakes (Jacobson, unpublished data).

There are no clinical signs specific for Pseudomonas
infection except for the cases in which a pigmented stain
imparts a specific yellow-green color and characteristically fruity odor to the involved tissues. Squamates suffering from ulcerative stomatitis may show a gaping of the
mouth in the area involved. The involved mucous membranes
are often edematous with petechial hemorrhages and
necrosis. Chronic involvement is seen as progressive
ulcerations with accumulations of caseous necrotic debris.
Often the reptile becomes anorectic and dehydrated with
a loss of body weight. A pneumonia resulting from
aspiration of caseous necrotic oral debris is a common
sequela to ulcerative stomatitis. The affected reptile
will be submitted exhibiting extreme gaping of the mouth
with cranial extension of a bubbling glottis. Harsh
sounds, indicating a fluid filled lung, may be ascultated.
Systemic disease shows no specific signs other than
lethargy and anorexia. Necrotic hemorrhagic body scales
may indicate systemic involvement. Blood samples submitted
for hematologic determinations often show a white blood
cell count greater than 20,000 per cubic millimeter with
increased numbers of heterophils and lymphocytes.

Integumentary lesions consist of hemorrhagic body
scales with edema and necrosis. Large areas of skin may

slough, exposing subcutaneous tissue. Severe cases of
Pseudomonas skin disease may result in a pneumonic
condition following inhalation of Pseudomonas microorganisms being shed into the surrounding atmosphere from the
lesion site. This problem is seen in animals kept in
small cages without adequate ventilation.

At necropsy many snakes examined with Pseudomonas
stomatitis show a green caseous exudate in the pharynx
which often extends into and totally occludes the
internal nares. Retrograde migration of bacteria up the
lacrimal duct may result in an inflammatory blockage of
the duct and accumulation of a caseous material in the
spectaculo-corneal space. Often this inflammatory response
extends down the esophagus and throughout the gastrointestinal system and is seen as small, hard hemorrhagic
nodules.

Internal lesions of systemic Pseudomonas infection
vary, but lung changes are present in most cases. Cooper
and Leakey (1976) described lung lesions in snakes varying
from mild congestion to the classical picture of severe
congestion with edema and a pseudomembranous lining of
white or yellow necrotic debris. Microscopic lesions of
coagulation necrosis can be seen in almost any organ and
are often surrounded by a mixed inflammatory response
consisting of heterophils, lymphocytes and monocytic phagocytes. The skin lesions often expose the dermis which is
usually covered by fibrin and cellular debris. A vasculitis is often seen associated with these skin lesions
and gram stains of histological sections may reveal clumps
of gram-negative microorganisms in the surrounding tissue.
Skin lesions may extend into deeper tissues. At necropsy
a severe necrotizing dermatitis in an Indonesian blue
tongue skink, Tiliqua gigas, was found connected to a
large intracoelomic perihepatic mass of necrotic debris
that yielded a pure culture of P. aeruginosa (Jacobson,
unpublished data).

DIAGNOSIS

The diagnosis of Pseudomonas infection is based upon
bacterial isolation on the appropriate media and characterization using appropriate biochemical tests. Swabs of
lesions are routinely cultured on sheep blood agar and
MacConkey's agar and incubated at 27 to 30 C. Large
greyish spreading colonies with irregular margins are
typical of P. aeruginosa and often the cultures have a
characteristic fruit-like odor (Carter, 1973). Greenish

and/or yellowish-green pigments may diffuse throughout clear media. On MacConkey's agar colonies are colorless, while on brilliant green agar they are red. P. maltophila colonies are round, smooth and nonpigmented with smooth margins. A greenish discoloration may be seen on blood agar.

Samples for diagnosis are easily secured from sick and debilitated animals. A percutaneous blood sample taken from the heart or caudal tail vein should be submitted for culture, in addition to hematological determinations. Vesicular skin lesions should be aspirated and cultured. Mouth lesions should be cleaned with sterile saline, exposing deeper tissues for culture. When appropriate, in the living specimen, biopsy specimens of skin lesions bordering on healthy tissue should be submitted for histological evaluation. Snakes suffering from pneumonic processes should be transtracheally washed and aspirates cultured for bacteria. With post-mortem specimens, bacterial isolates from lesions should always be correlated with histopathological lesions since Pseudomonas is commonly isolated from the oral cavity and gastrointestinal system of health squamates. The significance of bacterial isolates should always be considered with other findings to arrive at an accurate diagnosis.

CONTROL AND TREATMENT

Different authors have developed a variety of prophylactic programs and treatment regimes for healthy and diseased animals respectively. Often the problem in treating the sick reptile is not only treating the infection but also the underlying disease which predisposes to infection. The two problems, infection and underlying diseases, are inseparable. As in other animals, the control of the underlying disease may result in control of the infection. For the nutritionally compromised recent import, this is a most difficult task. Often the animal is off feed, on a low plane of nutrition and primed for invasion by opportunistic pathogens. Even when placed under ideal environmental conditions, these reptiles may continue to refuse food and steadily decline in body condition. The establishment of an active infection complicates the situation, further compromises the host, and a vicious cycle is created. Forced feeding, coupled with the administration of subcutaneous/intraperitoneal fluids and the appropriate antibiotics, is necessary to effectively treat these animals.

With oral lesions the necrotic debris should be cleansed daily and the mucous membrans irrigated with a 10% hydrogen peroxide solution. For cutaneous lesions, especially burn cases, the reptile should be soaked in a solution of 16 cc of 2% chlorhexidine added to 4 liters of water, twice per day until the disease has been controlled. Mafenide acetate is an ideal topical ointment for burn patients.

Each strain of Pseudomonas has its own sensitivity pattern for antibiotic therapy. The ability to quickly mutate complicates the problem of effectively treating and controlling this microorganism. In most cases, Pseudomonas spp. isolated from reptiles are sensitive to kanamycin, gentamicin, carbenicillin and chloramphenicol. The latter drug is routinely used when sensitivity permits since no detrimental side effects have been encountered in reptiles. Often gentamicin becomes the drug of choice and in a patient that is already compromised; gentamicin nephrotoxicity must be considered as a sequela to treatment. Reptiles generally are treated with 4 mg/kg body weight of gentamicin sulfate every 72 hours for 3 treatments. Administration of 44 cc/kg body weight of water either orally or as parenteral fluid is recommended to maintain adequate glomerular filtration. Combined gentamicin sulfate (4 mg/kg)/carbenicillin (400 mg/kg) therapy, administered independently, is commonly used in humans and is recommeded for the reptile patient suffering from a Pseudomonas infection. For suspected Pseudomonas spp. pneumonias, 2 mg of gentamicin/10 cc of saline is additionally nebulized to the sick animal twice per day for at least a week. Response to therapy, even in the most responsive animal, is a slow process and usually takes a minimun of 3 to 4 weeks to see clinical improvement. One python that was submitted with Pseudomonas burn sepsis ultimately died 3 months later from Pseudomonas pneumonia, although the initial skin infection was successfully controlled and healed.

Additional attempts at controlling Pseudomonas spp. infections have involved the use of bacterins. Although vaccines using formalized Pseudomonas isolates, grown at varying times and temperatures, did not appear to prolong life in affected snakes at an East African snake farm (Cooper and Leakey, 1976), an autogenous Pseudomonas bacterin was successful in controlling a chronic mouth infection in a reticulated python, P. reticulatus (Addison and Jacobson, 1974). In the latter study, the bacterin was prepared by suspending approximately 6×10^6 Pseudomonas cells/ml of 0.3% formalized saline.

The control of Pseudomonas levels in the animal's environment should be considered as a means of reducing infection, especially in the compromised reptile. Cage material and water bowls should be changed daily and the cage should be routinely cleaned with a sodium hypochlorite solution. Two effective techniques of eliminating pseudomonads from drinking water of laboratory rodents include: 1) chlorinating the water to 10 parts per million, and 2) acidifying the water with hydrochloric acid to pH 2.3 to 2.5. Neither of these treatments have been shown to be irritating to the gastrointestinal tract of rodents which continually receive water (McDougall et al., 1967). With regards to the second technique, Black (1979) found that acidifying the water given to snakes and allowing it to stand for 3 days in the animal's habitat, reduced the presence of P. aeruginosa. This application as well as good sanitation practices has definite application in the husbandry of captive reptiles, especially the animal affected with an ongoing Pseudomonas infection.

REFERENCES

Addison, B., and Jacobson, E., 1974, An autogenous bacterin for a chronic mouth infection in a reticulated python, J. Zoo Animal Med., 5:10-11.
Benedict, A.F., and Dawson, W.R., 1976, Metabolism, in: "Biology of the Reptilia," Vol. 5, C. Gans and W.R. Dawson, eds., Academic Press, New York.
Black, D.J., 1979, Use of acid water to control presence of Pseudomonas aeruginosa in the environment of captive snakes, Amer. Ass. Zoo Vet. Ann. Proc., 1978: 185-189.
Burtscher, J., 1931, Uber die mundfaule des schlangen. Zool. Garten, 4:235-244.
Buxton, A., and Fraser, G., 1977, "Animal microbiology," Vol. 1, Blackwell Sci. Publ., Oxford.
Caldwell, N.E., and Ryerson, P.L., 1940, A new species of the genus Pseudomonas pathogenic for certain reptiles, J. Bacteriol., 39:323-336.
Carter, G.R., 1973, "Diagnostic procedures in veterinary microbiology," 2nd ed., Charles C. Thomas Publ., Springfield.
Cooper, J.E., 1973, Treatment of necrotic stomatitis at the Nairobi Snake Park, Int. Zoo Yearbook, 13: 268-269.
Cooper, J.E., and Leakey, J.H.E., 1976, A septicaemic disease of East African snakes associated with enterobacteriaceae, Trans. Royal Soc. Trop. Med. Hyg., 70:80-84.

Davis, B.D., Dulbecco, R., Eisen, H., Gunsberg, H., and Wood, W.B., Jr., 1973, "Microbiology," 2nd ed., Harper and Row, Hagerstown.

Dieterich, R.A., 1967, What's wrong with your turtle?, Int. Turtle Tortoise Soc. J., 1:20-21.

Dogget, R.G., 1979, Microbiology of Pseudomonas aeruginosa in: "Pseudomonas aeruginosa: Clinical mainifestations of infection and current therapy," R.G. Dogget, ed., Academic Press, New York.

Evans, E.E., 1963, Comparative immunology. Antibody response in Dipsosaurus dorsalis at different temperatures, Proc. Soc. Exp. Biol. Med., 112: 531-533.

Folsch, D.W., and Leloup, P., 1976, Uber eine verlustreich verlaufene infektion in einem schlangenbestand, XVIII Internationalen Symposiums uber die Erkrankungen der Zootiere, Akademie der Wissenschaften der DDR, Berlin.

Gray, C.W., Davis, J., and McCarten, W.G., 1966, Treatment of Pseudomonas infections in the snake and lizard collection at Washington Zoo, Int. Zoo Yearbook, 6:278.

Jacobson, E., 1978, Diseases of the respiratory system of reptiles, Vet. Med./Small Animal Clin., 73:1169-1175.

Keydar, Y., Eylan, E., Mendelsohn, H., and Marder, U., 1971, Infektionen durch Pseudomonas aeruginosa bei der Palaestinaviper, Vipera xanthina palestinae, Salamandra, 7:101-116.

Ledbetter, E.O., and Kutscher, A.E., 1969, The aerobic and anaerobic flora of rattlesnake fangs and venom, Arch. Environ. Health, 19:770-778.

Levy, D., 1974, Pseudomonas infection in a rainbow boa, Bull. Philadelphia Herp. Soc., 22:35-36.

McDougall, P.T., Wolf, N.S., Stenback, W.A., and Trenton, J.J., 1967, Control of Pseudomonas aeruginosa in an experimental mouse colony, Lab. Animal Care, 17:204-214.

Murphy, J.B., and Armstrong, B.L., 1978, "Maintenance of rattlesnakes in captivity," Univ. Kansas Publ., Museum of Natural History, Lawrence.

Page, L.A., 1961, Experimental ulcerative stomatitis in king snakes, Cornell Vet., 51:258-266.

Page, L.A., 1966, Diseases and infections in snakes: A review, Bull. Wildlife Dis. Ass., 2:111-126.

Parrish, H.M., MacLaurin, A.W., and Tuttle, R.L., 1956, North American pit vipers: Bacterial flora of the mouths and venom glands, Virginia Med. Monthly, 83:383-385.

Partick, R., and Werkman, C.H., 1930, Notes on the bacterial flora of the snake, Proc. Iowa Acad. Sci., 37:330.

AEROMONAS

Emmett B. Shotts, Jr.

College of Veterinary Medicine

University of Georgia

INTRODUCTION

Sanarelli (1891) first noted this organism in 1891 from experimental frogs and reported it in the literature as Bacillus hydrophilus fuscus (Russell, 1898). In conjunction with this report was also information establishing the organism's pathogenicity for lizards, fish and an array of warm-blooded species. Additional reports by other investigators, notably Russell in 1898, described the organism as a polar monotrichous rod which produced gas from glucose. Older cultures produced an amber pigment (Sanarelli, 1891). Chester changed the name to Bacillus hydrophilus and its description appeared in the 1932 and 1934 editions of Bergey's Manual as Proteus hydrophilus (Bergey, 1923, 1934).

The dilemma of whether this organism should be in this genus continued until 1948 when it became known as Pseudomonas hydrophila. Prior to this edition of Bergey's Manual, Stanier (1943) had advocated the placement of the organism into a separate genus using the name Aeromonas proposed by Kleiyver and Niel (1936). However, it was not until the 7th edition of Bergey's Manual that the name Aeromonas hydrophila was adopted. During the ensuing time this organism has been referred to as Bacillus punctatus, Aerobacter liquefaciens, Bacterium punctatus, Achromobacter punctation, Pseudomonas punctata, Bacillus icthysosomium, Escherichia icthyosomium, Proteus icthyosomium, Pseudomonas fermentans and Pseudomonas icthyosomium. Ewing et al. (1980) concluded that all these organisms were in fact Aeromonas hydrophila.

Concepts regarding this organism were revised in the 8th edition of Bergey's manual by Schubert (1974) who described five subspecies of the genus Aeromonas, three as species of A. hydrophila and two as species of A. punctata (Schubert, 1971, 1974). Further suggestions as to change and the proposal of a new species, A. soberia, were advocated by Popoff and Veron (1976). Most recent work in this area would indicate that only one genotypic group of motile aeromonads exists based on DNA/DNA relationship and the name A. hydrophila was suggested (MacInnes et al., 1979).

DISTRIBUTION

A. hydrophila presents a challenge to both the clinician and the microbiologist because of its ubiquitous appearance in the the aquatic environment. This organism has been isolated from both diseased and healthy frogs (Hird et al., 1981). Isolations have been obtained from surface, tap, well and distilled water as well as from drainpipes, sink traps and the soil (Eurell et al., 1978; Ewing et al., 1960; Gilbert, 1970; Lindbert et al., 1973; Phillips, 1974).

Considered as a classic opportunistic pathogen, A. hydrophila establishes commonly in stressed or immuno-suppressed hosts. When reported from poikilothermic hosts common factors include waters of high organic content, handling, thermal stress or debilitation from bacterial infection or parasitic infestation (DeFigueiredo and Plumb 1977; Esch et al., 1976; Groberg et al., 1978; Hazen and Fliermans, 1979; Neilson, 1978; Plumb et al., 1976).

The range of species reported susceptible to this organism is large and includes: fish, crocodilians, frogs, salamanders, lizards, snakes, turtles, mollusks, earthworms, insects, pigs, bovines, dogs, cats, pigeons, mice, guinea pigs and humans (Boyer et al., 1971; Camin, 1948; Carr et al., 1976; Gordon et al., 1979; Graevenitz and Zinterhofer, 1970; Hibbs et al., 1971; Kleiyver and Niel, 1936; Marcus, 1971; Morse et al., 1974; Shotts et al., 1972).

In reptiles, bacterial diseases account for 74.1% of the infectious conditions encountered (Ippen and Schroder, 1977). Of these bacterial infections, Aeromonas accounts for 28.3% followed closely by Salmonella (27.7%) and Pseudomonas (10.2%). Aeromonas infections in general groups of reptiles have been implicated in 36.3% of the bacterial infections in turtles, 40.5% in alligators, 20.2% in lizards and 32.4% in snakes. While figures are not readily available, this organism has played a predominate role in mortality of frogs for many years (Russell, 1898).

SIGNS AND PATHOLOGY

Disease attributable to A. hydrophila may vary in signs from acute fulminating septicemia to a more benign latent infection. Clinical signs associated with this organism may include ecchymoses of mucous membranes, skin ulcerations, anemia and ascites.

The role of this organism in a disease of frogs referred to as "red leg" has been well documented in the literature since before the turn of the century (Caselitz, 1966; Russell, 1898). Classically an erythemic condition exists on the underside of the legs and abdomen of the frog. When opened the liver is dark and swollen and in most cases small necrotic areas may be noted in the musculature of the affected animal (Caselitz, 1966; Deesi, 1949). A. hydrophila also has been associated with ulceration and necrosis of the rostrum in Darwin's frogs, Rhinoderma darwini (Cooper et al., 1978). Aeromonas spp. are considered as a part of the normal flora of this species and varies with habitat, probably causing disease as a result of host stress (Kexel and Schubert, 1967).

In snakes, a condition known as "mouth rot" or ulcerative stomatitis is the most common type lesion attributed to A. hydrophila. Classically this chronic ulcerative inflammation of the oral cavity progresses and death results from a septicemia (Cowan, 1968; Marcus, 1971; Page, 1961; Punzo, 1975). At necropsy, hemorrhages are noted in all organs. Particularly characteristic are findings of hemorrhages on the mucosal lining of the mouth and of the serosal surfaces of the digestive tract. Usually the liver is mottled and brownish in color with varing sizes of necrotic foci ranging from pinpoint to 2 mm in diameter. The lungs are red and blood filled (Esterabadi et al., 1973). Very little is available regarding the epizootiology surrounding the spread of this disease in snake populations, however, it is well documented that the snake mite, Ophionyssus natricis, may be involved in the spread of this condition (Camin, 1948; Jacobson, 1978).

Boyer et al. (1971) have reported the occurrence of

Aeromonas infection in salamanders. This particular outbreak occurred in a colony of 3,000 Mexican axolotls, Siredon mexicanum. The signs most commonly noted were edema, reddening of subcutaneous tissues and anorexia. At necropsy, ascites, hemorrhages and pale livers with petechiae were the most common findings.

While no literature regarding specific clinical signs of disease in lizards is readily accessible, the occurrenc of disease in this group of animals has been documented (Ippen and Schroder, 1977). They state that Aeromonas spp. accounted for 20.2% of the bacterial diseases they noted in this group. Aeromonas was not noted as a part of the normal bacterial flora in a study of the household lizard, Gekko gecko (Tan et al., 1978).

Aeromonas spp. may cause mortality in turtles. When disease occurs it is most often seen as a septicemia accompanied by noticeable edema and subcutaneous bloody gelatinous exudate formation (Shotts et al., 1972).

Deaths from Aeromonas infection have been documented in crocodilians (Ippen and Schroder, 1977; Shotts et al., 1972). Most conclusive evidence is presented in work by Gordon et al. (1979) and reports available regarding outbreaks are confined to Alligator mississippiensis. The two best documentations of such disease in the wild come from the Southeastern United States; however, reports from captive populations are available in the literature (Ippen and Schroder, 1977). In zoo environments, it has been estimated that Aeromonas spp. are responsible for 40% of the bacterial disease seen in this group of animals. The dominant sign noted is sluggishness of the animal; in some cases external wounds may afford the organism entry.

In other situations the death is best described as a "sudden death syndrome". Death as a result of respiratory system involvement has been described (Shotts et al., 1972). At necropsy, swollen, blood engorged, darkened organs with petechiae on serous membranes are common findings. In most cases, death appears to be the result of acute septicemia. In the respiratory cases, a caseous exudate may be found blocking the bronchi. The pentastome, Sebekia oxycephala, has been involved in the respiratory form of the disease in alligators (Cosgrove et al., 1970; Shotts et al., 1972).

From a review of the literature and the cited information, it becomes apparent that this organism may infect and cause death in all groups of reptiles. There is some speculation as to whether it is a primary or secondary invader in some of the reported cases.

DIAGNOSIS

The recovery of this organism is relatively easy. *A. hydrophila* grows well on most ordinary media, at either 20 C or 37 C. Since this organism is an oxidase positive, fermentative rod, it is easily overlooked or mistaken for an enteric bacterium (Shotts and Bullock, 1975, 1976). Less chance of missing this organism is taken if some selective medium is used for clinical isolation; one such medium is RS medium (Shotts and Rimler, 1973). *A. hydrophila* grows as a characteristic yellow colony on this medium (Rimler et al., 1974). If possible, it would be desirable if isolates from questionable clinical material were proven by Koch's postulates to verify their role in the clinical problem under investigation. Commonly used broad spectrum antibiotics such as tetracycline and chloramphenicol are generally employed with varying results. Plasmid transfer associated with this genus makes it imperative that antibiotic sensitivity be determined in each clinical case prior to treatment.

CONTROL

Control of *Aeromonas* infection is best accomplished through avoidance predicated upon proper sanitation and environmental quality. This complex organism thrives in increased presence of organic matter found in the environment. Care should be used in attempting to control environmental quality through the prophylactic use of antibiotics since often this practice leads to development of antibiotic resistant bacterial populations.

REFERENCES

Bergey, D.H., 1923, "Manual of determinative bacteriology," 1st ed., Williams and Wilkins Co., Baltimore.
Bergey, D.H., 1934, "Manual of determinative bacteriology," 4th ed., Williams and Wilkins Co., Baltimore.
Boyer, C.I., Blacker, K., and DeLanney, L.E., 1971, *Aeromonas hydrophila* infection in the Mexican axolotl, *Siredon mexicanum*, Lab. Animal Sci., 21:372-375.

Breed, R.S., Murray, G.W.D., and Hitchens, A.P., 1948, "Bergey's manual of determinative bacteriology," 6th ed., Williams and Wilkins Co., Baltimore.

Camin, J., 1948, Mite transmission of a hemorrhagic septicemia in snakes, J. Parasitol., 34:345-354.

Carr, H.H., Amborski, R.L., Culley, D.D., and Amborski, G.F., 1976, Aerobic bacteria in the intestinal tracts of bullfrogs (Rana catesbeiana) maintained at low temperatures, Herpetologica, 32:239-244.

Caselitz, R.H., 1966, "Psudomonas-Aeromonas und ihre human medizinische Bedeutung," VEB Gustav Fisher Verlag, Jona.

Cooper, J.E., Needham, J.R., and Griffen, J., 1978, A bacterial disease of the Darwin's frog (Rhinoderma darwini), Lab. Animal, 12:91-93.

Cosgrove, G.E., Nelson, B.M., and Self, J.T., 1970, The pathology of pentastomid infection in primates, Lab. Animal Care, 20:354-360.

Cowan, D.F., 1968, Diseases of captive reptiles, J. Amer. Vet. Med. Ass., 153:843-859.

Deesi, J.L., 1949, The natural occurrence of "red leg" Pseudomonas hydrophila in a population of American toads, Bufo americanus, Ohio J. Sci., 49:70-71.

DeFigueiredo, J., and Plumb, J.A., 1977, Virulence of different isolates of Aeromonas hydrophila in catfish, Aquaculture, 11:349-354.

Esch, G.W., Hazen, T.C., Dimock, R.V., and Gibbons, J.W., 1976, Thermal effluent and the epizootiology of the ciliate Epistylis and the bacterium Aeromonas in association with centrarchid fish, Trans. Amer. Microscop. Soc., 95:687-693.

Esterabadi, A.H., Entessar, F., and Khan, M.A., 1973, Isolation and identification of Aeromonas hydrophila from an outbreak of haemorrhagic septicemia in snakes, Can. J. Comp. Med., 37:418-420.

Eurell, T.E., Lewis, D.H., and Grumbles, L.C., 1978, Comparison of selected diagnostic tests for detection of motile Aeromonas septicemia in fish, Amer. J. Vet. Res., 39:1384-1386.

Ewing, W.H., Hugh, R., and Johnson, J.G., 1960, "Studies on the Aeromonas group," DHEW, Center for Disease Control, Atlanta.

Gilbert, D.N., 1970, The apparent emergence of non-nosocomial-nosoccomial wound infections: A study of tornado casualities, J. Lab. Clin. Med., 76:999.

Gordon, R.W., Hazen, T.C., Esch, G.W., and Fleirmans, C.B., 1979, Isolation of Aeromonas hydrophila from the American alligator, Alligator mississippiensis, J. Wildlife Dis., 15:239-244.

Graevenitz, A., and Zinterhofer, L., 1970, The detection
of Aeromonas hydrophila in stool specimens,
Health Lab. Sci., 7:124-127.
Groberg, W.J., McCoy, R.H., Pilcher, K.S., and Fryer, J.L.,
1978, Relation of water temperature to infections
of coho salmon (Oncorhynchus kisutch), chinook
salmon (O. tshawytscha) and steelhead trout
(Salmo gairdneri) with Aeromonas salmonicida and
A. hydrophila, J. Fish Rev. Board Can., 35:1-7.
Hazen, T.C., and Fliermans, C.B., 1979, Distribution of
Aeromonas hydrophila in natural and man-made
thermal effluents, Appl. Environ. Microbiol.,
38:166-168.
Hazen, T.C., Esch, G.W., and Fliermans, C.B., 1977,
Distribution of Aeromonas hydrophila in a South
Carolina cooling reservoir, Abstrs. Ann. Meet.
Amer. Soc. Microbiol., 77:238.
Heywood, R., 1968, Aeromonas infections in snakes, Cornell
Vet., 58:236.
Hibbs, C.M., Merker, J.W., and Krickenberg, S.M., 1971,
Experimental Aeromonas hydrophila infection in
rabbits, Cornell Vet., 61:380-386.
Hird, D.W., Diesch, S.L., McKinnell, R.G., Gorham, E.,
Martin, F.B., Kurtz, S.W., and Dubrovolny, C.,
1981, Aeromonas hydrophila in wild caught frogs
and tadpoles (Rana pipiens) in Minnesota, Lab.
Animal Sci., 31:166-169.
Ippen, R., and Schroder, H.D., 1977, Zu den Erkrankungen
der Reptilien, XIX Internationalen Symposiums
uber die Erkrankungen der Zootiere, Akademie
der Wissenschaften der DDR, Berlin.
Jacobson, E., 1978, Diseases of the respiratory system
in reptiles, Vet. Med./Small Animal Clin.,
73:1169-1175.
Kexel, G., and Schubert, R.H.W., 1967, Die Darmflora von
froschen in ihrer abhangigkeit von Standort,
Arch. Hyg. Bakteriol., 151:436-445.
Kleiyver, A.J., and Niel, C.B., 1936, Prospects for a
natural system of classification of bacteria,
Abl. f. Bakteriol. Zabt., 94:369-403.
Lindbert, A.A., Nord, C.E., Hellgen M., and Sjoberg, L.,
1973, Identification of gram-negative aerobic
fermenters in a clinical bacteriological laboratory, Med. Microbiol, Immunol., 159:201-210.
MacInnes, J.J., Trust, T.J., and Crosa, J.H., 1979,
Deoxyribonucleic acid relationships among members
of the genus Aeromonas, Can. J. Microbiol.,
25:579-586.
Marcus, L.C., 1971, Infectious diseases of reptiles,
J. Amer. Vet. Med. Ass., 159:1626-1631.

Mead, A.R., 1969, Aeromonas liquifaciens in the leukodermi syndrome of Achatina fulica, Malacologia, 9:43.

Morse, E.V., Duncan, M.A., Krider, J.L., and Matteson, R.E., 1974, Bacterial enteritis in pigs following stress, J. Animal Sci., 39:158.

Neilson, A.H., 1978, The occurrence of aeromonads in activated sludge: Isolation of Aeromonas sobria and its possible confusion with Escherichia coli, J. Appl. Bacteriol., 44:259-264.

Page, L.A., 1961, Experimental ulcerative stomatitis in king snakes, Cornell Vet., 51:258-266.

Page, L.A., 1966, Diseases and infections of snakes: A review, Bull. Wildlife Dis. Ass., 2:111-126.

Phillips, J.A., Bernhart, H.E., and Rosenthal, S.G., 1974, Aeromonas hydrophila infections, Pediatrics, 53:110-112.

Plumb, J.A., Grizzle, J.M., and DeFigueiredo, J., 1976, Necrosis and bacterial infection in channel catfish (Ictalurus punctatus) following hypoxia, J. Wildlife Dis., 12:247-253.

Popoff, M., and Veron, M., 1976, A taxonomic study of the Aeromonas hydrophila-Aeromonas punctata group, J. Gen. Microbiol., 94:11-22.

Punzo, F., 1975, Ulcerative stomatitis in the Peruvian boa constrictor, Boa constrictor ortonii, J. Herpetol., 9:360-361.

Rimler, R.B., Shotts, E.B., and Ghittino, P., 1974, Infectious a Aeromonas hydrophila chez les poissons, diagnostic rapide a l'aide du milieu, R. S. Cah. Med. Vet., 43:47-52.

Roger, M., 1893, Une epizootie obseroll chez des grenouilles, C. R. Soc. Biol. Paris, 5:709.

Russell, F.H., 1898, An epidemic septicemic disease among frogs due to the Bacillus hydrophilus fuscus, J. Amer. Med. Ass., 30:1442-1449.

Sanarelli, G., 1891, Ueber einen neuen Mikroorganismus des Wassers, welcher fur Thiere mit veraenderlicher und konstanter Temperatur pathogen ist, Zentralbl. Bakteriol., 9:193-199; 222-228.

Schubert, R.H.W., 1971, Status of the names Aeromonas and Aerobacter liquefaciens, Beijerinck and designation of a neotype strain for Aeromonas hydrophila, Stanier, Int. J. Syst. Bacteriol., 21:87-90.

Schubert, R.H.W., 1974, Genus II Aeromonas, in: "Bergey's manual of determinative bacteriology," 8th ed., R.E. Buchanan and N.E. Gibbons, eds., Williams and Wilkins Co., Baltimore.

Shotts, E.B., and Bullock, G.L., 1975, Bacterial diseases of fish: Diagnostic procedures for gram-negative pathogens, J. Fish Res. Board Can., 32:1243-1247.

Shotts, E.B., and Bullock, G.L., 1976, Rapid diagnostic approaches in the identification of gram-negative bacterial diseases of fish, Fish Pathol., 10:187-190.

Shotts, E.B., and Rimler, R.B., 1973, Medium for the isolation of Aeromonas hydrophila, Appl. Microbiol., 26:550-553.

Shotts, E.B., Gaines, J.L., Martin, C., and Prestwood, A.K., 1972, Aeromonas induced death among fish reptiles in an eutrophis inland lake, J. Amer. Vet. Med. Ass., 161:603-607.

Stanier, R.Y., 1943, A note on the taxonomy of Proteus hydrophilus, J. Bacteriol., 46:213-214.

Tan, R.J.S., Lin, E.W., and Ishak, B., 1978, Intestinal bacterial flora of the household lizard, Gecko gecko, Res. Vet. Sci., 24:262-263.

Wohlgemuth, K.R., Pierce, R.L., and Kilbride, C.A., 1972, Bovine abortion associated with Aeromonas hydrophila, J. Amer. Vet. Med. Ass., 160:1001-1002.

SERRATIA

Gerald L. Hoff

Office of Epidemiological Services

Kansas City Health Department

INTRODUCTION

The enterobacterial genus Serratia has been recognized since ancient times as the cause of red spots on food. The red color resulting from the production of prodigiosin pigment was considered to be blood, and the appearance of blood spots on bread and consecrated wafers played on the superstitions of the populace (Grimont and Grimont, 1978). With the development of bacteriology, the organisms became regarded as saprophytes, although by the turn of the 20th century the pathogenic nature of Serratia began to be appreciated. Once the non-pigmented strains of the bacterium became recognized along with the risk of infection in surgery, physicians could no longer regard Serratia as saprophytic.

The earliest report of Serratia infection in a reptile was that of Duran-Reynals and Clausen (1937). Their subsequent experimental studies revealed a wide host range for the bacterium. Since these initial studies, however, there have been few reports concerning Serratia either in disease or as part of the reptilian enteric flora.

DISTRIBUTION

While bacteria of the genus Serratia are cosmopolitan in distribution, the ecological niche of the various members is confused due to taxonomic problems. Serratia spp. have been recovered from fresh and salt water, plankton, plants, insects, molluscs, herptiles, birds and mammals (Grimont and Grimont, 1978). Generally considered non-pathogens, the bacteria have been associated with clinical disease in insects and vertebrates. In man, disease caused by these organisms occurs almost entirely in the already compromised host, e.g. burn patients. On the other hand, Serratia spp. are recovered frequently from healthy, diseased and dead insects. This has led to attempts to utilize the bacteria as microbial insecticides. The relationship of Serratia with insects may be an important source of infection for reptiles.

Among herptiles, Serratia spp. have been associated only with reptiles, however, experimentally, Rana pipiens and Bufo americanus were found to be susceptible to infection (Clausen and Duran-Reynals, 1937). Serratia have been recovered from Anolis equestris, Basiliscus vittatus, Holbrookia texanus, Iguana iguana, Phrynosoma cornutum, Sceloporus poinsetti, Tupinambis teguixin, Urosaurus ornatus, undesignated geckos, Crotalus triseriatus aquilus, C. atrox, Chrysemys picta, C. scripta elegans and several undesignated turtle species (Ackerman et al., 1971; Boam et al., 1970; Clausen and Duran-Reynals, 1937; Duran-Reynals and Clausen, 1937; Jackson and Fulton, 1970; Ledbetter and Kutscher, 1969; Mathewson, 1979; McCoy and Seidler, 1973; Murphy and Armstrong, 1978). In free-ranging, apparently healthy reptiles in Texas, the enteric carriage rate for iguanid lizards was 7% (Mathewson, 1979), while greater than 10% of C. atrox had Serratia spp. isolated from their fangs or venom (Ledbetter and Kutscher, 1969).

ETIOLOGY

Bacteria of the genus Serratia, family Enterobacteriaceae are motile, peritrichously flagellated, gram-negative, faculatively anaerobic rods; some strains of which are encapsulated. When present, the characteristic feature of the genus is a non-diffusible pink, red or magenta pigment, prodigiosin. However, pigmentation is a variable characteristic of strains and is influenced by cultural conditions and medium. Many strains fail to produce pigment. Both pigmented and non-pigmented strains have been associated with disease in reptiles (Ackerman et al., 1971; Boam et al., 1970; Duran-Reynals and Clausen, 1937; Jackson and Fulton, 1970).

The taxonomy of the genus is confused. From the 1st to the 7th editions of Bergey's Manual, the number of species in the genus Serratia dropped from 23 to 5. The 8th edition lists only one species, S. marcescens, with 46 serotypes (Buchanan and Gibbons, 1974). Grimont and Grimont (1978) presented evidence for the existence of four species, S. marcescens, S. liquefaciens, S. plymuthica and S. marinoruba, while Ewing and Martin (1974) favor three species, S. marcescens, S. liquefaciens and S. rubidaea (equivalent to S. marinoruba).

More needs to be known about the ecology of the different species or biotypes of Serratia. Based on the Grimont and Grimont (1978) classification, certain ecological relationships are apparent. The habitat of S. plymuthica is predominately water, whereas S. liquefaciens and pigmented S. marcescens are commonly responsible for infections of reared insects and are widespread in nature. The habitat of non-pigmented biotypes A8 and TCT of S. marcescens seems limited to hospitalized patients, whereas biotypes A3 and A4 seem ubiquitous. Knowledge of the habitat of S. marinoruba is still incomplete.

All reported isolates of Serratia from reptiles are referable to S. marcescens (Grimont and Grimont, 1978).

TRANSMISSION

The mode of transmission for naturally acquired Serratia in reptiles is unknown. Given the ecological distribution of the bacteria, reptiles most likely acquire the infection through ingestion or via contamination of breaks in the integument. Experimentally, the infection can be induced by subcutaneous injection or grafting of Serratia contaminated materials (Clausen and Duran-Reynals, 1937).

PATHOGENESIS AND SIGNS

In reptiles, typically the natural or experimentally induced disease has been reported to manifest itself as subcutaneous abscesses which generally resolve over a period of several months (Boam et al., 1970; Clausen and Duran-Reynals, 1937; Jackson and Fulton, 1970). Infected animals may become lethargic, reduce or cease eating activities and some individuals die. Arthritis has been observed in T. teguixin and A. equestris (Ackerman et al., 1971; Clausen and Duran-Reynals, 1937). The pyogenic arthritis resolved in A. equestris over a period of months, but did cause a permanent deformity of the bones. In an experimentally infected R. pipiens which had a broken tibia, there was degeneration of bone and invasion of the marrow by S. marcescens biotype A4 (S. anolium) (Clausen and Duran-Reynals, 1937).

Experimental infection studies with S. marcescens biotype A4 have been conducted utilizing A. equestris, A. carolinensis, Tarentola mauritanica, Hemidactylus brookii, Sternotherus odoratus, Thamnophis butleri, Storeria dekayi, R. pipiens and B. americanus (Clausen and Duran-Reynals, 1937). Following subcutaneous injection, animals maintained at 18 to 24 C developed subcutaneous abscesses at the site of injection. The time interval between injection and observable lesions was variable. In lizards and amphibians, the abscesses were evident in 3 to 4 days, in snakes, not until 3 weeks post-inoculation, and in the turtle, abscesses were not evident until the third month. The abscesses persisted for extended periods of time and eventually disappeared. An abscess in a B. americanus ulcerated through the overlying integument.

Environmental temperatures have been shown to influence the outcome of the infection (Clausen and Duran-Reynals, 1937). Under ambient temperatures of 18 to 24 C, the disease was generally a chronic, well localized process. A prolonged bacteremia occurred, however, abscesses rarely developed at other body sites. Death, if it occurred, was never observed prior to 6 weeks post-inoculation. However, when animals were infected and held at 37 C or originally held at the lower temperatures and then moved to the higher temperature, the bacteremia became septicemic. The infection then became generalized and invariably death occurred within a few days to several weeks post-inoculation.

Jackson and Fulton (1970) have suggested a synergistic relationship between Serratia and the bacterial genus Citrobacter. This hypothesis arose from epizootics observed among turtles in which mortality was attributed to Citrobacter. It was felt that lypolytic and proteolytic action by Serratia on exposed skin surfaces facilitated subsequent entry into the body by Citrobacter, an organism capable of widespread systemic damage when it occurs internally outside the lumen of the intestine. Mixed cultures of Citrobacter-Serratia were recovered from dead turtles and Citrobacter is one of the most common enteric bacteria of the turtles (Jackson et al., 1969; Mayer and Frank, 1974; Roggendorf and Muller, 1976).

PATHOLOGY

The subcutaneous granulomatous abscesses are loosely attached to the surrounding tissues, which may be somewhat hemorrhagic. Ovoid in shape, the nodules vary in size from 2 X 2 mm to 10 X 25 mm in A. equestris (Duran-Reynals and Clausen, 1937). The fibrous capsule is infiltrated by mononuclear cells. In cross section, the nodules are filled with caseous pus, the central part of which is typically yellowish in color and necrotic.

Radiographically, the arthritic condition observed in T. teguixin was characterized by periarticular non-dense swelling and diffuse lytic lesions of the epiphyseal ends and articular surfaces of the proximal tibia and distal femur, with evidence of new bone growth in the regions of the metaphyses of the femur and tibia (Ackerman et al., 1971). An inspissated purulent material surrounded the joint, filling the synovial cavity. The articular surfaces of the femur and tibia were replaced by a soft pannus-like formation which extended along the metaphysis of the femur approximately 0.5 cm. S. marcescens was recovered from the joint space.

Histologically, the major portion of the articular cartilages of the femur and tibia were replaced with granulomatous tissue and fibrillar cartilage. The epiphyseal marrow cavity of the femur was reduced because of collapse of the articular surface and extension of the granulomatous tissue into the cavity. The synovial membrane, joint capsule and periosteum of the distal portion of the femur also were replaced by granulomatous tissue containing scattered foci of necrosis and cellular debris. The synovial cavity contained desquamated cellular debris and inflammatory cells. Similar material was in the tissues surrounding the joint. Gram-negative, rod-shaped bacteria were present in these tissues.

DIAGNOSIS

The diagnosis of Serratia infection is dependent upon bacterial isolation and identification. A number of non-inhibitory, differential and selective media are available. While the specific media utilized may vary from laboratory to laboratory, the basic scheme is the same (Lennette et al., 1974). Basically, three types of specimens for culture can be collected: sterile fluids; non-sterile fluids and swabs; and, tissues. Primary isolation techniques can then be adjusted for the type of specimen.

For blood and other sterile fluids, a differential plating medium is not necessary until growth is detected on the primary media such as blood agar. Primary growth should then be sub-cultured on an enteric differential plate by steaking isolated colonies and incubating at 35 C for 18 to 24 hours. Because any organism grown from these sterile sources is potentially clinically significant, at least one of each colony type on the enteric plate must be studied, whether pigmented or non-pigmented. According to Ackerman et al. (1971), 75% of the Serratia isolated may be non-chromogenic.

When dealing with non-sterile fluids and swabs of wounds, abscesses or the throat, an enteric differential plate should be included in the primary isolation procedure. Tissues and feces should be macerated in 0.65% saline. Aliquots of the resultant suspensions should be inoculated lightly onto a plate of differential medium, and more heavily onto a plate of selective medium

The identification of the isolates is dependent upon a series of biochemical tests. These may be accomplished with traditional procedures (Lennette et al., 1974) or by the use of commercially available kits for the identification of Enterobacteriaceae. The identification accuracy of the commercial kits for Serratia as compared to the conventional laboratory procedures ranges from 80 to 100% (Bruckner et al., 1982; Smith, 1975).

For information on infrasubspecific divisions of Serratia, Grimont and Grimont (1979) should be consulted.

TREATMENT AND CONTROL

Little information is available on treatment or control of Serratia infections in herptiles. Most natural or experimentally induced infections are self-limiting, resolving within a period of a few months. However, occasional mortality does occur, but whether death is a result of the Serratia infection or another opportunistic pathogen has not been determined (Jackson and Fulton, 1970).

The fact that infected captive animals may become lethargic and reduce or cease food consumption, would tend to suggest that in free-ranging animals, Serratia infection may prove detrimental for survival. However, free-ranging animals have the opportunity to thermoregulate and the infection might not be as severe. With captive specimens, a dramatic improvement in behavior was noticed within hours of surgical procedures to cleanse the abscesses (Boam et al., 1970). The typical reptilian pus in response to any normally pyogenic organism is caseous (Cowan, 1968), and as a result the abscesses will not drain spontaneously. Boam et al. (1970) felt that simple incision of the abscess was inadequate and that extensive "unroofing" was preferable. The abscess cavity should be flushed with hydrogen peroxide (3% by volume) and povidone iodine (Frye, 1973). The cavity can be packed and dressings applied if applicable. Anesthesia may or may not be required.

The use of antibiotics to treat the individual animal or in the water of aquatic species has not been advocated in the literature and used indiscriminately may induce resistant Serratia. Jackson and Fulton (1970) found that several hours of ultraviolet irradiation each day and the addition of 250 mg chloramphenicol per 20 gallons of water, two or three times per week immediately prior to feeding, seemed to bring an epizootic among turtles under control. The death rate decreased sharply, but individual turtles still possessed cutaneous lesions. As this was an outbreak in which several potential reptilian pathogens were involved, the effect of these measures on the Serratia is unknown.

REFERENCES

Ackerman, L.J., Kishimoto, R.A., and Emerson, J.E., 1971, Nonpigmented Serratia marcescens arthritis in a teju (Tupinambis teguixin), Amer. J. Vet. Res., 32:823-826.
Boam, G.W., Sanger, V.L., Cowan, D.F., and Vaughan, D.P., 1970, Subcutaneous abscesses in iguanid lizards, J. Amer. Vet. Med. Ass., 157:617-619.
Bruckner, D.A., Clark, V., and Martin, W.J., 1982, Comparison of Enteric-Tek with API 20E and conventional methods for identification of Enterobacteriaceae, J. Clin, Microbiol., 15:16-18.
Buchanan, R.E., and Gibbons, N.E., 1974, "Bergey's manual of determinative bacteriology," 8th ed., Williams and Wilkins Co., Baltimore.
Clausen, H.J., and Duran-Reynals, F., 1937, Studies on the experimental infection of some reptiles, amphibia, and fish with Serratia anolium, Amer. J. Pathol., 13:441-451.
Cowan, D.F., 1968, Diseases of captive reptiles, J. Amer. Vet. Med. Ass., 143:848-853.

Duran-Reynals, F., and Clausen, H.J., 1937, A contagious tumor-like condition in the lizard (Anolis equestris) as induced by a new bacterial species, Serratia anolium (SP.N.), J. Bacteriol., 33: 369-379.

Ewing, W.H., and Martin, W.J., 1974, Enterobacteriaceae, in: "Manual of clinical microbiology," 2nd ed., E.H. Lennette, E.H. Spaulding, and J.P. Truant, eds., Amer. Soc. Microbiol., Washington.

Frye, F.L., 1973, "Husbandry, medicine and surgery in captive reptiles," V.M. Publ. Inc., Bonner Springs.

Grimont, P.A.D., and Grimont, F., 1978, The genus Serratia, Ann. Rev. Microbiol., 32:221-248.

Grimont, P.A.D., and Grimont, F., 1979, Serratia, in: "Prokaryotes. A handbook on habitats, isolation, and identification of bacteria," M.P. Starr and H. Stolp, eds., Springer-Verlag, Heidelberg.

Jackson, C.G., and Fulton, M., 1970, A turtle epizootic apparently of microbial origin, J. Wildlife Dis., 6:446-468.

Jackson, M.M., Jackson, C.G., and Fulton, M., 1969, Investigation of the enteric bacteria of the Testudinata I: Occurrence of the genera Arizona, Citrobacter, Edwardsiella, and Salmonella, Bull. Wildlife Dis. Ass., 5:328-329.

Ledbetter, E.O., and Kutscher, A.E., 1969, The aerobic and anaerobic flora of rattlesnake fangs and venom, Arch. Environ. Health, 19:770-778.

Lennette, E.H., Spaulding, E.H., and Truant, J.P., 1974, "Manual of clinical microbiology," 2nd ed., Amer. Soc. Microbiol., Washington.

Mathewson, J.J., 1979, Enterobacteriaceae isolated from iguanid lizards of west-central Texas, Appl. Environ. Microbiol., 38:402-405.

Mayer, H., and Frank, W., 1974, Bacteriological investigations on reptiles and amphibians, Zentralbl. Bakteriol. Parasitenkd. Hyg. Abt. I Orig. A, 229:470-481.

McCoy, R.H., and Seidler, R.J., 1973, Potential pathogens in the environment: Isolation, enumeration and identification of seven genera of intestinal bacteria associated with small green pet turtles, Appl. Microbiol., 25:534-538.

Murphy, J.B., and Armstrong, B.L., 1978, "Maintenance of rattlesnakes in captivity," Univ. Kansas Museum Natural History, Spec. Publ. No. 3, Lawrence.

Roggendorf, M., and Muller, H.E., 1976, Enterobacteria from reptiles, Zentralbl. Bakteriol. Parasitenkd. Hyg. Abt. I Orig. A, 236:22-35.

Smith, P.B., 1975, "Performance of six bacterial identification systems," DHEW, Center for Disease Control, Atlanta.

SALMONELLA AND ARIZONA

Gerald L. Hoff and Diane M. Hoff

Office of Epidemiological Services

Kansas City Health Department

INTRODUCTION

Despite an extremely voluminous international literature relating to herptiles and bacteria of the genera Salmonella and Arizona, there are few reports which suggest these bacteria are pathogenic for amphibians or reptiles. Extensive listings of serotypes recovered from live or dead herptiles exist, with the greater proportion of isolates coming from vivarium collections or animals destined for the pet trade (Hoff and White, 1977). However, the emphasis for examining these animals has come from two sources, curiosity and public health concern, rather than herptilian husbandry. The reptiles, especially, have been shown to be a rich source of Salmonella and Arizona organisms for bacteriological study. The public health concern derives from the fact that both genera of bacteria are known to embrace human pathogens.

Isolates of Salmonella from herptiles are felt to be more virulent for man than Salmonella derived from birds or mammals (Schroder and Karasek, 1977). Consequently, there was great emphasis given to controlling the turtle-tortoise trade, particularly in North America where over 15×10^6 animals were sold yearly (Hoff and White, 1977), and more than 3×10^5 human salmonellosis cases were attributed to contact with turtles and their maintenance water (Chiodini and Sundberg, 1981; Lamm et al., 1972). As the trade in these animals was eliminated a significant decline in turtle associated cases of salmonellosis in man has been noted (Cohen et al., 1980;

D'Aoust and Lior, 1978). More recently, there has been a shift in emphasis to the relation of pet amphibians in human salmonellosis (Bartlett et al., 1977; Trust et al., 1981).

Increased emphasis is being given to Salmonella in free-ranging herptiles and the role these animals play as direct or indirect sources of human or other animal salmonellosis (Hoff and White, 1977; Mathewson, 1979; Sharma, 1979; Wuthe et al., 1979). Traditionally this concern has been more obvious in tropical and subtropical areas with their diverse fauna of synanthropic herptiles (Hoff and White, 1977; Kourany and Telford, 1981; Sharma, 1979).

Arizona hinshawii is a recognized pathogen of birds and man. Reports of transmission from Pituophis melanoleucus to turkey polts, and Graptemys sp. to man exist (Hinshaw and McNeil, 1944; Plow et al., 1968), however, the literature suggest little veterinary or public health interest in herptiles as a source of the bacterium. Human infections with A. hinshawii derived from pet turtles and tortoises undoubtedly occurred and likewise decreased with the regulation of the pet trade, but there are no published data from which to estimate the magnitude of the problem.

DISTRIBUTION

Salmonella spp. and A. hinshawii are ubiquitous in nature, being found in water, soil, manure and intestinal tracts of animals. They have great propensities to exist in the extrahost environment for considerable periods, with the aquatic environment the most favorable medium (Morse and Duncan, 1974). Under suitable environmental conditions, the bacteria may multiply in moist organic materials undergoing putrefaction. Although multiplication can occur between 6.7 and 45 C, optimal growth temperatures range from 35 to 37 C. Freezing reduces the total number of organisms, but the survivors may remain viable and infective for months. The acidity of the environment also affects the longevity of the bacteria. The pH in which growth occurs ranges from 4.1 to 9.0, with an optimum of 6.5 to 7.5. Weak organic acids have an inhibitory effect as does increased hydrogen ions.

The vast majority of Salmonella and Arizona serotypes show no particular host preference, however, a few Salmonella serotypes demonstrate definite adaptation to

specific hosts such as S. typhi and man or S. enteritidis
serotype pullorum and birds. Also a close correlation
exists between the frequency of isolation of certain serotypes from man and from other animals. In addition,
particular serotypes tend to occur in definite regional
patterns (Buchanan and Gibbons, 1974; Miller, 1962).

Reports of Salmonella isolates from herptiles indicate
a wide host range among lizards, snakes, turtles and
tortoises, with relatively fewer isolates from toads,
frogs and crocodilians (Ang et al., 1973; Bartlett et al.,
1977; Everard et al., 1979; Hoff and White, 1977; Ozek
et al., 1969; Sharma, 1979; Sharma et al., 1977). A.
hinshawii appears to be somewhat more limited in host
range, with the overwhelming majority of isolates coming
from snakes (Edwards et al., 1947; Kaura et al., 1972;
Muller, 1972; Roggendorf and Muller, 1976; Sharma et al.,
1977; Wuthe et al., 1979). Lizards yield a number of
A. hinshawii, but isolates from turtles, tortoises, frogs
and toads are not commonly reported (Ang et al., 1973;
Habermalz and Pietzch, 1973; Lie, 1968; Mathewson, 1979;
Mayer and Frank, 1974; Roggendorf and Muller, 1976).

ETIOLOGY

The genera Salmonella and Arizona belong to the tribe
Salmonelleae, family Enterobacteriaceae. The genus
Citrobacter is the third member of the tribe. The
bacteria are gram-negative, aerobic, non-capsulated, non-
spore forming, generally motile bacilli which grow readily
on simple culture media.

The taxonomy of the genus Salmonella is unsettled.
Two predominat classification systems currently exist in
practice (Buchanan and Gibbons, 1974; Ewing, 1972a).
For the purposes of this presentation, the classification
system of Ewing will be followed, recognizing only three
species: S. typhi, S. choleraesuis and S. enteritidis.
The genus Arizona is monospecific, with A. hinshawii
as the type species. Other names which have been applied
to A. hinshawii include Salmonella sp. Dar-es-salaam
type var. arizona, S. arizonae, A. arizonae, Paracolon-
bacterium arizonae and paracolon type 10 (Buchanan and
Gibbons, 1974; Edwards et al., 1947). Depending upon
the classification system being utilized, the current
literature identifies the bacterium as A. hinshawii or
S. arizonae, with the former being more common.

Based on somatic (O) and flagellar (H) antigens,

isolates of both genera have been characterized into hundreds of distinct serogroups and serotypes (Edwards and Ewing, 1972; Lennette et al., 1974). Although names have been assigned to the Salmonella serotypes, a numerical designation in the form of an antigenic formula would be more appropriate (Ewing, 1972a). From an extensive review of the literature by Hoff and White (1977), all isolates from reptiles as well as those from amphibians attributable to the genus Salmonella could be assigned to either S. enteriditis or A. hinshawii. Recently, S. choleraesuis was recovered from a snake, Nerodia sipidon (Cambre et al., 1980).

TRANSMISSION, PATHOGENESIS, SIGNS AND PATHOLOGY

The source of Salmonella or Arizona for herptiles is presumably through ingesting or imbiding contaminated substances or by transovarial transmission (Kourany and Telford, 1982). Salmonella can penetrate turtle eggs with subsequent production of infected hatchlings (Feeley and Treger, 1969; Lins, 1970). Penetration and infection of bird eggs and embryos by A. hinshawii has been documented (Williams, 1965), but whether this occurs with amphibians or reptiles is undocumented. Generally, infected herptiles are free of overt signs of disease, however, studies measuring clinical parameters of infection have not been reported. Roggendorf and Muller (1976) advanced the hypothesis that Salmonella and Arizona bacteria and reptiles evolved together moving from a host-parasite relationship to one of insession (Hall, 1980).

The few reports suggesting a pathogenic role for either Salmonella or Arizona in reptiles present a diverse spectrum of conditions. Ante-mortem signs are either variable or not given by the authors (Boam et al., 1970; Boever and Williams, 1975; Fey et al., 1956; Frye, 1981; Hinshaw and McNeil, 1946; Rewell et al., 1948). Subcutaneous abscesses, intraorbital abscesses, anorexia, necrotic stomatitis and pneumonia have been reported in various animals, however, cause and effect relationships were not established. Subcutaneous abscesses in Ctenosaura acanthura have yielded pure cultures of S. enteriditis serotype marina (Boam et al., 1970), but the investigators also recovered pure cultures of Serratia marcescens and Micrococcus sp. from subcutaneous abscesses of other lizards at the same vivarium.

Pathological conditions observed during post-mortem examinations of snakes and lizards, from which Salmonella or Arizona have been recovered include: hepatitis, splenitis, pancreatitis, nephritis, pneumonitis, mesenteritis, enteritis, gastritis, epicarditis and myocarditis (Boever and Williams, 1975; Cambre et al., 1980; Fey et al., 1956; Frye, 1981; Hinshaw and McNeil, 1946; Pagon et al., 1976; Rewell et al., 1948). Focal abscesses and granulomata are observed in the extra-intestinal tissues. The observed lesions, however, should not be considered pathognomonic nor even diagnostic of infection with these organisms (Cambre et al., 1980). Similar lesions in reptiles have been associated with other gram-negative bacteria. Over half of the reptiles at the National Zoological Park which had lesions associated with Arizona or Salmonella had underlying disease conditions such as cryptosporidiosis, mycobacteriosis, hepatocellular carcinoma, trauma associated with cagemate interaction, hyperthermia and eggbound oviduct (Cambre et al., 1980). It would appear from available data that in reptiles, Arizona and Salmonella are opportunistic pathogens (Boever and Williams, 1975; Cambre et al., 1980; Stoll, 1962).

Experimental exposure studies with Salmonella have been reported for Vipera a. ammodytes, Natrix natrix, Lacerta muralis, Testudo graeca and T. hermanni (Dimow, 1966a,b; Dimow and Slawtschew, 1967; Stoll, 1962). In all cases, oral exposure resulted in 1) lack of overt illness, 2) colonization of the intestinal tract with fecal excretion of bacteria within 24 hours, 3) no colonization of other body organs or blood, and 4) no humoral antibody response. Subcutaneous, intraperitoneal and intracardial inoculation produced similar results except that bacteria could be recovered from blood and liver, and that a specific humoral O and H agglutinin antibody response developed. Once colonized, reptiles apparently shed Salmonella in their feces throughout their lifetime. The ability of reptiles inoculated subcutaneously to develop an antibody response to Salmonella has been useful in the study of immunologic responses of Diposaurus dorsalis, Sphenodon punctatus and Alligator mississippiensis (Evans and Cowles, 1959; Marchalonis et al., 1969; Saluk et al., 1970).

The response of V. a. ammodytes, N. natrix and L. muralis to oral infection with A. hinshawii was identical to that of S. enteritidis oral exposure (Dimow, 1966a; Dimow and Slawtschew, 1967; Stoll, 1962). Subcutaneous or intraperitoneal inoculation of A. hinshawii in these species, as well as in Heloderma suspectum, Phyrnosoma solare and Sauromalus obesus (Caldwell and Ryerson, 1939), again produced results similar to the Salmonella exposure studies, with one major difference. Variable mortality rates occurred among the exposed animals, with A. hinshawii being recovered from the blood, peritoneal fluid, liver and feces. No signs of illness were observed prior to death and pathological lesions, if present in the viscera, were limited to abscesses and granulomata in the liver.

Exposure studies for amphibians have not been reported, however, the sparse data available suggests some variation from the reptilian situation. While intestinal colonization and shedding is well established (Ang et al., 1973; Bartlett et al., 1977; Everard et al., 1979; Ozek et al., 1969; Sharma, 1979; Sharma et al., 1977), isolations from the liver occur with greater frequency than do isolations from intestinal contents. In studies on Rana ridibunda, Ang et al. (1973) recovered 77% of the Arizona and Salmonella isolates from livers as opposed to 11% from intestinal contents. The isolations from the liver were not made from frogs which yielded either bacterium from the intestinal contents. The significance of this observation is not known.

Quantitative information on the amount of Salmonella or Arizona in the intestinal contents of herptiles is very limited, despite the great interest in excretion of the bacteria and the risk to humans. Studies by Sharma (1979) indicate that 10^4 to 10^{10} Salmonella per gram of feces can be found in Hemidactylus flavivirdis, Uromastix hardwicki and Bufo sp., with levels in toads being ten to one hundred times higher than in lizards. Salmonella levels per 100 ml of water in tanks containing individual infected Chrysemys scripta elegans ranged from 10^0 to 10^5 (Kaufmann et al., 1967). These levels are lower than those measured for Klebsiella sp. and Aeromonas sp. excreted by C. scripta elegans, 10^5 to 10^6 and greater than 10^6 respectively (McCoy and Seidler, 1973). Naja naja and Oligodon arnenis have been found harboring 10^7 to 10^8 A. hinshawii per gram of feces (Kaura et al., 1972).

From studies of free-ranging lizards there is some data to suggest that age of the animals examined may influence the percentage found to be harboring Salmonella. Prevalence rates for immature lizards in India and Florida, were lower than those for adult animals (Hoff and White, 1977; Sharma, 1979). Additionally, the amount of Salmonella per gram of fecal contents is lower in immature lizards (Sharma, 1979).

Stress in the form of dehydration can induce the

excretion of Salmonella and Arizona by C. scripta elegans
which previously were not shedding detectable levels of
bacteria (DuPonte et al., 1978). However, this form of
stress has not induced turtles certified free of Salmonella
to excrete either of these organisms (McKibben et al.,
1978). The effects of stress caused by crowding, shipping,
nutritional imbalance, etc., on Salmonella or Arizona
excretion by herptiles has not been examined.

DIAGNOSIS

The diagnosis of Salmonella or Arizona colonization
or infection is dependent upon bacterial isolation and
identification. Reports in the literature have linked
these bacteria and herptiles by recovery of the bacteria
from individual body tissues, homogenates of entire
animals, intestinal contents, rectal swabs, body washings
and water harboring aquatic species. Salmonella have
been recovered also from the fangs and venom of Crotalus
atrox (Ledbetter and Kutscher, 1969), the oral cavities
of Thamnophis spp. (Goldstein et al., 1981) and from
commercial turtle food (Knights and Swieczkowski, 1972).
A. hinshawii has been recovered from the oral cavities
of rattlesnakes and garter snakes (Goldstein et al., 1979,
1981). One problem with sampling the aquatic environment
is the possible confounding effect of Salmonella excretion
by other organisms (Bartlett and Trust, 1976; Bartlett
et al., 1977; Trust et al., 1981).

Unfortunately, there is little consensus as to the
best method of isolating Salmonella or Arizona from
herptiles. Wells et al. (1974) found that with C. scripta
elegans, the excretion method and homogenization method
(blending the entire animal) were equal in efficiency.
These two methods were superior to results obtained by
culturing individual organs. When turtles which were
actively excreting bacteria were administered antibiotics,
the homogenization method proved to be more sensitive than
the excretion method in detecting bacteria (Siebling et
al., 1975a). With amphibians, Ang et al. (1973) found
the culturing of individual organs, especially the liver,
far superior to the culturing of intestinal contents.

The laboratory methods for recovering and identifying
Salmonella and Arizona follow the basic scheme utilized
for all Enterobacteriaceae (Lennette et al., 1974).
Variations in the specific types of media employed may
occur among institutions. It always is advisable to employ
enrichment media in the examination of various kinds of

specimens, and their use is practically essential when dealing with fecal specimens or with herptiles treated with antibiotics. Many isolates of Arizona from reptiles are lactose negative (Koopman and Janssen, 1973; Roggendorf and Muller, 1976) and this must be taken into account when characterizing isolates. Once characterized biochemically isolates should be characterized completely by serologic procedures (Ewing, 1972b; Lennette et al., 1974).

TREATMENT AND CONTROL

Salmonella and Arizona rarely have been implicated in diseases of herptiles, therefore, the routine administration of antibiotics to the animals or their aquatic environment is both unnecessary and undesirable. Antibiotics may cause cessation of excretion but the animal may remain colonized (Siebeling et al., 1975a). A significant number of herptiles in vivarium and private collections are harboring Salmonella and/or Arizona potentially hazardous to the keepers. However, the risk from these captive animals is probably minimal because of husbandry practices and the older age of the keepers as opposed to the situation of children and pet herptiles (Zwart, 1960). Also, good personal hygienic practices are extremely effective in preventing transmission of these bacteria. The historic problem of turtle-associated Salmonella and probably Arizona in man has been resolved to a large extent through regulation and restriction of the trade in turtles and tortoises (D'Aoust and Lior, 1978). Consequently, the risk of infection in children from herptiles has been reduced with the virtual elimination of this source of exposure. The risk of infections acquired from native, free-ranging herptiles or from the new pet fad of aquarium amphibians, however, has not been completely evaluated (Bartlett et al., 1977; Hoff and White, 1977).

The growing popularity of the ornamental aquarium presents increased public health risk of salmonellosis not only from amphibians, but also from invertebrates (Bartlett and Trust, 1976). The widespread use of antibiotics in breeding, shipping, storage and in the home to control potential pathogens can induce the development of antibiotic resistant strains of Salmonella or Arizona. In a study of aquarium frogs, Hynocharus sp., Trust and Bartlett (1979) demonstrated multi-drug-resistance in Salmonella isolates. Each serotype was resistant to between 9 and 18 antibacterials with a number of R plasmids being involved. Resistance by all isolates to gentamicin, naladixic acid and novobiocin is particularly disturbing as were high rates of resistance to cephalothin, kanamycin, ampicillin, streptomycin and triple sulfa. Infection in man with these multi-drug-resistant Salmonella serotypes would obviously be a problem, especially in those septicemic and severe focal infections requiring antibiotic therapy (Trust and Bartlett, 1979).

One method proposed to control Salmonella and Arizona in pet turtles is the maintenance of a dry-environment in the home (Haga, 1972). This method requires that the turtle be kept in a dry bowl for all but 30 minutes of each day, during which time the turtle is transferred to a tank of water where it can swim and feed. After the wet phase is completed, the turtle is returned to the dry environment and the water properly disposed. This method has been demonstrated to be detrimental to the health and survival of the turtle (McKibben et al., 1978) and the dehydration induced stress may cause excretion of bacteria from turtles previously not excreting (DuPonte et al., 1978).

Siebeling et al. (1975b) utilized terramycin to treat fresh turtle eggs infected with either Salmonella or Arizona. The eggs were held at 30 C for 3 to 4 hours and immersed into a solution of the antibiotic for 30 minutes. The solution contained 1,500 or 2,000 micrograms of terramycin per ml and was used at a temperature of 6 to 12 C. The bacteria could not be recovered from the eggs or from the hatchlings for the 180 day period of the study. The procedure, however, is dependent upon the use of fresh turtle eggs and therefore has limited application.

REFERENCES

Ang, O., Ozek, O., Cetin, E.T., and Toreci, K., 1973, Salmonella serotypes isolated from tortoises and frogs in Instanbul, J. Hyg., 71:85-88.
Bartlett, K.H., and Trust, T.J., 1976, Isolation of salmonellae and other potential pathogens from the fresh water aquarium snail Ampullaria, Appl. Environ. Microbiol., 31:635-639.
Bartlett, K.H., Trust, T.J., and Lior, H., 1977, Small pet aquarium frogs as a source of Salmonella, Appl. Environ. Microbiol., 33:1026-1029.
Boam, G.W., Sanger, V.L., Cowan, D.F., and Vaughan, D.P., 1970, Subcutaneous abscesses in iguanid lizards, J. Amer. Vet. Med. Ass., 157:617-619.
Boever, W.J., and Williams, J., 1975, Arizona septicemia in three boa constrictors, Vet. Med. Small Animal Clin., 70:1357-1359.

Buchanan, R.E., and Gibbons, N.E., 1974, "Bergey's manual of determinative bacteriology," 8th ed., Williams and Wilkins Co., Baltimore.

Caldwell, M.E., and Ryerson, D.L., 1939, Salmonellosis in certain reptiles, J. Infect. Dis., 65:242-245.

Cambre, R.C., Green, D.E., Smith, E.E., Montali, R.J., and Bush, M., 1980, Salmonellosis and arizonosis in the reptile collection at the National Zoological Park, J. Amer. Vet. Med. Ass., 177:800-803.

Chiodini, R., and Sundberg, J.P., 1981, Salmonellosis in reptiles: A review, Amer. J. Epidemiol., 113:494-499.

Cohen, M.L., Potter, M., Pollard, R., and Feldman, R.A., 1980, Turtle-associated salmonellosis in the United States: Effect of public health action, 1970 to 1976, J. Amer. Med. Ass., 243:1247-1249.

D'Aoust, J.Y., and Lior, H., 1978, Pet turtle regulations and abatement of human salmonellosis, Can. J. Public Health, 69:107-108.

Dimow, I., 1966a, Versuche zur kunstlichen Infektion von Eideschsen (Lacerta muralis) mit Salmonella und Arizona-bakterien, Zentralbl. Veterinar-Medizin Reihe B, 13:587-590.

Dimow, I., 1966b, Versuche Landschildkroten der Arten Testudo graeca und Testudo hermanni mit Salmonella-bakterien zu infizieren, Zentralbl. Bakteriol. Parasitenkd. Hyg. Abt. I Orig. A, 199:181-184.

Dimow, I., and Salwtschew, R., 1967, Versuche der Experimentalinfizierung von Schlangen Vipera ammodytes ammodytes mit Salmonella und Arizona-bacterien, Pathol. Microbiol., 30:495-497.

DuPonte, M.W., Nakamura, R.M., and Chang, E.M.L., 1978, Activation of latent Salmonella and Arizona organisms by dehydration in red-eared turtles, Pseudemys scripta elegans, Amer. J. Vet. Res., 39:529-530.

Edwards, P.R., and Ewing, W.H., 1972, "Identification of Enterobacteriaceae," 3rd ed., Burgess Publishing Co., Minneapolis.

Edwards, P.R., West, M.G., and Bruner, D.W., 1947, "Arizona group of paracolon bacteria," Kentucky Agri. Exper. Station Bull. 499, Lexington.

Evans, E.E., and Cowles, R.B., 1959, Effect of temperature on antibody production in the reptile, Diposaurus dorsalis, Proc. Soc. Exp. Biol. Med., 101:482-483.

Everard, C.O.R., Tota, B., Bassett, D., and Ali, C., 1979, Salmonella in wildlife from Trinidad and Grenada, W.I., J. Wildlife Dis., 15:213-219.

Ewing, W.H., 1972a, The nomeclature of Salmonella, its
    usage and definitions of the three species,
    Can. J. Microbiol., 18:1629-1637.
Ewing, W.H., 1972b, "Isolation and identification of
    Salmonella and Shigella," DHEW, Center for
    Disease Control, Atlanta.
Fey, H.V., Edwards, P.R., and Stunzl, H., 1956, Arizona-
    Infektionen bei Reptilien mit Isolirung von 4
    neun Arizonatypen, Schwiez. Zietschr. allg.
    Pathol., 20:27-40.
Feeley, J.C., and Treger, M.D., 1969, Penetration of turtle
    eggs by Salmonella braenderup, Public Health
    Rep., 84:156-158.
Frye, F.L., 1981, "Biomedical and surgical aspects of
    captive reptile husbandry," V.M. Publishing
    Co., Bonner Springs.
Goldstein, E.J.C., Agyare, E.O., Vagvolgyi, A.E., and
    Halpern, M., 1981, Aerobic bacterial oral flora
    of garter snakes: Development of normal flora
    and pathogenic potential for snakes and humans,
    J. Clin. Microbiol., 13:954-956.
Goldstein, E.J.C., Citron, D.M., Gonzalez, H., Russell,
    F.E., and Finegold, S.M., 1979, Bacteriology
    of rattlesnake venom and implications for
    therapy, J. Infect. Dis., 140:818-821.
Habermalz, D., and Pietzsch, O., 1973, Identification of
    Arizona bacteria. A contribution to the problem
    of Salmonella infections among reptiles and
    amphibians in zoological gardens, Zentralbl.
    Bakteriol. Parasitenkd. Hyg. Abt. I Orig. A,
    225:323-342.
Haga, J.B., 1972, Baby green turtles after certification,
    Pets/Supplies/Marketing, H.B. Jovanovich, New
    York.
Hall, S.A., 1980, Incession: A suggestion for the
    epidemiologic anomasticon, Amer. J. Epidemiol.,
    111:132-134.
Hinshaw, W.R., and McNeil, E., 1944, Gopher snakes as
    carriers of salmonellosis and paracolon infec-
    tions, Cornell Vet., 24:248-254.
Hinshaw, W.R., and McNeil, E., 1946, Paracolon type 10
    from captive rattlesnakes, J. Bacteriol., 51:
    397-398.
Hoff, G.L., and White, F.H., 1977, Salmonella in reptiles:
    Isolation from free-ranging lizards (Reptilia,
    Lacertilia) in Florida, J. Herpetol., 11:123-129.
Kaufmann, A.F., Feeley, J.C., and Dewitt, W.E., 1967,
    Salmonella excretion by turtles, Public Health
    Rep., 82:840-842.
Kaura, Y.K., Sharma, V.K., Singh, I.P., Sakazaki, R., and

Rohde, R., 1972, Snakes as reservoirs of Arizona and Salmonella, Zentralbl. Bakteriol. Parasitenkd. Hyg. Abt. I Orig. A, 219:506-513.

Knights, E.M., and Swieczkowski, D., 1972, A new look at the turtle problem, Michigan Med., 71:441-442.

Koopman, J.P., and Janssen, F.G.J., 1973, The occurrence of salmonellas and lactose negative arizonas in reptiles in the Netherlands, and a comparison of three enrichment methods used in their isolation, J. Hyg., 71:363-371.

Kourany, M., and Telford, S.R., 1981, Lizards in the ecology of salmonellosis in Panama, Appl. Enriron. Microbiol., 41:1248-1253.

Kourany, M., and Telford, S., 1982, Salmonella and infections of alimentary and reproductive tracts of Panamanian lizards, Infect. Immun., 36:432-434.

Lamm, S.H., Taylor, A., Gangarosa, E.J., Anderson, H.W., and Young, W., 1972, Turtle-associated salmonellosis, I. An estimation of the magnitude of the problem in the United States, 1970-1971, Amer. J. Epidemiol., 95:511-517.

Ledbetter, E.O., and Kutscher, A.E., 1969, The aerobic and anaerobic flora of rattlesnake fangs and venom, Arch. Environ. Health, 19:770-778.

Lennette, E.H., Spaulding, E.H., and Truant, J.P., 1974, "Manual of clinical microbiology," 2nd ed., Amer. Soc. Microbiol., Washington.

Lie, P., 1968, Untersuchungen uber den Salmonellabefall von Kaltbluten, Arch. Hyg., 152:139-155.

Lins, Z.C., 1970, Studies on enteric bacterias in lower Amazon region, I. Serotypes of Salmonella isolated from wild forest animals in Para State, Brazil, Trans. Royal Soc. Trop. Med. Hyg., 64: 439-443.

Marchalonis, J.J., Ealey, E.H.M., and Diener, E., 1969, Immune response of the tuatara, Sphenodon punctatum, Australian J. Exp. Biol. Med. Sci., 47:367-370.

Mathewson, J.J., 1979, Enterobacteriaceae isolated from iguanid lizards of west-central Texas, Appl. Environ, Microbiol., 38:402-405.

Mayer, H., and Frank, W., 1974, Bacteriological investigations on reptiles and amphibians, Zentralbl. Bakteriol. Parasitenkd. Hyg. Abt. I Orig. A, 229:470-481.

McCoy, R.H., and Seidler, R.J., 1973, Potential pathogens in the environment: Isolation, enumeration and identification of seven genera of intestinal bacteria associated with small green pet turtles, Appl. Microbiol., 25:534-538.

McKibben, J.S., Porterfield, O.D., and Westergaard, J.M., 1978, Effect of dry versus wet bowl environment on pet turtles, Amer. J. Vet. Res., 39:109-114.

Miller, A.P., 1962, "Water and man's health," Community Water Supply Tech. Ser. No. 5, Agency for International Development, Washington.

Morse, E.V., and Duncan, M.A., 1974, Salmonellosis-An environmental health problem, J. Amer. Vet. Med. Ass., 165:1015-1019.

Muller, H.E., 1972, The aerobic faecal flora of reptiles with special reference to the enterobacteria of snakes, Zentralbl. Bakteriol. Parasitenkd. Hyg. Abt. I Orig. A, 222:487-495.

Ozek, O., Cetin, E.T., Ang, O., Toreci, K., and Sanli, Z., 1969, Salmonella serotypes isolated from frogs (Rana ridibunda), Zentralbl. Baketeriol. Parasitenkd. Hyg. Abt. I Orig. A, 210:557-559.

Pagon, S., Rohde, R., and Schweitzer, R., 1976, Occurrence of Salmonella in healthy snakes and snake cadavers: Isolation of a new Salmonella species belonging to the sub-genus IV (S. IV 18:Z36, Z38:-), Zentralbl. Bakteriol. Parasitenkd. Hyg. Abt. I Orig. A, 236:464-471.

Plows, C.D., Fretwell, G., and Parry, W.H., 1968, An Arizona serotype isolated from a case of gastroenteritis in Britain, J. Hyg., 66:109-115.

Rewell, R.E., Taylor, J., and Douglas, S.H., 1948, a new Salmonella type (Salm. takorod) isolated from a python, Monthly Bull. Ministry Health, Public Health Lab. Ser., London, pg. 266.

Roggendorf, M., and Muller, H.E., 1976, Enterobacteria from reptiles, Zentralbl. Bakteriol. Parasitenkd. Hyg. Abt. I Orig. A, 236:22-35.

Saluk, P.H., Krauss, J., and Clem, L.W., 1970, The presence of two antigentically distinct light chains in alligator immunoglobulins, Proc. Soc. Exp. Biol. Med., 133:365-369.

Schroder, H.D., and Karasek, E., 1977, Toxicity of salmonellae isolated from reptiles, XIX Internationalen Symposiums uber die Erkrankungen der Zootiere, Akademie der Wissenschaften der DDR, Berlin.

Siebeling, R.J., Neal, P.M., and Granberry, W.D., 1975a, Evaluation of methods for the isolation of Salmonella and Arizona organisms from pet turtles treated with antimicrobial agents, Appl. Microbiol., 29:240-245.

Siebeling, R.J., Neal, P.M., and Granberry, W.D., 1975b, Treatment of Salmonella-Arizona infected turtle eggs with terramycin and chloromycetin by the temperature-differential egg dip method, Appl. Microbiol., 30:791-799.

Sharma, V.K., 1979, Enterobacteriaceae infections in man and animals and detection of their natural reservoirs in India, Zentralbl. Bakteriol. Parasitenkd. Hyg. Abt. I Orig. A, 243:381-391.

Sharma, V.K., Rohde, R., Garg, D.N., and Kumar, A., 1977, Toads as natural reservoirs of Salmonella, Zentralbl. Bakteriol. Parasitenkd. Hyg. Abt. I Orig. A, 239:172-177.

Stoll, L., 1962, Experimentelle Infektionen mit keimen der Salmonella und Arizona-Gruppe bei Schlangen, Nord. Vet. Med., 14:225-232.

Trust, T.J., and Bartlett, K.H., 1979, Aquarium pets as a source of antibiotic resistant salmonellae, Can. J. Microbiol., 25:535-541.

Trust, T.J., Bartlett, K.H., and Lior, H., 1981, Importation of salmonellae with aquarium species, Can. J. Microbiol., 27:500-504.

Wells, J.G., Clark, G.Mc., and Morris, G.K., 1974, Evaluation of methods for isolating Salmonella and Arizona organisms from pet turtles, Appl. Microbiol., 27:8-10.

Williams, J.E., 1965, Paratyphoid and Arizona infections, in: "Diseases of poultry," 5th ed., H.E. Biester and L.H. Schwarte, eds., Iowa State Univ. Press, Ames.

Wuthe, H.H., Rohde, R., Aleksic, S., Schubert, C., and Wuthe, S., 1979, Salmonella in free-living snakes of northern Germany, Zentralbl. Bakteriol. Parasitenkd. Hyg. Abt. I Orig. A, 243:412-418.

Zwart, P., 1960, Salmonella and Arizona infections in reptiles in the Netherlands, Antionie Leeweunhoek, 26:250-254.

EDWARDSIELLA TARDA

Franklin H. White

College of Veterinary Medicine

University of Florida

INTRODUCTION

Since 1965, Edwardsiella tarda has been isolated from many different animal species and from the environment. It appears that the pathologic effects of E. tarda are similar to those produced by Salmonella spp. in the nature of the disease produced, both intestinal and extraintestinal, and in the carrier status of many animals where stress may be the triggering mechanism for active disease.

E. tarda has been isolated from diseased fish (Hawke, 1979; Meyer and Bullock, 1973; White et al., 1973), birds (Berg and Anderson, 1972; Chamoiseau, 1967; Forrester et al., 1976; Reichel et al., 1974; White et al., 1973), marine mammals (Coles et al., 1978; Forrester et al., 1975; Frye and Herald, 1969), domestic animals (Arambulo et al., 1967, 1968; Centi et al., 1977; Elazhary et al., 1973; Owens et al., 1974), wild mammals (Kourany and Vasquez, 1975; Kourany et al., 1976; White et al., 1975), ornamental fish water (Trust and Bartlett, 1974), freshwater aquarium snails (Bartlett and Trust, 1976), and surface waters (White et al., 1973). Numerous isolations of E. tarda from man have been reported since King and Adler (1964) described a case of enteric fever and acute gastroenteritis. Many reports of intestinal and extraintestinal infections in man have been reviewed (Bockemuhl et al., 1971; Clarridge et al., 1980; Jordan and Hadley, 1969; Koshi and Lalitha, 1976; Makula et al., 1973).

DISTRIBUTION

Snakes

The first reported isolations of the organisms now called E. tarda were made from numerous snakes in Japan during a survey to determine the prevalence of Salmonella and Arizona in reptiles (Sakazaki and Murata, 1962). These authors considered the organisms to be normal intestinal inhabitants of reptiles. D'Empaire (1969) used 15 isolates of E. tarda from snakes in Chad in growth studies. Iveson (1971) also used E. tarda isolates from tiger snakes, Notechis scutatus, of Western Autralia for growth studies. Muller (1972) reported the isolation of E. tarda from 5 of 15 snakes cultured in zoos in Germany, including Dendroaspis angusticeps, Lampropeltis getulus, Echis carinatus, and a false cobra. Roggendorf and Muller (1976) isolated E. tarda from 12% of 24 captive snakes in Germany. In Panama during 1965 to 1972, E. tarda was isolated from 5% of the snakes cultured for enteric bacteria. Twenty-seven genera were represented, and the organism was isolated from 5 different genera, Xenedon sp., Leimadophis sp., Chironius sp., Pseudoboa nevwiedi and Erythrolamprus bionus (Kourany et al., 1977). In India, E. tarda was isolated from only 1 of 33 snakes cultured, but this isolate was a new serotype (Sharma, 1979). There was no reported evidence of disease in any of the above reports on snakes as the result of E. tarda infection.

Lizards

In a study of the enterobacteria of reptiles, only 1 of 39 lizards was found to harbor E. tarda in Germany (Roggendorf and Muller, 1976). In Singapore, 43 household lizards, Gekko gecko, were randomly caught from 12 households and E. tarda was isolated from the intestinal contents of 10 of the reptiles (Tan and Lim, 1977). In the United States, no isolations of E. tarda were made from a total of 124 lizards captured from widespread locations in Florida and cultured for enteric bacteria (Hoff and White, 1977). Anolid lizards accounted for 96% of those examined. E. tarda was recovered from a cloacal swab specimen taken from an Australian skink, Tiliqua scincoides (White et al., 1969). The skink was one of several species cultured at a zoological park after E. tarda was found in the small intestine of an ostrich which died after a severe enteritis.

Turtles

In a study of growth requirements for E. tarda, an

isolate used was recovered from a turtle (species not given) in 1957 (D'Empaire, 1969). This would be the earliest date for the isolation of E. tarda from any species. Jackson et al. (1969a), in a survey of enteric bacteria of captive turtles, recovered E. tarda from Rhinoclemys annulata, Chrysemys scripta, C. nelsoni and C. concinna. Jackson et al. (1969b) added five additional species of turtles from which E. tarda was isolated, including two species before their possible contamination in captivity. E. tarda was found in the large intestine of 15 of 38 turtles cultured for enteric bacteria in the New York Zoological Park (Otis and Behler, 1973). All of these turtles also carried Salmonella durham. Among the turtle species represented were Sternotherus odoratus, C. scripta elegans, C. picta, Mauremys caspica, Melanochelys trijuga coronata, Graptemys kohni, Malaclemys terrapin terrapin and Terrapene carolina carolina. No evidence of disease due to E. tarda was found in any of the infected turtles.

Crocodilians

In Florida, E. tarda was isolated from the kidneys of a listless and unresponsive alligator, Alligator mississippiens, after it died at a zoological garden. The kidneys were congested and contained several necrotic foci in the cortex. A generalized fibrinous peritonitis was found in the alligator, and Proteus vulgaris was isolated from the necrotic oviducts. The contribution of E. tarda to the observed kidney lesions was not proven (Wallace et al., 1966). During an investigation of a die-off of fish and other aquatic species in a eutrophic lake in Florida, five apparently normal alligators, 1 to 1.2 m in length, were presented for necropsy. No lesions were found in the alligators, however, E. tarda was isolated from the contents of the large intestine of three animals. E. tarda also was isolated from cloacal swabs of 2 of 22 apparently normal alligators from another area in Florida (White et al., 1973). E. tarda was isolated from the cloacal contents of three crocodiles (species not given) in western Australia (Iveson, 1971).

Frogs and Toads

E. tarda was isolated from the intestinal contents of 7 of 78 frogs (species not given) in India (Sharma et al., 1974). One isolate was a new serotype. Also in India (Hissar), the intestinal contents of 329 toads, Bufo spp., were cultured for enteric bacteria, and although 36% were carriers of Salmonella spp., E. tarda was not isolated (Sharma et al., 1977). Subsequently, in the same area, 14 of 66 toads were found to be carriers of E. tarda (Kumar and Sharma, 1978). A summary of the Indian studies on enteric infections in man and animals was given by Sharma (1979). In Panama, E. tarda was found in the intestinal contents of various species of animals, including 2 of 34 giant toads, B. marinus (Kourany et al., 1977). Ninety-two frogs of nine unnamed genera were free of this organism. None of the aforementioned reports found evidence of disease or lesions in the frogs or toads

ETIOLOGY

Sakazaki and Murata (1962) reported the isolation of gram-negative enteric organisms in the feces of numerous snakes in Japan and referred to them as a new group in the family Enterobacteriaceae, which they called the Asakusa group. Sakazaki (1965) officially proposed this name for the new group. In the United States, King and Adler (1964) isolated a new member of the Enterobacteriaceae from the feces of a man hospitalized with enteric fever and acute gastroenteritis. They were unaware of the report of Aakazaki and Murata (1962) and suggested the name "Bartholomew group" for these organisms. During the period 1959 to 1965, the Center for Disease Control, in the United States, received 37 strains of an organism with the same characteristics as the Asakusa and Bartholomew groups; all but one strain were isolated from man, the exception came from a cow with diarrhea. They referred to these organisms as bacterium 1483-59. Ewing et al. (1965) proposed a new species and genus for these organisms, to be included in the family Enterobacteriaceae. The generic name Edwardsiella (Ewing and McWhorter) and the species name E. tarda were proposed. This new genus containing one species was described by Sakazaki (1974).

Most isolations of E. tarda have been made during routine enteric cultural attempts, using differential and selective media commonly employed for Salmonella spp., as described by Edwards and Ewing (1972).

Ewing et al. (1965) reported biochemical findings with 37 strains of E. tarda and compared the reactions to those of certain other Enterobacteriaceae, namely Proteus, Salmonella, Arizona, Citrobacter and Escherichia coli. There were many reactions that separated E. tarda from the other members of the family. Sakazaki (1967) also noted that the E. tarda isolated in Japan differed from Salmonella. He reported that the newly described organisms produced indol, and did not ferment mannitol, arabinose, xylose and trehalose. Of 18 carbohydrates tested, only glucose and maltose were fermented. Extensive biochemical characteristics of E. tarda compared to the reactions of other Enterobacteriaceae are given by Cowan (1974).

Sakazaki (1967) reported the results of serologic studies on 256 cultures of E. tarda, 249 from snake feces, 2 from seal intestinal contents and 5 from human patients with gastroenteritis. From the results of his agglutination and agglutinin-absorption studies, a scheme was presented consisting of 17 O groups and 11 H antigens, suggesting the existence of 18 serotypes. However, five of Sakazaki's strains failed to produce indol and eight did not decarboxylate ornithine, and probably were not E. tarda. Sakazaki found no significant antigenic relationships between E. tarda and Salmonella, Escherichia, Citrobacter, Proteus, Enterobacter and Hafnia. Ewing et al. (1965) studied 37 strains of E. tarda and found 8 O antigen groups and 10 H antigens, forming 21 serotypes. McWhorter et al. (1967) expanded these studies, reporting 42 O groups and 28 H antigens among 213 cultures, resulting in 103 serotypes. The strains were received from various laboratories in the United States and elsewhere from many sources. These studies are an indication of the serological diversity among E. tarda isolates. Iveson (1973) found 50 serotypes among 500 isolates from man and animals in western Australia.

DIAGNOSIS

Many media have been developed for the isolation of enterobacteria. The most often used enrichment media for the culture of fecal specimens is selenite F and tetrathionate broths, with selenite F probably most often used. However, studies by Iveson (1973) suggest that the isolation of E. tarda was greatly enhanced by the use of strontium chloride B enrichment broth. These media are very useful by allowing the growth of lactose negative enteric pathogens while inhibiting the growth of the usually more numerous coliform organisms. Of the many differential plate media used for primary culture of enteric specimens, and for subculturing from enrichment media, MacConkey's and Salmonella-Shigella (SS) media are often used. Lactose negative colonies are typically subcultured to Triple Sugar Iron (TSI) slants and from this medium to differential tubed media for final identification by means of biochemical reactions. Cultures may be identified serologically and confirmed by biochemical tests (Edwards and Ewing, 1972). More recently, many laboratories have utilized rapid identification methods once a pure culture is obtained and determined to be a cytochrome-oxidase negative organism. These methods permit the rapid differentiation of E. tarda from other enteric pathogens.

SIGNIFICANCE

Although often isolated from amphibians and reptiles, disease conditions or lesions due to E. tarda infections in these species have not been proven. It is possible that these animals are only asymptomatic carriers of the organisms; however, it may be that active infections simply have not been found, or that affected individuals may die and not be discovered or may be removed by predators/scavengers.

The original description of E. tarda was based largely on isolates from man (Ewing et al., 1965). Since then the most clear evidence of pathogenicity of E. tarda has been in human infections where both intestinal and extra-intestinal disease has been well documented (Bockemuhl et al., 1971; Clarridge et al., 1980; Jordan and Hadley, 1969; Makula et al., 1973). Proof of E. tarda as the causative agent of disease in domestic or wild species has not been as firmly established. The organism was associated with bovine diarrhea (Ewing et al., 1965), produced "emphysematous putrifactive disease" in catfish, Ictaturus punctatus (Meyer and Bullock, 1973), and was considered the cause of hemorrhagic disease in a large-mouth bass, Micropterus salmoides (White et al., 1973). E. tarda clearly was associated with enteric infection in an ostrich, Struthio camelus (White et al., 1969), and was associated with hemorrhagic enteritis in brown pelicans, Pelecannus occidentalis carolinensis, and common loons, Gavia immer (White et al., 1973).

It has been suggested that E. tarda can produce disease patterns in man similar to those caused by Salmonella, probably including enteric fever, and that the asymptomatic carrier state can occur (Jordan and Hadley, 1969). This may be true of other species infected with E. tarda as well, with active disease produced under stressful conditions. This agent could represent a zoonotic disease hazard to individuals working with amphibians and reptiles, and the same precautions should be followed as with Salmonella and Arizona infected animals.

REFERENCES

Arambulo, P.V., Westerlund, N.C., and Sarmiento, R.V., 1968, On the isolation of human enteric organisms from the bile of pigs and cattle, Acta Medica Phil., 5:84-86.

Arambulo, P.V., Westerlund, N.C., Sarmiento, R.V., and Abaga, A.S., 1967, Isolation of Edwardsiella tarda: A new genus of Enterobacteriaceae from pig bile in the Phillipines, Far East Med. J., 3:385-386.

Bartlett, K.H., and Trust, T.J., 1976, Isolation of salmonellae and other potential pathogens from the freshwater aquarium snail Ampullaria, Appl. Environ. Microbiol., 31:635-639.

Berg, R.W., and Anderson, A.W., 1972, Salmonellae and Edwardsiella tarda in gull feces: A source of contamination in fish processing plants, Appl. Microbiol., 24:501-503.

Bockemuhl, J., Pan-Urai, R., and Burkhardt, F., 1971, Edwardsiella tarda associated with human disease, Pathol. Microbiol., 37:393-401.

Centi, P., Cavazzini, G., and Corradini, L., 1977, Sull'-inquinamento microbiologico dell'ambiente da parte degli allevamenti, Nota I. Enterobacteriaceae da allevamenti bovini, Boll. Ist. Sieroter., 56:351-361.

Chamoiseau, G., 1967, Note sur le pouvoir pathogene d'Edwardsiella tarda. Un cas de septicemie mortelle du pigeon, Rev. Elev. Vet. Pays Trop., 20:493:495.

Clarridge, J.E., Musher, D.M., Fainstein, V., and Wallace, R.J., Jr., 1980, Extraintestinal infection caused by Edwardsiella tarda, J. Clin. Microbiol., 11: 511-514.

Coles, B.M., Stroud, R.K., and Sheggeby, S., 1978, Isolation of Edwardsiella tarda from three Oregon sea mammals, J. Wildlife Dis., 14:339-341.

Cowan, S.T., 1974, Family 1. Enterobacteriaceae, in: "Bergey's manual of determinative bacteriology," 8th ed., R.E. Buchanan and N.E. Gibbons, eds., Williams and Wilkins Co., Baltimore.

D'Empaire, M., 1969, Les facteurs de croissance des Edwardsiella tarda, Ann. Inst. Pasteur, 116: 63-68.

Edwards, P.R., and Ewing, W.H., 1972, "Identification of Enterobacteriaceae," 3rd ed., Burgess Publ. Co., Minneapolis.

Elazhary, M.A.S.Y., Tremblay, A., Lagace, A., and Roy, R.S., 1973, A preliminary study on the intestinal flora of cecum and colon of eight, ten and 12 week old swine, Can. J. Comp. Med., 37:369-374.

Ewing, W.H., McWhorter, A.C., Escobar, M.R., and Lubin, A.H., 1965, Edwardsiella, a new genus of Enterobacteriaceae based on a new species, E. tarda, Int. Bull. Bacteriol. Nomenclature Taxanom., 15:33-38.

Forrester, D.J., White, F.H., and Simpson, C.F., 1976, Parasites and diseases of sandhill cranes in Florida, Proc. Int. Crane Workshop, 1:284-290.

Forrester, D.J., White, F.H., Woodard, J.C., and Thompson, N.P., 1975, Intussusception in a Florida manatee, J. Wildlife Dis., 11:566-568.

Frye, F.L., and Herald, E.S., 1969, Osteomyelitis in a manatee, J. Amer. Vet. Med. Ass., 155:1073-1076.

Hawke, J.P., 1979, A bacterium associated with disease of pond cultured channel catfish, Ictalurus punctatus, J. Fish Res. Board Can., 36:1508-1512.

Hoff, G.L., and White, F.H., 1977, Salmonella in reptiles: Isolation from free-ranging lizards (Reptilia, Lacertilia) in Florida, J. Herpetol., 11:123-129.

Iveson, J.B., 1971, Strontium chloride B and EE enrichment broth media for the isolation of Edwardsiella, Salmonella and Arizona species from tiger snakes, J. Hyg., 69:223-230.

Iveson, J.B., 1973, Enrichment procedure for the isolation of Salmonella, Arizona, Edwardsiella and Shigella from faeces, J. Hyg., 71:349-361.

Jackson, M.M., Fulton, M., and Jackson, C.G., 1969a, A survey of the enteric bacteria (Enterobacteriaceae) of chelonians: Preliminary findings, ASB Bull., 16:55.

Jackson, M.M., Jackson, C.G., and Fulton, M., 1969b, Investigation of the enteric bacteria of the Testudinata, I. Occurrence of the genera Arizona, Citrobacter, Edwardsiella and Salmonella, Bull. Wildlife Dis. Ass., 5:328-329.

Jordon, G.W., and Hadley, W.K., 1969, Human infections with Edwardsiella tarda, Ann. Intern. Med., 70:283-288.

King, B.M., and Adler, D.L., 1964, A previously undescribed group of Enterobacteriaceae, Amer. J. Clin. Pathol., 41:230-232.

Koshi, G., and Lalitha, M.K., 1976, Edwardsiella tarda in a variety of human infections, Indian J. Med. Res., 64:1753-1759.

Kourany, M., and Vasquez, M.A., 1975, A survey to assess potential disease hazards along proposed sea level canal routes in Panama and Columbia, VIII. Survey of enterobacterial pathogens in wild caught vertebrates, Military Med., 140:22-25.

Kourany, M., Bowdre, L., and Herrer, A., 1976, Panamanian forest mammals as carriers of Salmonella, Amer. J. Trop. Med. Hyg., 25:449-455.

Kourany, M., Vasquez, M.A., and Saenz, R., 1977, Edwardsiellosis in man and animals in Panama: Clinical and epidemiological characteristics, Amer. J. Trop. Med. Hyg., 26:1183-1190.

Kumar, A., and Sharma, V.K., 1978, Enterobacteria of emerging pathogenic significance from clinical cases in man and animals and detection of toads and wall lizards as their reservoirs, Antonie Leeuwenhoek, 44:219-228.

Makula, A., Gatti, F., and Vandepitte, J., 1973, Edwardsiella tarda infections in Zaire, Ann. Soc. Belge Med. Trop., 53:165-172.

McWhorter, A.C., Ewing, W.H., and Sakazaki, R., 1967, Provisional antigenic schema for Edwardsiella tarda, Bacteriol. Proc., p.89.

Meyer, F.P., and Bullock, G.L., 1973, Edwardsiella tarda, a new pathogen of channel catfish (Ictalurus punctatus), Appl. Microbiol., 25:155-156.

Muller, H.E., 1972, Uber die aerobe Fakalflora von Reptilien, insbesondere uber die Enterobakterien von Schlangen, Zentralbl. Bakteriol. Parasitenkd. Hyg. Abt. I Orig. A, 222:487-495.

Otis, V.S., and Behler, J.L., 1973, The occurrence of salmonellae and Edwardsiella in the turtles of the New York Zoological Park, J. Wildlife Dis., 9:4-6.

Owens, D.R., Nelson, S.L., and Addison, J.B., 1974, Isolation of Edwardsiella tarda from swine, Appl. Microbiol., 27:703-705.

Reichel, W.L., Locke, L.N., and Prouty, R.M., 1974, Peregrine falcon suspected of pesticide poisoning, Avian Dis., 18:487-489.

Roggendorf, M., and Muller, H.E., 1976, Enterobakterien bei Reptilien, Zentralbl. Bakteriol. Parasitenkd. Hyg. Abt. I Orig. A, 236:22-35.

Sakazaki, R., 1965, A proposed group of the family Enterobacteriaceae, the Asakusa group, Int. Bull. Bacteriol. Nomenclature Taxonom., 15:45-47.

Sakazaki, R., 1967, Studies on the Asakusa group of Enterobacteriaceae, (Edwardsiella tarda), Jap. J. Med. Sci. Biol., 20:205-212.

Sakazaki, R., 1974, Genus II. Edwardsiella, in: "Bergey's manual of determinative bacteriology," 8th ed., R.E. Buchanan and N.E. Gibbons, eds., Williams and Wilkins Co., Baltimore.

Sakazaki, R., and Murata, Y., 1962, The new group of the Enterbacteriaceae, the Asakusa group, Jap. J. Bacteriol., 17:617-618.

Sharma, V.K., 1979, Enterobacteriaceae infections in man and animals and detection of their natural reservoirs in India, Zentralbl. Bakteriol. Parasitenkd. Hyg. Abt. I Orig. A, 243:381-391.

Sharma, V.K., Kaura, Y.K., and Singh, I.P., 1974, Frogs as carriers of Salmonella and Edwardsiella, Antonie Leeuwenhoek, 40:171-175.

Sharma, V.K., Rohde, R., Garg, D.N., and Kumar, A., 1977, Toads as natural reservoir of Salmonella, Zentralbl. Bakteriol. Parasitenkd. Hyg. Abt. I Orig. A, 239:172-177.

Tan, R.J.S., and Lim, E.W., 1977, Occurrence of Edwardsiella tarda in the household lizard, Gekko gecko, Jap. J. Med. Sci. Biol., 30:321-323.

Trust, T.J., and Bartlett, K.H., 1974, Occurrence of potential pathogens in water containing ornamental fishes, Appl. Mirobiol., 28:35-40.

Wallace, L.J., White, F.H., and Gore, H.L., 1966, Isolation of Edwardsiella tarda from a sea lion and two alligators, J. Amer. Vet. Med. Ass., 149: 881-883.

White, F.H., Neal, F.C., Simpson, C.F., and Walsh, A.F., 1969, Isolation of Edwardsiella tarda from an ostrich and an Australian skink, J. Amer. Vet. Med. Ass., 155:1057-1058.

White, F.H., Simpson, C.F., and Williams, L.E., 1973, Isolation of Edwardsiella tarda from aquatic species and surface waters in Florida, J. Wildlife Dis., 9:204-208.

White, F.H., Watson, J.J., Hoff, G.L., and Bigler, W.J., 1975, Edwardsiella tarda in Florida raccoons, Procyon lotor, Arch. Environ. Health, 30:602-603.

LEPTOSPIROSIS

[1]Gerald L. Hoff and [2]Franklin H. White

[1]Office of Epidemiological Services, Kansas City
[2]Health Department and College of Veterinary
Medicine, University of Florida

INTRODUCTION

Leptospirosis is a group of infectious diseases of man and animals, caused by various serovarities of the spirochetes *Leptospira interrogans* and *L. biflexa* (Alexander, 1974). However, *L. interrogans* is the species generally associated with disease manifestations, while *L. biflexa* is considered to be saprophytic, being found predominately in fresh water and soil. Isolations of *L. interrogans* have been made from clinical specimens, carriers and fresh water. Thus the ubiquitous nature of leptospires provides ample exposure of amphibians and reptiles to these organisms through contact with infected water or through ingestion of infected prey.

DISTRIBUTION

Isolations of leptospires have been made from *Chrysemys scripta elegans* (Glosser et al., 1974), *Emys orbicularis* (Combiesco et al., 1964), *Mauremys caspica* (Hoeden, 1968), *Heterodon platyrhinos* (Ferris et al., 1961), *Bothrops pradoi* (Hyakuta et al., 1980), *Lacerta agilis* (Plesko et al., 1962), *Rana pipiens* (Diesch et al., 1966) and toads (Babudieri, 1972). The isolates from *E. orbicularis* and *M. caspica* represented serovarities of *L. biflexa*, while the other reptilian isolates were *L. interrogans*. A new species, *L. ranarum*, was proposed for the amphibian isolates (Babudieri, 1972).

A number of serological surveys have reported agglutinins to leptospires among herpetofauna from various parts of the world (Andrews et al., 1965; Combiesco et al. 1958; Ferris et al., 1961; Glosser et al., 1974; Hoeden, 1968; Hyakutake et al., 1980; Thiel, 1948; Turner et al., 1959; White, 1963). However, there are difficulties with interpretation of serologic findings. Non-specific agglutinins have been recorded in the sera of free-ranging R. esculenta and R. fusca (Thiel, 1948) and of various turtle species (Combiesco et al., 1958; Shenberg et al., 1970; Hoeden, 1968). As a result, it has been proposed that no significance should be attached to the agglutination of leptospires by the sera of herptiles (Hoeden, 1968; Thiel, 1948).

ETIOLOGY

Weil (1886) studied four cases of infectious jaundice which he described as being distinct from other known diseases. This disease became known as "Weil's disease", a febrile illness of man characterized by nervous symptoms, enlarged liver and spleen, jaundice and renal involvement. Subsequently, the disease was found in certain occupational groups such as rice field, canal, canefield and abattoir workers, and others exposed to wet environments and animals.

The causative organism was not discovered until Inada et al. (1916) isolated, described and named it Spirochaeta icterohemorrhagiae. Ido et al. (1916) found virulent organisms in the kidneys of house and ditch rats. Stimson (1907) found an organism in kidney sections of a patient who was believed to have died from yellow fever, and named the spirochete, S. interrogans. In retrospect, his description of the organisms and drawings and evaluations of the original sections by Sellards (1940), showed that the organisms were leptospires. Noguchi (1918) studied the strains of S. icterohemorrhagiae from Japan, from soldiers in Flanders and strains isolated from rats in the United States, and is responsible for creating the geunus Leptospira, to be included in the order Spirochaetales.

Since the discovery of the causative agent of leptospirosis, many different serological types have been isolated from man and many other animal species. The pathogenic leptospires have been placed into 18 serogroups, containing 161 serovarieties (Turner, 1976).

PATHOGENESIS

Several experimental studies have suggested that frogs are refractory to infection with L. interrogans and L. ranarum (Diesch et al., 1967; Uhlenhurth and Fromme, 1919; Thiel, 1948). Only when frogs were inoculated with large concentrations of virulent leptospires would the spirochetes be present in the blood, kidney and liver. The presence of leptospires in these tissues was transitory, lasting from 1 to 7 days post-inoculation (Thiel, 1948). There was no excretion of leptospires in the urine. Therefore, the isolation of L. ranarum from the kidney tissue of free-ranging R. pipiens and toads (Babudieri, 1972; Diesch et al., 1966) may be fortuitous incidents or may represent an as yet unproven short term carrier-shedder state. Low level agglutinin responses of a transitory nature were detected in most inoculated frogs (Diesch et al., 1967; Thiel, 1948).

Inoculation of the turtles, E. orbicularis, Emydoidea blandingi and Chelydra serpentina with L. interrogans did not induce morbidity and leptospires were not recovered from the urine (Abdulla and Karstad, 1962; Combiesco et al., 1958). A leptospiremia was observed in E. blandingi between post-inoculation days 5 and 12, but organisms could not be recovered from the kidneys (Abdulla and Karstad, 1962). The failure to recover leptospires from the kidney tissue may have been due to the presence of large numbers of other bacteria, a problem encountered by other investigators working with reptiles (Hoeden, 1968; White, 1963). A low level agglutinin response was elicited in all inoculated turtles, while uninoculated cage mates remained seronegative (Abdulla and Karstad, 1962).

Garter snakes, Thamnophis sirtalis, responded to inoculation with L. interrogans with a leptospiremia, tissue infection of the liver and kidney, and agglutinins (Abdulla and Karstad, 1962). The leptospiremia occurred between post-inoculation days 5 and 14, while tissue infection persisted up to post-inoculation day 195. Although renal excretion of leptospires was not demonstrated, it undoubtedly occurred as uninoculated cage mates developed agglutinin responses and tissue infection with the same L. interrogans serovar. The agglutinin response of the inoculated snakes was of higher titer and longer duration than that of the uninoculated cage mates. The infections in three of ten inoculated snakes persisted through a 70 day induced hibernation, as evidenced by recovery of leptospires from the kidney tissues.

DIAGNOSIS

The diagnosis of leptospirosis is most often made from the results of serologic tests, but other methods are available, i.e., direct culture of urine, blood or tissues indirect culture by means of hamster or guinea pig inoculation, or direct microscopic examination of specimens by darkfield, silver impregnation or immunofluorescent techniques. A definitive diagnosis requires isolation of the organism, followed by serologic identification of the serovariety. Laboratory diagnostic techniques are reviewed by Alexander (1974), Shotts (1976) and Sulzer and Jones (1974).

Although many different serologic methods have been developed for the diagnosis of leptospirosis, the standard test is the microscopic agglutination test in which live leptospiral cultures are used as antigens. The improved microtechnique of Cole et al. (1973) utilizing microplates is widely used. In this procedure, live standardized leptospiral cultures are used as the antigens and are reacted with serial serum dilutions in plastic microtiter plates. The plates are read over a darkfield condenser and are examined for characteristic micro-agglutination.

Media containing rabbit serum enrichment have been used to culture blood, urine and tissues for leptospires. Limitations of these media are recognized, particularly when used to attempt recovery of fastidious serovarities of leptospires. The media gaining wide acceptance and which are capable of growing fastidious serovarities are those containing bovine albumin and polysorbate-80 (Ellinghausen and McCullough, 1965). Detailed cultural procedures are given by Sulzer and Jones (1974).

With darkfield microscopy, leptospires may be observed in clinical specimens if present in sufficient numbers, and if examined promptly. Also, silver impregnation stains may be used to identify leptospires in tissue section (Thompson, 1966). The immunofluorescent technique may be used to detect leptospires in urine and tissues (White Ristic, 1959; White et al., 1961).

PROGNOSIS AND IMMUNITY

All available evidence indicates that leptospirosis is not a morbidity or mortality factor for herptiles. While tissue infection can occur when large inocula of leptospires are administered, isolations of *Leptospira* spp. from free-ranging herptiles are very rare. In experimental studies, leptospiremia preceeded tissue infection. However, sera from free-ranging C. serpentina, C. picta and R. pipiens possessed leptospiricidal activity against both L. biflexa and L. interrogans (Charon et al., 1975). This complement mediated leptospiricidal activity is temperature dependent and similar to the bactericidal activity reported for the sera of Tiliqua rugosa and Bufo marinus (Schwab and Reeves, 1966). This leptospiricidal activity probably is overwhelmed by the dosage of organisms administered during experimental studies.

The significance of agglutinins to leptospires in the sera of herptiles is a confusing issue. In animals inoculated with L. interrogans serovars, agglutinins specific to the inoculated serovar appear in the sera. However, studies have shown that the agglutinins to leptospires detected in serological surveys are for the most part non-specific (Combiesco et al., 1958; Hoeden, 1968; Thiel, 1948; Shenberg et al., 1970). The agglutinins are located in the globulin fraction and seem to depend upon the age of the animal rather than on contact with L. interrogans serovars. Whether these agglutinins represent response to contact with leptospires, i.e., L. biflexa, or represent cross reactions stimulated by other antigens, remains to be determined (Charon et al., 1975). Consequently, the interpretation of serologic surveys among herpetofauna requires careful analysis.

CONTROL

There is no need for control procedures for leptospirosis among herptiles in terms of maintaining the health of these animals. However, since L. interrogans is a zoonotic disease agent, care should be taken when handling infected animals, especially snakes. The presence of long tissue infection in T. sirtalis and the fact that transmission to cage mates has been documented (Abdulla and Karstad, 1962) make these animals potentially dangerous to the keeper.

REFERENCES

Abdulla, P.K., and Karstad, L.H., 1962, Experimental infections with Leptospira pomona in snakes and turtles, Zoonoses Res., 1:295-306.
Alexander, A.D., 1974, Leptospira, in: "Manual of clinical microbiology," 2nd ed., E.H. Lennette, E.H.

Spaulding and J.P. Truant, eds., Amer. Soc. Microbiol., Washington.

Andrews, R.D., Reilly, J.R., Ferris, D.H., and Hanson, L.E., 1965, Leptospiral agglutinins in sera of southern Illinois herpetofauna, Bull. Wildlife Dis. Ass., 1:55-59.

Babudieri, B., 1972, Systematics of a leptospire strain isolated from a frog, Experientia, 28:1252-1253.

Charon, N.W., Johnson, R.C., and Muschell, L.H., 1975, Antileptospiral activity in lower vertebrate sera, Infect. Immun., 12:1386-1391.

Cole, J.K., Sulzer, C.R., and Pursell, A.R., 1973, Improved microtechnique for the leptospiral microscopic agglutination test, Appl. Microbiol., 25:976-980.

Combiesco, D., Sturdza, N., Elian, M., and Nicolesco, M., 1964, Study on the animal sources of infection in leptospirosis, Proc. 2nd Int. Symp. Leptospirae and Leptospirosis in Men and Animals, Lublin (1962), Part 1.

Combiesco, D., Sturdza, N., Sefer, M., and Radu, I., 1958, Leptospirenforschungen in Rumanien, Zentralbl. Bakteriol. Parasitenkd. Hyg. Abt. I Orig. A, 173:103-106.

Diesch, S.L., McCulloch, W.F., and Braun, J.L., 1967, Experimental leptospirosis in frogs, Nature, 214: 1139-1140.

Diesch, S.L., McCulloch, W.F., Braun, J.L., and Ellinghausen, H.C., 1966, Leptospires isolated from frog kidneys, Nature, 209:939-940.

Ellinghausen, H.C., and McCullough, W.G., 1965, Nutrition of Leptospira pomona and growth of 13 other serotypes: Fractionation of oleic albumin complex (OAC) and a medium of bovine albumin and polysorbate-80, Amer. J. Vet. Res., 26:45-51.

Ferris, D.H., Rhoades, H.E., Hanson, L.E., Galton, M., and Mansfield, M.E., 1961, Research into the nidality of Leptospira ballum in campestral hosts including the hog-nosed snake (Heterodon platyrhinos), Cornell Vet., 51:405-418.

Glosser, J.W., Sulzer, C.R., Eberhardt, M., and Winkler, W.G., 1974, Cultural and serologic evidence of Leptospira interrogans serotype tarassovi infection in turtles, J. Wildlife Dis., 10:429-435.

Hoeden, J., van der, 1968, Agglutination of leptospirae in sera of fresh water turtles, Antonie van Leeuwenhoek, 34:458-464.

Hyakutake, S., Biasi, P.D., Belluomini, H.E., and Santa Rosa, C.A., 1980, Leptospirosis in Brazilian snakes, Int. J. Zoonoses, 7:73-77.

Ido, Y., Hoki, R., Ito, H., and Wani, H., 1916, The prophylaxis of Weil's disease (spirochaetosis icterohemorrhagiae), J. Exp. Med., 24:471-483.

Inada, R., Ido, Y., Hoki, R., Kaneko, R., and Ito, H., 1916, The etiology, mode of infection, and specific therapy of Weil's disease (spirochaetosis icterohaemorrhagicae), J. Exp. Med., 23:377-402.

Noguchi, H., 1918, Morphological characteristics and nomenclature of Leptospira (Spirochaeta) icterohaemorrhagiae (Inado and Ido), J. Exp. Med., 27:575-592.

Plesko, L., Janovicova, E., and Lac, J., 1962, Beitrag zur Bedeutung von Kaltblutern fur die Zirkulation der Leptospiren in der Natur, Zentralbl. Bakteriol. Parasitenkd. Hyg. Abt. I Orig. A, 192:482-484.

Shenberg, E., Friedlander, A., Torten, M., and Ben-Efraim, S., 1970, Leptospiral agglutinin factor in turtles, Israel J. Med. Sci., 6:408-412.

Schwab, G.E., and Reeves, P.R., 1966, Comparison of bactericidal activity of different vertebrate sera, J. Bacteriol., 91:106-112.

Sellards, A.W., 1940, The interpretation of (?Spirochaeta) interrogans of Stimson in the light of subsequent development, Trans. Royal Soc. Trop. Med. Hyg., 33:545.

Shotts, E.B., Jr., 1976, Laboratory diagnosis of leptospirosis, in: "Biology of parasitic spirochetes," R.C. Johnson, ed., Academic Press, New York.

Stimson, A.M., 1907, A note on an organism found in yellow fever tissues, Public Health Rep., 22:541.

Sulzer, C.R., and Jones, W.L., 1974, "Leptospirosis: Methods in laboratory diagnosis," DHEW Center for Disease Control, Atlanta.

Theil, P.H., van, 1948, The role of frogs in the epidemiology of Weil's disease, Antonie van Leeuwenhoek, 14:129-144.

Thompson, S.W., 1966, "Selected histochemical and histopathological methods", Charles C. Thomas, Springfield.

Turner, L.H., 1976, Provisional list of serotypes, in: "Biology of parasitic spirochetes," R.C. Johnson, ed., Academic Press, New York.

Turner, L.H., Elisberg, B.L., Smith, C.E.G., and Broom, J.C., 1959, Acute febrile illnesses in Malaya: Leptospirosis, Med. J. Malaya, 14:83-86.

Uhlenhuth, P., and Fromme, W., 1919, Experimentelle Untersuchungen uber der Infektionsmodus, die Epidemiologie und Serumhandlung der Weilschen Krankheit (Icterus infectiosus), Z. Imm. forsch., 28:1.

Weil, A., 1886, Uber eine Eigentumliche, mit Milztumor, Icterus, und Nephritis einhergehende akute Infektious-Krankheit, Dtsch. Arch. Klin. Med., 39: 209-232.

White, F.H., 1963, Leptospiral agglutinins in snake serums Amer. J. Vet. Res., 24:179-182.

White, F.H., and Ristic, M., 1959, Detection of Leptospira pomona in guinea pig and bovine urine with fluorescein-labeled antibody, J. Infect. Dis., 105:118-123.

White, F.H., Stoliker, H.E., and Galton, M.M., 1961, Detection of leptospires in naturally infected dogs, using fluorescein-labeled antibody, Amer. J. Vet. Res., 22:650-654.

Q FEVER

Gerald L. Hoff

Office of Epidemiological Service

Kansas City Health Department

INTRODUCTION

Among the known rickettsial diseases, Q fever or coxiellosis is considered to have the most widespread distribution, being found essentially worldwide in the temperate and tropical climates. Coupled with this extensive geographic distribution is an equally impressive host range of arthropods, mammals, birds and reptiles. However, as a disease coxiellosis is most notable for its general lack of clinical illness in the majority of host species studied (Bell, 1970). Were it not for the fact that coxiellosis is a minor zoonosis of man (Burgdorfer, 1975), little interest probably would be given to Coxiella burneti.

In contrast to the vast literature concerning C. burneti in mammals (Bell, 1970), only a handful of reports of Q fever in herptiles or their ectoparasites exist. Tendeiro (1952) reported C. burneti in Amblyomma nuttali, Aponoma halla and Hyalomma truncatum ticks collected from reptiles in Portuguese Guinea, although this report was questioned by Babudieri (1959). The organism was isolated from Python molurus in India (Yadav and Sethi, 1980). Blanc et al. (1959) and Blanc (1961) experimentally infected Testudo gracea with C. burneti and effected haematophagous transmission to the tick, H. aegyptium. Serologic surveys have detected antibodies to C. burneti in Natrix natrix, Ptyas korros, P. mucosus, Naja naja, Ophiophagus hannah, P. molurus, Lycodon striatus and Kachuga sp. (Stephen and Roa, 1979; Yadav and Sethi, 1979). Antibodies were not detected in Crotalus viridus, Thamnophis sp., Rana tigrina and Bufo sp. (Enright et al., 1971; Stephen and Roa, 1979; Yadav and Sethi, 1979).

ETIOLOGY

C. burneti rickettsia are rod-shaped organisms, however occasionally they are diplobacilli or spheres (Buchanan and Gibbons, 1974). It resembles organisms of the genus Rickettsia in most staining properties, dependence on host cells for growth, and close natural association with arthropod and vertebrate hosts. Unlike Rickettsia spp., C. burneti is gram-positive, capable of passing through filters that retain other rickettsiae, resistant to drying and relatively elevated temperatures, and resistant to many physical and chemical agents. The ability to withstand dessication, heat and exposure to ultraviolet irradiation plays an important role in the epizootiology of C. burneti.

TRANSMISSION

Ticks play a significant role in maintaining and distributing C. burneti among their wildlife hosts. Expermentally, C. burneti infection occurs readily in ticks, with massive invasion of all tissues, particularly the epithelial cells of the gut (Burgdorfer, 1975). One gram of tick feces may contain up to 10^{10} infectious guinea pig doses, and the organism can survive in dried tick feces at room temperature for at least 586 days (Philip, 1948). Since ticks defecate periodically during engorgement, they are potent sources for contaminating skin and hair of their hosts. In addition, transovarian and transstadial transmission of C. burneti occurs (Burgdorfer, 1975). C. burneti infection in seven animal caretakers who were involved in deticking 500 ball pythons, P. regius, has been documented (Kim et al., 1978). No isolates of C. burneti were recovered from a small sample of ticks and the sera of two pythons were negative for antibodies. While no unequivocal direct link between the caretakers' illnesses and the pythons or parasites was established, the incident emphasizes the need to control ectoparasites of captive animals. The ticks involved were A. nuttalli, A. latum and A. flavomaculatum. While numerous other haematophagous arthropods are susceptible to experimental or natural infection with C. burneti, the role of these arthropods as vectors remains questionable (Burgdorfer, 1975).

Livestock and man can acquire the disease via inhalation of aerosolized particles containing infectious C. burneti. Infected placentas and post-partum discharges provide the major sources of environmental contamination (Burgdorfer, 1975). Dissication and disintegration of these massively infected tissues produce rickettsia-laden particles which are subject to dissemination by wind, man and animals. The importance of this cycle of transmission among wildlife species is unknown.

PATHOGENESIS

Available information on the pathogenesis of Q fever in reptiles is limited to the studies of Blanc et al. (1959) and Blanc (1961). Following intracardiac inoculation of T. graeca, a rickettsemia developed which persisted for at least 80 days. The infection was inapparent, with no temperature elevation and no agglutinin antibody response. The rickettsemia was sufficient to infect the tick, H. aegyptium. There were no comments on behavioral changes in infected tortoises.

DIAGNOSIS

The most convincing evidence of infection is recovery of C. burneti from the tissues of infected animals. After suitable preparation (Bell, 1970), a 10% suspension of inoculum is injected intraperitoneally into young adult male guinea pigs, Cavia porcellus. The body temperatures of the guinea pigs should be monitored daily. In the event of infection with C. burneti, a febrile response of 40 C or more will be noted after an incubation period of 5 to 12 days. It should be noted, however, that the isolate of C. burneti from P. molurus did not induce a febrile response in guinea pigs (Yadav and Sethi, 1980). After 2 or 3 days of fever, the guinea pigs should be killed for demonstration of the rickettsia from impression smears or slides from a cut spleen surface. Alternately, tissue or blood samples could be taken and used to inoculate other animals or 5 to 7 day old chicken embryos. The blood is injected into the yolk sac and stained smears are prepared from the yolk sacs of embryos which die between 3 and 8 days post-inoculation. If no deaths occur by the 8th day, blind passage to other embryonated eggs should be made. Hamsters, Mesocricetus auratus, may be used instead of guinea pigs and both are preferrable to mice, Mus musculus (Burgdorfer, 1975).

Preliminary identification of isolates from laboratory animals may be done on smears stained by Giemsa, Machiavello and fluorescent antibody techniques (Elisberg and Bozeman, 1969). Confirmatory evidence is obtained by development of specific antibodies in inoculated animals or by use of the embryo-grown organisms as complement-fixation antigens. Ticks may be initially screened by utilizing the hemolymph test (Burgdorfer, 1970). Hemolymph is collected on a slide by amputating the distal portion of one or more legs. The smear is heat fixed, stained by Gimenez method and examined microscopically. Preliminary identification of rickettsia can be obtained by fluorescent-antibody staining, with confirmation obtained through animal inoculation.

Burgdorfer (1975) cautions on the interpretation of results from inoculation of laboratory animals. The escape of viable C. burneti and infection of laboratory animals and investigators should be regarded as a distinct possibility. Only pretested animals should be used for primary isolation and sentinel animals should be distributed in the animal quarters and tested at regular intervals. Reisolation from a portion of the original material held in the frozen state affords confidence in the isolation results.

Unlike the Rickettsia spp., C. burneti undergoes a host-dependent phase shift in antigenic structure and serologic activity (Elisberg and Bozeman, 1969). Strains recovered from naturally infected ticks and vertebrates are in phase I and remain in this state if propagated in susceptible laboratory animals. When phase I organisms are cultivated serially in chick embryos, conversion to phase II occurs after a variable number of passages. This shift is readily reversed when yolk-sac grown organisms are injected into susceptible laboratory animals. These phases are important in certain serologic procedures. In guinea pigs, phase II antibodies are produced early in infection, while phase I antibodies do not appear until after 4 weeks of infection. While a number of serological tests for detecting C. burneti infection exist (Burgdorfer, 1975; Elisberg and Bozeman, 1969), the capillary or micro-agglutination and microcomplement-fixation procedures appear to be the most useful in dealing with small volumes of sera obtained from herptiles (Stephen and Rao, 1979).

CONTROL

Due to the limited information available on Q fever in reptiles, no recommendations on control of C. burneti in vivarium collections have been put forth. However, logic would dictate the control of ectoparasites, especially ticks, in the collection as a means of reducing the risk of potential spread of C. burneti between animals or to the people associated with the vivarium (Kim et al., 1978). Reichenbach-Klinke and Elkan (1965) reported the importation into Europe of H. aegyptium on tortoises. This tick species is known to be capable of becoming infected with C. burneti and maintaining transovarial and transstadial transmission (Blanc et al., 1959; Blanc, 1961). Suspension of dichlorvos impregnated plastic pest strips above the cages will eradicate ticks and mites (Frye, 1973).

REFERENCES

Babudieri, B., 1959, Q fever: A zoonosis, Adv. Vet. Sci., 5:81-182.
Bell, J.F., 1970, Q (Query) fever, in: "Infectious diseases of wild mammals," J.W. Davis, L.H. Karstad and D.O. Trainer, eds., Iowa State Univ. Press, Ames.
Blanc, G., 1961, Comportement de Rickettsia burneti Derrick chez la tique Hyalomma aegyptium (LIN) et al tortue terrestre Testudo graeca (LIN), Pathol. Microbiol., 24:21-26.
Blanc, G., Ascione, L., and Besiat, P., 1959, Rickettsieme experimentale de Testudo (Mauritanica) graeca avec R. burneti et infection de la tique Hyalomma aegyptium, Bull. Soc. Pathol. exotique, 52:564.
Buchanan, R.E., and Gibbons, N.E., 1974, "Bergey's manual of determinative bacteriology," 8th ed., Williams and Wilkins Co., Baltimore.
Burgdorfer, W., 1970, Hemolymph test: A technique for detection of rickettsiae in ticks, Amer. J. Trop. Med. Hyg., 19:1010-1014.
Burgdorfer, W., 1975, Q fever, in: "Diseases of animals transmitted to man," 6th ed., W.T. Hubbert, W.F. McCulloch and P.R. Schnurrenberger, eds., Charles C. Thomas, Springfield.
Elisberg, B.L., and Bozeman, F.M., 1969, Rickettsieae, in: "Diagnostic procedures for viral and rickett-sial infections," 4th ed., E.H. Lennette and N.F. Schmidt, eds., Amer. Public Health Ass., Inc., New York.
Enright, J.B., Franti, C.E., Behymer, D.E., Longhurst, W.M., Dutson, V.J., and Wright, M.E., 1971, Coxiella burneti in a wildlife-livestock environment: Distribution of Q fever in wild mammals, Amer. J. Epidemiol., 94:79-90.

Kim, S., Guirgis, S., Harris, D., Keelan, T., and Mayer, M., 1978, Q fever-New York, Center for Disease Control MMWR, 27:321-323.

Frye, F.L., 1973, "Husbandry, medicine and surgery in captive reptiles," V.M. Publishing Co., Bonner Springs.

Philip, C.B., 1948, Observations on experimental Q fever, J. Parasitol., 34:457-464.

Reichenbach-Klinke, H., and Elkan, E., 1965, "Principle diseases of lower vertebrates," Academic Press, New York.

Stephen, S., and Rao, K.N.A., 1979, Coxiellosis in reptile of South Kanara district, Karnataka, Indian J. Med. Res., 70:937-941.

Tendeiro, J., 1952, "Febre Q," Publ. Centro estudos de Guine, Portuguesa, Bissau.

Yadav, M.P., and Sethi, M.S., 1979, Poikilotherms as reservoirs of Q-fever (Coxiella burneti) in Uttar Pradesh, J. Wildlife Dis., 15:15-17.

Yadav, M.P., and Sethi, M.S., 1980, A study on the reservoir status of Q fever in avifauna, wild mammals and poikilotherms in Uttar Pradesh (India), Int. J. Zoonoses, 7:85-89

ARBOVIRUSES

[1]Kennedy F. Shortridge and [2]Akira Oya

[1]Department of Microbiology, Univ. of Hong Kong
[2]Department of Virology and Rickettsiology
National Institute of Health, Japan

INTRODUCTION

The study of arbovirus infections in amphibians and reptiles is still in its infancy. It seems to have arisen, not so much from fundamental investigations into the causation of overt disease as in the case of bacterial and parasitic infections, but rather from an attempt to explain the role of poikilothermic animals in the survival of viruses in nature.

An arbovirus by definition multiplies in a blood sucking arthropod and is transmitted by bite to a vertebrate. It is acquired from the infected blood of a vertebrate, multiplies in the tissue of the arthropod, becomes established in the salivary glands, and is then transmitted by bite to another susceptible vertebrate.

When we consider the large number of arboviruses that have been isolated it is perhaps not too surprising that so little is known about their vertebrate hosts. Each arbovirus must be submitted to comprehensive ecological observations and rigorous laboratory investigation in order to understand its natural history, an exceedingly difficult task. At present there are more than 360 recognized or candidate arboviruses (Berge, 1975; Karabatsos, 1978) but information on many is meagre to say the least. Although mammals and birds appear to be natural vertebrate hosts for a number of viruses, it is often difficult to place their importance in perspective. Such animals are usually investigated first as a

consequence of their relative ease of collection and
handling. It is only in recent years that poikilothermic
vertebrates have been subject to greater study because of
the failure of other animals to yield convincing information on arbovirus natural history. Indeed, there are a
number of arboviruses isolated from arthropods for which
no vertebrate host has been found to date in nature in
spite of extensive virological and serological investigations.

Concommitant with this search for vertebrate hosts
has been an attempt to explain the long term survival
of arboviruses in nature. These viruses occur in
virtually all regions of the earth encompassing widely
different climatic conditions. They probably circulate
all year round in tropical regions, but in temperate
areas this not apparent as the activity of host mosquitoes
often ceases for a few months. Two main hypotheses have
been advanced to explain the maintenance of the virus
where there is interruption to continuous transmission:
1) transovarial transmission which can occur in ticks and
in mosquitoes (Balfour et al., 1975; Rosen et al., 1978);
and, 2) overwintering in poikilothermic and homeothermic
vertebrate hosts (Danielova, 1975; Sulkin and Allen,
1974). The studies on poikilotherms have been largely
responsible for the emergence of this field of virology.

ETIOLOGY, TRANSMISSION AND PATHOGENESIS

Arthropod vectors

In order to maintain continuity of an arbovirus cycle
a hematophagous arthropod must be attracted to an animal
with circulating virus and feed on it. The majority of
arboviruses are mosquito-borne, several tick-borne and
phlebotomine-borne (sandfly), and a few are transmitted
by Culicoides spp. (midges and gnats).

Apart from mechanical transmission, mosquitoes act
as vectors of a number of pathogens including arboviruses.
Their importance as arbovirus vectors can be best gauged
from the human aspect, the one for which the most concrete
information is available. Viruses known or thought to
infect man have been recovered from more than 150 species
of mosquitoes belonging to 14 different genera: Aedeomyia,
Aedes, Anopheles, Culex, Culiseta, Deinocerites, Eretmapo-
dites, Haemagogus, Limatus, Mansonia, Psorophora, Sabethes,
Trichoprosopon and Wyeomia (Mattingly, 1973).

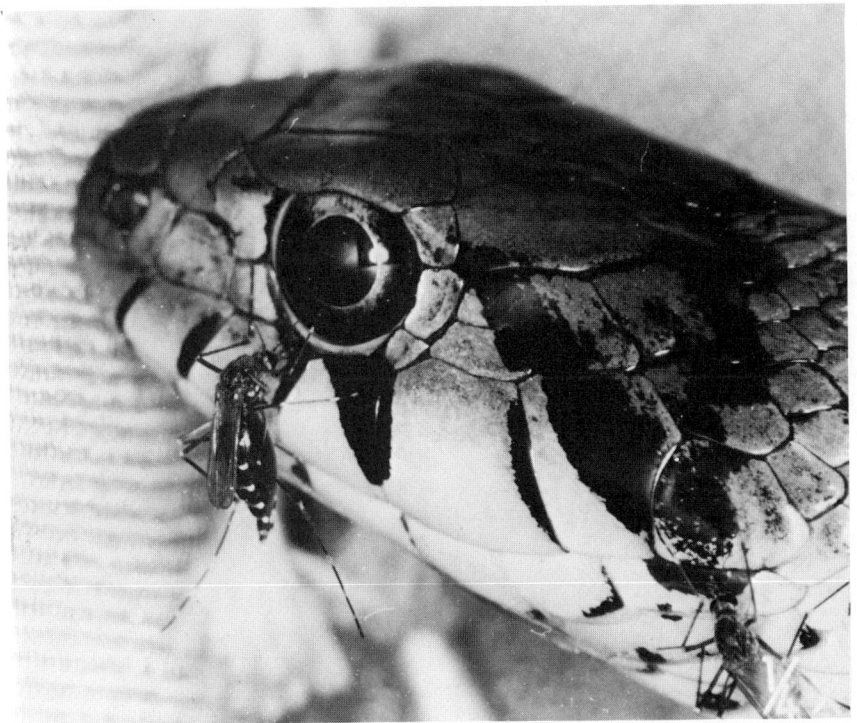

Fig. 10.1. Aedes aegypti feeding on the snake, Rhabdophis tigrina, in a cage (photo courtesy of Prof. I. Miyagi).

Many of the arboviruses also have been detected in terrestrial vertebrates including amphibians and reptiles. Much of the pertinent information on the association between arthropods and these animals is based on experimental studies employing mosquitoes and at least 26 species have been shown to feed on these animals (Table 10.1; Figs. 10.1-10.4).

Besides feeding on man and other animals, at least five of the genera given above, namely Aedes, Anopheles, Culex, Culiseta and Mansonia, also feed on poikilotherms. Although many arthropod species may be able to support arbovirus multiplication, feeding preferences are important in determining the range of potential vertebrate hosts for arboviruses. The isolation of western equine encephalitis (WEE) virus from mammals, birds and reptiles (Burton et al., 1966; Gebhardt et al., 1964) more than likely reflects the diverse feeding habits of Culex tarsalis, the principal vector of the virus. This is in

Table 10.1. A List of Mosquito Species and Amphibian and Reptilian Hosts.[a]

Mosquito Species	Host Species	Reference
Aedes aegypti	Lizards	Yuill, 1969
A. albopictus	Frogs, snakes	Miyagi, 1972
A. atlanticus	Turtles	Crans and Rockel, 1968
A. canadensis	Turtles, snakes	Crans and Rockel, 1968; DeFoliart, 1967; Hayes, 1961; Nolan et al., 1965
A. sollicitans	Turtles, snakes	Murphy et al., 1967
A. sticticus	Turtles, snakes	Wright and DeFoliart, 1970
A. togoi	Frogs, snakes	Miyagi, 1972
A. triseriatus	Turtles	Nolan et al., 1965
A. trivittatus	Turtles	Wright and DeFoliart, 1970
A. vexans	Frogs, turtles, snakes	Miyagi, 1972
Anopheles quadrimaculatus	Turtles, snakes	Murphy et al., 1967
Armigeres subalbatus	Frogs, turtles, snakes	Miyagi, 1972
Culex hayashi	Newts, frogs	Miyaga, 1972

C. infantulus	Frogs, turtles, lizards, snakes	Miyagi, 1972
C. pipiens	Frogs, turtles, snakes	Hayes, 1961; Miyagi, 1972; Wright and DeFoliart, 1970
C. resturans	Turtles, snakes	Hayes, 1961
C. salinanius	Turtles, snakes	Hayes, 1961
C. tarsalis	Snakes	Gebhardt et al., 1966; Thomas and Eklund, 1962
C. territans	Turtles, snakes	Murphy et al., 1967
C. tritaeniorhynchus	Frogs, turtles, snakes	Miyagi, 1972
Culesita melanura	Snakes	Hayes, 1961
C. minnesotae	Turtles	Hayes, 1961
C. morsita	Snakes	Hayes, 1961
Mansonia perturbans	Snakes	Hayes, 1961; Murphy et al., 1967; Wright and DeFoliart, 1970
Tripteroides bambusa	Turtles, snakes	Miyagi, 1972
Uranotaenia bimaculata	Frogs	Miyagi, 1972

[a]After Hoff and Trainer, 1973.

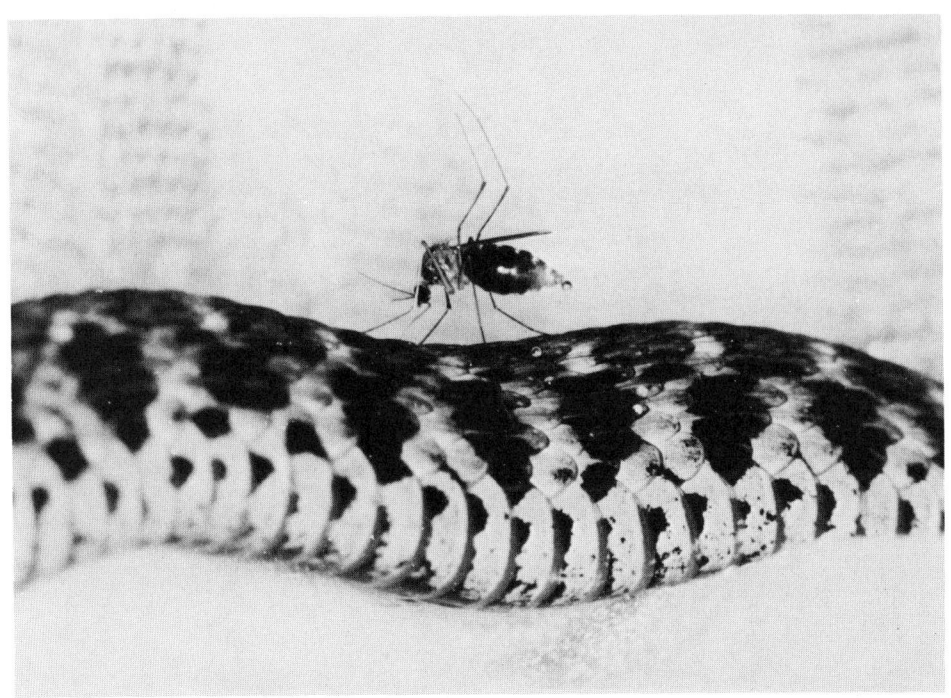

Fig. 10.2. Culex infantulus feeding on the snake, Rhabdophis tigrina, in a cage (photo courtesy of Prof. I. Miyagi).

contrast to groups such as Urotaenia whose feeding habits are largely unknown. However, there is evidence that U. bimaculata is capable of feeding on frogs (Miyagi, 1972) but its role as a vector is unknown. Other factors including flight habits and local geography contribute to the nature of the vector-host relationship.

As pointed out by Mattingly et al. (1973), vector relationships are complex and rarely more than partially understood. Many factors are involved and interpretations based on experimental studies must always be viewed with caution. Captive, hungry mosquitoes may readily feed on cold-blooded animals but may not necessarily do so in the field (Miyagi, 1978). Although C. tritaeniorhynchus is generally considered to be an important vector of Japanese encephalitis (JE) in the Far East (Matsuyama et al., 1960; Self et al., 1973) and the mosquito occurs in geographical areas where there is evidence of JE virus activity in snakes (Shortridge et al., 1974), there is no clear-cut proof that vector and host are significantly

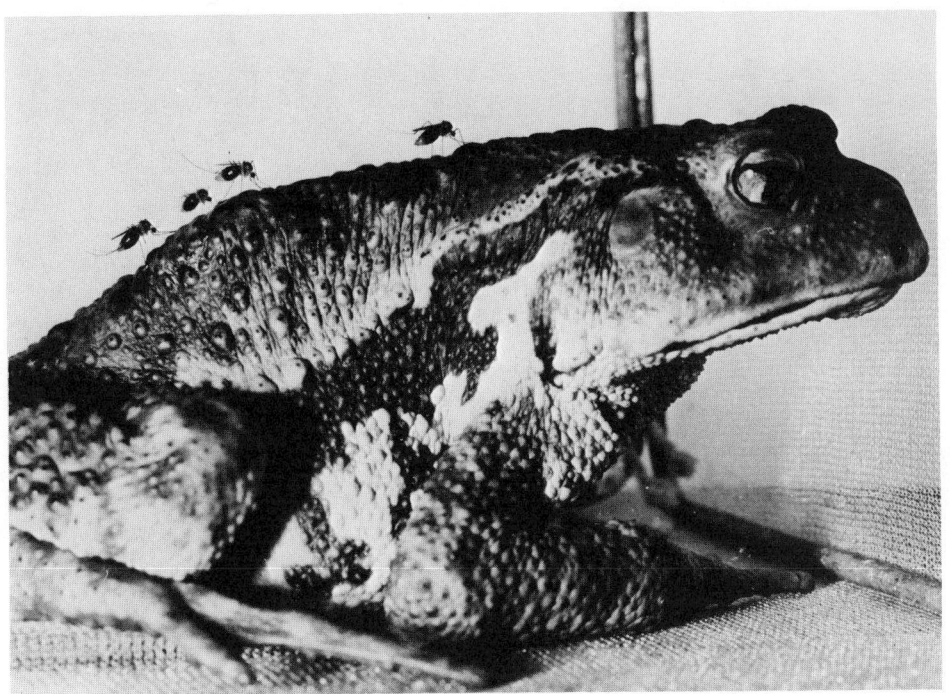

Fig. 10.3. Culex hayashii feeding on the toad, Bufo japonicus, in a cage (photo courtesy of Prof. I. Miyagi).

associated. Indeed, although C. tritaeniorhynchus is capable of feeding on such vertebrates it seems to do so reluctantly (Miyagi, 1972) suggesting that there may be inadequate contact for successful transmission of virus. This is perhaps not too surprising in that most culicine mosquitoes feed extensively on birds rather than mammals and cold-blooded animals. Miyagi (1972) showed this to be the case with C. kyotoensis, C. pallidothorax and C. vorax, but noted that two species C. infantulus and C. pipiens were exceptions, feeding readily on a variety of cold-blooded animals.

Ticks are well documented vectors and reservoirs of a number of pathogens including arboviruses (Berge, 1975; Sheals, 1973) and many are capable of parasitizing a wide range of reptiles (Balashov, 1972). Although upwards of 60 arboviruses infecting about 20 argasid and 60 ixodid species involve every major terrestrial vertebrate animal group (Hoogstraal, 1973), there is little evidence to suggest that there is a significant association. Yunker

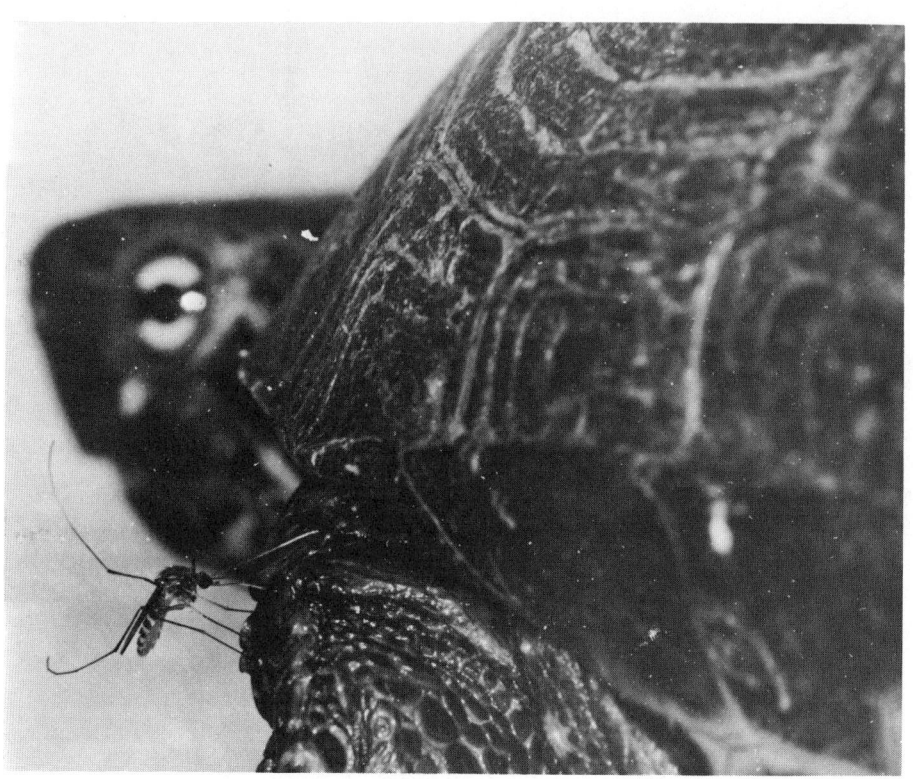

Fig. 10.4. Culex infantulus feeding on the turtle, Chinemys reevesi, in a cage (photo courtesy of Prof. I. Miyagi).

et al. (1975) were unable to isolate virus from parasitic Acarina found on a variety of Panamanian reptiles. Limited field studies to date on snakes and their ticks in New South Wales, Australia, also have been negative (Marshall, 1978).

Mention was made earlier that the feeding habits of mosquitoes seemed to be important in determining the distribution of arboviruses. Although many ticks might appear to parasitize a limited range of hosts, there is increasing evidence of a broader host range. For example, Hyalomma aegyptium which was thought to parasitize tortoises, and less often other reptiles, is a proven feeder on many mammals, particularly in the immature stages (Hoogstraal and Kaiser, 1960). In this connection, the millieu in which the viruses survive in ticks is seemingly more complex and perhaps more favourable than that of mosquitoes. Transstadial passage of virus from larval to nymph to adult ticks, a long life often two years or more, the relatively long feeding periods and enormous meals, and the association with dissimilar hosts often during successive host breeding cycles lend the arbovirus an enhanced potential for transmission. Thus, the isolation from Ixodes persulcatus and I. ricinus of a large number of arboviruses particularly those of the tick-borne group B complex found predominantly in Asia and Europe, may be a reflection of the long life of these ticks and a wide range of hosts which include a variety of lizards (Hoogstraal, 1973).

In spite of the paucity of information, it might not be unreasonable to expect amphibians and reptiles to be significant vertebrate hosts for tick-borne arboviruses, particularly where the habitat is restricted, say, to that of a burrow and its surrounding environment. Such investigations are surely warranted and may provide an insight into the ecology of arboviruses, particularly that of some of the lesser known ones isolated from specialized ticks in restricted habitats.

Some phlebotomine species, especially those of Sergentomyia, are attracted to cold-blooded animals, notably lizards, providing an apparently acceptable ecological association for the maintenance of an arbovirus (Lewis, 1973). This may be the case with Charleville virus which was first isolated from Phlebotomus spp. and later from the heart, liver and lung of the gecko, Gehyra australis (Doherty et al., 1973).

Arboviruses also have been isolated from Culicoides spp. (Doherty et al., 1973; Murray, 1970). Whether these arthropods feed on poikilotherms to any appreciable extent is unclear (Freeman, 1973). The relevance of hematophagus tabanid and glossina flies in virus transmission either mechanically or as vectors is even more obscure.

Thus, the association between arthropods and cold-blooded animals discussed above can at best only be considered as a guide to their possible role in the maintenance of arbovirus cycles. It is, however, possible that failure to demonstrate clearly a significant association between vector and host may be a consequence of the rarity of the phenomenon. A high infection rate may be detrimental to virus survival by exhausting the supply of susceptible hosts particularly if they carry virus for long periods of time. A similar hypothesis has been advanced by Rosen et al. (1978) to explain the apparent rarity of transovarial transmission as an overwintering mechanism of JE virus. Establishment of vector status will require long-term intensive study.

Reptilian and amphibian hosts

The largest number of arboviruses isolated from vertebrates has been from man and rodents, followed by birds and miscellaneous hosts (Berge, 1975; Karabatsos, 1978). Insofar as the last category is concerned, there have been relatively few isolations from amphibians and reptiles although there is considerable serological and experimental evidence to suggest that these animals are capable of being hosts for arboviurses (Table 10.2). It is perhaps unfortunate that although the largest number of arboviruses has been isolated in Africa, there have been few studies on that continent to explore the role of lower vertebrates in the natural history of arboviruses. Much of the information readily available is derived from experimental studies on WEE and eastern equine encephaliti (EEE) viruses, two viruses found in North America. These studies have highlighted the complex ecology that may exist and indicate a potential role for amphibians and reptiles in the maintenance cycles of arboviruses.

The bulk of virus isolations from free-ranging cold-blooded animals has been from reptiles. Whereas EEE and WEE viruses predominate in the isolations made from snakes and turtles, the isolates from lizards appear to be more varied although it is unclear whether this is the result of sampling or geographical factors. Limited isolations have been made from frogs. No doubt many more studies of this kind have been made but may not have been recorded in the literature largely because of their negative nature It may be worthwhile for a central international register to be kept so that all results positive and negative can be recorded in order that this specialized area of knowledge might be placed in better perspective.

While it would seem reasonable to assert that amphibians and reptiles have a potential role in the maintenance of arboviruses in nature, it is far from clear just how significant that might be. The isolation rate from free-ranging animals is generally very low in most regions of the world irrespective of climatic and ecological differences. For example, Lee et al. (1972) obtained two isolates of JE virus from 694 Chinese rat snakes, Elaphe rufodorsata, in Korea which has a cold climate. Likewise, in the tropical Amazon jungle of Brazil, Causey et al. (1966) reported four isolations of Marco virus from Ameiva a. ameiva amongst 1526 lizards examined, and in a follow-up study of 4400 reptiles of various species no further isolations were made.

Failure to isolate virus may be related in some way to the ability of these animals to undergo torpor particularly in colder climates in the winter months when physiological activitiy is markedly reduced. Experimental studies with WEE virus infected garter snakes, Thamnophis sp., have shown that after coming out of torpor, the snakes should be maintained at room temperature for several days for viremia to develop before attempting to isolate virus from the blood (Gebhardt and Hill, 1960; Thomas and Eklund, 1962). Similar observations have been made on the tortoise (Bowen, 1977). The effect of temperature rise on the viremia in experimentally infected animals is illustrated in Figs. 10.5 and 10.6. Not all animals respond uniformly to experimental infection in that there is variation in the time of appearance of viremia and in quantitiy of virus produced. Whereas viremia exists in mammals for a relatively short period prior to antibody production and virus elimination, in poikilothermic animals it may last for weeks or months at environmental temperatures of 20 C and above (Bowen, 1977; Oya, 1978). Inability to isolate virus at a higher frequency from the blood of free-ranging animals is in direct contrast to the persistent viremia observed in

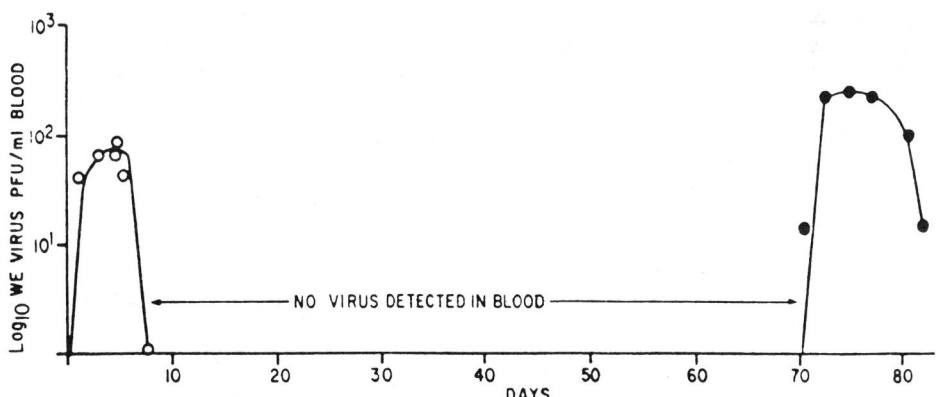

Fig. 10.5. Viremia response of representative snakes, Thamnophis sp., in torpor for 60 days at 5 C (± 0.3 C) beginning 18 hours after western equine encephalitis virus infection and then removed to room temperature (23 C ± 0.5 C) (from Gebhardt et al., 1973).

Table 10.2. A List of Arboviruses and Amphibian and Reptilian Host Literature.[a]

Order	Virus[b]	Evidence[c]	Reference
ORDER SQUAMATA			
Colubridae			
Coluber constrictor	EEE, WEE	ex, i, s	Dalrymple et al., 1972; Gebhardt and Stanton, 1967; Gebhardt et al., 1964; Hayes et al., 1964; Karstad, 1961
Diadophis punctatus	EEE	ex	Karstad, 1961
Haldea valeriae	EEE	ex	Karstad, 1961
Heterodon platyrhinos	EEE	ex	Karstad, 1961
Lampropeltis getulus	EEE, WEE	s	Dalrymple et al., 1972
Nerodia erythrogaster	VSV	s	Hoff and Trainer, 1973
N. sipedon	EEE, POW	ex, s	Bast et al., 1973; Hayes et al., 1964; Karstad, 1961
Opheodrys aestivus	EEE	ex	Karstad, 1961
Pituophis melanoleucus	SLE, WEE	i, s	Gebhardt and Stanton, 1967; Gebhardt et al., 1964; Spalatin et al., 1964
Ptyas korros	JE	s	Shortridge et al., 1977
Rhabdophis tigrina	JE	ex	Lee, 1968
Storeria occipito-maculata	EEE, POW, SLE	s	Whitney et al., 1968
Thamnophis elegans	WEE	ex, i, s	De St. Jeor, 1969; Gebhardt and Stanton, 1967
T. e. vargrans	WEE	i	Gebhardt and Hill, 1960

T. radix haydeni	WEE	ex, i, s	Burton et al., 1966; McLintock et al., 1967; Spalatin et al., 1964
T. sirtalis	EEE, WEE	ex, i	Gebhardt and Hill, 1960; Hayes et al., 1964
T. s. parietalis	WEE	i, s	Burton et al., 1966; McLintock et al., 1967
T. s. sirtalis	EEE, WEE, SLE, POW	s	Whitney et al., 1968
Thamnophis sp.	WEE	ex, i	Gebhardt et al., 1973; Prior and Agnew, 1971; Thomas et al., 1959, 1980
Elaphidae			
Bungarus fasciatus	JE	s	Shortridge et al., 1977
Elaphe guttata	EEE	ex, s	Karstad, 1961
E. obsoleta	WEE	s	Hoff and Trainer, 1973
E. rufodorsata	JE	ex, i	Lee et al., 1972
E. schrenckii	JE	ex	Lee, 1968
Naja naja	JE	s	Shortridge et al., 1974
Crotalidae			
Agkistrodon piscivorus	EEE	s	Karstad, 1961
Bothrops alternata	WEE	ex	Rosenbusch, 1939
Crotalus atrox	WEE, VEE	s	Hoff and Trainer, 1973; Smart et al., 1975
Lacertilidae			
Lacerta agilis	TBE, UUK	ex, s	Sekeyova et al., 1970; Sixl et al., 1971
L. viridis	TBE	ex	Rehacek et al., 1961; Sekeyova et al., 1970
Takydromus tachydromoides	JE	ex	Doi et al., 1968

Table 10.2. A List of Arboviruses and Amphibian and Reptilian Host Literature. (Continued)

Order	Virus	Evidence	Reference
Scincidae			
Ablepharus boutonni vergatus	ALM	i, s	Graf, 1967
Anolis carolinensis	EEE	ex	Karstad, 1961
Eumeces laticeps	EEE	ex	Karstad, 1961
Teiidae			
Ameiva a. ameiva	CHO, MAY, MCO, TIM^d	i	Causey et al., 1966; Woodall, 1967
Ameiva sp.	EEE	ex, s	Craighead et al., 1962
Cnemidophorus sp.	EEE	s	Craighead et al., 1962
Kentropyx calcaratus	CHO	i	Causey et al., 1966
Agamidae			
Calotes versicolor	GPB	s	Chastel, 1966
Anguidae			
Ophisaurus attenuatus	EEE	ex	Karstad, 1961
Gekkonidae			
Gecko gecko	GPB	s	Chastel, 1966
Gehyra australis	CHA	i	Doherty et al., 1973
Hemidactylus frenatus	JE	ex	Yuill, 1969
Platyurus platyurus	JE	ex	Yuill, 1969
Iguanidae			
Basiliscus sp.	EEE	s	Craighead et al., 1962
Tropidurus torquatus hispidus	MAY	i	Woodall, 1967

ARBOVIRUSES

ORDER TESTUDINATA

Testudinidae (including Emydidae)

Species	Viruses	Evidence	Reference
Chrysemys picta	EEE, WEE	ex, s	Dalrymple et al., 1972; Hayes et al., 1964
C. p. picta	BUN, EEE, WEE, SLE, POW	s	Whitney et al., 1968
C. scripta elegans	WEE	s	Hoff and Trainer, 1973
Clemmys caspica	GPA, GPB	s	Nir et al., 1972
C. guttata	EEE, WEE	ex, s	Dalrymple et al., 1972; Hayes et al., 1964; Smith and Anderson, 1980
C. insculpta	EEE	ex	Hayes et al., 1964
Gopherus berlandieri	WEE	ex, i	Bowen, 1977; Sudia et al., 1975
G. polyphemus	EEE	ex	Karstad, 1961
Malaclemys t. terrapin	WEE	i	Goldfield and Sussman, 1964
Sternotherus carinatus	EEE	ex	Karstad, 1961
Terrapene carolina	EEE, WEE	ex, i, s	Dalrymple et al., 1972; Goldfield and Sussman, 1964; Hayes et al., 1964; Karstad, 1961

Chelydridae

Species	Viruses	Evidence	Reference
Chelydra serpentina	BUN, EEE, WEE, SLE, POW	ex, i, s	Dalrymple et al., 1972; Goldfield and Sussman, 1964; Hayes et al., 1964; Whitney et al., 1968

Trionychidae

Species	Viruses	Evidence	Reference
Trionyx ferox	EEE	ex	Karstad, 1961
T. sinensis	JE	s	Shortridge et al., 1975
T. spinifer	VSV	s	Cook et al., 1965
T. s. emoryi	BUN, WEE	i, s	Hoff and Trainer, 1973

Table 10.2. A List of Arboviruses and Amphibian and Reptilian Host Literature. (Continued)

Order	Virus	Evidence	Reference
Kinosternidae			
Kinosternon subrubrum	EEE, WEE	ex, s	Dalrymple et al., 1972; Karstad, 1961
ORDER CRODIDILIA			
Crocodylidae			
Alligator mississippiensis	EEE	ex, s	Karstad, 1961
ORDER ANURA			
Ranidae			
Rana clamitans	EEE, WEE, POW	s	Bast et al., 1973; Dalrymple et al., 1972
R. catesbeiana	POW	s	Bast et al., 1973
R. nigromaculata	JE	ex	Kawasaki, 1972
R. pipiens	WEE	i, s	Burton et al., 1966
R. p. pipiens	SLE	s	Whitney et al., 1968
R. ridibunda	GPA, GPB	s	Nir et al., 1972
R. tigrina	JE	s	Shortridge et al., 1977

[a] After Hoff and Trainer, 1973.
[b] EEE=eastern equine encephalitis; WEE=western equine encephalitis; VEE=Venezuelan equine encephalitis; JE=Japanese encephalitis; SLE=St. Louis encephalitis;

VSV=vesicular stomatitis; POW=Powassan; BUN=Bunyamwera group; TBE=tick-borne encephalitis; UUK=Uukuniemi; ALM=Almpiwar; CHO=Chaco; MAY=Mayaro; MCO=Marco; TIM=Timbo; GPB=group B arbovirus; CHA=Charleville; GPA=group A arbovirus
[c]ex=experimental infection; i=isolation from natural infection; s=serological evidence
[d]Recent electron microscope studies have shown that Chaco, Marco and Timbo viruses are rhabdoviruses (Monath et al., 1979) as is vesicular stomatitis virus.

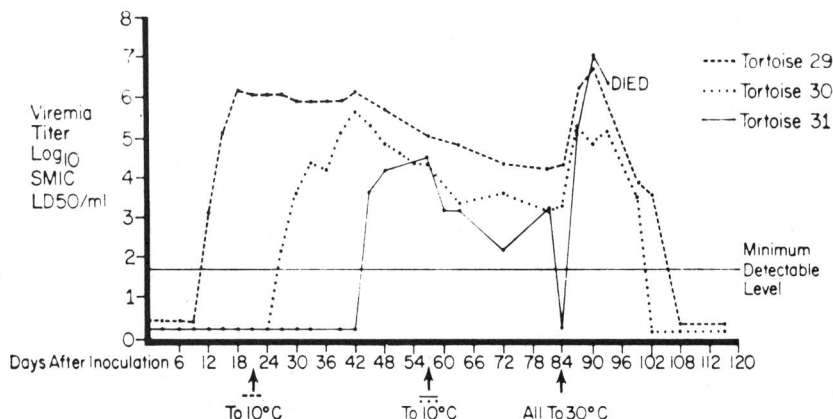

Fig. 10.6. Viremia response of three Texas tortoises, Gopherus berlandieri, held at 20 C until the appearance of viremia and then at 10 C and 30 C following inoculation with western equine encephalitis virus (from Bowen, 1977).

some of the experimental studies but just how valid it is to extrapolate from such exercises is a moot point. Admittedly, the majority of virus isolations from free-ranging animals, albeit limited, have been in the warmer months, but this may be nothing more than a consequence of the relative ease of collection in this period.

In evaluating the merits of experimental studies, it must be borne in mind that the stress of conducting such investigations in artifical environments may be greater than that in nature and may account for the higher frequency of isolation. In a review of the pathology of amphibians, Elkan (1976) pointed out that these animals as a group are highly specialized and narrowly adapted to their environment. If experimental studies are to be of any relevance they must be carried out under conditions which ensure that the animals thrive in the artifical habitat.

Experimental studies have, however, yielded valuable information from which it might be possible to extrapolate to events occurring in nature. Thus, in colder climates, the best time to isolate virus from the blood of free-ranging animals would seem to be in the spring. The situation in warmer is far from clear. If infection leads to a chronic state, then it might be inferred from the bulk of experimental findings that virus localizes in certain organs or tissues. It may well be that viremia is an infrequent event which might explain the relative rarity of isolations in tropical areas. Additionally, species with a high turnover in the wild may be less prone to viremia. At higher environmental temperatures, viremia may terminate faster and antibody appear earlier (Bowen 1977; Oya, 1978). Strss may also be a factor in the occurrence of viremia and it is possible that virus might be more readily isolated from the blood after holding the animal in a torpid state for some time. The practical difficulties of attempting to induce viremia in free-ranging animals by temperature manipulation could be considerable but might be undertaken in specialized laboratories. However, regardless of approach, the value of attempted virus isolation depends on the reliability and sensitivity of the culture techniques.

In most studies on free-ranging animals, virus isolation is attempted from the blood, however, it is uncertain whether or not this is the best source. Sparse information is available on the site of localization of virus other than in the blood. In what was perhaps one of the earliest experimental infection studies in this field, Rosenbusch (1939) was able to isolate WEE virus from the brain but not the blood of the snake, Bothrops alternata. A similar observation was made by Gebhardt and Hill (1960) who isolated the virus from the brain of one of four garter snakes following torpor at 4 C. In the case of free-ranging animals, Charleville virus was isolated from the heart, liver and lung of G. australis (Doherty et al., 1973) while Marco, Timbo and Chaco viruses were isolated from the liver and heart of A. a. ameiva (Causey et al., 1966). On the other hand, Hoff and Trainer (1973) were unable to isolate virus from the blood, heart, lung and liver of 47 snakes and two lizards collected in Texas in the summer, although they were able to show the presence of WEE virus antibody in these animals. Using the fluorescent antibody technique, Doi and Oya (1978) were unable to locate a focus of virus multiplication in experimentally infected lizards. It is of interest that WEE virus has been reported to be transmitted from naturally infected female garter snakes to their offspring (Gebhardt et al., 1964). Such a finding merits further study when viewed against the background that 1) reptiles are the most primitive vertebrates in which young develop within a protected environment created by the amnion (Manning and Turner, 1976), and 2) they appear to be subject to latent or sub-clinical infections.

It may be that in nature viremia is an infrequent event which, if otherwise, might be detrimental for virus survival. Indeed, when the limited information on amphibians and reptiles is considered in relation to the large number of arboviruses described, it is quite possible that these animals are involved in virus maintenance in limited ecological situations only. Alternatively, the low incidence of infection in free-ranging cold-blooded animal generally might be nothing more than the result of chance infection by vector arthropods. Thus, it is noteworthy that frogs, snakes and lizards were refractory to infection by Calovo and Tahyna viruses under various experimental conditions suggesting that poikilothermic vertebrates are not susceptilble to these viruses in nature (Aspock and Kunz, 1971).

Serology is a useful alternative to virus isolation for providing evidence of arbovirus infection. The production of antibody, like virus, is generally temperature dependent. Although the dynamics of virus-antibody interaction in lower vertebrates are largely unknown, virus appears to wax when antibody wanes.

Studies on the occurrence of JE virus antibody in amphibians and reptiles originating from the southern Chinese provinces of Guangdong and Guangxi indicate that there is 1) a seasonal difference in antibody level, and 2) some variation in the class of immunoglobulin responsible for this activity (Table 10.3). The titers are generally higher in the spring/summer months and this is most evident in the cobra, Naja naja. It was noted earlier that viremia was more apparent after temperature rise, particularly if the animals had been held in a torpid state. Karstad (1963) has suggested that such a phenomenon may lead to prolonged infection which, in colder climates, may give rise to cyclic viremia.

It is difficult to tell whether antibody detected in cold-blooded animals is due to recent infection, prolonged infection and/or reinfection, and this poses a problem in evaluating epidemiological data derived from serological studies. Experimental studies on the immune response of this category of animal have been carried out mainly with non-virus antigens (see Chapter 26). Their relevance in understanding the response to natural arbovirus infections is questionable especially as the animals do not appear to be adversely affected. These difficulties are compounded by the uncertainty of the ages of the animals. In zoological collections, snakes, particularly the large ones, have been known to live as long as 30

Table 10.3. Seasonal Characteristics of Japanese Encephalitis Virus Hemagglutination Inhibition (HI) Antibody in the Sera or Plasma of Representative Amphibians and Reptiles.[a]

Species	Season[b]	Mean[c] HI titers	Immunoglobulin detected[d] IgG	Macroglobulin
Naja naja	Spring/Summer	712 +̲ 651	+	−
	Autumn/Winter	127 +̲ 181	+	+
Bungarus fasicatus	Spring/Summer	145 +̲ 111	+	+
	Autumn/Winter	137 +̲ 70	+	+
Ptyas korros	Spring/Summer	31 +̲ 38	+	−
	Autumn/Winter	36 +̲ 16	+	+
Trionyx sinensis	Spring/Summer	35 +̲ 39	+	−
	Autumn/Winter	29 +̲ 50	+	−
Rana tigrina regulosa	Spring/Summer	68 +̲ 58	+	−

[a] Abridged from Shortridge et al., 1974, 1975, 1977.
[b] Spring/Summer=April-September; Autumn/Winter=October-March.
[c] Based on a positive titer of 10 or greater.
[d] Based on pools of serum collected mid-season and submitted to sucrose density gradient centrifugation.

years, toads 50 years and large turtles 100 years (Romer, 1978). Quite possibly, reinfection occurs all year round in the tropics, and in the temperate/cold climates in the warmer summer months. Nevertheless, it is difficult to reconcile this view with the general lack of serological information, particularly from the tropics, and other factors such as the influence of virus localization mentioned earlier may be relevant. Lack of serological evidence does not necessarily indicate a non-infected animal. Alternative approaches in virus isolation technique may provide a partial answer for demonstrating the occurrence of virus.

DIAGNOSIS

Much of the information about disease in amphibians and reptiles comes from studies on captive animals; debilitated ones may be ready prey. Thus, infections able to be studied in free-ranging animals are often ones causing little or no apparent manifestations. Those due to arboviruses would seem to fit into this pattern of behavior. Examination of animals for pathological effects consequent to arbovirus infection is unlikely to yield significant information. Thus far, there are no reports of the occurrence of specific lesions in experimentally infected amphibians and reptiles having a low or high grade viremia Other approaches are often more rewarding. These are diagnoses based on the isolation and identification of arboviruses from specific tissues or fluids of the animal or, alternatively, by the detection of specific antibody in its serum. Detection of specific antibody by serological tests employing known viruses, although an indirect approach, is a practical alternative in lieu of virus isolation for evaluating the extent of arbovirus infections in the population.

The recognition of arbovirus infection is important for two reasons: 1) collection of data for evaluating the role of amphibians and reptiles in the natural history of arboviruses with particular reference to virus maintenance, and 2) detection of new or novel arboviruses.

Intracerebral inoculation of mice is a commonly employed technique for the isolation of arboviruses from a variety of sources. Two to four day-old suckling mice are used in preference to adults because of their higher susceptibility to infection (Fig. 10.7). This is usually fatal although it may be necessary to passage infected brain material a number of times before paralysis and death occur.

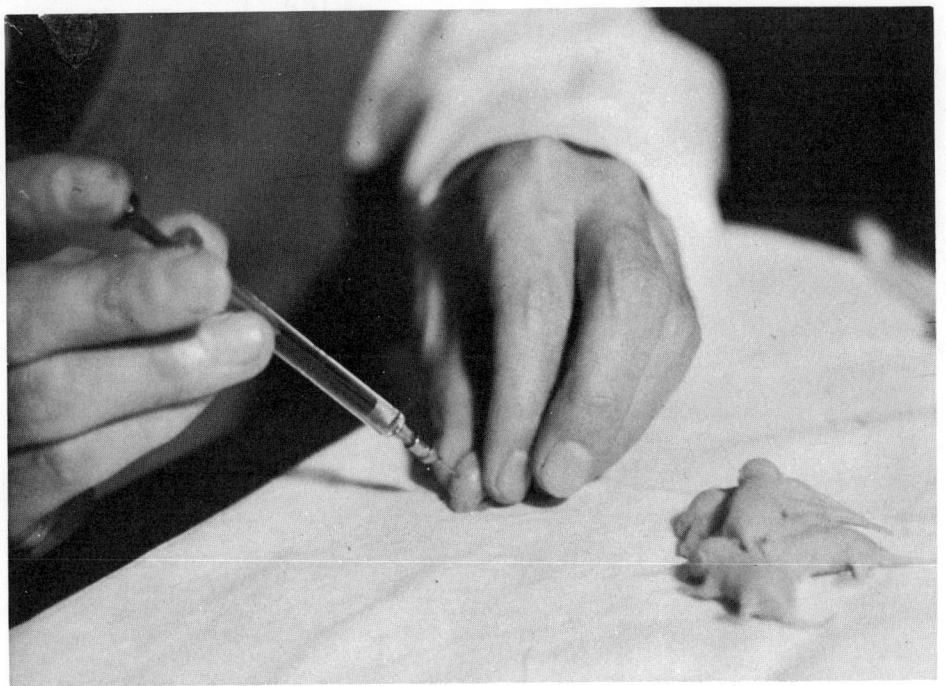

Fig. 10.7. Intracerebral inoculation of two to four day-old suckling mice for the isolation of arboviruses.

Most of the attempts to isolate virus from cold-blooded animals have been in suckling mice, but these laboratory hosts have some disadvantages. Temperature sensitive mutants which may preferentially grow in the free-ranging animal may do so poorly, if at all, in homeothermic mice. Slow growing viruses such as dengue may elicit an immune response in the suckling mice strong enough to prevent a fatal outcome of the infection.

The latter problem may be overcome by the use of cultured cells, a point emphasized by the isolation of JE virus from snakes (Lee et al., 1972). Continuous mammalian cell lines such as baby hamster kidney (BHK-21) (Karabatsos and Buckley, 1967), African green monkey kidney (Vero) (Yasumura and Kawakita, 1963) and grivet monkey kidney (BSC-1) (Halstead et al., 1964) have been used as susceptible cells for arboviruses. Virus multiplication in cultured cells can be recognized by 1) degeneration of the infected cells known as cytopathic effect or CPE, 2) detection of plaques on a cell monolayer, or

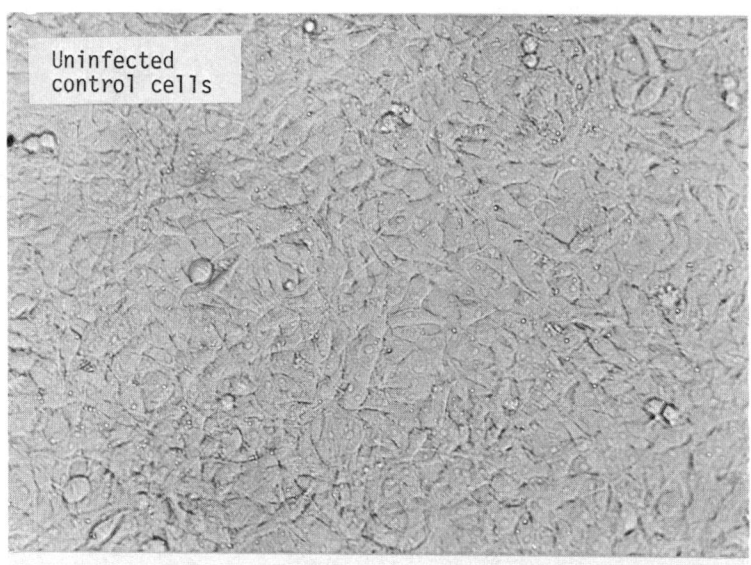
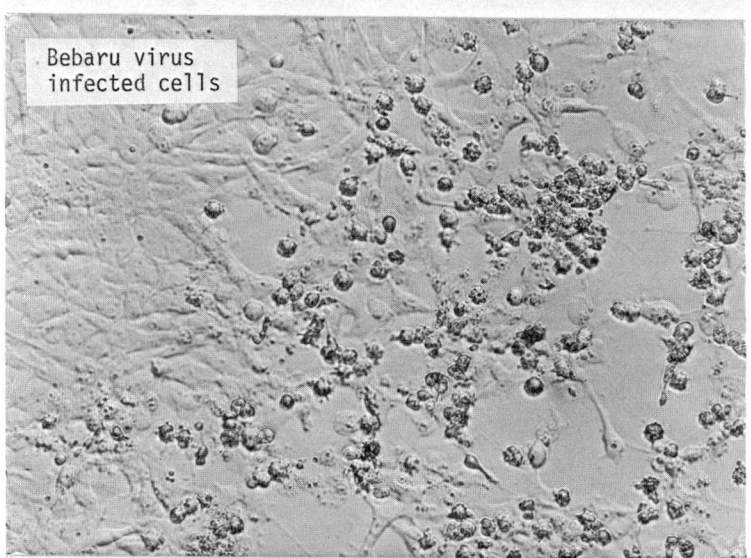

Fig. 10.8. Cytopathic effect by Bebaru virus in a continuous cell line (XTC-2) from the toad, Xenopus laevis. Cells become rounded and granular to form small aggregates as early as two days after addition of virus to the cell monolayer. Complete destruction of the monolayer ensues by the fourth to fifth day when the cells float freely in the liquid medium. X150 (photo courtesty of Dr. M. Pudney).

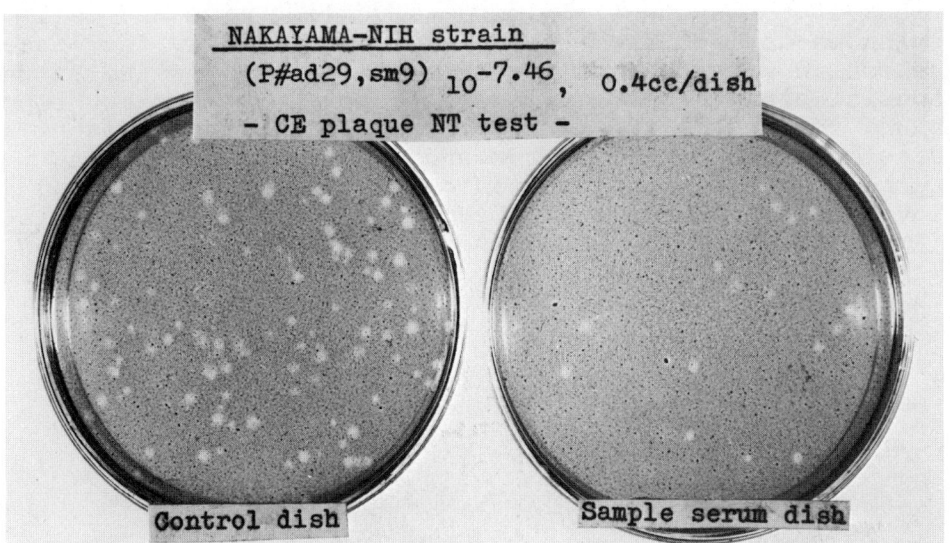

Fig. 10.9. Plaque production by the Nakayama-NIH strain of Japanese encephalitis virus in chick embryo fibroblast monolayers. A virus suspension is added to the cell monolayer and after the virus has had time to absorb, the liquid medium is replaced with an agar gel overlay to restrict the virus to the immediate vicinity of the originally infected cell. Each infective virus gives rise to a localized focus of infected cells that is visible to the naked eye. Visualization is enhanced by staining the monolayer with a vital dye. Virus may be readily quantitated in this manner (control). Alternatively, if virus and immune serum are mixed before adding to the monolayer, there is a reduction in the number of plaques and this forms the basis of the neutralization test for quantitating antibody (sample serum).

3) detection of viral antigens by the fluorescent antibody technique. Examples of CPE and plaques are shown in Figs. 10.8 and 10.9 respectively. Identification of virus isolates is performed by routine techniques employing physical (Fig. 10.10), chemical and serological procedures.

Failure to isolate arboviruses from free-ranging amphibians and reptiles could lie in the inherent limitations of the systems employed. Suckling mice and cell cultures derived from homeothermic animals may introduce selective pressures on virus populations. Because of the special biological relationship arboviruses and arthropods share in nature, the tissues of the mosquito represent a viable alternative. Dengue and JE viruses have been successfully propagated and detected in vivo following intrathoracic inoculation of Toxorhynchites amboinensis (Rosen and Gubler, 1974; Rosen et al., 1978). Thus, as was pointed out by Buckley (1969), mosquito cells growing in culture at 28 C might find ready application for the

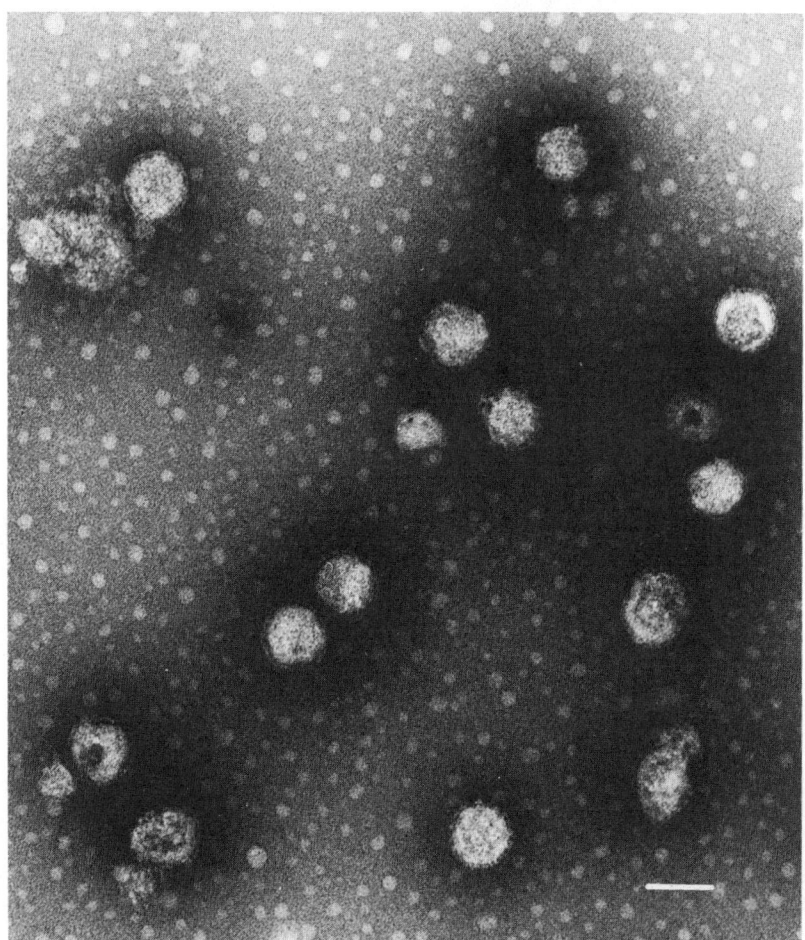

Fig. 10.10. Electron micrograph showing particles of Japanese encephalitis virus isolated from suckling mouse brain (bar = 20 nm).

isolation of arboviruses including temperature sensitive mutants. Varma et al. (1975/76) found a cell line established from Aedes pseudoscutellaris more sensitive than suckling mice and marginally better than Vero cells for the primary isolation of yellow fever virus. Mosquito cells are able to support the growth of a number of arboviruses and have the advantage that they are relatively easy and less expensive to maintain than mammalian cells. On the other hand, arbovirus multiplication generally does not cause CPE (Pudney et al., 1979). This particularly limits their usefulness for isolating "unknown" viruses. Additionally, some mosquito cell lines may be contaminated with virus-like particles (Pudney et al., 1973, 1979). Those particles resembling togaviruses have been causatively linked with the production of CPE under stress of multiplication by the arbovirus inoculum. The recent production of several cell lines from mosquitoes has not been paralleled by a similar degree of success in the case of other arthropods. Cell lines have been established from ticks (Varma et al., 1975) and bugs (Pudney and Lanar, 1977), but their potential for arbovirus isolation has not been established.

Poikilothermic vertebrate cell lines represent a second phylogenetically attractive alternative to mammalian systems for attempted isolation of arboviruses from free-ranging amphibians and reptiles. A variety of lines have been established (Lunger and Clark, 1978), some of which are able to support the multiplication of a range of viruses including arboviruses, although this is not always accompanied with the production of CPE. The XTC-2 line established from the clawed toad, Xenopus laevis, seems to have been the most successful of the poikilothermic cell lines investigated to date (Pudney et al., 1973). CPE or plaque production occurred following infection by a wide range of arboviruses, the only exception being some flaviviruses which failed to replicate (Leake et al., 1977).

A major advantage of these cell lines over mammalian ones is that they have an extremely wide temperature growth range. In the case of reptilian cells, this is approximately 18 to 37 C. Although the susceptibility of poikilothermic cells to arbovirus infection over this range has not been evaluated to any extent, the importance of temperature in attempted virus isolation may be adduced from the ease with which Fer de Lance virus, a probable paramyxovirus, grew and produced CPE in reptilian cell cultures maintained at 30 C but not at 37 C (Clark et al., 1979). This virus was initially isolated from tropical

American pit vipers, Bothrops atrox, after inoculation
of diseased lung tissue into 25 day-old embryonated eggs
of the snake, Cyclagras gigas, incubated at 27 C. Clearly
the potential of the embryonated snake egg system needs
to be evaluated further. A problem frequently encountered
with suckling mice and many cell lines is that the fluids
and tissues of snakes are often toxic and in such cases
dilution of the inoculum is necessary. This may reduce
the chances of isolating virus which is often present in
the infected animal at low titer. Embryonated snake eggs
may circumvent this. On the other hand, the system may
prove to be very expensive and it should be borne in mind
that its application would need to be kept in perspective
in the event that arboviruses are confirmed to be transmitted congenitally in reptiles (Gebhardt et al., 1966).

Thus, the rarity of virus isolations from free-ranging amphibians and reptiles may be a reflection of the
inherent restrictions of the host systems employed. Alternative approaches described here may be useful.

Many arboviruses contain surface projections called
hemagglutinins which are able to bind red blood cells.
Hemagglutination has proved highly valuable for virus
quantification. Conversely, the antibody that is produced
against this antigen as a consequence of infection can
be quantitated serologically by hemagglutination inhibition
(HI) of the arbovirus (Fig. 10.11).

As indicated earlier, arbovirus isolation from animals
and even from man under optimal conditions is difficult.
This has meant that greater emphasis has had to be placed
on arbovirus serology. This is particularly so in the
case of amphibians and reptiles from which relatively few
agents have been isolated. Naturally, the real proof of
the presence of virus in an animal lies in its isolation,
but it must not be forgotten that the validity of virus
isolation is dependent on its being carried out under
laboratory conditions which exclude the presence of
contaminating virus. Detection of antibody merely reflects
a series of events which indicate that the animal has been
in contact with virus. Nevertheless, the HI test, chiefly
because of its relative ease of operation, has been widely
used in epizootiological studies. It has been particularly
useful in the elucidation of the natural history of some
of the better known arboviruses. The difficulties that
affect the reliable and confident interpretation of human
arbovirus serology apply even more so to cold-blooded
animals.

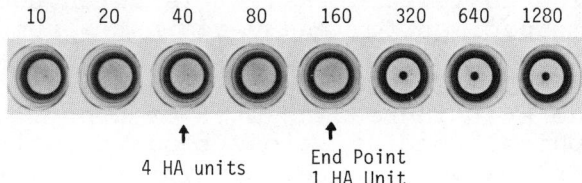

Fig. 10.11. Examples of hemagglutination (HA) and hemagglutination inhibition (HI) titrations. HA is seen as a widespread pattern on the bottom of the well of a plastic tray. When there is insufficient virus to agglutinate the erythrocytes, the cells settle at the bottom of the well as a button. In the HI test, dilutions of an animal serum sample 1) previously treated to remove lipoprotein non-specific inhibitors of HA, and 2) untreated, are challenged with 4 HA units of virus determined from the HA titration. The removal of non-specific inhibitors is seen in the reduction in HI titers from 160 to 10 in untreated and treated sera, respectively, the latter titer being suggestive of a low level of presumptive antibody. The hemagglutinin content of the challenging virus is checked by further titration.

At present there are approximately 360 arboviruses or arbovirus-like agents distributed among 50 antigenic groups (Karabatsos, 1978). Because the hemagglutinins of the members of each group may often share some degree of antigenic relatedness, it is often necessary to submit a serum specimen for assay against a number of agents before the nature of the infecting agent can be established. This is clearly a problem and is becoming more comple with the ever increasing list of arboviruses, although geographical considerations tend to limit selection of agents to be used in the assay. Herein lies one of the difficulties of this type of work in that the assays employ known agents. Knowledge of the arboviruses that are associated with amphibians and reptiles is minimal and it will be some time before the serological investigation of these animals is on the same footing as human or veterinary arbovirus serology.

Another complication in the interpretation of arbovirus serology is that an animal may be infected by a number of closely related arboviruses and in such cases the antibodies produced by the first virus may dominate over others. Experimentally, *C. tritaeniorhynchus* is capable of feeding on a number of cold-blooded animals (Miyagi, 1972). This mosquito is generally considered to be the most significant vector in the Far East of JE virus, a group B arbovirus, but it may also carry the antigenically related Tembusu virus (Russell, 1972). Thus, should a snake or frog in this region be infected by the two viruses at different times, confident identification of the antibodies by HI tests may prove difficult.

In addition to antibody, the sera of many vertebrates contain naturally occurring substances called non-specific inhibitors (NSI) which inhibit virus hemagglutination although unrelated to "classical" antibody. Whereas antibody arises as a consequence of antigenic stimulation from virus infection, NSI's are present in serum independent of such stimuli.

The NSI's of arbovirus hemagglutination reside in the lipoprotein fraction and comprise high density lipoprotein (HDL), low density lipoprotein (LDL) and very low density lipoprotein (VLDL) according to their ultracentrifugation characteristics (Bidwell and Mills, 1968; Shortridge and Ho, 1976). In order to detect specific antibody, these lipoproteins must be selectively removed from the serum. The earliest and perhaps the most widely used method is kaolin treatment, but there is evidence that this and other agents may additionally remove high molecular weight immunoglobulins of the IgM class (Schmidt et al., 1971). As this is the predominant immunoglobulin in lower vertebrates it is likely that false negative HI tests for arbovirus antibody may occur as the result of these treatments.

However, the evaluation of arbovirus serology in amphibians and reptiles is more complex and unfortunately many of the guidelines are based on human serum lipoprotiens. The condition under which serum is stored prior to assay markedly influences the efficiency of lipoprotein removal apparently as a result of reorientation of the lipid and protein moieties of the inhibitory lipoprotein complex (Shortridge, 1977). There is a tendency for the lipoproteins in aged or deteriorated sera to behave in the manner of HDL and such lipoproteins are incompletely removed giving rise to false positive antibody findings. This would seem to be particularly important in lower vertebrates where HDL is responsible for considerable NSI activity (Bidwell and Mills, 1968) which does not seem to be the case in man (Shortridge and Ho, 1974).

While HDL is no doubt an important factor in the HI test, LDL would seem to play a significant role due to its variable distribution in lower vertebrate sera. For example, Mills and Taylaur (1971) found in a study of the serum lipoproteins of 34 vertebrates, that the LDL levels ranged from the highest value observed in an animal, 1168 mg/100 ml in the green snake, _Liopeltis vernalis_, to undetectable levels in the tortoise, _Testudo graeca_, and the water monitor, _Varanus salvator_.

Considerable comment on NSI's is made against the background that much of the data listed in Table 10.2 has been based on the HI test. The validity of certain arbovirus-amphibian and arbovirus-reptile associations must, therefore, be treated with caution. It would seem necessary for the presence of presumptive antibody to be confirmed by addational tests such as virus neutralization or the demonstration that it is associated with the immunoglobulin fraction (Fig. 10.12). Yuill et al. (1971) in a study on five species of turtle captured during a period of EEE virus dissemination in Maryland, could not draw any conclusion on the role of these animals in the natural history of the virus precisely for these reasons. These difficulties are exacerbated even futher with lesser known viruses.

It should be borne in mind that a number of arboviruses do not hemagglutinate and these comments only

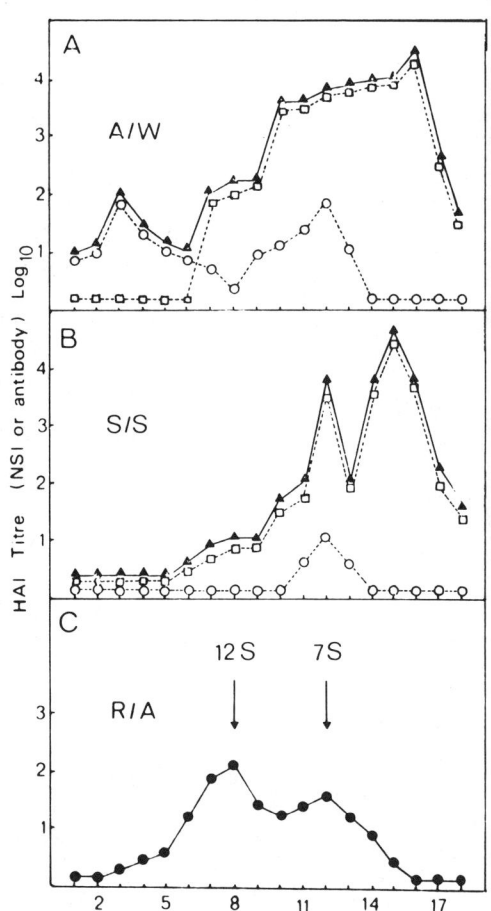

Fig. 10.12.
Density gradient centrifugation of pooled cobra plasma from snakes collected in autumn/winter (A/W) and spring/summer (S/S) seasons and a rabbit antiserum (R/A) containing markers of established sedimentation coefficient. The HI activity for Japanese encephalitis virus was tested in the gradient fractions which were untreated (▲——▲), treated with 2-mercaptoethanol to inactivate IgM (□---□) or with kaolin to remove non-specific inhibitors (o---o). It can be seen that HI activity in A/W occurs in the IgM and 7S IgG positions and in S/S, in the 7S IgG position only. The demonstration that presumptive antibody detected by HI has sedimentation characteristics similar to those of immunoglobulins provides useful complementary information for the interpretation of serological findings (from Shortridge et al., 1974).

apply to those that do. In spite of the difficulties in interpretation, the HI test is very useful, particularly because of its relative ease of operation and economy as well as the orientating information it provides for natural history studies. The difficulties cited above may be overcome by the application of sensitive second generation techniques such as radioimmunoassay (RIA) and enzyme-linked immunosorbent assay (ELISA). Conversely, they can be used for virus identification. However, while still being essentially experimental in the arbovirus field generally, these techniques do have the limitation that they may only be applied using known antigen or antibody.

Neutralization of virus infectivity is accomplished by mixing infectious virus with an antiserum or serum from an immune animal. This is usually carried out in suckling mice or suitable cell culture. The neutralization test is widely used for virus identification and serological surveillance. In general, it is thought to be the most specific of the conventional serological tests in spite of the fact that a number of arboviruses show some degree of cross-reactivity. Obviously this causes difficulty in the interpretation of serological data, but less than that encountered with the HI test.

Sera for assay are heated at 56 C for 30 minutes with a view of destroying neutralization accessory factors (Whitman, 1947) and inhibitory substances that are known to occur in normal animal sera. For the effective neutralization of arbovirus infectivity, complement may be required (Ozaki and Tabeyi, 1967; Westaway, 1965). However, little is known about the behavior of sera from lower vertebrates such as the effects of heating on IgM or the occurrence of antibody of low avidity. The presence of such antibody could lead to false-negative results and may be a contributing factor to the largely negative findings obtained in some serological studies. Considering the possible existence of break-through phenomenon and low titer antibody, plaque reduction appears to be the most sensitive neutralization test for the routine assay of sera (Shortridge et al., 1974, 1975, 1977).

A newly described serological procedure for which there is little experience is the snake globulin precipitation (SGP) test (Thomas et al., 1980). The test relies on the ability of antibody to combine with virus, but not necessarily to neutralize the virus. SGP has been conducted only with experimentally infected and free-ranging, Thamnophis sirtalis and T. ordinoides, and appear to be an extremely sensitive and reliable procedure. Antibody was detected in snakes over 4.5 years following virus inoculation. While the applicability of SGP to sera from other reptiles and from amphibians remains to be demonstrated, it could represent a major step forward in the study of the relationship between arboviruses and amphibians and reptiles.

PROGNOSIS

Amphibians and reptiles may be subject to arbovirus infections, however at present, there is no definite information to indicate that these infections are detrimental to the animals. Given the long-term association with virus, amphibians and reptiles may prove to have a unique niche in the maintenance of arboviruses in nature. The field is still relatively unexplored. Further progress is largely dependent on the refinement of virus isolation and serological techniques for the confident interpretation of epidemiological data.

REFERENCES

Aspock, H., and Kunz, C., 1971, Untersuchungen uber die Uberwinterung von Tahyna- und Calovo-virus in Amphibien und Reptilien, Zentralbl. Bakteriol. Parasitenkd. Hyg. Abt. I Orig. A, 216:1-8.

Balashov, Y.S., 1972, Bloodsucking ticks (Ixodoidea)- vectors of diseases of man and animals, Entomol. Soc. Amer., 8:159-376.

Balfour, H.H., Jr., Edelman, C.K., Cook, F.E., Barton, W.I., Buzicky, A.W., Siem, R.A., and Bauer, H., 1975, Isolates of California encephalitis (La Crosse) virus from field-collected eggs and larvae of Aedes triseriatus: Identification of the overwintering site of California encephalitis, J. Infect. Dis., 131:712-716.

Bast, T.F., Whitney, E., and Benach, J.L., 1973, Considerations on the ecology of several arboviruses in eastern Long Island, Amer. J. Trop. Med. Hyg., 22:109-115.

Berge, T.O., 1975, "International catalogue of arboviruses," 2nd ed., DHEW Publ. No. (CDC) 75-8301, United States Government Printing Office, Washington.

Bidwell, D.E., and Mills, G.L., 1968, Serum non-specific inhibitors of arbovirus haemagglutination, J. Comp. Pathol., 78:469-476.

Bowen, G.S., 1977, Prolonged western equine encephalitis viremia in the Texas tortoise (Gopherus berlandieri), Amer. J. Trop. Med. Hyg., 26:171-175.

Buckley, S.M., 1969, Susceptibility of the Aedes albopictus and A. aegypti cell lines to infection with arboviruses, Proc. Soc. Exp. Biol. Med., 131: 625-630.

Burton, A.N., McLintock, J., and Rempel, J.G., 1966, Western equine encephalitis virus in Saskatchewan garter snakes and leopard frogs, Science, 154: 1029-1031.

Causey, O.R., Shope, R.E., and Bensabeth, G., 1966, Marco, Timbo and Chaco, newly recognized arboviruses from lizards of Brazil, Amer. J. Trop. Med. Hyg., 15:239-243.

Chastel, C., 1966, Infections a arbovirus au Cambodge. Enquete serologique chez les reptiles, Bull. World Health Organ., 34:701-707.

Clark, H.F., Lief, F.S., Lunger, P.D., Waters, D., Leloup, P., Foelsch, D.W., and Wyler, R.W., 1979, Fer de Lance virus (FDLV): A probable paramyxovirus isolated from a reptile, J. Gen. Virol., 44: 405-418.

Cook, R.S., Trainer, D.O., Glazener, W.C., and Nassif, B.D., 1965, A serological study of infectious diseases of wild populations in South Texas, Trans. North Amer. Wildlife Natur. Res. Conf., 30:142-155.

Craighead, J.E., Shelekov, A., and Peralta, P.H., 1962, The lizard: A possible host for eastern equine encephalitis virus in Panama, Amer. J. Hyg., 76:82-87.

Crans, W.J., and Rockel, E.G., 1968, The mosquitoes attracted to turtles, Mosq. News, 28:332-337.

Dalrymple, J.M., Young, O.P., Eldridge, B.F., and Russell, P.K., 1972, Ecology of arboviruses in a Maryland freshwater swamp, Amer. J. Epidemiol., 96: 129-140.

Danielova, V., 1975, Overwintering of mosquito-borne viruses, Med. Biol., 53:282-287.

DeFoliart, G.R., 1967, Aedes canadensis (Theobald) feeding on Blanding's turtle, J. Med. Entomol., 4:31.

De St. Jeor, S.C., 1969, Experimental and natural western equine encephalitis virus infections in reptiles, Ph.D. Thesis, Univ. Utah, Salt Lake City.

Doherty, R.L., Carley, J.G., Standfast, H.A., Dyce, A.L., Kay, B.H., and Snowdon, W.A., 1973, Isolation of arboviruses from mosquitoes, biting midges, sandflies and vertebrates collected in Queensland, 1969 and 1970, Trans. Royal Soc. Trop. Med. Hyg., 67:536-543.

Doi, R., and Oya, A., 1978, Unpublished data, National Institute of Health, Tokyo.

Doi, R., Oya, A., and Telford, S.R., 1968, A preliminary report on infection of the lizard, Takydromus tachydromides, with Japanese encephalitis virus, Jap. J. Med. Sci. Biol., 21:205-207.

Elkan, E., 1976, Pathology of the Amphibia, in: "Physiology of the Amphibia," B. Lofts, ed., Academic Press, New York.

Freeman, P., 1973, Ceratopogonidae, in: "Insects and other arthropods of medical importance," K.G.V. Smith, ed., Trustees of the British Museum, London.

Gebhardt, L.P., and Hill, D.W., 1960, Overwintering of western equine encephalitis virus, Proc. Soc. Exp. Biol. Med., 104:695-698.

Gebhardt, L.P., and Stanton, G.J., 1967, The role of poikilothermic hosts as virus reservoirs, Jap. J. Med. Sci. Biol., 20:30-34.

Gebhardt, L.P., Stanton, G.J., and Year, S., 1966, Transmission of WEE virus to snakes by infected Culex tarsalis mosquitoes, Proc. Soc. Exp. Biol. Med., 123:233-235.

Gebhardt, L.P., De St. Jeor, S.C., Stanton, G.J., and Stringfellow, D.A., 1973, Ecology of western encephalitis virus, Proc. Soc. Exp. Biol. Med., 142:731-733.

Gebhardt, L.P., Stanton, G.J., Hill, D.W., and Collett, G.C., 1964, Natural overwintering hosts of the virus of western equine encephalitis, New England J. Med., 217:172-177.

Goldfield, M., and Sussman, O., 1964, Ecologic studies of eastern equine and western equine encephalitis viruses in New Jersey (non-avian vertebrate studies), Report presented at Center for Disease Control, Atlanta, Aug. 6, 1964.

Graf, P.A., 1967, in: "International catalogue of arboviruses," 2nd ed., T.O. Berge, ed., DHEW Publ. No. (CDC) 75-8301, United States Government Printing Office, Washington.

Halstead, S.B., Sukhavachana, P., and Nisalak, A., 1964, Assay of mouse adapted dengue viruses in mammalian cell cultures by an interference method, Proc. Soc. Exp. Biol. Med., 115:1062-1068.

Hayes, R.O., 1961, Host preferences of Culiseta melanura and allied mosquitoes, Mosq. News, 21:179-187.

Hayes, R.O., Daniels, J.B., Manfield, H.K., and Wheeler, R.E., 1964, Field and laboratory studies on eastern encephalitis in warm- and cold-blooded vertebrates, Amer. J. Trop. Med. Hyg., 13:595-606.

Hoff, G.L., and Trainer, D.O., 1973, Arboviruses in reptiles: Isolation of a bunyamwera group virus from a naturally infected turtle, J. Herpetol., 7:55-62.

Hoogstraal, H., 1973, Viruses and ticks, in: "Viruses and invertebrates," A. Gibbs, ed., North Holland Publ. Co., Amsterdam.

Hoogstraal, H., and Kaiser, M.N., 1960, Some host relationships of the tortoise tick, Hyalomma (Hyalommasta) aegyptium (L.) (Ixodoidea, Ixodidae) in Turkey, Ann. Entomol. Soc. Amer., 53:457-458.

Karabatsos, N., 1978, Supplement to international catalogue of arboviruses including certain other viruses of vertebrates, Amer. J. Trop. Med. Hyg., 27:372-440.

Karabatsos, N., and Buckley, S.M., 1967, Susceptibility of the baby hamster kidney cell line (BHK-21) to infection with arboviruses, Amer. J. Trop. Med. Hyg., 16:99-105.

Karstad, L., 1961, Reptiles as possible reservoir hosts for eastern encephalitis virus, Proc. North Amer. Wildlife Natur. Res. Conf., 26:186-202.

Karstad, L., 1963, Influence of low body temperature on establishment of prolonged infection in animal reservoirs, J. Amer. Vet. Med. Ass., 100:186-193.

Kawasaki, M., 1972, Hemagglutination inhibitory substance in Japanese encephalitis infected frogs during and after hibernation, Med. Biol., 84:113-116.

Leake, C.J., Varma, M.G.R., and Pudney, M., 1977, Cytopathic effect and plaque formation by arboviruses in a continous cell line (XTC-2) from the toad, Xenopus laevis, J. Gen. Virol., 35:335-339.

Lee, H.W., 1968, Multiplication and antibody formation of Japanese encephalitis virus in snakes: Proliferation of the virus, Seoul J. Med., 9:157-161.

Lee, H.W., Min, B.W., and Lim, Y.W., 1972, Isolation and serologic studies of Japanese encephalitis virus from snakes in Korea, J. Korean Med. Ass., 15:69-74.

Lewis, D.J., 1973, Phlebotomidae and psychodidae, in: "Insects and other arthropods of medical importance," K.G.V. Smith, ed., Trustees of the British Museum, London.

Lunger, P.D., and Clark, H.F., 1978, Reptilia-related viruses, Adv. Virus Res., 23:159-204.

Manning, M.J., and Turner, R.J., 1976, "Comparative immunology," Blackie and Son, Glasgow.

Marshall, I.D., 1978, Personal communication, Microbiology Dept., Australian National Univ., Canberea.

Matsuyama, T., Oya, A., Kobayoshi, I., Nakamura, I., Takahashi, M., and Kitaoka, M., 1960, Isolation of arbor viruses from mosquitoes collected at live-stock pens in Gumma Prefecture in 1959, Jap. J. Med. Sci. Biol., 13:191-198.

Mattingly, P.F., 1973, Culicidae, in: "Insects and other arthropods of medical importance," K.G.V. Smith, ed., Trustees of the British Museum, London.

Mattingly, P.F., Crosskey, R.W., and Smith, K.G.V., 1973, Summary of arthropod vectors, in: "Insects and other arthropods of medical importance," K.G.V. Smith, ed., Trustees of the British Museum, London.

McLintock, J., Burton, A.N., and Rempel, J.G., 1967, Inter-epidemic hosts of western encephalitis virus in Saskatchewan, Proc. Ann. Meet. New Jersey Extermination Ass., 54:97-104.

Mills, G.L., and Taylaur, C.E., 1971, The distribution and composition of serum lipoproteins in eighteen animals, Comp. Biochem. Physiol., 40B:489-501.

Miyagi, I., 1972, Feeding habits of some Japanese mosquitoes on cold-blooded animals in laboratory Trop. Med., 14:203-217.

Miyagi, I., 1978, Personal communication, Univ. Ryukyus, Japan.

Monath, T.P., Cropp, C.B., Frazier, C.L., Murphy, F.A., and Whitfield, S.G., 1979, Viruses isolated from reptiles: Identification of three new members of the family Rhabdoviridae, Arch. Virol., 60:1-12.

Murray, M.D., 1970, Identification of blood-meals in biting midges (Culicoides: Ceratopogonidae), Ann. Trop. Med. Parasitol., 64:187-206.

Murphy, F.J., Burbutis, P.P., and Bray, D.F., 1967, Bionomics of Culex salinarius Coquillet. II Host acceptance and feeding by the adult females

of C. salinarius and other mosquito species, Mosq. News, 27:366-374.
Nir, Y.R., Avivi, A., Lasovski, Y., Margalit, J., and Goldwasser, R., 1972, Arbovirus activity in Israel, Israeli J. Med. Sci., 8:1695-1701.
Nolan, M.P., Moussa, M.A., and Haynes, D.E., 1965, Aedes mosquitoes feeding on turtles in nature, Mosq. News, 25:218-219.
Oya, A., 1978, Unpublished data, National Institute of Health, Tokyo.
Ozaki, Y., and Tabeyi, K., 1967, Studies on the neutralization of Japanese encephalitis virus. I Application of kinetic neutralization to the measurement of the neutralizing potency of antiserum, J. Immunol., 98:1218-1223.
Prior, M.G., and Agnew, R.M., 1971, Antibody against western equine encephalitis virus occurring in the serum of garter snakes (Colubridae: Thamnophis) in Saskatchewan, Can. J. Comp. Med., 35:40-43.
Pudney, M., and Lanar, D., 1977, Establishment and characterization of a cell line (BTC-32) from the triatomine bug, Triatoma infestans (Klug) (Hemiptera: Reduviidae), Ann. Trop. Med. Parasitol., 71:109-118.
Pudney, M., Leake, C.J., and Varma, M.G.R., 1979, Replication of arboviruses in arthropod in vitro systems, in: "Arctic arboviruses," E. Kurstak, ed., Academic Press, New York.
Pudney, M., Varma, M.G.R., and Leake, C.J., 1973, Establishment of a cell line (XTC-2) from the South African clawed toad, Xenopus laevis, Experientia, 29:466-467.
Pudney, M., Varma, M.G.R., and Shortridge, K.F., 1973, Rod-shaped virus-like particles in cultured Anopheles cells and in an Anopheles laboratory colony, in: "Proceedings of the 3rd international colloquium on invertebrate tissue culture," J. Rehacek, D. Blaskovic, and W.F. Hink, eds., Publ. House Sovak Acad. Sci., Bratislava.
Rehacek, J., Nosek, J., and Gresikova, M., 1961, Study of the relation of the green lizard (Lacerta viridis Lavr.) to natural foci of tick-borne encephalitis, J. Hyg. Epidemiol. Microbiol. Immunol., 5:366-371.
Romer, J.D., 1978, Personal communication, Pest Control, Urban Services Dept., Hong Kong.
Rosen, L., and Gubler, D., 1974, The use of mosquitoes to detect and propagate dengue viruses, Amer. J. Trop. Med. Hyg., 23:1153-1160.

Rosen, L., Tesh, R.B., Lien, J.C., and Cross, J.H., 1978, Transovarial transmission of Japanese encephalitis virus by mosquitoes, Science, 199:909-911.

Rosenbusch, F., 1939, Equine encephalomyelitis in the Argentine and its experimental aspects, Proc. Pacific Sci. Congress, 6:209-214.

Russell, P.K., 1972, in: "International catalogue of arboviruses," 2nd ed., T.O. Berge, ed., DHEW Publ. No. (CDC) 75-8301, United States Government Printing Office, Washington.

Schmidt, N.J., Gee, P.S., Dennis, J., and Lennette, E.H., 1971, Enzymes produced by a Pseudomonas species which inactivate inhibitors of certain viral hemagglutinins. II Effect of proteinase and phospholipase C on viral hemagglutinin inhibitor present in human sera, J. Immunol., 106:1615-1623.

Self, L.S., Shin, H.K., Kim, K.H., Lee, K.W., Chow, C.Y., and Hong, H.K., 1973, Ecological studies on Culex tritaeniorhynchus as a vector of Japanese encephalitis, Bull. World Health Organ., 49:41-47.

Sekeyova, M., Gresikova, M., and Leska, J., 1970, Formation of antibody to tick-borne encephalitis virus in Lacerta viridis and L. agilis lizards, Acta Virol., 14:87-90.

Sheals, J.G., 1973, Arachnida, in: "Insects and other arthropods of medical importance," K.G.V. Smith, ed., Trustees of the British Museum, London.

Shortridge, K.F., 1977, Rubella virus serology: Detection of residual lipoprotein inhibitors of haemagglutination using sensitive indicator arboviruses, J. Clin. Pathol., 30:409-416.

Shortridge, K.F., and Ho, W.K.K., 1974, Human serum lipoproteins as inhibitors of haemagglutination for selected togaviruses, J. Gen. Virol., 23:113-116.

Shortridge, K.F., and Ho, W.K.K., 1976, Comparison of the activities in inhibition of haemagglutination by different togaviruses for human serum lipoproteins and their constituents, J. Gen. Virol., 33:523-527.

Shortridge, K.F., Oya, A., Kobayashi, M., and Duggan, R., 1977, Japanese encephalitis antibody in cold-blooded animals, Trans. Royal Soc. Trop. Med. Hyg., 71:261-262.

Shortridge, K.F., Ng, M.H., Oya, A., Kobayashi, M., Munro, R., Wong, F., and Lance, V., 1974, Arbovirus infections in reptiles: Immunological evidence for a high incidence of Japanese encephalitis virus in the cobra, Naja naja, Trans. Royal Soc. Trop. Med. Hyg., 68:454-460.

Shortridge, K.F., Ng, M.H., Oya, A., and Yip, D.Y., 1975, Arbovirus infections in reptiles: Studies on the presence of Japanese encephalitis antibody in the plasma of the turtle, Trionyx sinensis, Southeast Asian J. Trop. Med. Public Health, 6:161-169.

Sixl, W., Sekeyova, M., and Riedl, H., 1971, Discovery of antibodies to arboviruses in Lacerta agilis, Arch. Hyg. Bakteriol., 154:609.

Smart, D.L., Trainer, D.O., and Yuill, T.M., 1975, Serologic evidence of Venezuelan equine encephalitis in some wild and domestic populations of southern Texas, J. Wildlife Dis., 11:195-200.

Smith, A., and Anderson, C.R., 1980, Susceptibility of two turtle species to eastern equine encephalitis virus, J. Wildlife Dis., 16:615-617.

Spalatin, J., Connell, R., Burton, A.N., and Gollop, B.J., 1964, Western equine encephalitis in Saskatchewan reptiles and amphibians, 1961-1963, Can. J. Comp. Med. Vet. Sci., 28:131-142.

Sudia, W.D., Newhouse, V.F., Beadle, L.D., Miller, D.L., Johnson, G.J., Jr., Young, R., Calisher, C.H., and Maness, K., 1975, Epidemic Venezuelan equine encephalitis in North America in 1971: Vector studies, Amer. J. Epidemiol., 101:17-35.

Sulkin, S.E., and Allen, R., 1974, Virus infection in bats, Monogr. Virol., 8:27-103.

Thomas, L.A., and Eklund, C.M., 1962, Overwintering of western equine encephalomyelitis virus in garter snakes experimentally infected by Culex tarsalis, Proc. Soc. Exp. Biol. Med., 109:421-424.

Thomas, L.A., Eklund, C.M., and Rush, W.A., 1959, Susceptibility of garter snakes (Thamnophis spp.) to western equine encephalomyelitis virus, Proc. Soc. Exp. Biol. Med., 99:698-701.

Thomas, L.A., Patzer, E.R., Cory, J.C., and Coe, J.E., 1980, Antibody development in garter snakes (Thamnophis spp.) experimentally infected with western equine encephalitis virus, Amer. J. Trop. Med. Hyg., 29:112-117.

Varma, M.G.R., Pudney, M., and Leake, C.J., 1975, The establishment of three cell lines from the tick, Rhipicephalus appendiculatus (Acari: Ixodidae) and their infection with some arboviruses, J. Med. Entomol., 11:698-706.

Varma, M.G.R., Pudney, M., Leake, C.J., and Peralta, P., 1975/1976, Isolations in a mosquito (Aedes pseudoscutellaris) cell line (Mos. 61) of yellow fever virus from original field material, Intervirology, 6:50-56.

Westaway, E.G., 1965, The neutralization of arboviruses. I Neutralization in homologous virus-serum mixtures with two group B arboviruses, Virology 26:517-527.

Whitman, L., 1947, The neutralization of western equine encephalomyelitis virus by human convalescent serum. The influence of heat labile substances in serum on the neutralization index, J. Immunol., 56:97-108.

Whitney, E., Jamnback, H., Means, R.G., and Matthew, T.H., 1968, Arthropod-borne-virus survey in St. Lawrence County, New York: Arbovirus reactivity in serum from amphibians, reptiles, birds and mammals, Amer. J. Trop. Med. Hyg., 17:645-650.

Woodall, J.P., 1967, in: "International catalogue of arboviruses including certain other viruses of vertebrates," 2nd ed., T.O. Berge, ed., DHEW Publ. No. (CDC) 75-8301, United States Government Printing Office, Washington.

Wright, R.E., and DeFoliart, G.R., 1970, Associations of Wisconsin mosquitoes and woodland vertebrate hosts, Ann. Entomol. Soc. Amer., 63:777-786.

Yasumura, Y., and Kawakita, Y., 1963, Studies on SV40 in relationship with tissue culture, Nippon Rinsho, 21:1201-1209.

Yuill, T.M., 1969, Mosquitoes for drawing blood from small reptiles, Trans. Royal Soc. Trop. Med. Hyg., 63:407-408.

Yuill, T.M., Brandt, W.E., and Buescher, E.L., 1971, Non-specific arbovirus hemagglutinin inhibitors in turtle sera, J. Immunol., 106:1413-1415.

Yunker, C.E., Brennan, J.M., Hughes, L.E., Philip, C.B., Clifford, C.M., Peralta, P.H., and Vogel, J., 1975, Isolation of viral and rickettsial agents from Panamanian acarina, J. Med. Entomol., 12:250-255.

REPTILIAN RHABDOVIRUSES

C. Bruce Cropp

Bureau of Laboratories

Centers for Disease Control

INTRODUCTION

Reptilian-associated viruses have received relatively little attention, partly because of the lack of recognized medical and economic importance. Virological studies with mammalian and avian host systems, rather than those with poikilothermic vertebrates, have dominated animal virology. Infectious processes in homothermic vertebrates are more similar to those in man than are those in reptiles, and thus they provide more analogous information. Moreover, in many instances, lower homothermic animals are involved as primary and secondary hosts or reservoirs in the infectious chain of vertebrate viruses (Lunger and Clark, 1978).

A few studies have, nevertheless, implicated reptiles as a potential vertebrate host for medically important viruses of the family Togaviridae (Thomas and Eklund, 1960). Attention has been focused on the role of snakes (Gebhart et al., 1964) and turtles (Bowen, 1977) in transmission and overwintering of western equine encephalitis virus in North America, on lizards as hosts for eastern equine encephalitis virus in Central America (Craighead et al., 1962), and on snakes and turtles as reservoirs of Japanese encephalitis virus in Asia (Shortridge et al., 1975). Despite these studies, the evidence that reptiles contribute significantly to natural transmission cycles of any of the togaviruses remains inconclusive. Even less information is available concerning the involvement of poikilothermic animals in the natural history of viruses of the family Bunyaviridae (Hoff and Trainer, 1973).

Recently, taxonomically unclassified arboviruses which utilize reptiles as their primary vertebrate hosts have been identified as members of the rhabdovirus family (Monath et al., 1979).

ETIOLOGY

The Rhabdoviridae constitute a genus that is based on structural similarity (surface projections, membranous envelope and coiled nucleocapsid). These viruses are of special interest because of the broad diversity of their ecological relationships, which include infection of various vertebrates, invertebrates and plants. All member viruses that infect vertebrates investigated thus far contain single stranded RNA as the genome and at least three distinct protein components (Hummeler and Tomassini, 1973). Marco, Timbo and Chaco viruses are the group members associated with reptiles.

In thin sections of infected green monkey kidney (Vero) and terrapin heart (TH-1) cells, Marco viral particles exhibited all the structural details of typical rhabdoviruses, but the overall particle shape was conical with a mean length of 180 nm. Budding was found primarily upon the plasma membranes but also occurred upon the endoplasmic reticulum. No inclusion bodies were observed. Because of its conical shape, Marco virus most closely resembled three other rhabdoviruses: Kotonkan, Obodhiang and bovine ephemeral fever viruses (Fig. 11.1).

In contrast, the Chaco viral particle is cylindrical with a mean particle length of 202 nm. Budding occurs only upon intracytoplasmic membranes. The formation of viral inclusion bodies could not be evaluated. Chaco resembles other rhabdoviruses with particles longer than those of the prototype vesicular stomatitis virus (Fig. 11.2). These viruses include Flanders, Hart Park, Mt. Elgon bat, Kamese, Joinjakaka, Navarro, Kwatta, BeAn 157575, Mossuril, New Minto and Sawgrass.

Timbo virus particles are morphologically similar to those of Chaco virus, as expected from the serological relationship between these viruses (Causey et al., 1966).

The wide geographic distribution of the Rhabdoviridae the source of the isolates, the diseases produced in nature and in experimental animals, plus the ultrastructural characteristics have been reviewed by Murphy (1979). The distribution of Marco, Chaco and Timbo viruses is

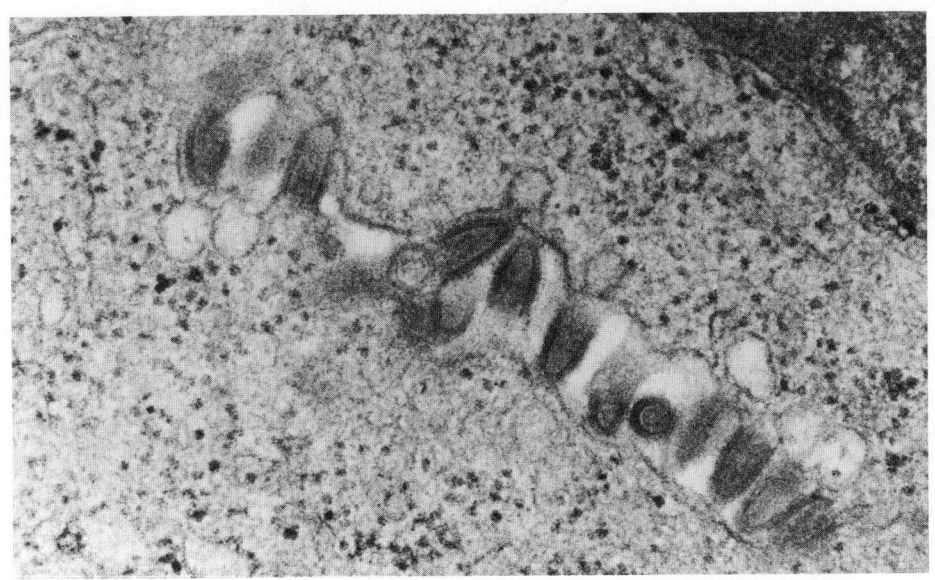

Fig. 11.1. Marco virus in TH-1 cell culture. The conical shaped virus particles are budding upon complex structures of the plasma membrane. X84,000

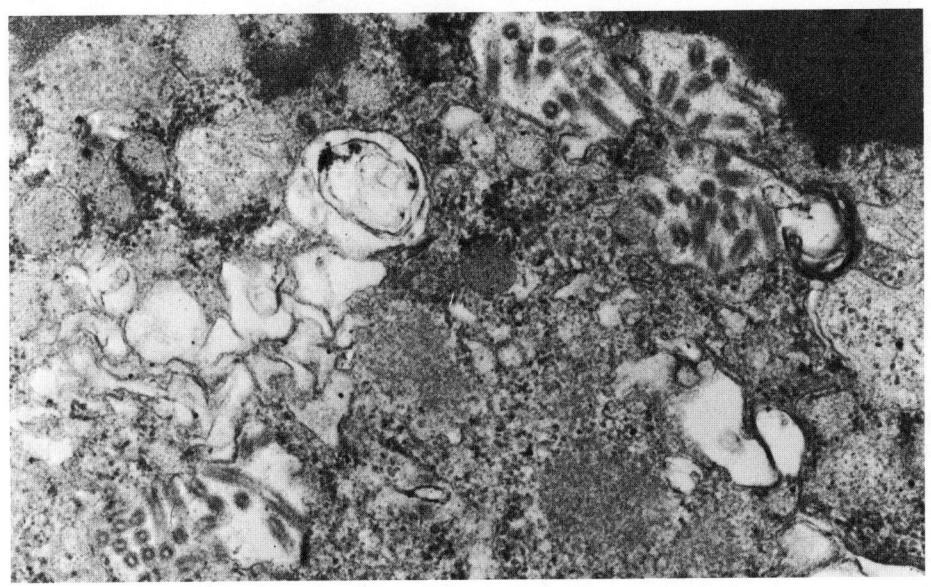

Fig. 11.2. Chaco virus in Vero cell culture. Long virus particles are budding upon membranes of the endoplasmic reticulum. X49,200

limited to the Amazon basin and naturally occurring disease associated with these viruses remains to be defined. It is not known at this time whether lizard species develop adequate viremias to be important in viral transmission.

TRANSMISSION

In 1966, Causey et al. described three arboviruses, Marco, Chaco and Timbo, isolated from lizards in Brazil. Six strains of Timbo virus, four of Marco and three of Chaco virus were isolated from Ameiva a. ameiva and one strain of Chaco virus was recovered from Kentropyx calcaratus lizards. Most of the 4,766 lizard specimens tested, belonging to at least 14 species, were obtained in 1962 and 1963 during intensive studies on the role of lizards in viral transmission in the Amazon region. The initial viral isolations were made by intracerebral (IC) inoculation of organ suspensions into suckling mice. No strains of Marco, Timbo and Chaco viruses were recovered from over 3,000 lizards of species other than A. a. ameiva and K. calcaratus, or from many thousands of birds, bats, rodents, marsupials, human beings, sentinel mice and pools of arthropods tested by the Belem Virus Laboratory. All of the virus-positive specimens in 1962-1963 were captured at the edges of the Utinga and Instituto Agronomico do Norte forest near Belem. Since 1963, few investigations of lizards as hosts for viruses have been done. A single isolate was obtained from A. a. ameiva collected in 1976 in the southwest Amazon region (Acre State); this virus is closely related to Timbo virus (Pinheiro, F., quoted in Monath, 1979). Neutralizing antibodies to Timbo virus have been found in 5 of 225 A. a. ameiva and 5 of 162 other reptiles tested from Para State, Brazil (Berge, 1975).

Multiple serial passages of Marco and Chaco viruses were done in Aedes aegypti mosquitoes by intrathoracic inoculation of salivary gland material (Berge, 1975; Causey et al., 1966). Transfer of Marco virus in Anopheles quadrimaculatus and of Chaco virus in An. quadrimaculatus and Culex fatigans failed after two passages.

On the basis of these limited observations, few conclusions can be drawn regarding the ecology of the agents. Their association with lizards and in particular with the teiid species A. a. ameiva, appears well-founded, but it is not known whether this vertebrate develops a viremia sufficient to serve as a source for arthropod infection. Mosquito transmission is suggested by the experimental studies; members of many tropical mosquito species, especially those belonging to the abundant subgenus Culex (melanoconion), feed extensively on reptiles. The capacity of these viruses to infect man or economically important animals remains unknown (Berge, 1975; Monath, 1979, Monath et al., 1979).

DIAGNOSIS

Laboratory strains of Marco and Chaco viruses are pathogenic for Swiss mice IC, whereas Timbo virus is relatively nonpathogenic (Table 11.1). The illness in infant mice is characterized by signs of central nervous system dysfunction, including ataxia, lethargy, tremors, paraspinal muscle contraction and coma. The encephalitic process is not rapidly progressive, and mice with signs of profound illness often survive for several days.

All three viruses grow equally well in a mammalian cell line (Vero). In both mammalian and poikilotherm vertebrate cell cultures, the three viruses replicate to highest titer at 30 C (Table 11.2), which indicates that they are naturally temperature-sensitive agents. The optimum temperature for virus replication may be a useful marker of the vertebrate class to which the virus is ecologically related (Monath et al., 1979).

Cytopathic effect (CPE) has been shown to be minimal or absent in various poikilothermic cell lines infected with the reptilian rhabdoviruses (Monath et al., 1979). Only Marco virus produces subtle, focal CPE (vacuolation) in TH-1 cells. Since CPE was absent with Chaco and Timbo viruses in poikilothermic cells, infectivity must be detected by a subpassage into a susceptible host (mice or Vero cells) or by demonstration of resistance to challenge with vesicular stomatitis virus. Thus a number of factors limit the usefulness of poikilothermic cell lines for isolation or assay of these viruses. The problems involved are in propagation of some poikilothermic cell lines, the absence of CPE and the requirement for subpassage to a susceptible host or for challenge with vesicular stomatitis virus for the detection of the agent (Monath, 1979). At present, no information is available on animal pathology.

Marco, Chaco and Timbo virus antigens and ascitic fluids have been tested by complement-fixation test against 34 other rhabdoviruses (Causey et al., 1966,

Table 11.1. Growth of Reptilian Viruses in Mice and in Cell Cultures (from Monath, 1979).

Virus	Suckling Mice			Vero Cells		TH-1 Cells
	$ICLD_{50}/ml$[a]	AST[b] (days)	Pathogenicity LD_{50}/PFU	PFU/ml[c]	Plaque Morphology	ID_{50}/ml[d]
Marco	$10^{7.4}$	3.2	5	$10^{6.7}$	Distinct, small, 0.5–1.0 nm	4.7
Chaco	$10^{7.0}$	7.6	5	$10^{6.3}$	Faint, pin-point	4.5
Timbo	$10^{3.5}$	8.5	0.0005	$10^{6.4}$	Distinct, small, 0.5–1.0 nm	NT

[a]$ICLD_{50}$ = Intracerebral inoculation lethal dose which kills 50% of the mice.
[b]AST = Average survival time after inoculation of 100 $ICLD_{50}$.
[c]PFU = Plaque forming units of virus.
[d]ID_{50} = Determined by protection against challenge with vesicular stomatitis virus.

Table 11.2. Growth of Reptile Rhabdoviruses in Cell Lines of Homeothermic and Poikilothermic Origin. Maximal Replication in all Cell Lines was at 30 C (from Monath et al., 1979).

Cell Line	Marco			Chaco			Timbo		
	CPE	Max. Yield[a]	Day	CPE	Max. Yield	Day	CPE	Max. Yield	Day
Vero African green monkey kidney	4+	5.3	6	4+	3.5	6	4+	3.8	6
BHK-21 (C-13) baby hamster kidney	3+	5.9	4-5	3+	5.7	5	3-4+	5.0	3
VSW Russell's viper spleen	0	5.4	4	0	6.0	6	0	Trace	
TH-1 (Subline B1) turtle heart	1+ Focal	5.1	3	0	0		0	0	
8625 Rattlesnake fibroma	0	2.3	9	0	Trace		0	0	
VH-2 Russell's viper heart	0	2.3	8	0	0		0	0	

[a] Log PFU or LD_{50}

Monath et al., 1979). Timbo and Chaco viruses are clearly related but distinct from one another; neither reacted with any other rhabdovirus. No relationship was found between Marco virus and other rhabdoviruses, including Chaco and Timbo, which share the same lizard host in Brazil.

REFERENCES

Berge, T.O., 1975, "International catalogue of arboviruses," 2nd ed., DHEW Publ. No. (CDC) 75-8301, United States Government Printing Office, Washington.

Bowen, G.S., 1977, Prolonged western equine encephalitis viremia in the Texas tortoise (Gopherus berlandieri), Amer. J. Trop. Med. Hyg., 26:171-175.

Causey, O.R., Shope, R., and Bensabath, G., 1966, Marco, Timbo, and Chaco, newly recognized arboviruses from lizards in Brazil, Amer. J. Trop. Med. Hyg., 15:239-243.

Craighead, J.E., Shelokov, A., and Peralta, P., 1962, The lizard: A possible host for eastern encephalitis virus in Panama, Amer. J. Trop. Med. Hyg., 11:82-87.

Gebhart, L.P., Stanton, G., Itill, D., and Collett, G., 1964, Natural overwintering host of the virus of western equine encephalitis, New England J. Med., 271:172-176.

Hoff, G.L., and Trainer, D.O., 1973, Arboviruses in reptiles: Isolation of a Bunyamwera group virus from a naturally-infected turtle, J. Herpetol., 7:55-62.

Hummeler, K., and Tomassini, H., 1973, Rhabdoviruses, in: "Ultrastructure of animal viruses and bacteriophages," J. Dalton and F. Haguenau, eds., Academic Press, Inc., New York.

Lunger, P.D., and Clark, F., 1978, Reptilia-related viruses, Adv. Virus Res., 23:159-179.

Monath, T.P., 1979, Reptile rhabdoviruses, in: "Rhabdoviruses," D.H. Bishop, ed., CRC Press, West Palm Beach.

Monath, T.P., Cropp, C., Frazier, C., Murphy, F., and Whitfield, S., 1979, Viruses isolated from reptiles: Identification of three new members of the family Rhabdoviridae, Arch. Virol., 60:1-12.

Murphy, F.A., 1979, Electron microscopy of the rhabdoviruses of animals, in: "Rhabodoviruses," D.H. Bishop, ed., CRC Press, West Palm Beach.

Shortridge, K.F., Oya, A., Kobayashi, M., and Yip, D., 1975, Arbovirus infections in reptiles: Studies on the presence of Japanese encephalitis virus antibody in plasma of the turtle, Trionyx sinensis, Southeast Asian J. Trop. Med. Public Health, 6:161-169.

Thomas, L.A., and Eklund, C., 1960, Overwintering of western equine encephalomyelitis virus in experimentally infected garter snakes and transmission to mosquitoes, Proc. Soc. Exp. Biol. Med., 105: 52-55.

HERPESVIRUSES OF REPTILES

Gerald L. Hoff and Diane M. Hoff

Office of Epidemiological Services

Kansas City Health Department

INTRODUCTION

Knowledge concerning the viral infections of amphibians and reptiles is extremely limited with a few exceptions. The herpesvirus causing renal adenocarcinoma in frogs (Chapter 22), the herpesvirus causing grey-patch disease in sea turtles, and the arthropod-transmitted viruses of reptiles (Chapters 10 and 11) are probably the best studied herptilian viral agents in terms of the virus-host-environment relationships. Information on other viral agents tends to be restricted to case reports (Cooper et al., 1982; Jacobson, 1980; Julian and Durham, 1982; Lunger and Clark, 1979; Wolf et al., 1968) or to virological studies of the agents themselves (Andersen et al., 1979; Granoff, 1969; Stehbens and Johnston, 1966).

Consequently, viruses infecting amphibians and reptiles can be categorized according to the scheme of Clark and Lunger (1981), remembering that as the data base on each agent expands the categorization may change. These categories are: 1) viruses circumstantially associated with herptilian disease; 2) viruses associated with herptilian tumors; 3) viruses non-pathogenic for herptiles, in the maintenance cycles of which the animals may play a reservoir or amplifying role; and 4) viruses restricted to herptiles of unknown disease producing potential. The herpesviruses of snakes and chelonians appear to fall in category 1, while the data on lizard herpesviruses is so confused that they should be placed in category 4 for the present.

Virions resembling herpesviruses have been observed in skin papillomas of Lacerta viridis (Raynaud and Adrian, 1976), however the role of the virus as the etiologic agent of the disease is uncertain. Reovirus and papovavirus-like virions also were observed in the lesions. More recently, Cooper et al. (1982) observed papovavirus-like particles in other papillomatous L. viridis. Consequently, the Lacerta herpesvirus must be placed in category 4. Within this category also must be placed the herpesvirus isolated from organ explants of an apparently health Iguana iguana (Clark and Karzon, 1972). Inoculation of this agent into young iguanas, Anolis carolinensis, Gekko gecko, Thamnophis sirtalis, Storeria dekayi, Elaphe obsoleta, Terrapene carolina, Chrysemys scripta, Caiman crocodylus, Rana pipiens and Bufo americanus produced no clinical disease. Virus was recovered, however, by tissue explant from the iguanas, G. gecko and T. carolina. Serologic studies of the virus indicated that it was different from mammalian and avian herpesviruses and represented a new member of the herpesvirus group (Clark and Karzon, 1972). Frye et al. (1977) reported the presence of herpes virus in organs of I. iguana, which presented with a variety of clinical signs, however a cause and effect relationship was not established.

Herpesviruses have been observed in the venom of Naja naja, N. n. kaouthia and Bungarus fasciatus (Monroe et al., 1968; Simpson et al., 1979), but attempts to isolate these agents have been unsuccessful probably due to venom toxicity to the assay systems (Lunger and Clark, 1979; Simpson et al., 1979). The virions in the venom of N. naja and B. fasciatus were discovered during studies of the action of snake venom on Rauscher virus (Monroe et al., 1968), whereas the virions in the venom of N. n. kaouthia were revealed during an investigation of low-grade venom production in snakes maintained for antivenin production (Simpson et al., 1979). Histologic studies demonstrated an active herpesvirus infection of the venom gland of the snakes with resulting structural damage to the glands. Based on this limited information the venom-associated herpesviruses of snakes may be tentatively placed in category 1.

Herpesviruses have been associated with clinical disease in three species of turtles, but only have been demonstrated as the etiologic agent in one species. There are no data to indicate whether these viruses are a single entity or represent multiple agents. Hepatic necrosis and pulmonary infection have observed in Clemmys marmorata and Chrysemys picta with herpesvirus virions being present in the affected cells (Cox et al., 1980; Frye et al., 1977). At present it is not clear whether the observed herpesviruses were the etiologic agents of the diseases or were merely latent agents reactivated by the ongoing disease process in the turtles. Hence these viruses should be placed in category 4 until further information is available.

In category 1 can be placed the herpesvirus causing grey-patch disease in aquaculture raised Chelonia mydas (Rebell et al., 1975). Epizootics of this skin disease among turtles 56 to 80 days post-hatching have occurred in multiple groups of reared turtles. The virus is present in the affected epidermal cells and has been experimentally transmitted to susceptible turtles. Environmental factors have been demonstrated to play a contributing role in the epizootics (Haines and Kleese, 1977).

ETIOLOGY

The herpesviruses of reptiles belong to an as yet undetermined sub-family(ies) of the family Herpesviridae (Roizman et al., 1981). As members of the family, they possess a double stranded, linear DNA genome. There is an icosahedral capsid with a reported diameter for the reptilian viruses of 85 to 125 nm. The virus is enveloped. Replication occurs in the nucleus of the infected cell with the envelope being acquired by budding through the inner lamella of the nuclear membrane. Virus particles accumulate in the space between the inner and outer lamellae of the nuclear membrane and in cisternae of the endoplasmic reticulum. They are released by transport to the cell surface through the modified endoplasmic reticulum.

TRANSMISSION

The mechanism of transmission of reptilian herpesviruses is unknown and it may differ for the various reptile groups as well as for terrestrial and aquatic species. For lizards direct contact seems to be the mechanism involved (Raynaud and Adrian, 1976). Among aquaculture reared C. mydas shedding of virus from skin lesions into the water with subsequent transmission to susceptible turtles seems probable. The shedding of virus and severity of disease is affected by water temperature (Haines and Kleese, 1977) and possibly other stress factors associated with overcrowding (Rebell et al., 1975). This mechanism of transmission would be analogous to that of the renal adenocarcinoma herpesvirus of R. pipiens (Chapter 22). Bacteria free material from lesions of infected turtles will cause infection in susceptible turtles when scratched on the skin (Rebell et al., 1975). Thus, trauma to the skin of susceptible animals in herpesvirus contaminated water could provide the portal of entry for the virus.

SIGNS, PATHOGENESIS AND PATHOLOGY

Herpesvirus infection in reptiles has been manifested by inapparent to clinical disease. No signs of disease were noted in I. iguana, G. gecko and T. carolina when inoculated with iguana herpesvirus, although the virus could be recovered by organ explant techniques (Clark and Karzon, 1972). Herpesvirus also has been recovered from I. iguana with a variety of clinical signs (Frye et al., 1977). Each of these iguanas had severe lymphocytosis and most had an acute onset of anorexia, lethargy and loss of the normal brilliant green coloration. All these animals were found to be affected with severe splenic lymphoid hyperplasia and most had significant histiocytic lymphoid infiltration of liver, spleen, myocardium and bone marrow. While herpesvirus was recovered from the affected tissues it was not determined if the virus represented the etiological agent or a fortuitous recovery of a latent virus.

Papillomatous skin lesions occurred in L. viridis infected with herpesvirus, however the presence of other viruses in the lesions obscures the etiologic relationship (Raynaud and Adrian, 1976).

In N. n. kaouthia the only sign of disease was the production of a tenacious, cell-contaminated low grade venom (Simpson et al., 1979). The venom glands were found to be enlarged with the lumina of some of the tubular glands containing considerable cellular debris. Patches of the epithelial lining of such lumina were desquamated. Microvilli were absent from the surfaces of degenerated epithelial cells and there was mononuclear cell infiltration of the subepithelium of glands lined by degenerated epithelium. Intranuclear herpesvirus capsids were occasionally observed in attached epithelial cells, whereas the nuclei of ruptured or necrotic cells in the lumina contained numerous capsids. Enveloped cell-free virions were found in the lumina along with cellular debris, coated vesicles containing venom, lymphocytes and plasma cells.

Clinical signs of disease in C. marmorata were characterized by the sudden onset of lethargy, anorexia and muscular weakness (Frye et al., 1977). The turtles weakly responded to pinching of the limbs by feebly attempting to withdraw into their shells, but would almost immediately go limp again. Numerous petechial and small ecchymotic hemorrhages were present beneath the skin of the limbs, neck and plastron. The infections terminated fatally. Upon necropsy, the livers and spleens of the turtles appeared to be slightly swollen, the kidneys pale and the remainder of the parenchymatous organs normal. Erythrocytic vacuolization and moderate lymphocytosis were seen on stained blood films and eosinophils were diminished in number. Eosinophilic intranuclear herpesvirus inclusion bodies were observed in hepatocytes from areas of acute hepatic necrosis.

In a C. picta, which died subsequent to surgery for another medical condition, Cox et al. (1980) found that the liver was friable and greenish-brown in color, kidneys were pale, spleen congested and lungs edematous. Eosinophilic intranuclear herpesvirus inclusion bodies were found in hepatocytes adjacent to areas of coagulation necrosis in the liver as well as in the bronchial epithelium.

Two types of skin lesions occur in grey-patch disease of C. mydas: nonspreading papules and spreading grey patches, with superficial epidermal necrosis (Rebell et al., 1975). These lesions appeared when the aquaculture reared turtles were 56 to 80 days old. The lesions increased in size at the rate of approximately 5 mm/week. After a period of several months during which 90 to 100% of each group of reared turtles developed signs of disease, the characteristic lesions of grey-patch disease resolved naturally. During the active disease period, a mortality rate of 5 to 20% was observed in turtles with extensive lesions.

The papular lesions are small and sharply circumscribed, with marked hyperkeratosis and acanthosis of the epidermis. In the upper half of the epidermis, the nuclei contain inclusion bodies with the remaining nuclear chromatin being condensed into clumps at the periphery of the inclusions. Nuclei containing these inclusions are enlarged. The upper layers of the epidermis are infiltated by eosinophilic granulocytes and the dermis contains an infiltrate of mononuclear cells and eosinophilic granulocytes predominately around the blood vessels.

Spreading lesions generally are similar to papular lesions, but are much more extensive and less sharply circumscribed. There is marked hyperkeratosis. Deeper portions of the keratin contain residual nuclei with intranuclear inculusions. The underlying epidermis is acanthotic with papillary hyperplasia throughout the upper half of the epidermis. The nuclei contain inclusions identical to those in the papular lesions. There is increased vascularity of the underlying dermis with an infiltrate made up of mononuclear cells and eosinophilic granulocytes. In later stages of the disease, the entire epidermis is replaced by a necrotic crust, fibrin and inflammatory cells.

With rising water temperature, the incubation period for grey-patch disease is decreased while the severity of the lesions is increased (Haines and Kleese, 1977). Hence the disease appears to represent a heat-stressed induction of a latent herpesvirus infection. Experimentally, the most dramatic development of grey-patch disease was in turtles subjected to a sudden temperature change (25 C to 30 C) and in those maintained at high temperatures (30 C). This situation is similar to that described for channel catfish, Ictalurus punctatus, infected with herpesvirus (Wolf, 1973), but the reverse of that which occurs with frogs and the renal adenocarcinoma herpesvirus (Chapter 22).

DIAGNOSIS

Little information is available on the best method of diagnosing herpesvirus infection in reptiles. The majority of reports have relied on light microscopic detection of eosinophic intranuclear inclusion bodies in affected cells, followed by visualization of intranuclear and intracytoplasmic virions by electron microscopy.

Actual recovery of the virus has been accomplished by explants of affected tissues (Clark and Karzon, 1972). Once giant cell formation and subsequent development of cytopathic effect (CPE), the supernant fluids can be harvested and the virus maintained in poikilothermic cell lines. For iguana herpesvirus, Clark and Karzon (1972) found that various Iguana and Terrapene cell lines were susceptible to infection. The type of CPE induced was affected by incubation temperature as was the rate of CPE progression. At 36 C the CPE consisted entirely of irregularly shaped syncytia containing a few to several hundred nuclei. In cells incubated at 30 C or lower, the predominant CPE was more cell destructive, consisting of pycnosis and cytoplasmic retraction of individual cells accompanied by the formation of giant cells. Virtually no virus was released from the cultures incubated at 36 C, whereas virus was released from cultures incubated at lower temperatures. Plaque assay is possible once the virus is recovered in cell culture.

IMMUNITY AND CONTROL

In all probability the herpesviruses of reptiles behave in the host as do the better studied herpesviruses of mammals and birds. The initial infection may be associated with an acute localized or generalized disease of varying severity, followed by the establishment of a latent infection which may or may not remain quiescent for the life of the animal. Stressful conditions may reactivate the virus and lead to clinical disease with viral shedding (Haines and Kleese, 1977). Little is known about the immune response of reptiles to herpesvirus infection, however, iguana herpesvirus did not induce a detectable virus-neutralization titer in experimentally inoculated amphibians and reptiles (Clark and Karzon, 1972).

While the incidence of grey-patch disease among sea turtles may be controlled through the manipulation of the water temperature during aquaculture (Haines and Kleese, 1977), there are no data indicating that this procedure will influence the incidence of infection in the population, despite the fact it should reduce the rate of transmission.

REFERENCES

Andersen, P.R., Barbacid, M., Tronick, S.R., Clark, H.F., and Aaronson, S.A., 1979, Evolutionary relatedness of viper and primate endogenous retroviruses, Science, 204:318-321.
Clark, H.F., and Karzon, D.T., 1972, Iguana virus, a herpes-like virus isolated from cultured cells of a lizard, Iguana iguana, Infect. Immun., 5: 559-569.
Clark, H.F., and Lunger, P.D., 1981, Viruses of reptiles, in: "Diseases of the Reptilia," J.E. Cooper and O.F. Jackson, eds., Academic Press, New York.
Cooper, J.E., Gschmeissner, S., and Holt, P.E., 1982, Viral particles in a papilloma from a green lizard (Lacerta viridis), Lab. Animal, 16:12-13.

Cox, W.R., Rapley, W.A., and Barker, I.K., 1980, Herpesvirus-like infection in a painted turtle, J. Wildlife Dis., 16:445-449.

Frye, F.L., Oshiro, L.S., Dutra, F.R., and Carney, J.D., 1977, Herpesvirus-like infection in two Pacific pond turtles, J. Amer. Vet. Med. Ass., 171:882-884.

Granoff, A., 1969, Viruses of Amphibia, Curr. Topics Microbiol. Immunol., 50:108-137.

Haines, H., and Kleese, W.C., 1977, Effect of water temperature on a herpesvirus infection of sea turtles, Infect. Immun., 15:756-759.

Jacobson, E.R., 1980, Viral agents and viral diseases of reptiles, in: "Reproductive biology and diseases of captive reptiles," J.B. Murphy and J.T. Collins, eds., Soc. Study Amphibians Reptiles Contrib. Herpetol., 1.

Julian, A.F., and Durham, P.J.K., 1982, Adenoviral hepatitis in a female bearded dragon (Amphibolurus barbatus), New Zealand Vet. J., 30: 59-60.

Lunger, P.D., and Clark, H.F., 1979, Reptilia-related viruses, Adv. Virus Res., 23:159-204.

Monroe, J.H., Shibley, G.P., Schidlovsky, G., Nakai, T., Howatson, A.F., Wivel, N.W., and O'Connor, T.E., 1968, Action of snake venom on Rauscher virus, J. Nat. Cancer Inst., 40:135-140.

Raynaud, M.M.A., and Adrian, M., 1976, Lesions cutanees a structure papillomateuse associees a des virus chez le lezard vert (Lacerta viridis Laur.), C.R. Acad. Sci. Paris, 283:845-847.

Rebell, G., Rywlin, A., and Haines, H., 1975, A herpesvirus-type agent associated with skin lesions of green sea turtles in aquaculture, Amer. J. Vet. Res., 36:1221-1224.

Roizman, B., Carmichael, L.E., Deinhardt, F., de-The, G., Nahmias, A.J., Plowright, W., Rapp, F., Sheldrick, P., Takahashi, M., and Wolf, K., 1981, Herpesviridae, Intervirology, 16:201-217.

Simpson, C., Jacobson, E., and Gaskin, S., 1979, Herpes virus associated venom gland infection of Siamese cobras, J. Amer. Vet. Med. Ass., 175: 941-943.

Stehbens, W.E., and Johnston, M.R.L., 1966, The viral nature of Pirhemocyton tarentolae, J. Ultrastructure Res., 15:543-554.

Wolf, K., 1973, Herpesviruses of lower vertebrates, in: "The herpesviruses," A.S. Kaplan, ed., Academic Press, New York.

Wolf, K., Bullock, G.L., Dunbar, C.E., and Quimby, M.C., 1968, Tadpole edema virus: A viscerotropic pathogen for anuran amphibians, J. Infect. Dis., 118:253-262.

AMPHIBIAN CHROMOMYCOSIS

Robert E. Schmidt

School of Aerospace Medicine

Brooks Air Force Base

INTRODUCTION

Chromomycosis of amphibians is a fungal disease characterized by the occurrence of ulcerative or granulomatous skin lesions and/or disseminated granulomas in internal organs. The reported history of the disease in amphibians began with the report of Carini (1910) on a case in the South American bullfrog, <u>Leptodactylus</u> <u>pentadactylus</u>. This antedates the first reported human cases by <u>Lane</u> (1915) and Medlar (1915). Experimental production of the disease in several animals, including frogs, was first accomplished by DeArea Leao et al. (1947) and extended to toads by Trejos (1953).

The name "chromomycosis" was proposed by Moore and DeAlmeida (1935). They believed the older name "chromoblastomycosis" was misinformative because of histopathologic differences and because the causative organisms were not blastomycetes. Carrion (1950), however, felt that the name "blastomycosis" should be preserved because the name had been extensively used in the literature.

DISTRIBUTION

Chromomycosis has a world-wide distribution, although occurring more frequently in tropical or subtropical areas (Emmons et al., 1970). Most of the early reports of amphibian chromomycosis came from South America (Correa et al., 1968; DeArea Leao et al., 1947; Trejos, 1963).

Table 13.1. Species of Amphibians with Reported Chromo-

Species	System Affected
Ambystoma tigrinum mavortium	Skeletal muscle granuloma
Bufo alvarius	Skin and internal organs
B. blombergi	Numerous internal organs
B. bufo	Skin and internal organs
B. marinus	Numerous internal organs
	Skin and internal organs
B. melanostictus	Skin and internal organs
Hyla caerulea	Skin and internal organs
H. suptentrionalis	Skin and internal organs
Leptodactylus ocellatus	Mesenteric granulomas
L. pentadactylus	Mesenteric granulomas
Phyllobates trinitatis	Skin and internal organs
Pternohyla fodiens	Skin and internal organs
Rana pipiens	Skin and internal organs
R. temporaria	Skin and internal organs
Rhacophorus sp.	Skin and internal organs

By 1950 cases in man had been reported from everywhere except continental Asia (Carrion, 1950). The first reports of chromomycosis in amphibians in Asia were those of Dhaliwal and Griffiths (1963; 1964).

During the past eight years several reports of multiple cases of chromomycosis have appeared (Cicmanic et al., 1973; Elkan and Philpot, 1973; Goodwin, 1974; Rush et al., 1974) involving toads and frogs in zoological collections and research laboratories. The disease has been seen in a tiger salamander, Ambystoma tigrinum mavortium (Migaki and Frye, 1975). Amphibian cases have been reported primarily from North and South America, Europe and South Asia. Table 13.1 lists species of amphibians with reported chromomycosis.

ETIOLOGY

Although chromomycosis is a clinical and pathologic entity, it is caused by several fungi of the family Dematiaceae. These fungi produce simple conidiophores and have dark brown or black conidia, spores or hyphae. The problem in reading the literature concerning chromomycosis (Natural and Experimental Infection).

Organism Isolated	Reference
Undetermined	Migaki and Frye, 1975
Hormodendrum sp.	Frank and Roester, 1970
None	Schmidt and Hartfiel, 1977
Hormodendrum sp.	Frank and Roester, 1970
Fonsecaea pedrosoi	Cicmanic et al., 1973
F. pedrosoi	Trejos, 1953
Undetermined	Dhaliwal and Griffiths, 1964
Phialophora-like	Elkan and Philpot, 1973
Phialophora-like	Elkan and Philpot, 1973
Phialophora pedrosoi	DeArea Leao et al., 1947
P. pedrosoi	DeArea Leao et al., 1947
Phialophora-like	Elkan and Philpot, 1973
Phialophora-like	Elkan and Philpot, 1973
Undetermined	Rush et al., 1974
Hormodendrum sp.	Frank and Roester, 1970
Phialophora-like	Elkan and Philpot, 1973

mycosis is that a great deal of taxonomic confusion is present. Moore and DeAlmeida (1935) and Carrion (1950) presented historical reviews of the various names given to fungi isolated from cases of chromomycosis. Emmons et al. (1970) stated that P. verrucosa, P. compacta, P. dermatididis, P. pedrosoi and Cladiosporium carrionii are the principal causes. An explanation of why the various species of Phialophora at one time or another have been placed in several genera is given by Emmons et al. (1970) and detailed descriptions of the fungi and their growth characteristics can be found in an article by Silva (1960) and in Emmons et al. (1970).

TRANSMISSION

Transmission of the disease agent to amphibians is speculative. In man, the disease most commonly involves the skin of the feet and legs. The site of infection is correlated with cutaneous lesions allowing introduction of spores of one of the etiologic fungi. The mode of infection in amphibians is probably very similar to that in man. In one report, no toad with internal lesions was seen unless there was at least one skin lesion (Dhaliwal and Griffiths, 1964). Other reports, however,

have described amphibians with internal lesions and no
skin lesions (Cicmanic et al., 1973; Schmidt and Hartfiel,
1977). Successful culture feeding experiments indicate
the possibility that the alimentary tract may be a portal
of entry for the organism (Goodwin, 1974).

PATHOGENESIS

The pathogenesis of chromomycosis in amphibians
remains speculative, just as is the mode of transmission.
The problem is how to explain the occurrence of disseminated infections without a primary cutaneous lesion. The
answer may lie in one of three possibilities: 1) that
the cutaneous lesion was inocuous and overlooked; 2) that
infection resulted from the inoculation of fungus directly
into the body cavity via a contaminated wood splinter;
or 3) that infective material was ingested.

Experimentally, amphibian chromomycosis has resulted
from inoculation of organisms intraperitoneally, into
the dorsal lymph sac and by subcutaneous transplants of
infected tissue (Cicmanic et al., 1973; Dhaliwal and
Griffiths, 1964; Rush et al., 1974). Following inoculation
into the skin, inflammatory cells migrate to the site
with subsequent nodule formation and ulceration (Dhaliwal
and Griffiths, 1964). Disseminated lesions follow, imply-
ing spead via the vascular and/or particular organ affected, leading to functional problems related to the affected
organs. Studies with Bufo marinus demonstrated that
infection and death occurred only in the stressed group;
the unstressed group remained free of the disease (Cinmanic
et al., 1973). Thus infection and death may be correlated
with an overall depression of the immune system, rather
than a primary fungal infection.

SIGNS

No consistent clinical pattern has been described
in frogs and toads. In many cases the presenting sign
will be papular and ulcerative skin lesions, primarily
on the ventral body. At this stage, animals will be alert,
active and have normal appetites (Rush et al., 1974).
Gradual wasting occurs with debilitation, depression,
anorexia and death in 4 to 11 months. In some cases,
the skin lesions may present as vesicles or tumor-like
enlargements (Elkan and Philpot, 1973; Frank and Roester,
1970). In many cases, however, no external lesion is
seen. The presenting clinical sign will be nonspecific

debilitation or spontaneous death (Cicmanic et al., 1973; Schmidt and Hartfiel, 1977). In a tiger salamander, the presenting sign was described as a soft tissue mass involving the left lumbar area (Migaki and Frye, 1975).

PATHOLOGY

Gross lesions are seen in the skin and/or internal organs of toads and frogs, and have been reported in the muscle of a tiger salamander. Skin lesions are variable and may occur as hard, white tumor-like nodules 10 to 20 mm in diameter or as larger, soft, reddish masses which may ulcerate (Fig. 13.1). Papular and vesicular lesions can also be present. Fine black lines may appear on the surface of the papules (Rush et al., 1974). Ulcerative areas are usually sharply circumscribed (Fig. 13.2) and underlying soft tissue damage and occasional bone destruction have been seen. Skin lesions occur primarily on the ventral and rostral parts of the animal (Elkan and Philpot, 1973).

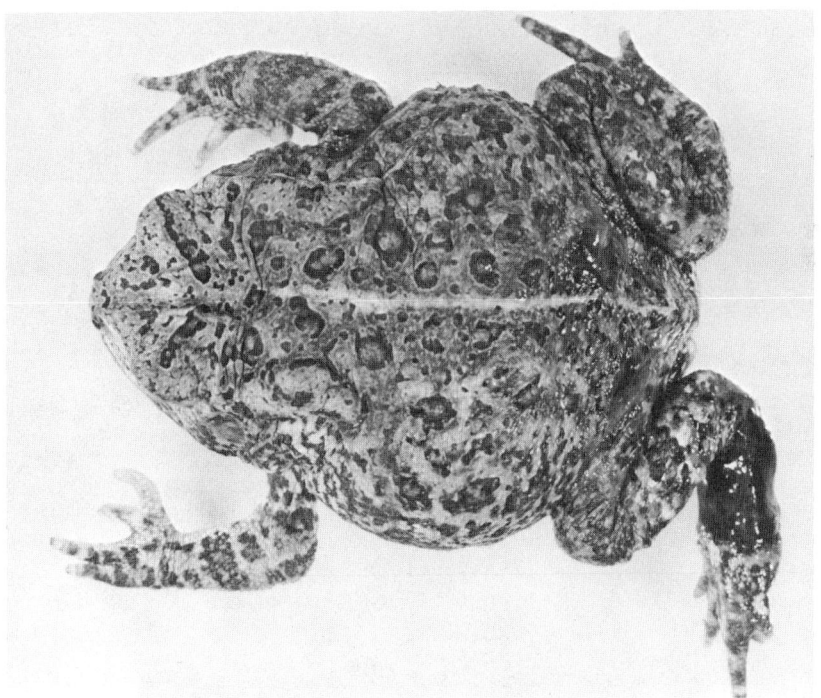

Fig. 13.1. Reddish necrotic areas on the back and leg of a toad, Bufo houstonensis.

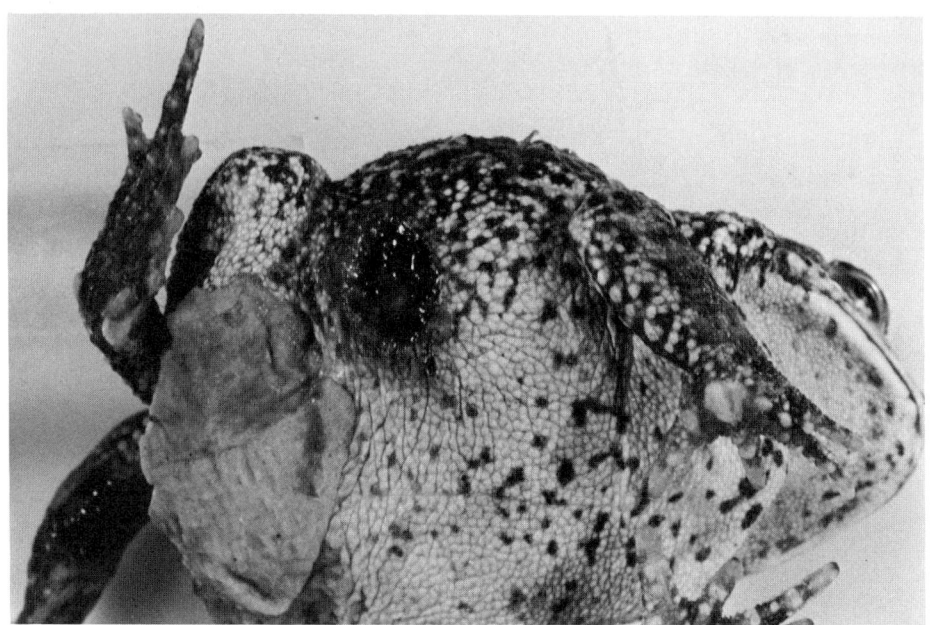

Fig. 13.2. Circumscribed ulcer on ventral body of a toad, Bufo houstonensis.

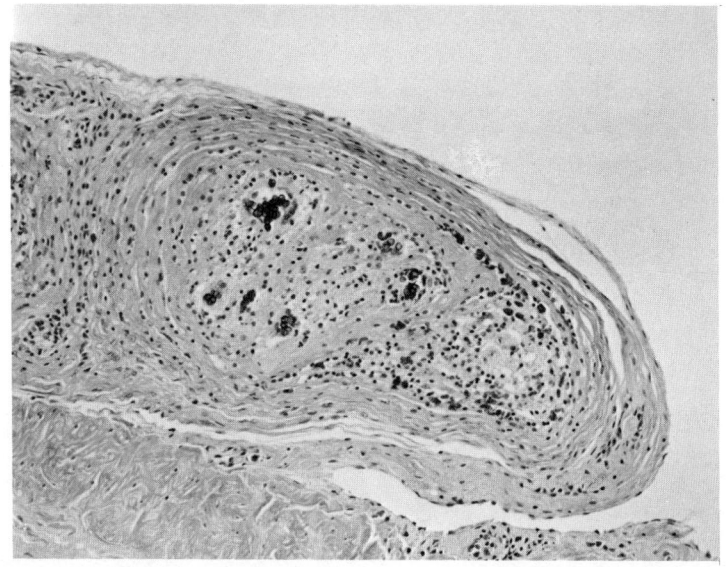

Fig. 13.3. Septate hyphae and scattered mononuclear inflammatory cells from infected toad skin. H&E X320

The histologic appearance of the skin ulcers is characterized by congestion and granulomatous inflammation with a pleocellular infiltrate, primarily macrophages and giant cells, some containing portions of fungus. Coagulative and caseous necrotic foci are often seen and pigmented septate hyphae or occasionally single to four-celled fungal cells may be present (Fig. 13.3). The inflammation may extend under intact areas of skin adjacent to the ulcers. When tumor-like nodules are seen in the skin, they often contain a dense mycelial mass.

Disseminated infections can affect one or many internal organs, with the heart, lung, kidney, meniges, skeletal muscle, bone marrow and spleen all being involved (Cicmanic et al., 1973; Schmidt and Hartfiel, 1977). The gross lesions are firm, white to gray-black nodules which may be single or coalesing and can vary from 0.3 to 3.0 cm, or occasionally occur as large masses replacing much of a particular organ. On section they appear as concentric rings with small dark brown or black foci randomly scattered throughout (Fig. 13.4).

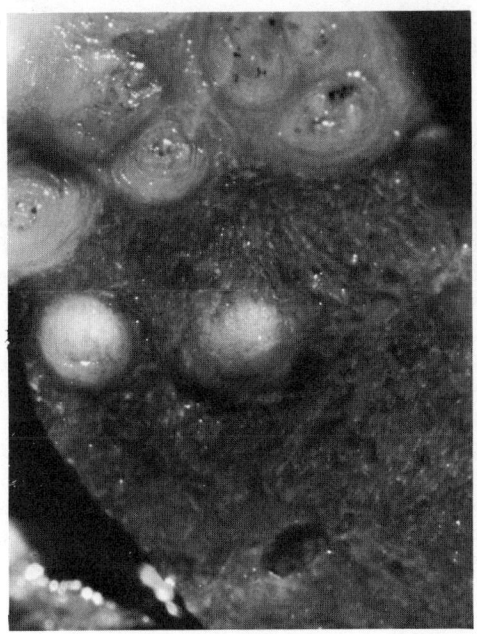

Fig. 13.4. Solitary and confluent granulomas in kidney of Blomberg's toad, Bufo blombergi. The scattered blsck foci (arrow) in sectioned lesions represent groups of pigmented fungi.

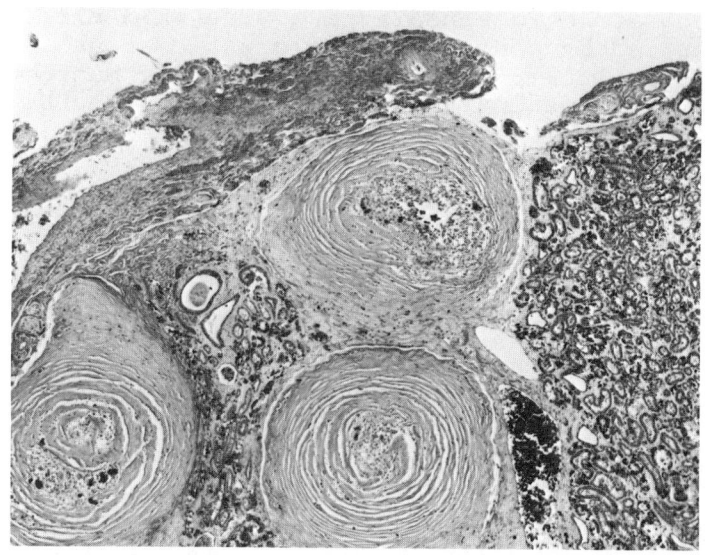

Fig. 13.5. Histologic appearance of kidney from <u>Bufo blombergi</u> Compare with gross appearance in Fig. 13.4. The lesions are primarily whorls of mature connective tissue with pigmented fungi and inflammatory cells at their center. H&E X44

Granulomas present in internal organs have basically the same histologic appearance regardless of the organ affected. They commonly have concentric lamellae composed of fibrous tissue interspersed with variable numbers of inflammatory cells and clumps of organisms (Figs. 13.5 and 13.6). Macrophages and multinucleated giant cells predominate in areas around the fungal cells, and fungal cells may be present within giant cells (Fig. 13.7). Occasionally the center of the granuloma will be necrotic. The organisms are dark brown and septate, occurring in variably sized groups (Fig. 13.8). Special stains are of no benefit as the pigmented fungi are adequately visualized in hematoxylin and eosin stains. Histologically a disseminated inflammatory lesion can occur in organs that were normal grossly. These are characterized by loss of normal architecture, the presence of septate hyphae and infiltration of macrophages (Fig. 13.9).

DIAGNOSIS

The initial objective in dealing with a sick amphibian or a group of sick amphibians is to make a rapid diagnosis

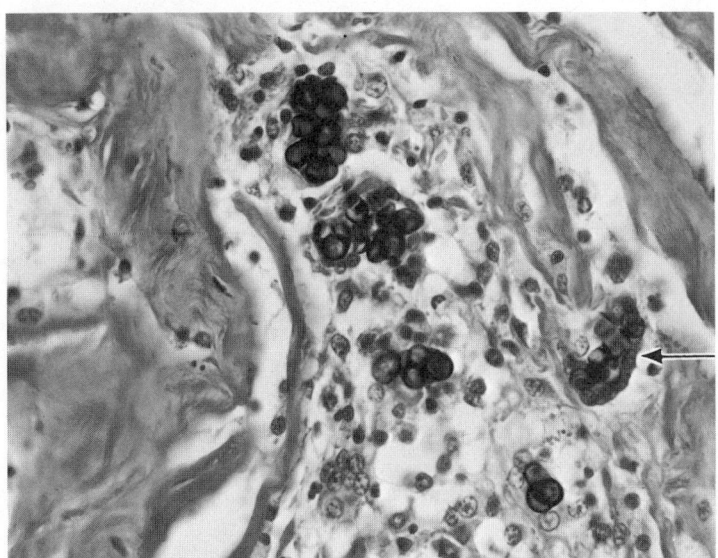

Fig. 13.6. Detail of lesion in capsule of the liver from Bufo blombergi. Well defined groups of fungal cells (arrow) are seen. H&E X130

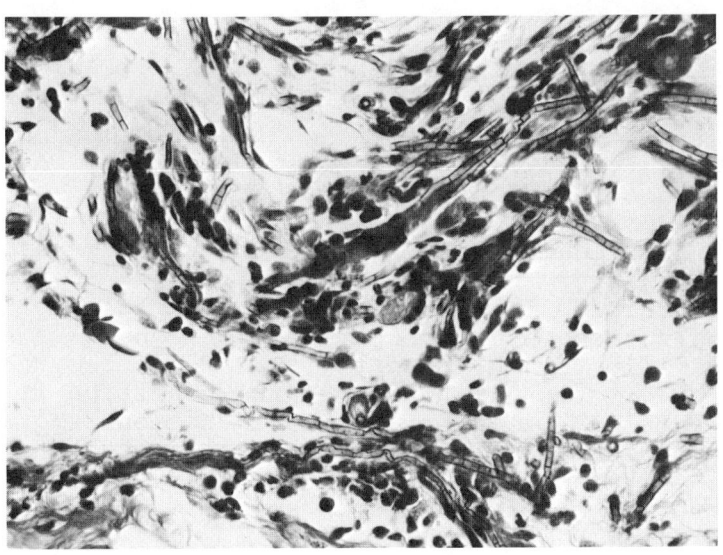

Fig. 13.7. Higher magnification of an area in Fig. 13.2 to illustrate fungal cells and inflammatory response consisting primarily of macrophages and giant cells. H&E X450

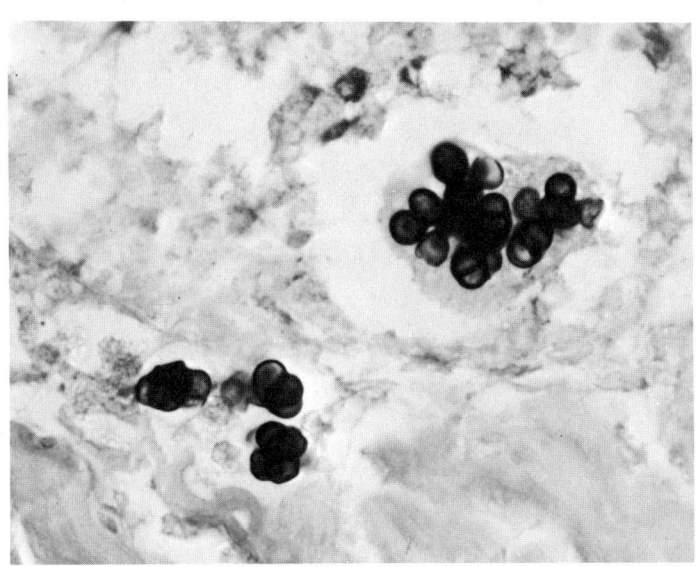

Fig. 13.8. Detail of fungal cells from a necrotic lesion in the kidney of a Bufo blombergi. Note the characteristic groups of septate cells. H&E X650

that will allow rational decisions as to treatment (if any), animal disposition, or preventive measures to be taken. A rapid, inexpensive method of diagnosis using scales from the cutaneous lesion has been described for man (Borelli, 1957), and the same principle can be used with cutaneous or deep lesions. Material can be scraped and spread on a slide, or direct impressions of the cut surface of a lesion made. The causative organisms are always dark brown or black and easily seen microscopically without staining the preparation. Borelli's method involves putting a few drops of xylene on scale material and coverslipping the preparation. He states that if the direct examination is negative, the condition is not chromomycosis. Differential considerations should include other mycotic infections (with non-pigmented fungal cells and hyphae) and tuberculosis, which can cause a disseminated granulomatous disease in amphibians.

Histopathologic examination of lesions will result in a definitive morphologic diagnosis, however final etiologic diagnosis can only be made by culture of the organism. Because of the problem and confusion involved

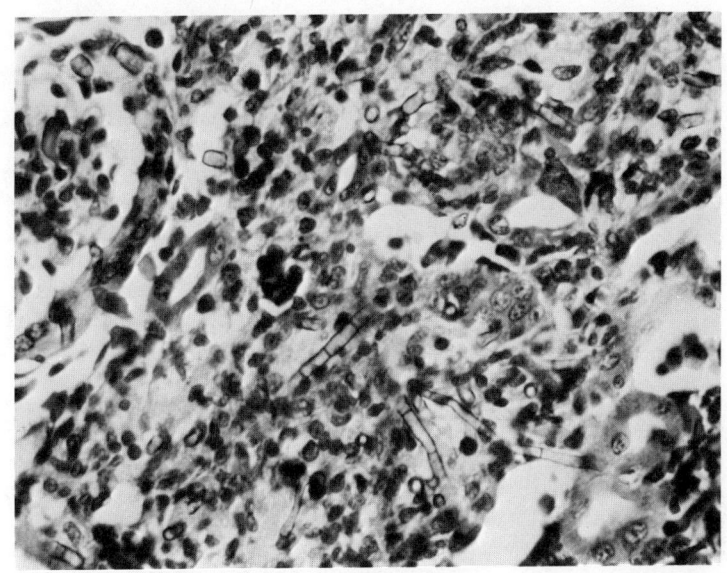

Fig. 13.9. Septate hyphae and macrophage infiltration in the kidney of a <u>Bufo</u> <u>houstonensis</u>. No gross lesion was noted, but inflammatory foci such as this were scattered throughout the parenchyma. H&E X510

in naming the organisms found in cases of chromomycosis, the culture interpretation may depend on the mycologist doing the cultures and the classification scheme used. Details of the laboratory procedures are given by Beneke and Rogers (1970). From a practical standpoint, the appearance of the fungi in tissue, their pathogenicity and usally their macroscopic cultural shape are the same. Since they produce one disease, specific identification is not useful either for rapid diagnosis or more rational treatment of the problem (Borelli, 1957).

PROGNOSIS AND IMMUNITY

There is not enough known about amphibian chromomycosis to determine if there are self-limiting infections or animals with a natural immunity. In cases where the diagnosis is made in a live animal or where sick animals are still present in a group following diagnosis, the prognosis is poor. No cases of recovery from amphibian chromomycosis have been reported.

CONTROL

Even if a clinical case was diagnosed early, there is no practical method to treat individuals or groups of amphibians. Control and prevention must rely on manageme factors and should be directed towards proper quarantine and quality control of newly arrived amphibians as well as prevention of nonspecific stress. Naturally occurring disease is more likely to be a problem in debilitated animals (Cicmanic et al., 1973). Since the causative organism is present in the environment, strict sanitation and periodic culture of material in the animals' living space are essential.

It should be remembered that chromomycosis is also a disease of man. Handlers of amphibians ought to be aware that they can be infected from the same environmentɛ sources that infect the animals. In addition, zoonotic spread of disease is possible, especially from animals with skin lesions where infective fungal spores may be present. Handlers of sick amphibians should wear gloves and exercise reasonable caution.

REFERENCES

Beneke, E.S., and Rogers, A.L., 1970, "Medical mycology manual," Burgess Publ. Co., Minneapolis.

Borelli, D., 1957, Diagnosis of chromomycosis, Arch. Dermatol., 76:789-790.

Carini, A., 1910, Sur une muisissure qui cause un maladie spontanee du "Leptodactylus pentadactylus," Ann. Inst. Pasteur, 24:157-162.

Carrion, A.L., 1950, Chromoblastomycosis, Ann. New York Acad. Sci., 50:1255-1282.

Cicmanic, J.L., Ringler, D.H., and Beneke, E.S., 1973, Spontaneous occurrence and experimental transmission of the fungus, Fonsecaea pedrosi, in the marine toad, Bufo marinus, Lab. Animal Sci., 23:43-47.

Correa, R., Correa, I., Garces, G., Mender, D., Morales, L.F., and Restrept, A., 1968, Lesiones micoticas (Chromomicosis)? observadas en sapos (Bufo sp.), Antig. Med., 18:175-184.

DeArea Leao, A.E., Mello, M.T., and Cury, A., 1947, Chromoblastomicose experimental, Rev. Brazil Biol., 7:5-24.

Dhaliwal, S.S., and Griffiths, D.A., 1963, Fungal disease in Malayan toads: An acute lethal inflammatory reaction, Nature, 197:467-469.

Dhaliwal, S.S., and Griffiths, D.A., 1964, Fungal disease of Malayan toads (Bufo melanostictus), Sabourdia,

Elkan, E., and Philpot, C.M., 1973, Mycotic infections in frogs due to a phialophora-like fungus, Sabourdia, 11:99-105.

Emmons, C.W., Binford, C.H., and Utz, J.P., "Medical mycology," Lea and Febiger, Philadelphia.

Frank, W., and Roester, V., 1970, Amphibien als troger von Hormiscium (Hormodendrum) dermatitidis KANO, Einem Erreger der Chromoblastomykose (Chromomykose) des Menschen, Z. Tropmed. Parasitol., 21:93-108.

Goodwin, L.G., 1974, Nuffield Institute of Comparative Medicine. The Zoological Society of London scientific report, 1971-1973, J. Zool. Lond., 173:127.

Lane, C.G., 1915, A cutaneous disease caused by a new fungus, Phialophora verrucosa, J. Cutaneous Dis., 33:840-846.

Medlar, E.M., 1915, A cutaneous infection caused by a new fungus, Phialophora verrucosa, with a study of the fungus, J. Med. Res., 32:507-522.

Migaki, G., and Frye, F.L., 1975, Mycotic granuloma in a tiger salamander, J. Wildlife Dis., 11:525-528.

Moore, M., and DeAlmeida, F., 1935, Etiologic agents of chromomycosis (Chromoblastomycosis of Terra, Tomes, Fonseca and Leao, 1922) of North and South America, Rev. Biol. Hyg., 7:94-97.

Rush, H.G., Anver, M.R., and Beneke, E.S., 1974, Systemic chromomycosis in Rana pipiens, Lab. Animal Sci., 24:646-655.

Schmidt, R.E., and Hartfiel, D.A., 1977, Chromomycosis in amphibians: Review and case report, J. Zoo Animal Med., 8:26-28.

Silva, M., 1960, Growth characteristics of the fungi of chromoblastomycosis, Ann. New York Acad. Sci., 89:17-29.

Trejos, A., 1953, Chromoblastomicosis experimental en Bufo marinus, Rev. Biol. Trop., 1:39-53.

FUNGAL DISEASES IN REPTILES

George Migaki, E.R. Jacobson and H.W. Casey

Registry of Comparative Pathology, Armed Forces
Institue of Pathology, and College of Veterinary
Medicine, University of Florida

INTRODUCTION

Mycotic diseases in reptiles encompass infection with any member of the kingdom Fungi. Approximately 100 species are considered pathogens or potential pathogens in mammals and birds. Reports of fungal disease in reptiles are rare compared to such reports in higher vertebrates. The integumentary, digestive and respiratory systems are most commonly affected. From a comparative standpoint, phycomycosis, aspergillosis, candidiasis, dermatophilosis and geotrichosis appear to be more common, while such systemic fungal diseases as histoplasmosis, North American blastomycosis, coccidioidomycosis, cryptococcosis and paracoccidioidomycosis have not been reported. However, some of the lesser known fungi such as the genera Trichosporon, Chrysosporium, Beauveria, Cephalosporium, Fusarium and Paecilomyces have been reported as causative agents of disease in reptiles.

ETIOLOGY

Phycomycosis

Phycomycosis is caused by a large number of related disease-producing fungi that are members of the class Phycomycetes. These include the genera Mucor, Absidia, Rhizopus, Mortierella, Basidiobolus, Hyphomyces and Entomophthora. In tissue sections the fungi are seen as irregularly branching, rarely septate, very broad hyphae of irregular width (up to 15 microns).

A common disease, phycomycosis has been reported in a variety of animals, and the lesions are most frequently observed in the skin, digestive, genital and respiratory tracts. The fungi have a predilection for invading blood vessels, thus resulting in necrosis of adjacent tissue.

The disease has been reported in various reptiles. Hunt (1957) states that most necrosis of the shell in turtles is mycotic in origin and that the plastron is more commonly involved than the carapace. Organisms resembling the order Mucorales have been found invading beneath the plates of the epidermal laminae. Blazek et al. (1968) found Basidiobolus ranarum in a granulomatous lesion located in the corner of the mouth of a giant tortoise, Geochelone gigantea. Zwart (1968) isolated Rhizopus arrhizus from lesions in the lungs and skin of a garter snake Thamnophis sirtalis. Werner et al. (1978) reported a granulomatous dermatitis over the mid-doso-

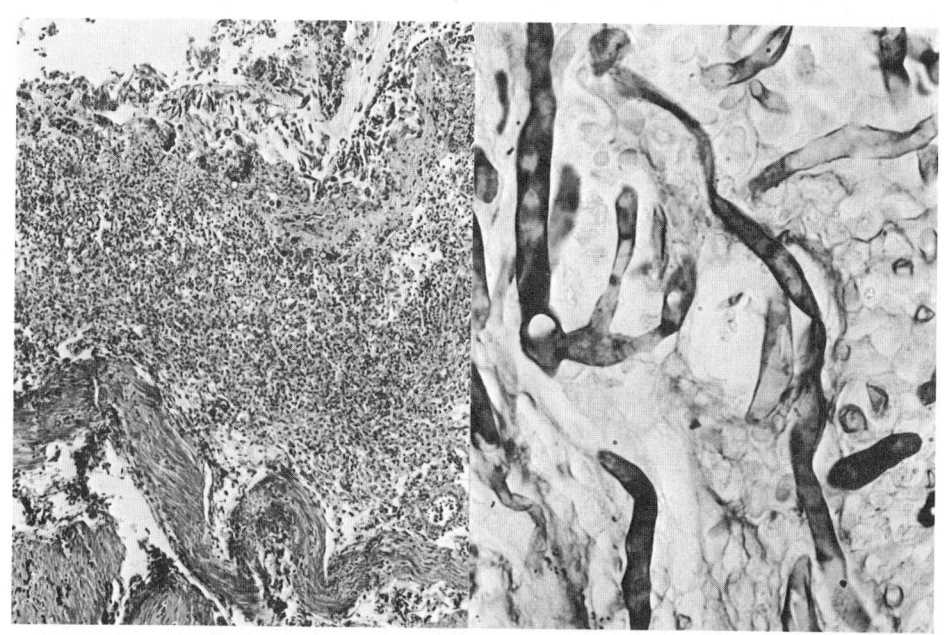

Fig. 14.1. Left. Phycomycosis in the colon of Chamaeleo jacksoni with necrosis and leukocytic infiltrates. H&E X114 AFIP neg. 78-4676 Photo courtesy of Dr. J.C. Murphy.
Right. Tissue stained by Gomori methenamine-silver method shows the fungus to be irregularly branching wide hyphae with occassional septations. X720 AFIP neg. 78-4679

lateral area of the body in an Eastern indigo snake, Drymarchon corais couperi. The fungi in the lesions resembled the organisms belonging to the family Mucoraceae. Sindler et al. (1978) found organisms resembling the class Phycomycetes in caseous nodules in the loose connective tissue adjacent to the trachea of a red milk snake, Lampropeltis triangulum syspila. Shalev et al. (1977) reported mycotic enteritis in an adult chameleon, Chamaeleo jacksoni, that had an intussusception of the terminal portion of the colon. Fungi resembling those of the class Phycomycetes were found in the necrotic areas of the colon (Fig. 14.1). Frank (1966) isolated Mucor from multiple cutaneous lesions in a bearded lizard, Amphibolurus barbatus. Jasmin et al. (1968) stated that Rhizopus, Aspergillus and Penicillium were isolated from normal appearing skin and scales of alligators, Alligator mississippiensis. Three species of crocodilians including Morelet's crocodile, Crocodylus moreleti, an American crocodile, C. acutus, and a Nile crocodile, C. niloticus, developed severe respiratory infections over a period of three months and eventually died (Silberman et al., 1977). Lesions were almost exclusively in the lungs and Mucor was isolated.

Phycomycosis was described in a western massasaugua rattlesnake, Sistrurus catenatus, with infection of the telencephalon, orbit and facial structures (Williams et al., 1979). The left olfactory bulb was replaced by a pyogranulomatous inflammatory lesion which extended into the forebrain on the left side. By the use of the Gomori methenamine-silver technique, the presence of fine septate branching hyphae in the center of the granulomatous mass were demonstrated. It was suspected that the fungus might have been a primary infection resulting from injury, perhaps the bite of a mouse or other penetrating trauma.

Aspergillosis

This disease is caused primarily by Aspergillus fumigatus; however, other species also have been incriminated as the causative agent. The hyphae are well developed, branched, septate and their cells as a rule are multinucleate. Conidiophores terminate in a bulbous head called a vesicle which produces sterigmata over its entire surface. Dichotomous branching, septations and uniformity in the diameter of the hyphae are the morphologic and diagnostic features of Aspergillus in tissue sections (Fig. 14.2).

Aspergillosis is perhaps one of the most common fungal infections in reptiles. The organism is common in the

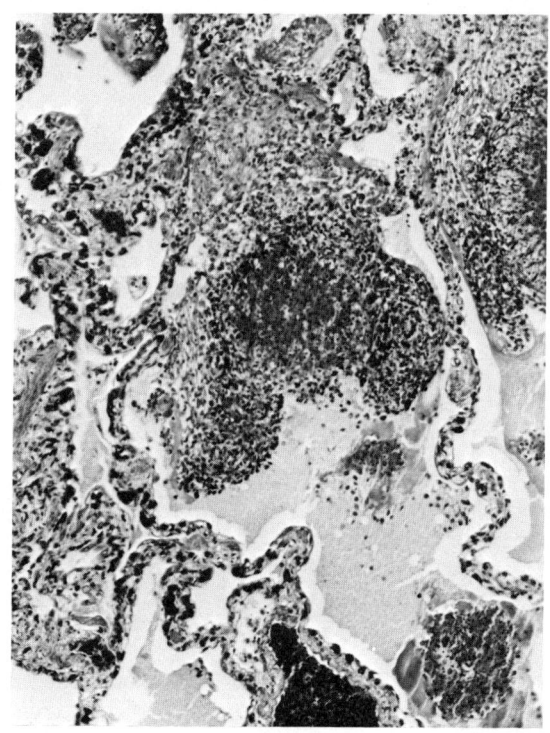

Fig. 14.2. Areas of necrosis in lung tissue of a common iguana, Iguana iguana, stained by Gomori methenamine-silver method. Hyphae are uniform in diameter, septations are numerous and prominent. X240 AFIP neg. 78-4542

air and the respiratory tract is the most common site of infection (Fig. 14.3). The skin and mucous membranes of body systems may become infected by direct contact. Hamerton (1934), in reviewing necropsy data at the London Zoological Society, found 12 deaths due to fungal infections in reptiles. The fungi in all of the cases were not identified, but the report included a St. Hilaire's terrapin, Hydraspis hilarii, and a black-pointed tegu, Tupinambis nigropunctatus, both of which died from generalized aspergillosis. Additionally, there was a puff adder, Bitis arietans, which died of fungal peritonitis due to Aspergillus. Hunt (1957) stated that pulmonary mycosis which accounted for 3% of the deaths in reptiles in a zoological collection resulted in consolidation and gangrene of the lungs of affected turtles. Aspergillus hyphae were identified in large numbers in lung tissue

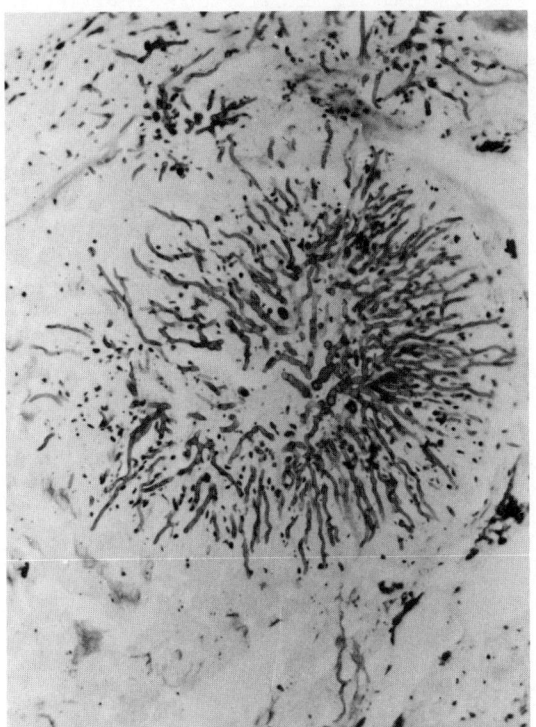

Fig. 14.3. Aspergillosis in the lung of a common iguana. Note multiple areas of necrosis. H&E X114 AFIP neg. 78-4684 Photo courtesy of the National Zoological Park.

specimens and was more common in the terrestrial species than in aquatic turtles. Georg et al. (1962) reported a fatal pneumonitis due to A. amstelodami in a Galapagos tortoise, G. elephantopus, that had lived at the Chicago Zoological Park for over 30 years. From the Copenhagen Zoo, Andersen and Eriksen (1968) described a fatal case of aspergillosis involving the lung of an Aldabra tortoise, G. gigantea elephantina, that had been ill for over one year. Frye and Dutra (1974) reported on a mature female musk turtle, Sternotherus odoratus, with chronic ulcerative lesions on both forefeet. Hyphal structures resembling Aspergillus were found in the granulomatous inflammatory process which consisted of histiocytes, fibroblasts and giant cells. Jasmin and Baucom (1967) cultured Mucor, Aspergillus and Rhizopus from cutaneous lesions due to Erysipelothrix insidiosa in a 100 year old American crocodile from a zoological park in Florida. Later Jasmin et al. (1968) isolated A. fumigatus and A. ustus from fatal pneumonic lesions in captive American alligators 2 to 6 weeks of age.

Cephalosporiosis

This disease is caused by the genus Cephalosporium, which is ordinarily a saprophyte, but which has been associated with cases of mycetoma and mycotic keratitis in man (Emmons, 1977). Colonies of this fungus will grow rapidly and are often white to yellow in color. Conidiophores may be lateral or terminal branches with the conidium bearing area usually localized at the extreme tip

The first report was of a viper, Natrix natrix, that died in a zoo in Antwerp with a large mass (3.5 x 3.5 cm) found along the trachea; Cephalosporium organisms were

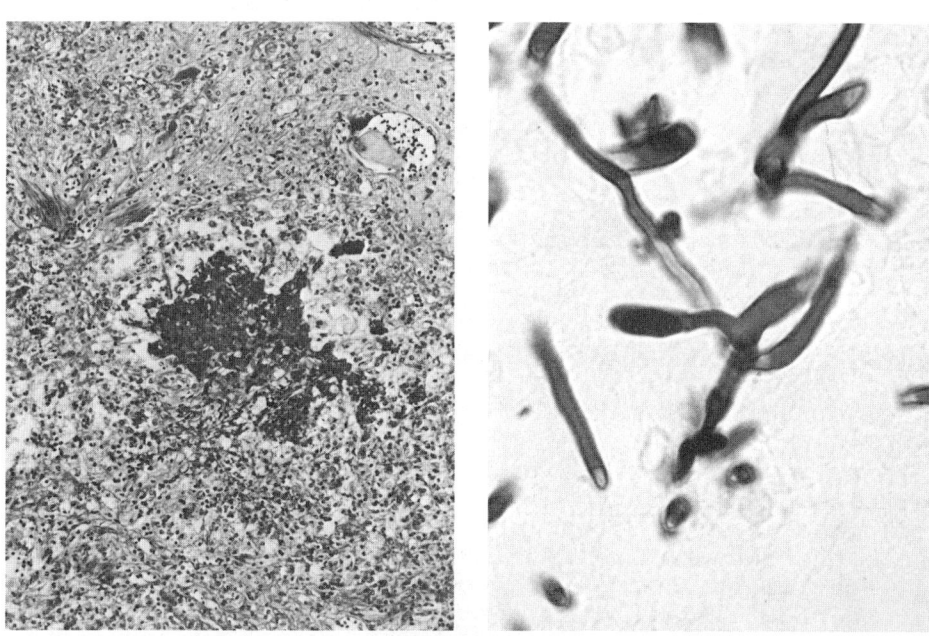

Fig. 14.4. Left. Cephalosporiosis in the lung of a caiman, Caiman sclerops, with a large discrete granulomatous abscess. H&E X140 AFIP neg. 78-4537 Photo courtesy of Dr. G.S. Trevino. Right. Gomori methenamine-silver stained tissue demonstrating septate, branching hyphae with spores on their tips. X1800 AFIP neg. 78-5110

cultured from the lesions (Rhodain and Mattlet, 1950). Later Trevino (1972) described multiple caseous granulomas in the lungs, liver and kidneys in three 6 month old caimans, Caiman sclerops (Fig. 14.4) from which Cephalosporium were grown in culture.

Penicilliosis

The penicillia are common and cosmopolitan fungi, the so-called green mold and blue molds. The mycelium produces simple, long, erect conidiophores which branch in broom-like fashion. The conidiophore, commonly called the brush, is technically known as the penicillus. The conidia are globose to ovoid.

Documented reports of infection due to the genus Penicillium are rare compared to those of infections caused by Aspergillus. The common blue-green molds of the genus Penicillium are ubiquitous in nature; therefore their role as pathogens must be substantiated by histopathologic examination. Hamerton (1934) at the London Zoological Garden described a severe generalized case of penicilliosis in a large blackish tortoise, G. nigrita, obtained from the Galapagos Islands. Multiple lesions were found in the lungs, stomach, liver and pancreas from which organisms of the genus Penicillium were cultured and also identified in tissue sections. Bemmel et al. (1960) reported the isolation of P. lilacinum from the lung of a yellow-legged tortoise, G. denticulata, from the Royal Rotterdam Zoo. They considered the fungus to be the principal cause of the pneumonia and death of the animal. P. lilacinum has been cultured from and identified in granulomatous nodules in the lung of a loggerhead turtle, Caretta caretta, and green turtle, Chelonia mydas (Goodwin, 1974). For several weeks before death both turtles swam with difficulty, near the surface of the water with the head and body tilted downwards. Pulmonary mycosis due to P. lilacinum was diagnosed in one ornate terrapin, Chrysemys ornata calirostris, and it was considered likely that this fungus was responsible for the lung lesions seen in another freshwater chelonian (Keymer, 1978).

Candidiasis

The fungus has both mycelial forms and yeast-like forms. Inoculation on Sabouraud's glucose agar maintained aerobically at 37 C will produce white to cream colored colonies in 24 to 48 hours. Circular or elliptical cells 2 to 6 microns in size (with or without buds) can be seen in young colonies. From older colonies and along colony edges mycelia with thick walled, round chlamydospores 7 to 9 microns in diameter can be demonstrated. Culture on cornmeal agar under reduced oxygen tensions and incubation at less than 37 C will promote chlamydospore formation.

In tissue sections the organisms appear as round to ovoid yeast-like cells (4 to 6 microns in diameter) arranged in chains, thus forming pseudohyphae. Known also as moniliasis and thrush, this disease is caused primarily by Candida albicans and C. tropicalis, which are common fungi with worldwide distribution.

Candidiasis is one of the most common fungal infections in man and animals. The fungi are considered true obligate saprophytes of the oral and gastrointestinal tracts. The pathogenesis is probably similar to that of other fungal infections in that debilitation, prolonged antibiotic therapy and use of immunosuppressive drugs are predisposing factors to infection. The lowered body resistance allows tissue invasion, which may remain localized or become disseminated.

In reptiles, Reichenbach-Klinke and Elkan (1965) reported a two-banded chameleon, C. bitaeniatus, with multiple necrotic areas in the liver, from which organisms morphologically similar to C. albicans were demonstrated in tissue sections. Zwart et al. (1968) reported the isolation of C. albicans from necrotic esophageal lesions in a dragon lizard, Crocodilurus lacertinus, from the Royal Rotterdam Zoo.

Geotrichosis

The disease is caused by the genus Geotrichum. In culture, well developed mycelia consisting of hyphae with terminal portions that break up into short arthrospores that are cuboid or short cylinders with flattened ends are produced. In tissue sections G. candidum appears as a yeast-like cell, about 5 microns in diameter, and also as short, septate mycelia resembling "pseudohyphae."

Infection associated with G. candidum, a ubiquitous fungus, is considered rare in animals; however, a disseminated case has been described in a dog (Lincoln and Adcock, 1968). Karstad (1961) isolated G. candidum from caseous subcutaneous nodules in a common water snake, Nerodia sipedon, and Page (1966) cites Karstad, who isolated G. candidum from pustules on the skin of a captive garter snake, T. sirtalis. Georg et al. (1962) reported a fatal pulmonary disease in a Galapagos tortoise in which both G. candidum and A. amstelodami were isolated from the lesions.

Experimentally, Sinclair and El-Tobshy (1969) produced generalized infections in snapping turtles, Chelydra s. serpentina, and red-eared turtles, Chrysemys scripta elegans, by using isolates from plant and human sources. Injections were made in the hindlegs and into the pleuroperitoneal cavity. Necrosis was produced at the injection sites and the fungi were readily demonstrated in tissue sections. Recently, McKenzie and Green (1976) described in several carpet pythons, Morelia spilotes variegata, necrotic skin lesions along the entire body. These snakes had been in captivity about four months. The lesions were found mostly over the ventral and lateral body surfaces, and in tissue sections the hyphae in the lesions were regularly branching, septate measuring about 3 microns in diameter. G. candidum was isolated.

Paecilomycosis

Species of Paecilomyces resemble those of Penicillium, but Paecilomyces never produce greenish-blue colonies when cultured and the margin of the colony often appears shredded rather than entire. Conidial structures are much more irregular than those of Penicillium and the phialides taper into long tubes.

The genus Paecilomyces is seldom reported as the cause of infection in man and animals (Patnaik et al., 1972). Georg et al. (1962) cultured P. fumoso-roseus from pulmonary abscesses in an Aldabra tortoise that had been in captivity at the Chicago Zoological Park for about five months prior to death. In tissue sections they found the fungi to be septate, branched mycelia measuring 3 to 4 microns in diameter. P. fumoso-roseus is considered a saprophyte, but it was thought to have acquired the ability to invade tissues because of lowered resistance of the tortoise due to its inability to adjust to the new environment (Georg et al., 1962). Histologic examination of 29 juvenile green sea turtles with a buoyancy abnormality revealed granulomatous lung lesions containing branching septate hyphae (Figs. 14.5 and 14.6) (Jacobson et al., 1979). Paecilomyces sp. (in addition to Sporotrichium and Cladosporium) was cultured from several turtles. Peak mortality occurred during the month with the coolest water temperature.

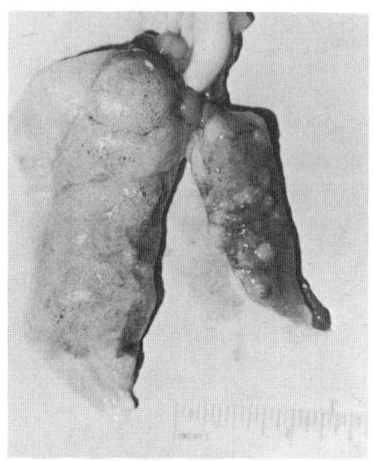 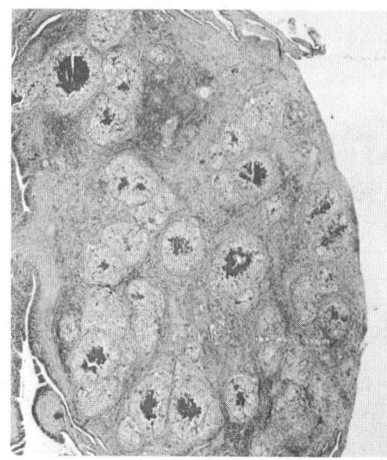

Fig. 14.5. Left. The right lung of a green turtle, Chelonia mydas, is consolidated with numerous nodules while the left lung is larger and emphysematous.
Right. Lung nodules consist of multiple granulomatous inflammatory reactions with a caseated center. H&E X63

Beauveriosis

Infection due to the genus Beauveria is apparently rare in man and animals, and the fungus is more widely known as a pathogen in insects. Colonies appear white or slightly pigmented, and are fluffy to powdery. The hyphae are narrow and conidiophores are simple or branched, rarely septate.

Georg et al. (1962) reported the isolation of this organism from a Galapagos tortoise with pulmonary abscesses, and from an Aldabra tortoise with numerous necrotic areas in the lungs. In tissue sections, the organisms are best demonstrated by the Gomori methenamine-silver method and appear as branched, septate mycelia (measuring about 4 to 5 microns in diameter) with flask-shaped conidiophores at their tips.

B. bassiana was isolated from pulmonary lesions in several alligators that died of fatal pulmonary disease (Fromtling et al., 1979). An extended period of hibernation caused by a severe winter and failure of a heating system at a zoological park was considered to have

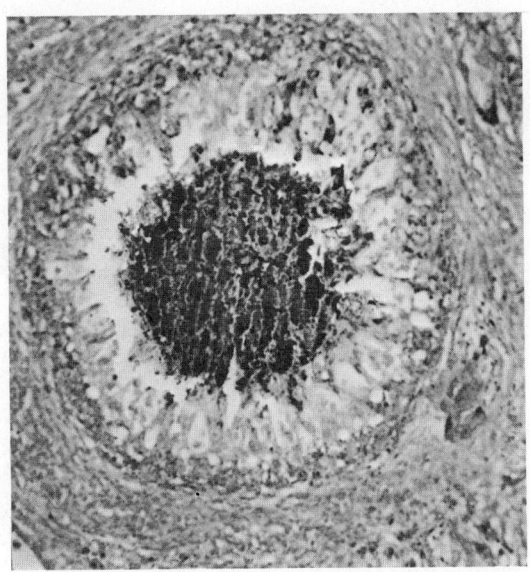

Fig. 14.6. A granulomatous inflammatory response around a caseated center containing several hyphae in lung tissue of the turtle in Fig. 14.5. Gomori methenamine-silver stain X160

predisposed the alligator to infection. The fact that B. bassiana does not grow at 37 C suggests why it infects insects and poikilotherms and has not been reported as a pathogen in homeotherms.

Chrysosporiosis

Colonies of Chrysosporium keratinophilum show a wide range of variability in pigment, but most are bright in color. Hyphae are hyaline and septate with conidiophores being poorly differentiated, branching irregularly. Conidia are aleurispores.

Reports of disease due to the genus Chrysosporium in man and animals are rare, however, the organism is frequently cultured from normal-appearing skin. Zwart et al. (1968) isolated C. keratinophilum from the lesions of two common iguanas, Iguana iguana, that had died at the Royal Rotterdam Zoo. One animal had a 1.5 cm broad necrotic lesion in the stomach, and the other had necrotic lesions in the gallbladder and miliary lesions in the lungs.

Fusariomycosis

Colonies are fluffy due to extensive aerial mycelia, often producing diffusible pink, purple or yellow pigment. Conidiophores can be either single or grouped into sporodochia, slender or stout with irregular branching.

Organsims of the genus Fusarium are common soil inhabitants, and reports of fusariomycosis are rare, however, some of the human cases of mycotic keratitis are caused by this fungal agent (Rippon, 1974). In reptiles, the first report of suspected Fusarium infection was in 1890 and involved a green lizard, Lacerta viridis with skin lesions (Reichenbach-Klinke and Elkan, 1965). Since then Fusarium has been isolated from under the scales of a radiated tortoise, Testudo radiata (Frank, 1966) and from skin lesions in a caiman, C. crocodilus fuscus, from a zoo in southern Germany (Kuttin et al., 1978). Zwart et al. (1973) reported a rainbow boa, Epicrates cenchris maurus, with a severe infection of the spectacle, which required enucleation. They isolated F. oxysporum from a lesion on the inner side of the spectacle and obtained a pure culture. They cited a report by Vroege who isolated F. oxysporum from the lacrimal fluid which had accumulated as a result of obstruction of the lacrimal duct in a boa constrictor, Boa constrictor, and they also report Poelma's finding of F. oxysporum in the skin lesion of a common chameleon, C. dilepis (Zwart et al., 1973).

Trichosporiosis

Infections with this fungal organism are most commonly due to Trichosporon beigelli (cutaneum). In culture colonies are cream colored yeast-like and will eventually become yellowish-gray and wrinkled. The colony consists of hyphae and many arthrospores and some blastospores.

The genus Trichosporon is rarely associated with disease. In man some of the species have been associated with white piedra (Emmons et al., 1977). Kuttin et al. (1978) isolated Trichosporon sp. from well-circumscribed lesions (about 3 cm in diameter) in the buccal mucosa and pharynx of a Nile crocodile, C. niloticus, and from circumscribed lesions (about 1 cm in diameter) on the corner of the mouth of a young male spectacled caiman, both of which resided in the same water basin in a zoo in southern Germany. Several Anolis carolinensis submitted from a research colony were found to have nuchal hematomas from which T. cutaneum and the bacterium Pseudomonas aeruginosa were isolated (Jacobson and Greenberg, unpubl. information).

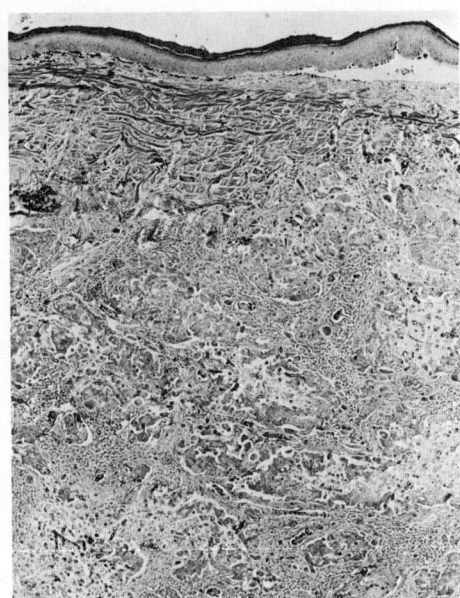 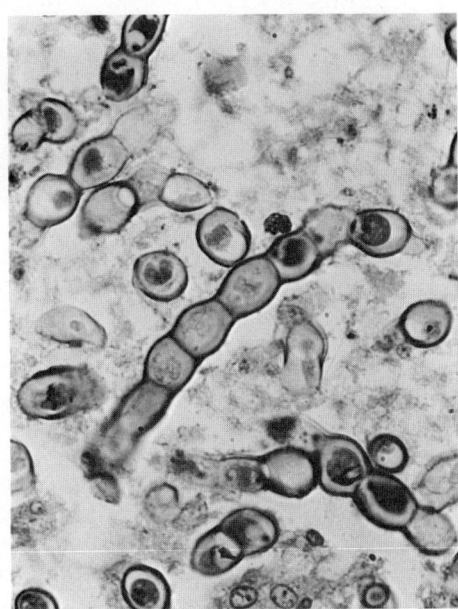

Fig. 14.7. <u>Left</u>. Cladosporiosis in the skin of an anaconda, <u>Eunectes murinus</u>, with multiple areas of granuloma containing necrotic centers and grown-pigmented fungi. H&E X45 AFIP neg. 78-4681 Photo courtesy of the National Zoological Park.
<u>Right</u>. Higher magnification demonstrating yeast-like branching of the fungi. H&E X720 AFIP neg. 78-4638

Chromomycosis

The fungi included under this heading are the pigmented or dematiacious forms varying in color from light brown to brown-black. Various genera are included and the principal ones are: <u>Phialophora</u>, <u>Hormodendrum</u>, <u>Cladosporium</u> and <u>Fonsecaea</u>. These fungi are similar morphologically in tissue section. They may occur singly, in pairs or in small clusters.

In man the lesions are most commonly found on the skin and cause a verrucous dermatitis. The disease is relatively rare in animals except in amphibians, in which the lesions are systemic and the animals die (see chapter 13).

Frank (1970) described a generalized case of chromomycosis in a radiated tortoise involving the lower jaw, liver, spleen, lungs, pancreas, tongue and thyroid glands. Dark-brown hyphae were found in the lesions, but the fungu was not identified. In addition, a similar fungus had caused a severe ulcerative dermatitis on the ventral skin of a reticulated python, Python reticulatus (Frank, 1970). The same author also found a dematiacious fungus that caused a skin lesion in a boa constrictor (Frank, 1976). Marcus (1971) reported an adult anaconda, Eunectes murinus affected with subcutaneous nodules (Fig. 14.7) and a severe ulcerative stomatitis that had extended into the mandible. Organisms resembling those of the genus Cladosporium were found in the granulomatous inflammatory lesions.

Actinomycosis

Although this represents a bacterial disease, the historical inclusion of this group of pathogens with true mycoses merit discussion here. The usual etiologic agents of actinomycosis are Actinomyces israelii (man) and A. bovis (cattle or swine). Both are anaerobic or microaerophilic. These gram-positive, occasionally branched filamentous microorganisms in situ form "sulfurgranules" which may reach a diameter of 1 or 2 mm, and are white to yellowish.

This is a chronic suppurative granulomatous infection and involves both soft and hard tissues. The disease is considered relatively common in man and animals. The organisms are probably inhabitants of the oral and gastrointestinal tracts and damage to the mucous membrane a them to become pathogenic. Two cases have been reported in reptiles. One involved a large subcutaneous abscess behind the head of a boa constrictor from the Leipzig Zoological Gardens (Meyn, 1942). The other (Wadsworth, 1960) was a firm nodule, containing a central area of caseation necrosis, located just behind the neck of a female African cobra, Naja sp. Organisms morphologically similar to Actinomyces were found in the necrotic areas.

Dermatophilosis

This bacterial microorganism is historically included with the fungi. Known also as cutaneous streptothricosis, this disease is caused by Dermatophilus congolensis and has been reported in a variety of animals. A diagnostic feature of this branching, filamentous organism is the presence of horizontal and vertical septations forming coccoid structures.

Simmons et al. (1972) reported the first case in a reptile, an Australian bearded lizard, Amphibolurus barbatus, that had subcutaneous nodules on the ventral body surface and on the forelimbs. From the isolate, the disease was experimentally transmitted by subcutaneous and intraperitoneal inoculations in four bearded lizards and one blue-tongue lizard, Tiliqua s. scincoides. The experimentally produced lesions resembled the spontaneous condition, and it was suggested that by mechanical transfer biting insects could transmit the organisms from animal to animal. Later, in 1975, Montali et al. reported three Australian bearded lizards that were received at the National Zoological Park from a zoo supplier in California. The animals arrived in poor condition and had multiple raised golden-brown cutaneous nodules (3 to 5 mm in diameter) on their heads, bodies and extremities. D. congolensis was demonstrated in tissue sections. One animal died a day following arrival, and the other two died 2 to 4 weeks later. The following year, Anver et al. (1976) reported cutaneous hyperkeratotic nodules containing D. congolensis on both dorsal and ventral surfaces of the trunk and extremities in two marble lizards, Calotes mystaceus. These animals were captured in Thailand and shipped to the University of Michigan. Experimentally, six marble lizards were inoculated subcutaneously with isolates from the natural cases. All had lesions at the injection sites, which indicated that lizards are susceptible hosts to D. congolensis.

Dermatophytosis

Dermatophytosis is caused by a group of keratinolytic fungi and affects keratinized tissues such as the hair, nails and stratum corneum of the skin. The disease is common in both man and animals, and many fungal organisms (including those of the genera Trichophyton, Microsporum and Epidermophyton) have been identified, some being host specific, while others are infectious to a wide variety of animals. In fact, infected animals may serve as reservoirs of infection for other animals, including man.

In reptiles the disease is apparently uncommon. There is a single report (Rees, 1967) in which Microsporum cookei was isolated from the epidermal scales of otherwise normal skin of a monitor, Varanus sp. A Trichophyton sp. was isolated from granulomatous lesions of the foot pads of a juvenile alligator submitted to the University of Florida. Hyphae were demonstrated in tissue sections.

PATHOGENESIS

As in higher vertebrates, fungi in reptiles may be primary or secondary invaders. Mycotic disease may be associated with predisposing factors including high humidity, malnutrition, overcrowding and debris buildup in the animal's environment. Mycotic disease may show species differences related to the animal's ecology. In one study, pulmonary mycosis was more common in terrestrial turtles than in aquatic species (Hunt, 1957). Primary viral and bacterial infections may predispose to secondary mycotic disease.

Low environmental temperature has been considered to be a predisposing factor in mycotic disease in a variety of reptilian species. Although P. fumoso-roseus cultured from pulmonary abscesses in an Aldabra tortoise was considered a saprophyte, the authors believed that lowered resistance of the tortoise due to an inability to adjust to the new environment was a predisposing factor (Georg et al., 1962).

In the same report, B. bassiana was isolated from pulmonary lesions in an Aldabra tortoise and a Galapagos tortoise. Experimentally, two box turtles were challenged via the intrapulmonary route with spores of this isolate and while a turtle maintained at 22 C remained normal, the second turtle maintained at 15.5 C died 4 days post-inoculation. This suggested to the authors that the low temperature may have predisposed to infection.

Mortality due to mycotic pneumonia in juvenile green sea turtles raised in mariculture was found to be highest during the coolest months of the year (Jacobson et al., 1979). It was postulated that the low environmental temperatures may have depressed the immune system of the sea turtles to allow saprophytic fungi to become pathogens. Seasonal variation in the lymphoid system of reptiles has been described (Hussein et al., 1978a,b) and immunoglobulin production in reptiles is influenced by environmental temperature (Evans, 1963). Thus, susceptibility to potential pathogens may vary with changes in body temperature. The immune system of the hatchling turtles may have been compromised by the cool water temperatures allowing infection with fungi in the environment.

Fatal pulmonary disease in two captive American alligators due to B. bassiana was associated with low environmental temperature (Fromtling, 1979). An extended hibernation period because of a severe winter and a failure of the zoo heating system may have predisposed the alligators to infection. Although the fungus was successfully cultured at 28 C repeated attempts to grow the organism on the same media at 37 C failed. This suggests why this organism infects insects and poikilotherms and has not been reported to produce disease in homeotherms.

In addition to temperature, other environmental factors may predispose to fungal disease. Overcrowding in a zoologic collection and debris buildup in the exhibit were considered contributing factors for a Mucor pneumonia in three species of crocodilians (Silberman et al., 1977). The stress of shipment may have contributed to the development of a mycotic enteritis in a Jackson's chameleon (Shalev et al., 1977). Skin lesions in carpet pythons were associated with high local humidity in the cage which may have reduced the capacity of the skin to resist infection (McKenzie and Green, 1976).

DIAGNOSIS

Fungal disease involving the integumentary system may show a fairly characteristic clinical appearance for a given species. Aquatic turtles will generally show circular multifocal grey patches on the carpace, plastron or extremities. Often the epithelial surface is ulcerated with hyphae extending into dermis. Snakes will most characteristically show multifocal proliferative necrotizing skin lesions which may be found anywhere on the integument. In one species of snake, the lesions were initially found in the hinge region between adjacent scales (McKenzie and Green, 1976).

Systemic involvement is most often identified on post-mortem examination. In almost all cases fungal agents will result in a granulomatous inflammatory reaction, often resulting in nodule formation. It must be stressed that granuloma formation is the characteristic response a reptile exhibits to a wide range of pathogens including numerous bacteria and parasites.

Ultimately identification of the causative agent will depend on laboratory diagnosis. Biopsy specimens can be easily secured from animals with skin disease. Specimens should be placed in neutral buffered 10% formalin and submitted for histopathologic evaluation. Post-mortem material should be similarly processed. The morphology of the fungus in tissue is important in its identification, although usually it is not so informative as morphology in culture. Special stains for identifying fungi in tissue section include Gridley's Fungus, Gomori methenamine-silver and Periodic Acid Schiff reaction. The technique of fluorescent antibody staining has been developed for mycoses in man, but lacks complete specificity. Its application to reptile mycoses has not been identified.

Whenever possible a tissue specimen should be submitted for mycologic culture. Skin samples often contain saprophytic organisms and fungi cultured should be correlated with organisms demonstrated in tissue section. Prior to biopsy, skin lesions should be cleaned with an organic iodine solution and 70% alcohol. Biopsy specimens should be thoroughly ground and subsequently cultured on the appropriate media. In cases of suspected mycotic respiratory disease, lung washings should be submitted for culture. Granulomatous inflammatory lesions found on necropsy should also be routinely cultured for fungi.

The agar media most commonly used are the Emmons' modification of Sabouraud's with or without antibiotics, cysteine glucose blood, thioglycollate semisolid, potato-glucose, corn meal, rice-Tween, trypticase glucose, Littman's ox-gall and yeast extract (Emmons et al., 1977). The temperature of incubation should not exceed 30 C for primary isolation cultures and for reptiles are routinely cultured at 20 to 24 C. The identification of cultured fungal organisms is beyond the scope of the chapter and identification procedures can be found in a variety of medical mycology texts (Ainsworth and Austwick, 1973; Emmons et al., 1977).

CONTROL AND TREATMENT

Many of the reports in the literature suggest interplay between low temperature and predisposition to mycotic disease. In captivity, reptiles should be offered a thermal gradient to allow proper thermoregulation. The enclosure should be at least within the preferred optimum range for the species. Enclosures and cages should be routinely cleaned and disinfected to prevent debris buildup in the environment. Overcrowding should be avoided, in particular for aquatic species. In such enclosures there should be continual circulating water with a filter system to adequately handle the detritus load. The number of deaths of captive American alligators due to a mycotic pneumonia was reduced by instigating sanitary procedures, which included chlorination of the water, disinfecting the

premises with a copper sulfate solution, providing more
sunlight and removing the clinically sick alligators
(Silberman et al., 1977). High humidity should be avoided
in the species that inhabit xeric and mesic habitats in
nature. Animals suspected of mycotic disease should be
isolated from cagemates.

The only report of treatment is that of eye enucleation in a rainbow boa diagnosed as having a Fusarium eye
infection (Zwart et al., 1973). Localized cutaneous
mycotic granulomas have been surgically removed in several
species of colubrid snakes. Additionally several cases
of mycotic skin disease have been treated successfully
by soaking in a dilute organic iodine solution twice
daily followed by the topical application of tinactin.
Two cagemate ball pythons, P. regius, diagnosed as having
a Trichoderma sp. dermatitis were unsuccessfully treated
with oral griseofulvin at 20 mg/kg body weight and 40
mg/kg body weight respectively every three days for five
treatments. Suspected mycotic pneumonias have been treated
with 5 mg of amphotericin B nebullized in 150 cc of saline
twice daily (for 1 hour each) for a week. Oral candidiasis
in a python was treated orally, via a stomach tube, with
mycostatin at 100,000 units/kg once daily for 10 days.

REFERENCES

Ainsworth, G.C., and Austwick, P.K.C., 1973, "Fungal
diseases of animals," 2nd ed., Rev. Series No.
6, Commonwealth Bur. Animal Health, Commonwealth
Agricultural Bur., Farnham Royal Slough, England.
Andersen, S., and Eriksen, E., 1968, Aspergillose bei einer
Elephantenschildkrote (Testudo gigantea
elephantina), X Internationalen Symposiums uber
die Erkrankungen der Zootiere, Akademie der
Wissenschaften der DDR, Berlin.
Anver, M.R., Park, J.S., and Rush, H.G., 1976, Dermatophilosis in the marble lizard (Calotes
mystaceus), Lab. Animal Sci., 26:817-823.
Bemmel, A.C.V., Van Peters, J.C., and Zwart, P., 1960,
Report on births and deaths occurring in the
Gardens of the Royal Rotterdam Zoo during the
year 1958, Tijdschr. Diergeneesk., 85:1203-1213.
Blazek, K., Jaros, Z., Otcenasek, M., and Konrad, J., 1968,
Zum Vorkommen und zur Histopathologie der tiefen
Organmykosen bei den Zootieren, X Internationalen
Symposiums uber die Erkrankungen der Zootiere,
Akademie der Wissenschaften der DDR, Berlin.

Emmons, C.W., Binford, C.H., Utz, J.P., and Kwon-Chung, K.J., 1977, "Medical mycology," 3rd ed., Lea and Febiger, Philadelphia.

Evans, E.E., 1963, Comparative immunology. Antibody response in Dipsosaurus dorsalis at different temperatures, Proc. Soc. Exp. Biol. Med., 112: 531-533.

Frank, W., 1966, Multiple Hypkeratose bei einer Bartagame, Amphibolurus barbatus (Reptilia, Agamidae), hervorgerufen durch eine Pilzinfektion; zugleich ein Bertag zur Problematik von Mykosen bei Reptilien, Salamandra, 2:6-12.

Frank, W., 1970, Mykotische Erkrankungen der Haut und der inneren Organe bei Amphibien und Reptilien, XII Internationalen Symposiums uber die Erkrankungen der Zootiere, Akademie der Wissenschaften der DDR, Berlin.

Frank, W., 1976, Mycotic infections in amphibians and reptiles, in: "Wildlife diseases," L.A. Page, ed., Plenum Publ. Corp., New York.

Fromtling, R.A., Jansen, J.M., Robinson, B.E., and Bulmer, G.S., 1979, Fatal mycotic pulmonary disease of captive American alligators, Vet. Pathol., 16: 428-431.

Frye, F.L., and Dutra, F.R., 1974, Mycotic granulomata involving the forefeet of a turtle, Vet. Med. Small Animal Clin., 69:1554-1556.

Georg, L.E., Williamson, W.M., Tilden, E.B., and Getty, R.E., 1962, Mycotic pulmonary disease of captive giant tortoises due to Beauvaria bassiana and Paecilomyces fumoso-roseus, Sabouraudia, 2:80-86.

Goodwin, L.G., 1974, Journal of zoology, Proc. Zool. Soc. London, 173:125.

Hamerton, A.E., 1934, Report on the deaths occurring in the Society's garden during the year 1933, Proc. Zool. Soc. London, 104:389-403.

Hunt, T.J., 1957, Notes on diseases and mortality in testudines, Herpetologica, 13:19-23.

Hussien, M.F., Badir, N., and El Ridi, R., 1978a, Differential effect of seasonal variation on lymphoid tissue of the lizard, Chalcides ocellatus, Dev. Comp. Immunol., 2:297-310.

Hussien, M.F., Badir, N., and El Ridi, R., 1978b, Effect of seasonal variation on lymphoid tissues of the lizards, Mabuya quinquetaeniata Licht and Uromastyx aegyptia, Dev. Comp. Immunol., 2:469-478.

Jacobson, E.R., Gaskin, J.M., Shields, R.P., and White, F.H., 1979, Mycotic pneumonia in mariculture reared green sea turtles, J. Amer. Vet. Med. Ass., 175:929-933.

Jasmin, A.M., and Baucom, J.N., 1967, Erysipelothrix insidiosa infections in the caiman (Caiman crocodilus) and the American crocodile (Crocodilus acutus), Amer. J. Vet. Clin. Pathol., 1:173-177.

Jasmin, A.M., Carroll, J.M., and Baucom, J.N., 1968, Pulmonary aspergillosis of the American alligator (Alligator mississippiensis), Amer. J. Vet. Clin. Pathol., 2:93-95.

Karstad, L., 1961, Reptiles as possible reservoir hosts for eastern encephalitis virus, Trans. North Amer. Natur. Resources Conf., 26:186-202.

Keymer, I.F., 1978, Diseases of chelonians: (2) Necropsy survey of terrapins and turtles, Vet. Rec., 103:577-582.

Kuttin, E.S., Muller, J., May, W., Albrecht, F., and Sigalas, M., 1978, Mykosen bei Krokodilen, Mykosen, 21:39-48.

Lincoln, S.D., and Adcock, J.L., 1968, Disseminated geotrichosis in a dog, Pathol. Vet., 5:282-289.

Marcus, L.C., 1971, Infectious diseases of reptiles, J. Amer. Vet. Med. Ass., 159:1626-1631.

McKenzie, R.A., and Green, P.E., 1976, Mycotic dermatitis in captive carpet snakes, J. Wildlife Dis., 12: 405-408.

Meyn, A., 1942, Actinomyces Infektion bei einer Schlange, Zool. Garten N.F., 14:251-253.

Montali, R.J., Smith, E.E., Davenport, M., and Bush, M., 1975, Dermatophilosis in Australian bearded lizards, J. Amer. Vet. Med. Ass., 167:553-555.

Page, L.A., 1966, Diseases and infections of snakes: A review, Bull. Wildlife Dis. Ass., 2:111-126.

Patnaik, A.K., Liu, S.K., Wilkins, R.J., Johnson, G.F., and Seitz, P.E., 1972, Paecilomycosis in a dog, J. Amer. Vet. Med. Ass., 161:806-813.

Rees, R.G., 1967, Keratinophilic fungi from Queensland: I. Isolation from animal hairs and scales, Sabouraudia, 5:165-172.

Reichenbach-Klinke, H., and Elkan, E., 1965, "The principal diseases of lower vertebrates," Academic Press, New York.

Rippon, J.W., 1974, "Medical mycology," W.B. Saunders, Philadelphia.

Rodhain, J., and Mattlet, G., 1950, Une tumeur mycosique chez la couleure viperine Tropidonotus natrix, Ann. Parasitol., 25:77-79.

Shalev, M., Murphy, J.C., and Fox, J.G., 1977 Mycotic enteritis in a chameleon and a brief review of phycomyceses of animals, J. Amer. Vet. Med. Ass., 171:872-875.

Silberman, M.S., Blue, J., and Mahaffey, E., 1977, Phycomycoses resulting in the death of crocodilians in a common pool, Ann. Proc. Amer. Ass. Zoo Vet. (Honolulu), Hill's, Topeka.

Simmons, G.C., Sullivan, N.D., and Green, P.E., 1972, Dermatophilosis in a lizard (Amphibolurus barbatus), Australian Vet. J., 48:465-466.

Sinclair, J.B., and El-Tobshy, A.M., 1969, Pathogenicity of plant and animal isolates of Geotrichum candidum in the turtle, Mycologia, 61:473-480.

Sindler, R.B., Plue, R.E., and Herman, D.W., 1978, Phycomycosis in a red milksnake (Lampropeltis triangulum syspila), Vet. Med. Small Animal Clin., 73:64-65.

Trevino, G.S., 1972, Cephalosporiosis in three caimans, J. Wildlife Dis., 8:384-388.

Wadsworth, J.R., 1960, Tumors and tumor-like lesions of snakes, J. Amer. Vet. Med. Ass., 137:419-420.

Werner, R., Balady, M.A., and Kolaja, G.J., 1978, Phycomycotic dermatitis in an Eastern indigo snake, Vet. Med. Small Animal Clin., 73:362-363.

Williams, L.W., Jacobson, E., Gelatt, K.N., Barrie, K.P., and Shields, R.P., 1979, Phycomycosis in a western massasagua rattlesnake (Sistrurus catenatus) with infection of the telencephalon, orbit and facial structures, Vet. Med. Small Animal Clin., 74:1181-1184.

Zwart, P., 1968, Parasitare und mykotishe Lungenaffektione bei Reptilien, X Internationalen Symposiums uber die Erkrankungen der Zootiere, Akademie der Wissenschaften der DDR, Berlin.

Zwart, P., Poelma, F.G., Strik, W.J., Peters, J.C., and Polder, 1968, Report on births and deaths occurring in the Gardens of the Royal Rotterdam Zoo "Blijdorp" during the years 1961 and 1962, Tijdschr. Diergeneesk., 93:348-365.

Zwart, P., Verwer, M.A.J., Devries, G.A., Hermanides-Nijhof, E.J., and Devries, H.W., 1973, Fungal infection of the eyes of the snake Epicrates chenchria maurus: Enucleation under halothane narcosis, J. Small Animal Pract., 14:773-779.

PENTASOMIASIS

Gerald E. Cosgrove, D.E. Deakins and J.T. Self

Pathology Department, Zoological Society of
San Diego and Department of Zoology, University
of Oklahoma

INTRODUCTION

In the class Pentastomida, there are about 50 species in 20 genera. The adults of the great majority of species are parasites of reptiles (Table 15.1). Immature forms occur in reptiles, other vertebrates, or rarely in invertebrates. Their complex migrations in hosts, encystment, muscular activity and their armature of hooks are potential causes of tissue lesions.

The adults are large and spectacular parasites (Fig. 15.1) and they have been known for centuries, but their zoological status has always been uncertain. They are obligate endoparasites with primitive arthropod affinities. Apparently at least four species occur in reptiles in northern North America: Porocephalus crotali, Kiricephalus coarctatus, Raillietiella bicaudata and Sebekia oxycephala. Hill (1963) records reports from North American reptiles. Reichenback-Klinke and Elkan (1965) list the species, indicating worldwide geographical and host distribution. An extensive review and bibliography of the Pentastomida is available (Self, 1969), as well as of the genus Porocephalus (Riley and Self, 1979).

DISTRIBUTION

In North America, pentastomes have been found in free-ranging reptiles in Mexico, the Southern Atlantic

Table 15.1. Worldwide Host Distribution of Adult Pentasor Genera in Orders of Reptiles.[a]

Genus	Snakes	Lizards	Crocodilians	Turtles
Raillietiella	2[b]	9	-	-
Cephalobaena	1	-	-	-
Kiricephalus	2	-	-	-
Porocephalus	6	-	-	-
Armillifer	3	-	-	-
Waddycephalus	1	-	-	-
Cubirea	2	-	-	-
Gigliolella	1	-	-	-
Ligamifer	1	-	-	-
Sambonia	-	4	-	-
Elenia	-	1	-	-
Sebekia	-	-	6	-
Leiperia	-	-	2	-
Subtriquetra	-	-	2	-
Alofia	-	-	5	-
Diesingia	-	-	-	1
Butantinella	-	-	-	1
Total genera	9	3	4	4

[a]After Self (1969).
[b]Number of species in each genus.

and Gulf States, Texas, Oklahoma and a few Midwestern states (Nicoli and Nicoli, 1966; Self, 1969). One species S. oxycephala, is found as an adult in Alligator mississippiensis, in the United States and caimans in Mexico, with larvae in fish and turtles. Adult P. crotali are found most commonly in several species of rattlesnakes, in Agkistrodon contortrix and in A. piscivorus (Riley and Self, 1979). K. coarctatus occurs in colubrid species including Thamnophis spp., Nerodia spp., Masticophis spp., and Drymarchon corais, with one report from an A. piscivorus. R. bicaudata occurs in colubrids in North America, but other species elsewhere are lizard parasites (Fain, 1966). There may be other species of Raillietiella in North American snakes and lizards, but this is not documented.

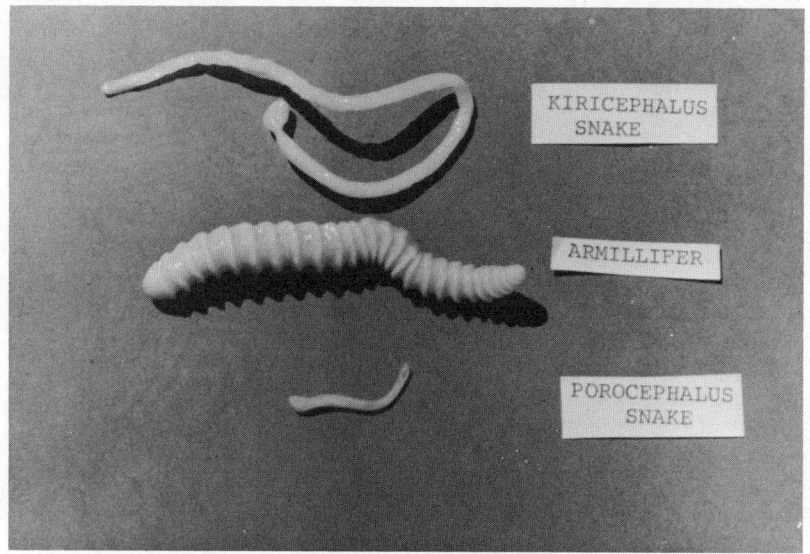

Fig. 15.1. Representatives of adult pentastomes of three genera commonly found in snake lungs.

TRANSMISSION

The basic cycle of transmission involves passage of eggs in sputum or feces, contamination of the environment, ingestion by an intermediate host or a series of intermediate hosts in a predator-prey relationship, and ingestion of an intermediate host by a final host (Esslinger, 1962; Penn, 1942). Migration and final development, with separate male and female worms, occur in the tissues and lungs of the final host. In reptiles, an auto-infection cycle is possible if fecal passage of eggs is so delayed that intra-intestinal hatching occurs (Deakins, 1973). In a specific cycle, that of P. crotali, the adults are present in the lungs of A. piscivorus (Penn, 1942). Sexes are separate, and fertilized females deposit eggs in the lungs, which are carried by the sputum to the mouth or exterior, contaminating the environment. The muskrat, Ondatra zibethica, ingests the eggs which hatch in the small intestine, liberating the larvae. The larvae penetrate the intestinal wall and potentially can migrate to many tissues, but most frequently to liver and lung, where they become encysted as nymphs, which grow tremendously and molt several times, becoming infective nymphs in about three months. When an A. piscivorous eats a muskrat, the nymphs are released from the cysts, migrate up the esophagus, down the trachea and into the lungs, where they develop into adults. Sometimes an entire female worm is coughed up and dies, with resulting massive localized egg contamination of the environment and massive infestation of the intermediate host.

Cycles for the other pentastomes, where known, are similar, except that appropriate intermediate hosts, suitable as prey to the final host, are utilized. For example S. oxycephala from alligators, utilizes fish as intermediate hosts. Species of Kiricephalus utilize lizards, snakes and occasionally amphibians as intermediate hosts. Species of Raillietiella utilize insects, lizards and amphibians as intermediate hosts (Self, 1969).

Pentastomid larva and nymphs do not appear to be highly host specific, being found in a wide variety of species of intermediate hosts, e.g. P. crotali has been reported from many mammalian species in several different orders. Some old world linguatulids occur frequently in man in the nymphal stages (Nicoli and Nicoli, 1966).

PATHOGENESIS AND PATHOLOGY

The preferred site of the adults is the lung, where mechanical trauma occurs from the four movable hooks on the anterior end. The lung tissue hemorrhages, becomes secondarily infected and the potential exists for perforation through the lung into ectopic sites. The trauma and infection may lead to lung irritation, excessive mucus production and alveolar wall thickening, thus producing interference with oxygenation. The presence of adults is sometimes associated with anemia, anoxia or hypoproteinemia (Deakins, 1973). Adults often move, being coughed up and swallowed, or wandering and reattaching. There is apparently a tendency to become active and move about in stressed hosts (Self and Kuntz, 1967).

In some cases, adults are found in other sites than the lungs. This is more common in certain genera, especially Kiricephalus, where dermal and sub-pleural infestations occur. From dermal locations, escape through rents in the skin is possible (Self and Kuntz, 1967). Coelomic walls and visceral organs may be the seat of adults.

Female adults migrating or in ectopic situations may deposit eggs in tissues which leads to a sequence of inflammatory reactions around the egg; acute, chronic or granulomatous, with forgeign body giant cells, until the egg is sequestered and destroyed.

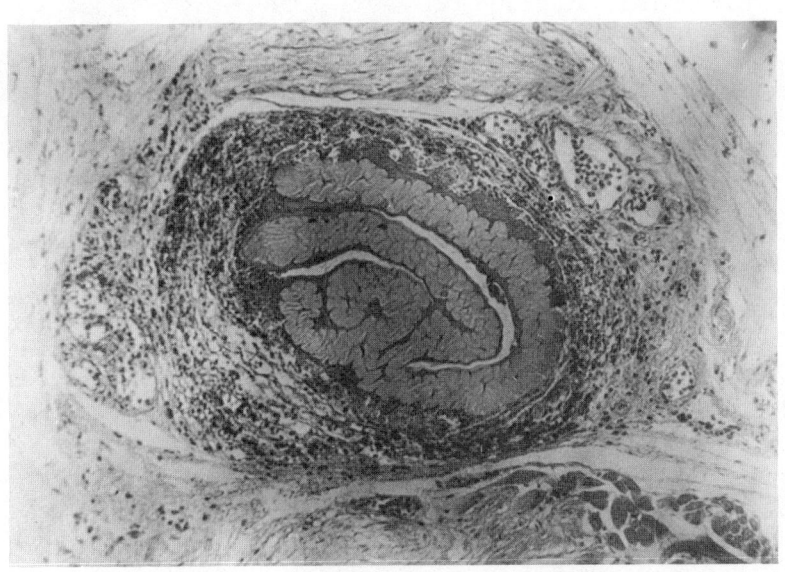

Fig. 15.2. Histologic section from the serosa of Naja sp. with Raillietiella nymphal cuticular remains surrounded by intense inflammatory reaction and a fibrous capsule. H&E X120

Natural and experimental infections reveal the following course of events (Deakins, 1973; Esslinger, 1962; Penn, 1942). The motile larva released from the egg works its way through the intestinal and other tissues with muscular activity by means of its own hooked appendages and an anterior penetration apparatus. This produces a visceral larval migrans burrow of tissue damage with hemorrhage, necrosis and mild inflammatory reaction. The severity depends largely on the numbers of invading larvae. If larvae survive, they moult and become nymphs during migration. If larvae or nymphs die, a surrounding inflammatory reaction results, with eosinophils, abscessation, granulomas, and healing by fibrosis and calcification (Fig. 15.2). Cuticular remnants in such lesions provide a clue to the cause. Live larvae or nymphs frequently penetrate the bowl with resulting peritonitis. They also may circulate as parasitic emboli in blood vessels. When they encyst in a tissue, feeding occurs with slight local pathology at a fixed feeding site opposite the mouth of the nymph where a papilla of host tissue is formed. While in tissue cysts, marked growth occurs. Excystation and new migration may occur or they remain in situ until ingested by an appropriate final host. They may be viable

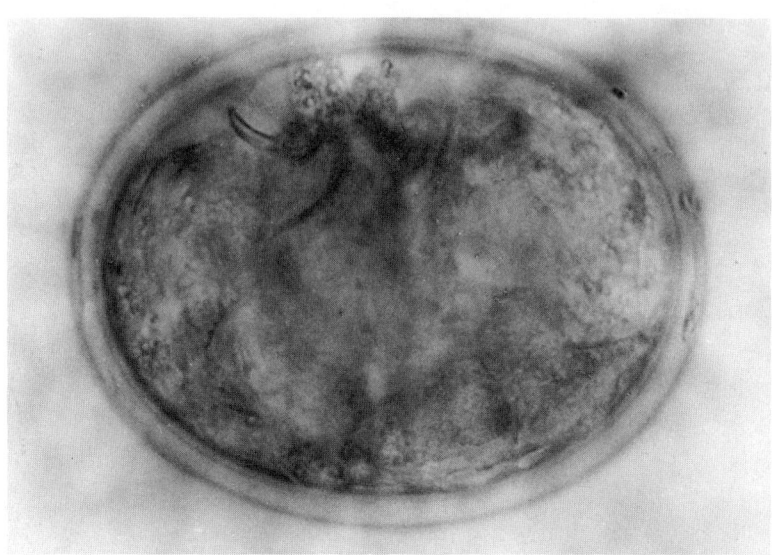

Fig. 15.3. Egg of *Raillietiella* sp. in a cobra, *Naja* sp. X710

for years in nymphal cyst stages (Deakins, 1973). After ingestion in the final host, nymphs released from cysts in the digestive tract invade the intestinal wall and eventually find their way to the lung, using mechanical means or natural passages, where they penetrate through with tissue damage. They attach impermanently to the alveolar wall as juveniles, which feed and grow to adults.

The effects of migration stages vary, depending on the numbers of organisms ingested and invading, previous presensitizing contact and sequential exposures to infective eggs (Deakins, 1973). There may be systemic eosinophilia and signs of toxemia or septicemia. Local organ reactions may include degenerative changes of hydropric or fatty type and evidences of nuclear damage in parenchymal cells.

DIAGNOSIS, TREATMENT AND PROGNOSIS

Many cases of pentastomiasis are associated with other diseases such as infections, parasitism, malnutrition, etc., which obscure the diagnosis. Blood studies may show leukocytosis and eosinophila. X-rays may show adult worms or calcified cyst remnants. Eggs may be found orally, nasally or in feces (Fig. 15.3). Adults and juveniles may be found while leaving the reptile and this may result in self cures or marked improvement of symptoms. Nymphs may exit through body walls or skin. Histologic studies of biopsies or necropsy specimens reveal the parasites or their remains.

No good treatment is known. Surgical removal of adults or nymphs is possible. Antibiotics are used to treat associated pneumonia or secondary infections. Reinfection should be prevented by hygienic measures and good husbandry. Auto-infection usually only occurs in captive snakes where elimination of feces is slowed or absent due to poor feeding, disease, weakness or dehydration, allowing eggs to hatch in the intestinal tract. Herpetologists should use ordinary hygienic precautions to prevent contamination by viable eggs, as man can serve as the intermediate host of reptilian pentastomes (Fain, 1966; Self and Kuntz, 1967).

REFERENCES

Deakins, D.E., 1973, Pentastome pathology in captive reptiles, Ph.D. thesis, Univ. Oklahoma, Norman.
Esslinger, J.H., 1962, Development of Porocephalus crotali (Humboldt, 1808) (Pentastomida) in experimental intermediate hosts, J. Parasitol., 48:452-456.
Fain, A., 1966, Pentastomida of snakes: Their parasitological role in man and animal, Mem. Inst. Butantan. Sim. Int., 33:167-174.
Hill, H.R., 1936, New host records of the linguatulid, Kiricephalus coarctatus (Diesing) in the United States, Bull. Southern California Acad. Sci., 34:226-227.
Nicoli, R.M., and Nicoli, J., 1966, Biologie des Pentastomides, Ann. Parasitol., 41:255-277.
Penn, G.H., Jr., 1942, The life history of Porocephalus crotali, parasite of the Louisiana muskrat, J. Parasitol., 41:255-277.
Reichenbach-Klinke, H.E., and Elkan, E., 1965, "The principal diseases of lower vertebrates," Academic Press, New York.
Riley, J., and Self, J.T., 1979, On the systematics on the pentastome genus Porocephalus (Humboldt, 1811) with descriptions of two new species, Systematic Parasitol., 1:25-42.
Self, J.T., 1969, Biological relationships of the Pentastomida: A bibliography of the Pentastomida, Exp. Parasitol., 24:63-119.
Self, J.T., and Kuntz, R.E., 1967, Host-parasite relations in some Pentastomida, J. Parasitol., 52:202-206.

LUNGWORMS

Roger E. Brannian

Kansas City Zoological Garden

Kansas City Parks Department

INTRODUCTION

Nematodes of the family Rhabdiasidae have long been known to parasitize the lungs of amphibians and reptiles (Yorke and Maplestone, 1926). Historically, these parasites have been regarded as being of low pathogenicity. More recent reports, however, have incriminated rhabdiasid nematodes as a significant cause of respiratory disease in snakes (Deakins and Cosgrove, 1978; Fantham and Porter, 1950; Fiennes, 1961; Jacobson, 1976; Zwart, 1968; Zwart and Jansen, 1969).

DISTRIBUTION

Lungworm parasitism has been reported in reptiles and amphibians from locations throughout the world. Although parasitism by rhabdiasids has been recorded in a variety of herptilian hosts, the anuran families of Ranidae and Bufonidae and the snake family Colubridae appear to be the most important host groups (Baker, 1978a).

In North America, colubrid snakes of the genera Elaphe, Lampropeltis, Nerodia, Thamnophis and Heterodon are commonly infected (Yamaguti, 1961). Rhabdias ranae was found to infect 71 to 75% of a population of wood frogs, Rana sylvatica, in Ontario (Baker, 1978b) and Lees (1962) recorded an overall infection rate of 48.7% for R. bufonis in an English frog population.

ETIOLOGY AND TRANSMISSION

The nematode family Rhabdiasidae includes the genera Rhabdias, Acanthorhabdias and Entomelas. A fourth genus, Shorttia, has been proposed by researchers in India (Singh and Ratnamala, 1975). Of these genera, Rhabdias is the most prevalent.

Life cycles in the family Rhabdiasidae involve both parasitic and free-living phases. The adult parasite is a parthenogenetic female or a protandrous hermaphrodite. Eggs are laid in the lung and carried up the respiratory tract to the oral cavity where they are then swallowed. Development proceeds in the gastrointestinal tract and embryonated eggs or larvae are passed in the feces. These larvae may develop into infective larvae directly, or may become free-living males and females. Bisexual mating occurs in the free-living forms with infective larvae resulting. Infective larvae gain entrance into a new host by being swallowed or by penetration of the skin. However, skin penetration of reptiles has not been demonstrated. The larvae undergo a tissue migration which terminates in the lungs. The life cycle is complete when the larvae develop into mature parasitic adults in the lungs (Baker, 1978c; Chu, 1936; Goodey, 1924; Hyman, 1951; Kaplan, 1973; Reichenback-Klinke and Elkan, 1965).

PATHOLOGY

Documented evidence of significant pathology in herptiles other than snakes is lacking. In snakes, the parasite can produce substantial inflammatory reactions (Deakins and Cosgrove, 1978). The lesions have been described as those of a verminous pneumonia with many areas of consolidation (Jacobson, 1976). Zwart and Jansen (1969) reported a pneumonia with a prominent granulomatous process. A gray sticky exudate is produced in quantity, often with embryonated eggs and larvae visibl microscopically (Fantham and Porter, 1950; Fiennes, 1961; Jacobson, 1976; Zwart, 1968). Bronchioles and alveoli may be occluded with adult worms (Jacobson, 1976). Secondary bacterial pneumonia often accompanies lungworm infection (Jacobson, 1976, 1978; Zwart, 1968).

DIAGNOSIS

Clinical signs of lungworm infection are similar to those of other respiratory diseases in snakes. Signs

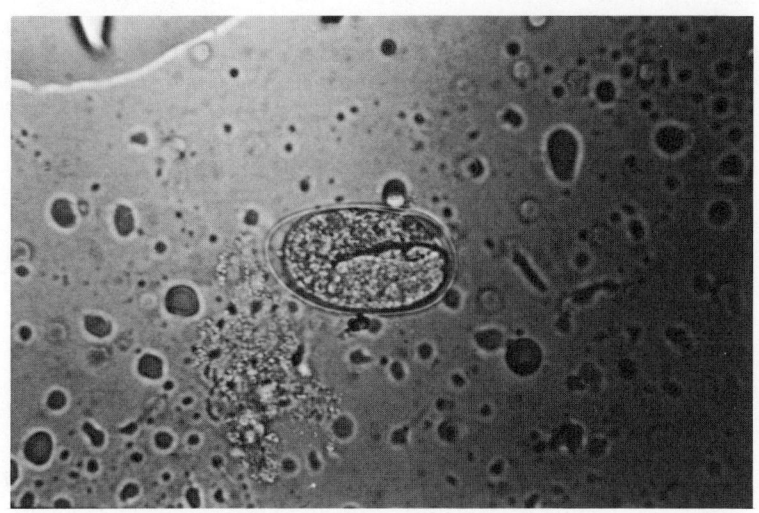

Fig. 16.1. Lungworm ovum from a rhinoceros viper, Bitis nasicornis.

include anorexia, open-mouth or labored breathing, crackling respiratory sounds, bubbles or exudate from the glottis and exaggerated gular movements (Jacobson, 1976; Zwart, 1968; Zwart and Jansen, 1969).

Diagnosis of infection by rhabdiasids is based on finding embryonated ova and/or larvae in the respiratory tract (Fig. 16.1). If exudate is not readily obtainable in suspect cases, tracheal or bronchial washings may be obtained by inserting a cannula through the glottis and into the respiratory tract (Jacobson, 1978). Sterile saline, 0.25 to 1.0 ml, is flushed into the trachea and aspirated out again. The washings are examined microscopically for lungworm larvae and ova. The ova measure 60 to 65 microns by 40 to 45 microns.

Rhabdiasid eggs and larvae are seen also in the feces, but may be confused with the eggs and larvae of the related intestinal parasite, Strongyloides.

TREATMENT AND CONTROL

Treatment and control of the parasite in wild populations are impractical. In captive snakes, lungworms can be effectively treated with levamisole at a dosage rate of 10 mg/kg, given intracoelomically (Jacobson, 1976, 1978; Zwart and Jansen, 1969). A second treatment two weeks after the first is recommended.

Because the life cycle of the rhabdiasids is direct, the parasite can be readily transmitted among captive snakes. Goodey (1924) found that the infective larvae of R. fuscovenosa resisted dessication on a dry glass surface for 24 hours. Chu (1936) found infective larvae of the same species to survive in sterile water for up to 82 days. Based on these observations and knowledge of the organism's life cylce, the best preventative measures in captivity would include prompt removal of feces from cages and thorough cleaning of the captive environment. Infected snakes should be treated to eliminate the source of the parasite.

REFERENCES

Baker, M.R., 1978a, Morphology and taxonomy of Rhabdias spp. (Nematoda: Rhabdiasidae) from reptiles and amphibians of southern Ontario, Can. J. Zool., 56:2127-2141.

Baker, M.R., 1978b, Seasonal population changes in Rhabdias ranae Walton, 1929 (Nematoda: Rhabdiasidae) in Rana sylvatica of Ontario, Can. J. Zool., 57:179-183.

Baker, M.R., 1978c, The free-living and parasitic development of Rhabdias spp. (Nematoda: Rhabdiasidae) in amphibians, Can. J. Zool., 57:161-178.

Chu, T., 1936, Studies on the life history of Rhabdias fuscovenosa var. catanensis (Rizzo, 1902) new rank, J. Parasitol., 22:140-160.

Deakins, D.E., and Cosgrove, G.E., 1978, Reptilian helminthiasis, Wildlife Disease Ass. Symp. on Diseases of Reptiles, Fort Collins, Colorado.

Fantham, H.B., and Porter, A., 1950, The endoparasites of certain South African snakes, together with some remarks on their structure and effects on their hosts, Proc. Zool. Soc. London, 120: 599-647.

Fiennes, R.N.T.W., 1961, Diseases of snakes caused by internal parasites, III Internationalen Symposiums uber die Erkankungen der Zootiere, Akademie der Wissenschaften der DDR, Berlin.

Goodey, T., 1924, The anatomy and life history of the nematode Rhabdias fuscovenosa from the grass snake, Tropidonotus natrix, J. Helminthol., 2:51-64.

Hyman, L.H., 1951, "The invertebrates: Acanthocephala, Aschelminthes, and Entoprocta," Vol. 3, McGraw-Hill, New York.

Jacobson, E., 1976, Use of Ripercol-L for the treatment of lungworms in snakes, J. Zoo Animal Med., 7:14-15.

Jacobson, E., 1978, Diseases of the respiratory system in reptiles, Vet. Med. Small Animal Clin., 73: 1169-1175.

Kaplan, H.M., 1973, Parasites of laboratory reptiles and amphibians, in: "Parasites of laboratory animals," R.J. Flynn, ed., Iowa State Univ. Press, Ames.

Lees, E., 1962, The incidence of helminth parasites in a particular frog population, Parasitology, 52:95-102.

Reichenbach-Klinke, H., and Elkan, E., 1965, "The principle diseases of lower vertebrates," Academic Press, New York.

Singh, S.N., and Ratnamala, R., 1975, On a new genus and new species of Rhabdiasoid nematode, Shorttia shorttia n.g., n.sp., infesting lungs of amphibians, Indian J. Helminthol., 27:132-138.

Yamaguti, S., 1961, "Systema Helminthum. The nematodes of vertebrates," vol. 3, Intersci. Publ., New York.

Yorke, W., and Maplestone, P., 1962(orig. 1926), "The nematode parasites of vertebrates," Hafner Publ. Co., New York.

Zwart, P., 1968, Parasitare und mykotische Lungenaffektionen bei Reptilien, X Internationalen Symposiums uber die Erkankungen der Zootiere, Akademie der Wissenschaften der DDR, Berlin.

Zwart, P., and Jansen, J., 1969, Treatment of lungworms in snakes with tetramisole, Vet. Rec., 84:374.

ASCARIDOID NEMATODES

J.F.A. Sprent

Department of Parasitology

University of Queensland

INTRODUCTION

Knowledge about ascaridoid nematodes of reptiles has gradually accumulated since the 18th century. No species in reptiles were listed by Linnaeus (1758) or Goeze (1782), but Rudolphi (1819) listed 17 species. The first work in which the reptilian species were listed together was that of Dujardin (1845).

Throughout most of the 19th century all ascaridoid species in reptiles were included in the genus Ascaris and a synopsis of this genus was compiled by Stossich (1896). There were 30 species listed from reptiles, many of these having been named and described in the second half of the 19th century, especially by R. Molin, O. von Linstow, A. Schneider, K. Wedl and C. Parona. The subgenus Polydelphis had been proposed already by Dujardin (1845), but it was in the early years of the 20th century that most of the genera were proposed into which the species in reptiles are now segregated; there are no longer any species from reptiles remaining in the genus Ascaris. Especially active in proposing new genera were H.A. Baylis, L. Gedoelst and K.I. Skrjabin. Yorke and Maplestone (1926) listed 11 genera containing species in reptiles. During the 1930's further additions to the known species in reptiles and amphibians were made, especially by Baylis, H.A. Kreis, J.H. Schuurmans-Stekhoven and L. Travassos.

Unfortunately knowledge about modes of infection, life history patterns and harmful effects has not kept pace,

with the result that there is little to report on these
aspects of infection with ascaridoid nematodes of reptiles
and amphibians.

At this point it is necessary to emphasize that this
is not a comprehensive review, but only a broad outline
of the subject, mainly at the generic level. For this
reason only literature references on general aspects are
included. For further references, especially at the
species level, the reader is referred to the review
articles on each genus containing species in amphibians
and reptiles compiled by the author and listed among the
references at the end of the chapter.

DISTRIBUTION

A perusal of the reptile hosts from which ascaridoid
species have been collected reveals that they do not occur
in Sphenodon and that they have a patchy distribution
throughout the different reptile groups. In general, it
may be said that they have dispersed widely among predatory
reptiles, such as snakes and crocodilians, but occur more
sparsely among other reptile groups, such as lizards and
chelonians, in which they occur only in certain families.
Thus, among the lizards, ascaridoids occur especially in
chameleons and larger predators, such as monitors and
tegu, Tupinambis spp., whereas herbivorous lizards
evidently escaped infection. It is interesting to note
that the two host genera, Varanus and Tupinambis, are in
different families and widely separated geographically,
yet they harbor closely related ascaridoids. Among the
chelonians, ascaridoids occur in marine turtles, freshwater
turtles and land tortoises. Ascaridoids occur in amphibian
hosts, but are reported only from a few families among
the Anura.

It must be emphasized that knowledge of the host range
is probably far from complete. On the other hand,
increasing scarcity of opportunity to examine animals in
their natural state may restrict definitive studies on
their host range.

As might be expected, the distribution of species in
marine reptiles, more or less coincides with that of their
hosts. Thus, Paraheterotyphlum spp. are found in sea
snakes in the Western Pacific Ocean and the seas off
Southeast Asia; they have not been found to occur in
other hosts or outside the regions frequented by sea
snakes. Sulcascaris sulcata has been collected from sea

turtles in the Mediterranean, Western Atlantic and Western Pacific Ocean and probably occurs only in those hosts and throughout their range.

In contrast, ascaridoids of freshwater and terrestrial reptiles show a distribution which varies in the different host groups. This may be limited by the availability of intermediate hosts. Some occur throughout almost the whole range of their host groups; this appears to be true for Dujardinascaris in crocodilians, Ophidascaris in snakes and Orneoascaris in monitor lizards. On the other hand, some ascaridoids appear to be restricted in distribution and not to extend to the whole geographic range of their hosts. Thus, in terrestrial tortoises Angusticaecum holopterum has been reported in Europe, Africa, Western Asia and South America, but there seems to be no record of its occurrence in tortoises in North America, Australia or Southeast Asia. Polydelphis anoura occurs in pythons in Africa, Asia and Australia, but so far natural infections have not been reported in boas in South America. Hexametra spp. occur in snakes in South America, Europe, Africa, Madagascar and Asia, but not in Australia. In anuran amphibians, species of the genus Orneoascaris have not been recorded so far in the New World, but are common in Africa, India and Southeast Asia and recent observations indicate that one species has reached Australia. Krefftascaris parmenteri has been found so far only in freshwater turtles of Eastern Australia.

ETIOLOGY

The genera of ascaridoid nematodes occurring in reptiles and amphibians fall within two families of the superfamily Ascaridoidea, namely the Ascarididae and the Anisakidae. The former contains most of the species occurring in terrestrial and fluviatile hosts, whereas species in marine hosts almost all belong in the latter family. These two families differ mainly in the form of the excretory system. In the Ascarididae, the system has a lateral filament running along each side of the body adjacent to the lateral chord; in the Anisakidae, the filament on the right side is reduced or absent.

In the ascaridoid group there are between 50 and 100 species so far known to occur in amphibians and reptiles. Estimation of the extent of speciation must, however, be regarded as subjective to some extent, because many of the named species represent no more than one observer's interpretation of apparent differences, often assessed in only a few specimens. The group as a whole comprises relatively few species in relation to the number of genera.

It is difficult to be precise about the characteristic features of ascaridoid nematodes without going into detail which would be tedious to the general reader. Details of morphology have been reduced, therefore, to the minimum necessary to appreciate general features such as feeding habits, life history patterns and identification. For detailed information on the morphology and taxonomy of the Ascaridoidea and their differentiation from other nematodes the reader is referred to Chabaud (1965).

Ascaridoid nematodes of reptiles vary in size to a considerable degree. In some species which incidentally occur in the largest hosts, the crocodilians, the males are mature at a length of less than 10 mm. In the largest species, which occur in pythons, females may measure over 200 mm. Most of the species in reptiles, irrespective of size, are found with their anterior end buried in the mucous membrane of the stomach. It is unlikely that they are feeding at this site, because when food is present in the host's stomach they are usually found to be living within the food mass and probably feed on the material which is being digested, rather than on the host.

In general, it may be stated that species in particular ascaridoid genera tend to occur in particular host groups. For example, species in Ophidascaris and Polydelphis have been collected only in snakes, Sulcascaris and Angusticaecum only in chelonians, Paraheterotyphlum only in sea snakes. Nevertheless, there are exceptions, such as Orneoascaris, Goezia and Terranova whose species occur in more than one host group of reptiles. Some genera in crocodilians are collected also in fish, for example Dujardinascaris and Brevimulticaecum.

TRANSMISSION

Male ascaridoids are slightly smaller and more slender than females and the sexes can be differentiated by the tail. Females have a straight tail, usually tapering to a conical tip; the male tail is curved ventrally. On the male tail there are a number of sessile papillae, some situated on the part of the tail behind the cloaca, others arranged in two subventral parallel rows in front of the cloaca (Fig. 17.1). In the males of some species there

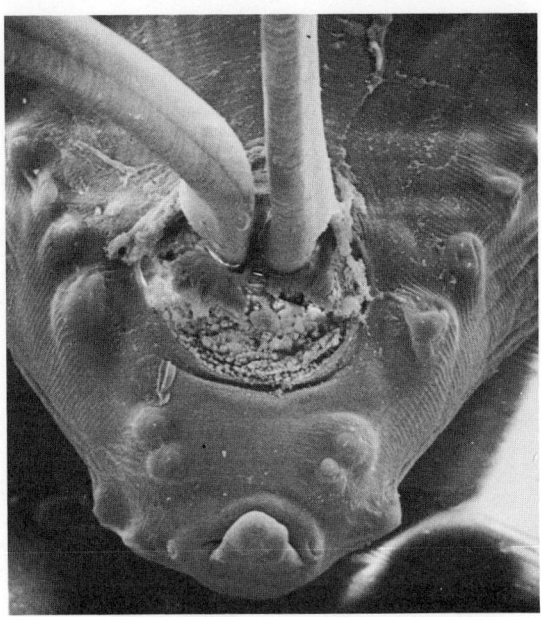

Fig. 17.1. Ventral region of the tail of a male Ophidascaris showing copulatory papillae and spicules protruding from cloaca. X200

are only four precloacal papillae on each side, whereas in other species there may be 100 or more. These papillae are assumed to be associated with copulation, during which the male coils the curved tail around the female in the region of the vulva, which is situated in the middle third of the body (Fig. 17.2), its position depending partly on the particular species, partly on the stage of growth. The larger the female the further forward is the vulva relative to the length of the body. The spermatozoa accumulate in the seminal vesicle and are injected into the female by the ejaculatory duct. This is facilitated by the spicules, a pair of gutter-shaped or rod-like structures which probably distend the vulva and vagina and aid in the passage of the disc-like spermatozoa into the female. The spicules in some species are guided by the gubernaculum, a cuticular structure on the dorsal aspect of the cloaca. The female reproductive system consists of the vulva leading into a cuticle-lined vagina which continues as the uterus. The latter usually divides into two uterine branches, but in some genera there are four (Fig. 17.3) and in others, six. In the female, sperm is stored in the seminal receptacle, a tubular structure located between the uterine branch and oviduct.

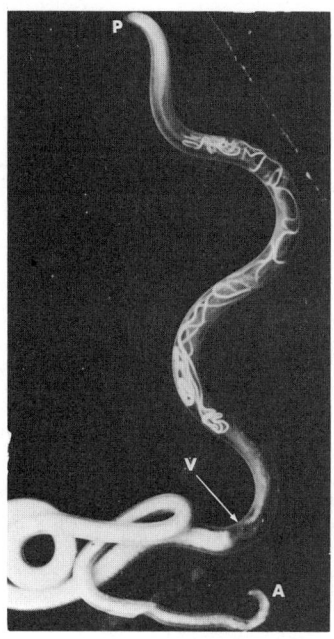

Fig. 17.2. Adult female Ophidascaris showing position of the vulva and ovarian filaments (A=anterior end, P=posterior end, V=vulva).

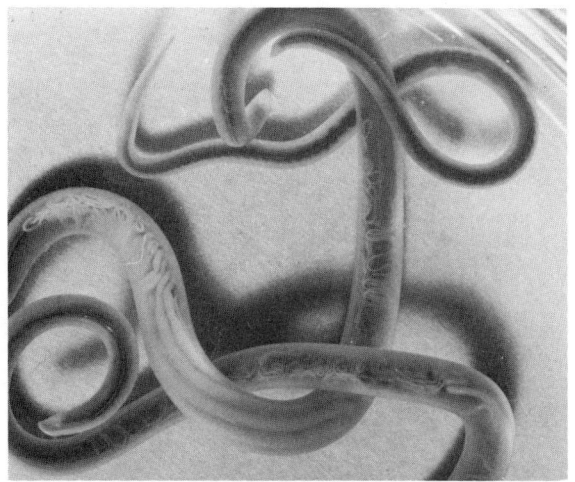

Fig. 17.3. Female Polydelphis anoura showing four uterine branches. X5

ASCARIDOID NEMATODES 225

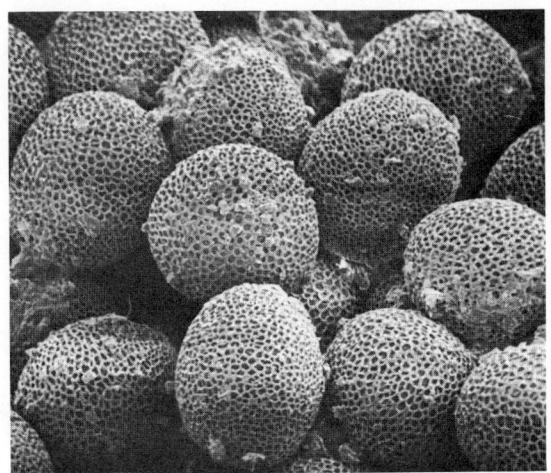

Fig. 17.4. Eggs showing pitted surface. X250

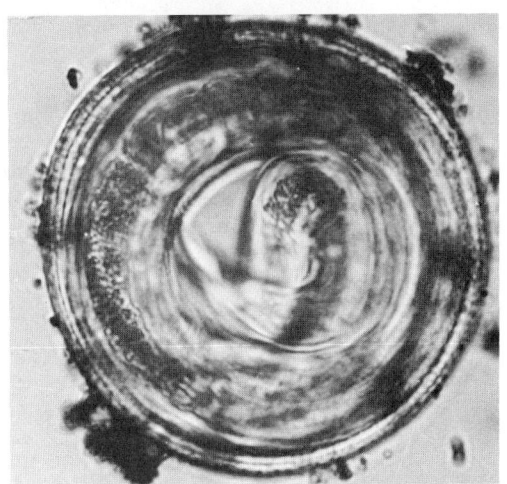

Fig. 17.5. Egg containing third stage larva. X1000

The fertilized eggs are covered with a shell which is usually pitted (Fig. 17.4). In most species the eggs are extruded in single file through the vulva. Development of the embryo commences after the egg is laid. The eggs pass out in the feces of the host and if temperature and humidity are optimal they contain a moving embryos in a few days (Fig. 17.5). After a week the first stage larva is formed. It is almost homogeneous in appearance, the

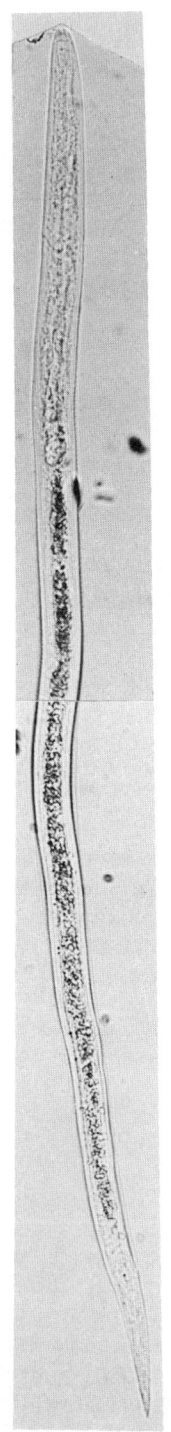

Fig. 17.6. Third stage larva after hatching. X600

body being filled with granules and globules which obscure the structure. In many species, and possibly all species, the first moult is quickly followed by the second moult, so that the larva is now a third stage larva (Araujo, 1971). It is possible now to observe structures, such as the esophagus, because the granules are by now aggregated within the cells of the intestine (Fig. 17.6).

The larva is now infective, but has not grown beyond 0.4 to 0.5 mm which is the length at which most species hatch from the eggs. In some species, especially those in aquatic hosts, eggs hatch spontaneously, but usually hatching does not occur until the egg has been swallowed.

It is not possible to give a general account of further events because, as previously indicated, relatively few studies have been conducted on life history patterns of these nematodes in reptiles. As most species occur in predatory reptiles, it is likely that an intermediate host is utilized. Among ascaridoids of terrestrial reptiles, certain species in snakes and monitor lizards have been observed to use frogs, lizards or mammals as intermediate hosts. Species in chameleons have been found to develop in insects (Chabaud et al., 1962). Among ascaridoids of aquatic reptiles, development may occur in crustacea, bivalve molluscs or fish. In some instances two intermediate hosts may be involved in the life history pattern, invertebrates being necessary to carry the larvae from the feces to the second intermediate host.

A. holopterum is unusual among ascaridoids of reptiles in that its hosts are herbivorous; they occur in the herbivorous land tortoises. Infection probably occurs directly by ingestion of eggs with the larvae undergoing two phases of development, one in the lungs where growth of the third stage larva occurs, and one in the alimentary tract where the third and fourth moult occurs (Sprent, 1980a).

In all ascaridoids of reptiles whose development is known, the third stage is a phase of growth rather than differentiation and is spent in tissues, such as lungs, body cavity or subcutaneous tissue, the larva being not adapted in the form of its lips for feeding in the alimentary tract (Fig. 17.7). This growth phase may be spent either in the definitive host or in an intermediate host. It is only when the fourth stage is reached that the lips begin to resemble those of the adult stage (Fig. 17.8) and a life in the alimentary tract can be commenced. It is in the fourth stage that the gonads undergo most of their development and the sexes become clearly diffentiated.

Irrespective of whether intermediate hosts are utilized, the third and fourth moults usually occur in the alimentary tract of the definitive reptile host, but one known exception appears to be S. sulcata in which species the fourth stage is reached in the mollusc intermediate host (Sprent, 1977c).

PATHOGENESIS AND PATHOLOGY

The harmful effects of ascaridoid nematodes are difficult to assess because of the paucity of knowledge of symptomatology in reptiles. It would seem likely that harmful effects might arise as a result of several features of infection with these nematodes.

Their size in relation to the host is considerable in some instances, so that in situations where food is scarce and a heavy infection prevails there must ensue some deprivation of nutriment from the stomach and small intestine, rather than any actual ingestion of host tissue.

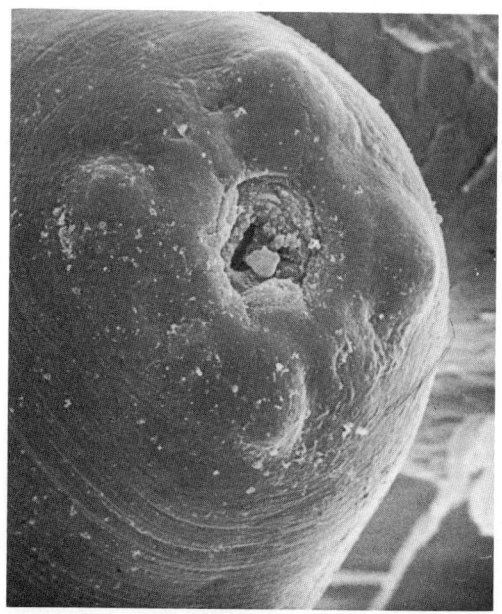

Fig. 17.7. Anterior tip of third stage larva showing mouth and labial papillae. X900

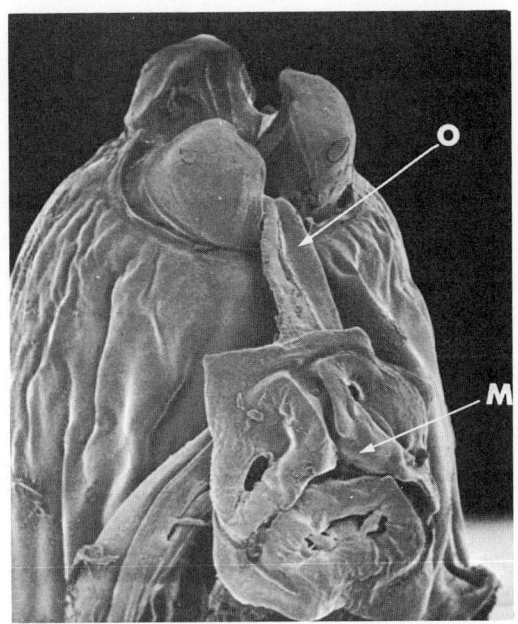

Fig. 17.8. Fourth moult of Ophidascaris sp. The fourth stage lips (M) are still attached by the esophagus (O) and the body is still covered with the fourth stage cuticle. X260

Heavy infections, where the worm mass is large relative to the host, have been reported in tortoises with A. holopterum.

Blockage may ensue in the alimentary tract from a large mass of worms. This appears to occur especially with dead worms in the large bowel and thus might be expected to follow anthelmintic treatment. Again this has been reported in infection with A. holopterum in tortoises (Sprent, 1980a).

Blockage in other organs occurs especially in snakes, as a result of immature stage of Ophidascaris spp. undergoing migrations prior to attaining maturity in the alimentary tract. Third stage larvae may be found to have invaded the heart, large blood vessels or the lungs. Migration from the alimentary tract is likely to occur when growth in the intermediate host has not reached a stage which is suitable for existence in the stomach. Usually after a period of development as third stage larvae, the third moult occurs when larvae reach the

Table 17.1. Key to the Identification of Ascaridoid Genera Occurring in Amphibians and Reptiles.[a]

ASCARIDINAE

Small worms, of even width, labial pulp divided
 into 2 rounded anterior lobes by deep cleft
 (frogs and frog-eating reptiles)....................Orneoascaris (Fig. 17.15)

Medium to large worms, labial pulp not divided
 by deep cleft, interlabia present in adult,
  uterus with 2 branches (in snakes)................Ophidascaris (Fig. 17.12)
  uterus with 4 branches (in snakes)..............Travassosascaris (Fig. 17.12)
 interlabia absent in adult,
  uterus with 2 branches (in tortoises)............Angusticaecum (Fig. 17.15)
  uterus with 4 branches (in snakes)................Polydelphis (Fig. 17.12)
  uterus with 6 branches (in snakes/lizards).........Hexametra (Fig. 17.12)

HETEROCHEILINAE

Interlabia absent (in freshwater turtles)..............Krefftascaris (Fig. 17.15)

Interlabia present (in crocodilians)
 ventriculus oval and smooth, lips flat with
  interlocking facets and rounded denticles......Dujardinascaris (Fig. 17.11)
 ventriculus with long finger-like appendices,
  lips rounded, smooth, with sharp denticles...........Multicaecum (Fig. 17.11)

ventriculus lobate or with short club-like
appendices, lips flat, notched, without
denticles
    ventriculus with short club-like
    appendices..............................<u>Brevimulticaecum</u> (Fig. 17.11)
    ventriculus lobate
        excretory pore less than halfway to
        nerve ring from anterior end........<u>Ortleppascaris</u> (Fig. 17.11)
        excretory pore more than halfway to
        nerve ring from anterior end........<u>Gedoelstascaris</u> (Fig. 17.11)

CONTRACAECINAE

Ventriculus globular with appendix (occasionally in
aquatic reptiles).....................................<u>Contracaecum</u>

ANISAKINAE

Ventriculus elongate, without appendix
    interlabia absent (in crocodilians/aquatic
    snakes)......................................<u>Terranova</u> (Fig. 17.11)
    interlabia present (in marine turtles)........<u>Sulcascaris</u> (Fig. 17.15)

RAPHIDASCARIDINAE

Body stout with rings of spine-like projections
(in sea snakes and crocodilians)..............................<u>Goezia</u> (Fig. 17.12)

Body slender and smooth (in sea snakes)...............<u>Paraheterotyphlum</u> (Fig. 17.12)

aSprent, in press a.

stomach of the definitive host. If for some reason the larvae are swallowed at a stage before this moult can occur, they tend to migrate into adjacent tissues, especially heart, lung and body cavity, where they may be found lying freely or encapsulated (Sprent and McKeown 1979).

Adult ascaridoid nematodes are frequently found with the anterior part of the body deeply buried in the mucous membrane of the esophagus, stomach or small intestine (Fig. 17.9). Some species are threaded through a tunnel in the wall so that the middle part of the worm is attached. It is likely that the worms are not feeding at this site, but use this for anchorage at times when there is no food. After the worm has been pulled out, there remains an indurated crater with a tunnel made of connective tissue and infiltrated with eosinophil leukocytes extending into the submucosa (Fig. 17.10). In some instances, many worms may be embedded together, sometimes sharing the same crater or forming a tumor-like granulomatous mass with many craters and intertwined tunnels. Such nodular masses can sometimes be palpated in the living snake.

Whether these nodules and their inhabitants are the cause of ill health it is difficult of state. Otherwise healthy-looking snakes caught in the wild may have a surprisingly large number of embedded worms and the stomac may be disfigured by several nodular masses.

In some instances, especially when the peritoneum has been pierced and there is communication via the tunnels between the body cavity and the lumen of the stomach, there is evidence of secondary bacterial infectio and the presence of cheesy pus. Such lesions may heal and produce chalky white nodules and tortuous casts. As indicated above, the larvae of some species migrate to the lungs or body cavity. The presence of larvae in the lungs may cause severe inflammation and hemorrhage and at a later stage nodules with a cheesy yellow pus may appear.

DIAGNOSIS

A key to the genera of ascaroids parasitizing amphibians and reptiles is presented in Table 17.1.

Crocodylia

Ascaridoid nematodes are commonly encountered in

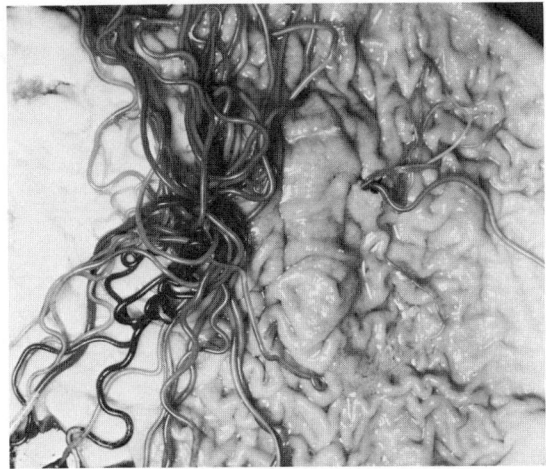

Fig. 17.9. Clump of Ophidascaris sp. in the stomach of a snake. X1

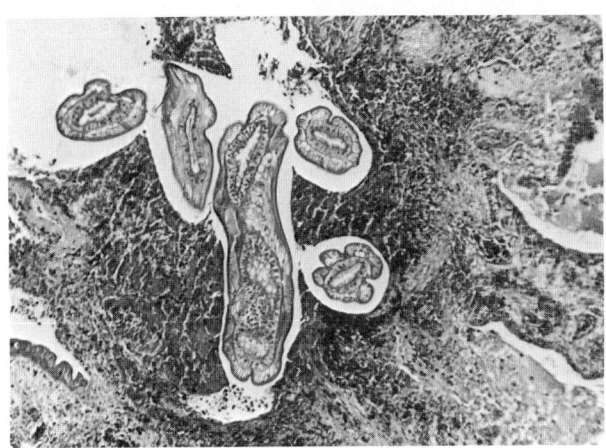

Fig. 17.10. Section of nodule in the stomach of a snake showing a lesion caused by Ophidascaris sp. X10

crocodilians throughout the extent of their geographical range (no data is available for Alligator sinensis). Indeed, the number of genera and species in crocodilians is more than in any other group of reptiles, indicating that the host-parasite relationship is relatively ancient Ascaridoids of crocodilians are relatively small in size compared with those in other reptiles. They are found attached by their anterior ends or loose in the stomach and small intestine.

There are two groups of species in crocodilians. One group of species belongs within the genus Terranova, a genus containing species in a wide spectrum of hosts, including sharks, rays, sawfish and snakes. The females attain a length of 55 mm and are of even width, with no interlabia; there is an elongate ventriculus and the tail end of the male is slightly expanded. T. lanceolata is found in the caimans of South America, T. crocodili is found in the crocodiles of Africa, Asia and Australia. For a key to identification of the species of Terranova in crocodilians see Sprent (1979a).

The other group of species is mainly restricted to crocodilians, but near relations are sometimes encountered in freshwater fish. These species, belonging within the Heterocheilinae, are segregated into several genera namely Dujardinascaris, Ortleppascaris, Gedoelstascaris, Multicaecum, Brevimulticaecum, Hartwichia and Trispiculascaris (Fig. 17.11). In several of the species in Dujardinascaris the females are robust in form measuring up to 40 mm in length and are coiled in the characteristic helicoid spiral resembling the shells of gastropod snails, whereas the males are much smaller, more slender and coiled in a flat watch-spring coil. In the other genera, the males are smaller than the females, but both sexes are sinuous and irregularly coiled. For keys to identification of species in these genera see Sprent (1977b, 1978c, 1979a, in press b).

The life history is not known for any of these species, but it seems likely that infection occurs at a very young age when crocodiles are feeding on small fish and crustacea harboring third stage larvae. At the time of their ingestion the larvae are only about 1 mm in length. They undergo two moults in crocodiles. Fourth stage larvae measure about 2 to 5 mm in length, adults range from less than 5 mm so it appears likely that the fourth moult occurs at about this length. Other ascaridoids occasionally found in crocodilians belong in the genera Goezia (Sprent, 1978a), Orneoascaris and Contracaecum.

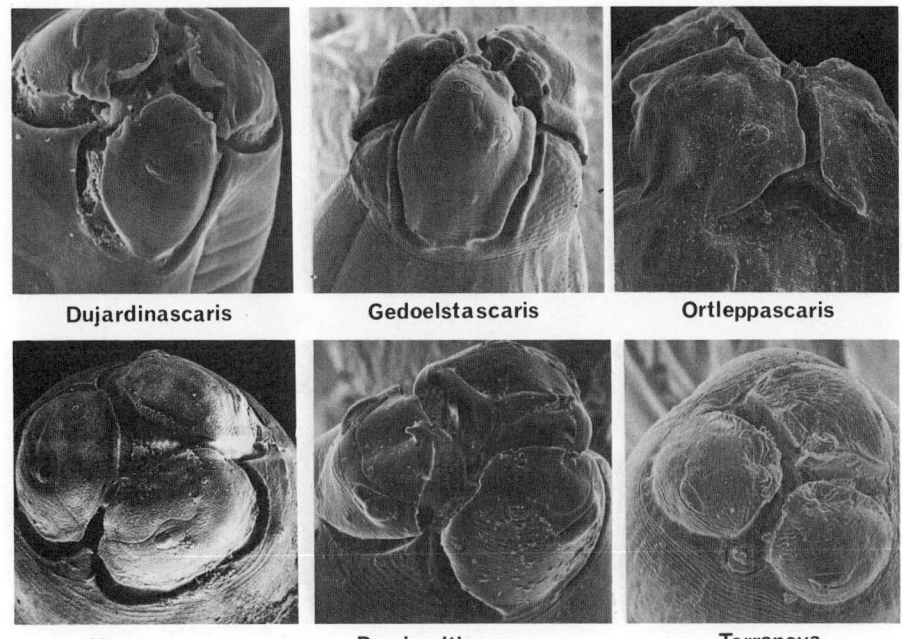

Fig. 17.11. Features of the mouth region in genera with species in crocodilians. Dujardinascaris X400, Gedoelstascaris X350, Ortleppascaris X400, Multicaecum X300, Brevimulticaecum X800, Terranova X650

Serpentes

In the Western Pacific Ocean sea snakes are infected with two species of Paraheterotyphlum, namely P. ophiophagus (in more northern waters around Taiwan) and P. australe (in the more southern region off the east coast of Australia). For differentiation of the two species see Sprent (1978b). Both species are large, smooth, slender worms; males measuring up to 95 mm and females up to 168 mm. They have elongate lips without interlabia (Fig. 17.12). They are easily differentiated from Goezia holmesi which also occurs in sea snakes. That species is small and grub-like, and has the body covered with spines. G. holmesi has been collected in sea snakes only along the northern coast of Australia. No pathological effects have been described and the infection is probably acquired from ingestion of fish.

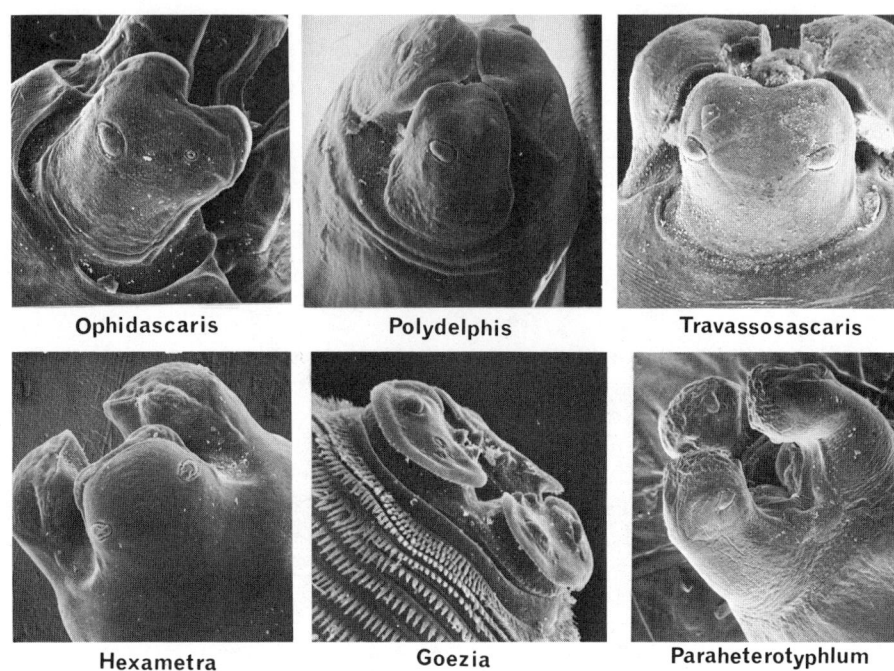

Fig. 17.12. Features of the mouth region in genera with species occurring in snakes. Ophidascaris X300, Polydelphis X300, Travassosascaris X250, Hexametra X200, Goezia X840, Paraheterotyphlum X200

The Cuban snake, Alsophis cathigerus pepei, as well as Nerodia spp., Agkistrodon piscivorous and several other North American snakes, harbor T. caballeroi. This is a medium-sized, slender, elongate species about 15 to 30 mm in length found attached in the stomach. It can be recognized by the rather small rounded lips and by the possession of a pair of cusp-like teeth on the oral margin of each subventral lip (Sprent, 1979b).

In the pythons which frequent the land masses bordering the Indian Ocean (except Madagascar) two species groups are found. The first group comprises only one species, namely P. anoura, which occurs throughout the geographic range of the hosts. It occurs in the anterior part of the small intestine, is a relatively robust worm, widest in the middle part of the body and a flesh-pink uniform color; the vulva is situated anterior to the middle of the

body and there are no interlabia. The life history of
this species involves encapsulation of third stage larvae
in the wall of the intestine, mesentery, liver and lungs
of rodents. The larvae do not grow beyond 7 mm in length
in rodents and are infective to pythons at this stage.
They undergo the third and fourth moults and attain the
adult stage without further migration in the python host
(Sprent, 1978d).

The second group comprises several species all
belonging to the genus Ophidascaris. One or more slightly
different species have been described from each of the
geographical areas in which pythons are found. They are
slender worms with distinct color patterns varying from
dark red to yellow. The posterior part of the body is
wider than the anterior part giving a whip-like appearance.
The vulva is situated behind the middle of the body.
Interlabia are present. These species are usually found
with the anterior end deeply buried in the mucosa of the
stomach. Sometimes clusters of worms may be found protruding from a single crater-like nodule. The following
species have been described: O. amucronata in Python sebae
in Africa, O. filaria in P. molurus molurus in India and
Sri Lanka, O. infundibulicola and O. baylisi in P. reticulatus and P. curtus in Thailand and Malaya, O. papuanus
and O. niuginiensis in Liasis amethystinus and Chondropython viridis in Papua New Guinea, O. robertsi and
O. moreliae in Morelia spilotes, Aspidites spp. and L.
amethystinus in Australia (Sprent, 1977a; Sprent and
McKeown, 1979). Ascaridoid nematodes of pythons utilize
mammals as intermediate hosts. These probably become
infected by eating smaller animals which feed on snake
feces containing eggs. The particular mammals serving
as intermediate hosts in each locality is not known,
except for Australia where marsupials, such as bandicoots
and opossums are found to be naturally infected. When
eggs of each species were experimentally fed to laboratory
mice, larvae of each Ophidascaris spp. were found to
undergo a characteristic degree of growth and migrate to
particular tissues of the mouse, e.g. subcutaneous tissue
(Fig. 17.13), liver, blood vessels or body cavity.

After a period of growth in the intermediate host
the extent of which varied from 5 mm to 90 mm among the
different species, the third stage larvae were infective
to pythons. Two or more different growth patterns were
observed among the eight species (Sprent and McKeown,
1979). The third stage larvae of O. filaria and O.
moreliae grew only to about 5 mm in subcutaneous tissue
of mice. When they were ingested by pythons these larvae

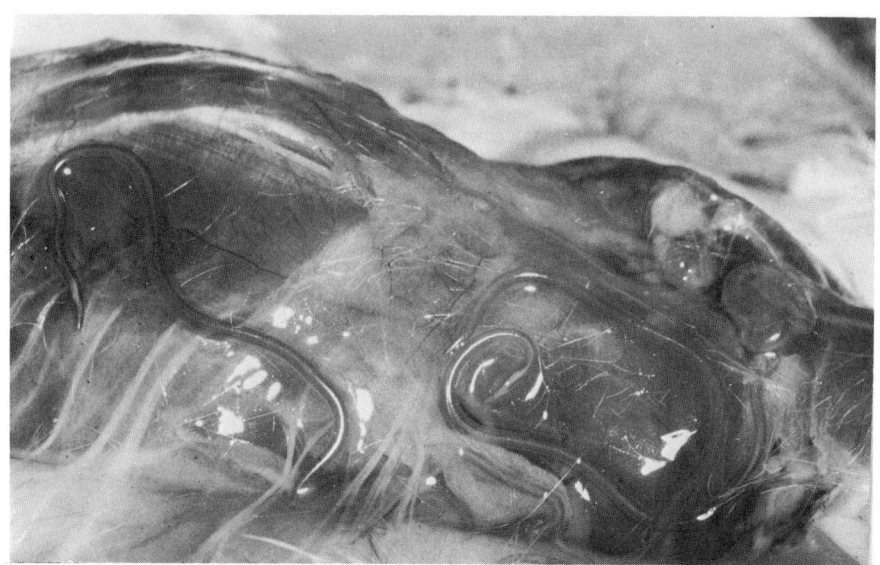

Fig. 17.13. Third stage larva of Ophidascaris infundibulicola in subcutaneous tissue of an intermediat host. X3

migrated to the lungs, grew there to a length of 30 mm or more, completed the third moult, migrated up the trachea and reached the stomach where the fourth moult to the adult stage occurred. In contrast, the third stage larvae of O. baylisi, O. infundibulicola, O. amucronata and O. niuginiensis grew to 30 mm or more in the subcutaneous tissue of mice. When they were ingested by pythons the larvae did not migrate to the lungs, but underwent the third and fourth moult and reached the adult stage in the stomach.

The third stage of the other two species, O. robertsi and O. papuanus, grew to a length of 50 mm or more for the former, 15 mm for the latter, in the liver and body cavity of rodents, but when ingested by pythons, they migrated into the body cavity (Fig. 17.14) where they underwent the third and fourth moults. They then moved into the stomach as adults (Sprent and McKeown, 1979).

The elapid snakes of Australia harbor O. pyrrhus, a species which resembles the species in pythons in general appearance, but the whip-like form of the body is more marked and the lips more shallow. It differs also in that the worm is looped through a fold of the

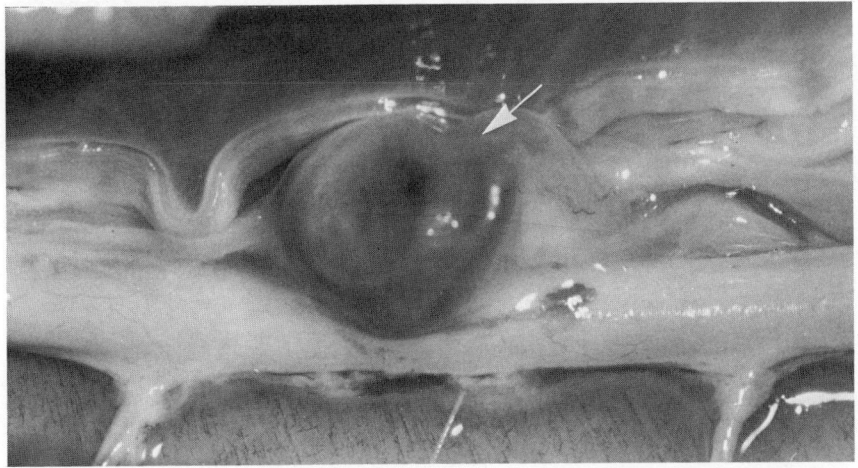

Fig. 17.14. Fourth stage larva of Ophidascaris robertsi in a nodule on the aorta of a snake. X2.5

stomach mucosa so that the middle of the body is free, the anterior and posterior ends protruding freely into the lumen. Immature forms, probably of this species, have been found encapsulated in the subcutaneous tissues of lizards and it is probable that infection occurs through ingesting lizards. Another species, O. cretinorum, has been described in coral snakes in South America (Freitas, 1968), but it is probably the same species as occurs in the colubrines of that region. The cobras of Africa and Asia harbor one or more species of Ophidascaris, but the species names are in a confused state; in Africa the name is O. najae, but in India it seems probable that cobras have a different species, possibly the same species as found in Asian colubrines. Cobras harbor H. quadricornis which also occurs in a wide range of other Asian and African snakes. The third stage larvae of this latter species are found in the body cavity of rodents where they grow to a length of 60 mm or more (Sprent, 1978d).

In the stomach of crotaline species of the New World, especially rattlesnakes, there occur three distinct ascaridoid genera. One possesses interlabia and four uterine branches and comprises the single genus and species, T. araujoi, extending from Mexico to Brazil. Another species possesses no interlabia and six uterine branches. This species, H. boddaertii, probably extends over the range of the rattlesnakes in both North and South America and occurs also in colubrine snakes. The third species has so far been found only in Brazilian crotalines. It is known by several species names, O. arndti, O. travassosi, and O. sprenti, but is probably a single species, O. arndti having priority (Sprent, in prep.). The life history of these species in rattlesnakes involves mammalian intermediate hosts, the larvae of T. araujoi and H. boddaertii migrate to the body cavity of rodents where the former grows to 30 mm in length, the latter to 80 mm (Sprent, 1978d). The life history and development of O. arndti has not been elucidated in detail but preliminary observations indicate that the larvae migrate to the liver, body cavity and scrotum of mice. Bitis arietans in Africa harbors O. radiosa and all the Old World vipers are commonly found to harbor H. quadricornis. Infection is acquired through eating rodents in which the third stage larvae occur in the body cavity.

Several species belonging within the genus Ophidascaris have been described from colubrine snakes, but they are not well known, some of them having been found only on a single occasion. In this category are O. mombasica and O. solenopoion in colubrine snakes in Africa and Madagascar respectively. Both these species resemble the previously mentioned Australian species, O. pyrrhus in elapids, in their mode of attachment to the mucous membrane of the stomach. In Asian colubrines there is O. solitaria distinguishable from other species in its possessing cervical alae, probably the same species as occurs also in Asian cobras. Two species, O. trichuriformis and O. sicki, occur in South American colubrines (Freitas, 1968). The former has a whip-like body with the posterior part markedly wider. The former species is threaded through the mucosa of the stomach with the anterior and posterior ends protruding. The latter species is of even width and attached by its anterior end. Both these species probably extend in their range through Mexico to North America, but are known by various other names. They are probably acquired through eating frogs. Colubrine snakes in the New World may harbor H. boddaertii, the same species referred to above in rattlesnakes. The African and Asian colubrines harbor H. quadricornis, a species very close to H. boddaertii. The former species is widely dispersed over the Old World, extending from Africa through Southern Europe, the Middle East and India, to the Indonesian Islands, but has not reached Australia. It occurs also in elapid and viperid snakes and occasionally in pythons (Sprent, 1978d).

Sauria

Ascaridoids have a patchy distribution in the lizards. They occur in three groups. The most isolated group comprises one species, O. alata, in the South American Tupinambis spp. in Surinam and Brazil. It is probable that this species should be placed in a genus of its own, as it shows basic differences from other species in Orneoascaris (Sprent, in press c).

Another group comprises at least two species in the genus Hexametra occurring in chameleons in Africa (H. hexametra) and Madagascar (H. angusticaecoides); infection of chameleons has been shown to occur through ingestion of insects (Sprent, 1978d).

The third group of species occurs in the monitor lizards, Varanus spp. These species were previously placed in Amplicaecum, but now are placed in the genus Orneoascaris (Le-Van-Hoa, 1960). The number of species is uncertain, but there is one species in Australia (O. mackerrasae), at least one species in Thailand and India (O. varani) and one species in Africa (O. schoutedeni) (Sprent, in press c).

Testudines

The chelonians do not appear to be a host group in which a primary radiation of ascaridoids has occurred, but rather has been invaded on separate occasions by ascaridoids derived from other host groups. Three such incursions may be considered, the first in marine turtles by forms derived from other marine animals, the second in the terrestrial tortoises by forms derived from anuran amphibians, and the third in the freshwater turtles by forms perhaps derived from other fluviatile hosts, such as fish or crocodilians.

The species occurring in marine turtles and probably extending throughout their range is S. sulcata (Fig. 17.15). This species is found with the anterior end embedded in the stomach near its junction with the esophagus. They attain a length of over 100 mm in the female. They are most commonly found in the loggerhead turtle, Caretta caretta, but have been collected from the green turtle, Chelonia mydas. Infection is acquired by eating various bivalves, particularly clams and scallops

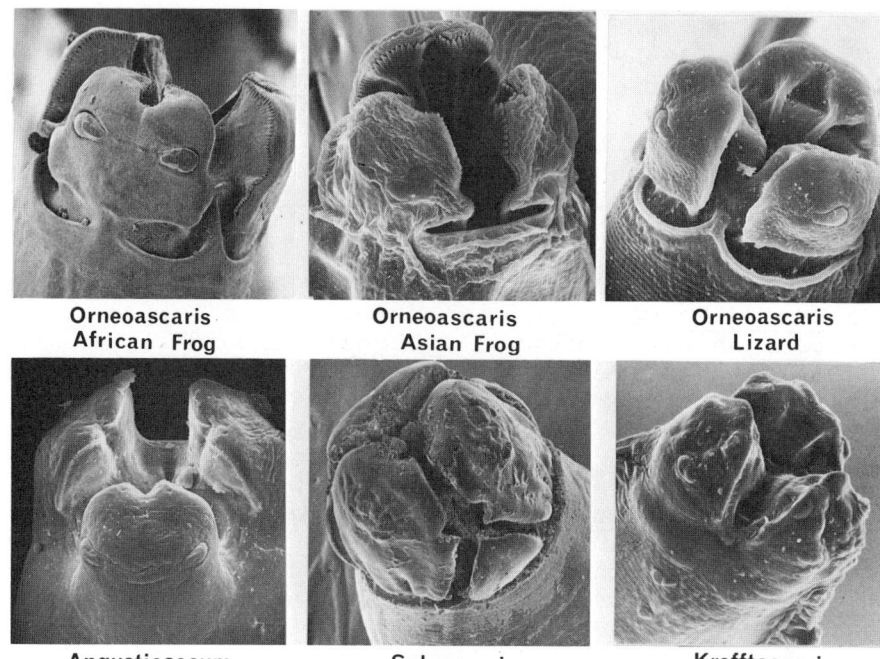

Fig. 17.15. Features of the mouth region in genera with species found in anurans, lizards and chelonians. Orneoascaris (African frog) X850, Orneoascaris (Asian frog) X550, Orneoascaris (lizard) X900, Angusticaecum X350, Sulcascaris X300, Krefftascaris X1000

in which the larval stages are encapsulated, especially in the adductor muscle. This parasite has considerable economic importance because the larvae attain a length of 40 mm or more in the adductor muscle of edible bivalves and their presence results in rejection by food inspectors (Sprent, 1977c).

A. holopterum occurs in several species of land tortoises, Testudo spp., as well as in the European pond turtle, Emys orbicularis, and the African hingeback, Kinixys belliana. They are large worms and occur in the stomach, small intestine, and occasionally in the large intestine where they have been reported to cause blockage. Signs of gastrointestinal disturbance have been reported. Infection probably occurs by ingestion of embryonated eggs with the food. The larvae migrate to the lungs and probably move into the stomach via the trachea and esophagus (Sprent, 1980a).

In Eastern Australia the long-necked water turtle, Chelodina longicollis, is infected with K. parmenteri. This species occurs in the stomach (Sprent, 1980a).

Amphibia

Several species belonging to the genus Orneoascaris occur in the stomach and small intestine of frogs and toads of the families Ranidae, Bufonidae and Brevicipitidae. They are probably all referable to three species, namely O. chrysanthemoides, O. numidicum and O. schoutedeni. They are found in equatorial Africa, Southern Europe, North Africa, India, Southeast Asia and New Guinea. One species has reached the northern shores of Australia, probably carried there by one species of Rana which has reached the Australian continent.

REFERENCES

Araujo, P., 1971, Considerations sur la deuxieme mue des larves d'Ascarides parasites de serpents, Ann. Parasitol. Humaine Comparee, 46:605-611.
Chabaud, A.G., 1965, Ordre des Ascaridida, in: "Traite de zoologie: Anatomie, systematique, biologie. Tome IV, Fasc. III. Nemathelminthes (Nematodes, Gordiaces), rotiferes, gastrotriches, kinorhynques," P.P. Grasse, ed., Masson, Paris.
Chabaud, A.G., Brygoo, E.R., and Petter, A.J., 1962, Cycle evolutif de l'Ascaride des Cameleons malgaches, Bull. Soc. Zool. France, 87:515-532.
Dujardin, F., 1845, "Histoire naturelle des helminthes ou vers intestinaux," Librairie Encyclopedique de Roret, Paris.
Freitas, J.F., 1968, Revisao do genero Ophidascaris Baylis, 1921 (Nematoda, Ascaridoidea), Mem. Instituto Oswaldo Cruz, 66:1-83.
Goeze, J.A.E., 1782, 'Versuch einer Naturgeschichte der Eingeweiderwurmer thierischer Korper," Blankenburg.
Le-Van-Hoa, 1960, Synonymie des genres Amplicaecum Baylis 1920 et Orneoascaris Skrjabin 1916, Ann. Parasitol. Humaine Comparee, 35:760-761.
Linnaeus, C., 1758, "Systema naturae per regna tria naturae, secundum classes, ordines, genera, species, cum characteribus, differentiis, synonymis, locis. Editio decima, reformata," Holmiae.
Rudolphi, C.A., 1819, "Entozoorum synopsis cui accedunt mantissa duplex et indices locupletissimi," Rucker, Berolini.

Sprent, J.F.A., 1977a, Studies on ascaridoid nematodes in pythons: A resume, in: "Excerta Parasitologi en memoria del doctor Eduardo Caballero y Caballero," Instituto de Biologia, Mexico, Publ. Especiales, 4:477-485.

Sprent, J.F.A., 1977b, Ascaridoid nematodes of amphibians and reptiles: Dujardinascaris, J. Helminthol., 51:253-287.

Sprent, J.F.A., 1977c, Ascaridoid nematodes of amphibians and reptiles: Sulcascaris, J. Helminthol., 51:379-387.

Sprent, J.F.A., 1978a, Ascaridoid nematodes of amphibians and reptiles: Goezia, J. Helminthol., 52:91-98.

Sprent, J.F.A., 1978b, Ascaridoid nematodes of amphibians and reptiles: Paraheterotyphlum, J. Helminthol. 52:163-170.

Sprent, J.F.A., 1978c, Ascaridoid nematodes of amphibians and reptiles: Gedoelstascaris n.g. and Ortleppascaris n.g., J. Helminthol., 52:261-282.

Sprent, J.F.A., 1978d, Ascaridoid nematodes of amphibians and reptiles: Polydelphis, Travassosascaris n.g. and Hexametra, J. Helminthol., 52:355-384.

Sprent, J.F.A., 1979a, Ascaridoid nematodes of amphibians and reptiles: Multicaecum and Brevimulticaecum, J. Helminthol., 53:91-116.

Sprent, J.F.A., 1979b, Ascaridoid nematodes of amphibians and reptiles: Terranova, J. Helminthol., 53:265-282.

Sprent, J.F.A., 1980a, Ascaridoid nematodes of amphibians and reptiles: Angusticaecum and Krefftascaris n.g., J. Helminthol., 54:53-73.

Sprent, J.F.A., 1980b, Ascaridoid nematodes of sirenians-the Heterocheilinae redefined, J. Helminthol., 54:309-327.

Sprent, J.F.A., in press a, Observations on the systematic of ascaridoid nematodes, in: "Concepts in nematode systematics," H. Platt, ed., Academic Press, New York.

Sprent, J.F.A., in press b, Ascaridoid nematodes of amphibians and reptiles: Typhlophorus, Hartwichia and Trispiculascaris, J. Helminthol.

Sprent, J.F.A., in press c, Ascaridoid nematodes of amphibians and reptiles: Orneoascaris, J. Helminthol.

Sprent, J.F.A., in prep., Ascaridoid nematodes of amphibians and reptiles: Ophidascaris.

Sprent, J.F.A., and McKeown, E.A., 1979, Studies on ascaridoid nematodes in pythons: Development in the definitive host, in: "Dynamic aspects of host-parasite relationships," Vol. 3, A. Zuckerman, ed., Israel Univ. Press, Jerusalem.

Stossich, M., 1896, Il genere Ascaris Linne. Lavoro monografico, Bollettino della Soc. Adriatica di Sci. Naturali in Trieste, 17:9-120.
Yorke, W., and Maplestone, P.A., 1926, "The nematode parasites of vertebrates," J.A. Churchill, London.

PLATYHELMINTHS

Daniel R. Brooks

Department of Zoology

University of British Columbia

INTRODUCTION

Amphibians and reptiles host a great variety of platyhelminth parasites, both adult and larval or juvenile stages (Tables 18.1 and 18.2). The association between amphibians and reptiles and their vast array of flatworms is long-standing judging from their geographical and host distribution. That the associations are successful may be confirmed by the marked paucity of reports linking platyhelminths as etiological agents of herptilian disease.

In general, the types and variety of adult platyhelminths parasitizing herptiles depends on 1) the feeding habits of the vertebrate host, and 2) the degree to which the vertebrate host is adapted to aquatic existence. Brandt (1936), Prokopic and Krivanec (1975) and Brooks (1976) all showed a marked correlation between the relative amount of time spent in association with aquatic habitats and the number of species of platyhelminths hosted by frogs. Because the majority of obligate intermediate hosts for platyhelminths are aquatic, those amphibians and reptiles preying on aquatic organisms are exposed more often to platyhelminth parasites than those preferring less aquatic prey. Amphibians and reptiles serve as ecological bridges (either by serving as second intermediate hosts or paratenic hosts) between invertebrate intermediate hosts and piscine, avian and mammalian definitive hosts. Thus, the types of larval or juvenile platyhelminths hosted by a particular herptile often reflects to a considerable degree the amount of predation upon that herptile

Table 18.1. Selected General Categories of Platyhelminth Parasites from Amphibians and Reptiles.

CESTODA

Order Proteocephalidea
    Genera: <u>Proteocephalus</u>, <u>Ophiotaenia</u>, <u>Testudotaenia</u>, <u>Batrachotaenia</u>, <u>Acanthotaenia</u>, <u>Kapsulotaenia</u>, <u>Crepidobothrium</u>, <u>Deblockotaenia</u>, <u>Tejidotaenia</u>
    Appearance and habitat: Small fragile worms in upper small intestine; larvae in viscera.
    Diagnosis: Finding eggs with onchospheres in feces.
    Transmission: Infection occurs when host ingests infected copepods or small fishes or amphibians. Larvae may become adults or penetrate stomach and encyst for a period in liver; they may then later excyst and penetrate intestine, becoming adults. Treatment regimes should consider the possibility of auto-infection into account because drugs aimed at eliminating intestinal forms may not eliminate larval forms in the liver.

Order Pseudophyllidea
    Genera: <u>Cephaloclamys</u>, <u>Duthiersia</u>, <u>Bothridium</u>, <u>Bothriocephalus</u>, <u>Spirometra</u> (sparganum)
    Appearance and habitat: Medium sized to large worms in small intestine; larvae in musculature or viscera.
    Diagnosis: Finding operculated eggs with ciliated larvae in feces.
    Transmission: Infection occurs when infected small fish or amphibians are ingested (adult forms) or when infected copepods are eaten (larval forms). No auto-infection phenomena have been documented for this group.

Order Anoplocephalidea
    Genera: <u>Oochoristica</u>, <u>Semenoviella</u>, <u>Diochetos</u>, <u>Pancerina</u>

Order Dilepididea
    Genus: <u>Ophiovalipora</u>
    Appearance and habitat: Small to medium sized worms in intestinal tract.
    Diagnosis: Finding anoperculate eggs with onchospheres in feces.
    Transmission: Infection occurs when infected mites (positively documented only for <u>Oochoristica</u>) are ingested. Two species of <u>Oochoristica</u> have been reported as occurring extra-intestinally on occasion.

Table 18.1. Selected General Categories of Platyhelminth Parasites from Amphibians and Reptiles. (Continued)

MONOGENEA

Order Gyrodactylidae
  Genus: Gyrodactylus
Order Polystomatidae
  Genera: Polystoma, Eupolystoma, Parapolystoma, Pseudopolystoma, Neopolystoma, Polystomoides, Polystomoidella, Beauchampia, Diplorchis, Neodiplorchis, Sphyranura
  Appearance and habitat: Microscopic to macroscopic worms attached to skin, gills, or in roof of mouth or urinary bladder.
  Diagnosis: Finding worms in situ, or finding onchomiracidia in feces.
  Transmission: Most monogeneans exhibit direct life cycles. Some polystomatids, however, display complex life cycles involving one generation of larval forms inhabiting the gills of larval anurans and a generation of adults occurring in the urinary bladders of adult anurans.

DIGENEA

Order (many, see Yamaguti, 1971)
  Appearance and habitat: Small soft-bodied worms in virtually any cavitied organ.
  Diagnosis: Finding operculate tanned eggs in feces.
  Transmission: Infection may occur in a variety of manners, all involving ingestion of a second intermediate host; the second intermediate host may be vegetation or a wide range of invertebrates or vertebrates.

ASPIDOGASTREA

Order Aspidogastridae
  Genera: Lophotaspis, Multicotyle, Cotylaspis, Lyssemysia
  Appearance and habitat: Small soft-bodied worms in small intestine.
  Diagnosis: Finding ciliated cotylocidia larvae in feces.
  Transmission: Infection occurs as a result of ingesting infected mollusks.

Table 18.1. Selected General Categories of Platyhelminth Parasites from Amphibians and Reptiles. (Continued)

AMPHILINIDEA

Order Austramphilinidae
    Genus: <u>Austramphilina</u>
        Appearance and habitat: Medium sized spatulate worms in body cavity.
        Diagnosis: Inapparent ante-mortem.
        Transmission: Unknown, possibly direct.

---

by a particular type of fish, bird or mammal. Factors intrinsic to phylogenetically related species of host also influence the kinds of platyhelminths infecting them. For instance, spirorchiid digeneans infect a variety of freshwater turtles. While a number of other types of amphibians and reptiles are sympatric with aquatic turtles having presumably similar degrees of exposure to the free-swimming infective spirorchiid larvae, only turtles are infected. Alternatively, there are no records of adult cestodes infecting crocodilians despite their aquatic and piscivorous habits which undoubtedly result in exposure to large numbers of larval and adult cestodes. Under the majority of natural circumstances, the relationship between amphibians or reptiles and the platyhelminths they host is one of functional co-accommodation. Just as in the case of predator-prey relationships, the loss of some individuals of either host or parasite is necessary for the continuing survival of both host and parasite populations. An individual case of maladaptation leading to such a loss may be of concern to a zoo curator, but it is not significant to natural populations.

DISTRIBUTION

The subject of distribution of platyhelminths infecting amphibians and reptiles covers three topics: geographical distribution, "among-host" distribution and "between-host" distribution. Each of these categories is examined separately.

Present geographical distributions of platyhelminths infecting herptiles apparently reflect cosmopolitan ancestral distributions achieved more than 200 million

Table 18.2. Major Monophyletic Groups of Amphibians and Reptiles Hosting Platyhelminth Parasites and Approximate Numbers of Species Hosted by Each Group. Numbers Refer Only to Platyhelminths Occurring as Adults in Amphibians and Reptiles.

	Digenea	Aspidogastrea	Monogenea	Cestoidea	Amphilinidea
Anura	400	0	30	30	0
Caudata	50	0	6	20	0
Gymnophiona	0	0	0	0	0
Chelonia	400	8	40	3	1
Crocodylia	60	0	0	0	0
Diapsida	0	0	0	0	0
Sauria	75	0	0	45	0
Ophidia	250	0	0	25	0

years ago (Brooks, 1977, 1978a, 1978b, 1979; Brooks and Overstreet, 1978). Many genera, such as the digenean genera Telorchis in freshwater turtles and Haematoloechus in frogs, are ubiquitous, occurring in nearly every locality of their vertebrate hosts. Other groups occur only in limited areas. Parasitic helminths are limited in their geographic range by the distribution and mobility of their least vagile obligate hosts. For many platyhelminths, that host is an aquatic mollusk or arthropod possessing a relatively limited distribution. Accordingly, many platyhelminth species infecting amphibians and reptiles are highly endemic. Therefore, it is possible to characterize such species without reference to their evolutionary histories.

For example, North American amphibians harbor species of the amphistome digenean genus Megalodiscus, South American amphibians host members of Catadiscus, and Old World amphibians host members of Diplodiscus. The most extensive compilations of host and locality data for described species include Yamaguti's (1959-1963) "Systema Helminthum" and his (1971) "Synopsis of Digenetic Trematodes of Vertebrates", plus the U.S. Department of Agriculture's "Index Catalogue of Medical and Veterinary Zoology". These references plus Tuff and Huffman (1977) contain little morphological information, but provide much useful information about parasites which might occur in a given host species in a given area.

For a particular species of platyhelminth to be host specific, it must be 1) tolerated by the host and tolerant of the host, and 2) exposed to the host in some manner relevant to its infective stages. The first reflects an historical phenomenon, i.e., the degree to which hosts and parasites have become co-accommodated with time. Most platyhelminths parasitize members of monophyletic groups at some level. For example, spirorchiid digeneans infect only turtles, although other reptiles are probably exposed to spirorchiid cercariae. Spirorchiids comprising the genus Vasotrema infect only soft-shelled turtles, Trionyx spp., even though other turtles are probably exposed to Vasotrema cercariae. Proteocephalid cestodes infecting salamanders are highly host-specific whereas Proteocephalus perspicua will survive in virtually any snake which ingests infected intermediate hosts (Brooks, 1978a).

The second aspect of "among-host" distribution includes the means by which herptilian hosts come into contact with infective stages of various platyhelminths. More of this will be presented below, but two general aspects pertain at this juncture. The degree of "aquaticness", or the relative amount of time a host spends in aquatic habitats bears directly on the number and variety of potential platyhelminth parasites to which it will be exposed; likewise, the feeding habits of those various hosts may enhance or diminish the probablity of exposure. A puzzling exception to this generalization is the absence of cestode, monogenean, aspidogastrid or amphilinidean parasites infecting crocodilians. Crocodilians are predominately aquatic, predominately piscivorous and voracious. Crocodilians do host a variety of digeneans (Brooks, 1979) which are highly specific for crocodilians.

Adult platyhelminths predominate in the alimentary canal from mouth to rectum, but not generally in the large intestine, and also occur in associated organs formed embryologically as gut (archenteron) outpocketings; lungs, bile ducts and gall bladder, urogenital system and gills. Blood flukes infecting turtles and a single amphilinidean occurring in turtle body cavities appear to be the only exceptions (Table 18.3). Carter and Etges (1973) and Shoop and Janovy (1978) reported adult cestodes, Oochoristica anolis and O. bivitellobata, respectively, occurring extraintestinally in lizard body cavities, but those are exceptional findings. Larval platyhelminths occur encysted in mesentery or muscle, or free or encysted in internal organs.

Digeneans are responsible for the bulk of the variety in infection sites. Cestodes and aspidogastrids rarely occur outside the intestine. Monogeneans occur on the gills, or in oral or urinary cavities; larval anurans may host Gyrodactylus spp. on their skins. The only known amphilinidean infecting an amphibian or reptilian host resides in the body cavity. Digeneans occur in every body region that platyhelminths are known to occur. However, each species exhibits marked site preference. Such site preference may be so specific that many different kinds of platyhelminths may co-exist in a given host. Schroeder and Ulmer (1959) demonstrated that five species of blood fluke, Spirorchis spp., occurred in turtles, but were spatially segregated by preferred site.

The specific geographical restrictions, host tolerances and infection-site preferences of platyhelminth parasites allow one to predict with great accuracy the types of flatworms likely to be hosted by a given herptile in natural conditions. Continuing surveys and faunal studies can only enhance those predictive abilities.

Table 18.3. Infection Sites Inhabited by Platyhelminths Infecting Amphibians and Reptiles According to Host Group.

Body Site	AN*	CA	CH	CR	SA	OP
Buccal cavity/gills	+	+	+	+	+	+
Esophagus				+		+
Stomach		+	+			
Small intestine	+	+	+	+	+	+
Gall bladder/bile ducts	+		+		+	+
Large intestine						
Rectum	+	+	+			+
Lungs	+	+	+			+
Urinary bladder/renal ducts	+	+	+			+
Oviducts			+			+
Circulatory system			+			
Body cavity			+			
Mesenteries (larvae)	+	+	+	+	+	+
Organs (larvae)	+	+	+	+	+	+
Musculature (larvae)	+	+	+	+	+	+

*AN=anura; CA=caudata; CH=chelonia; CR=crocodylia; SA=sauria; OP=ophidia

ETIOLOGY

Combes (1972) presented a study of the etiology of amphibian helminths, emphasizing the behavior of the amphibian host, primarily the degree of aquaticness and feeding habits. His model pertains directly to the etiology of platyhelminths infecting reptiles as well. Platyhelminth life cycles are considered to represent one of five classes according to mode of infection, i.e., direct or indirect, and type of food chain, i.e., totally aquatic, partially aquatic, partially terrestrial, and wholly terrestrial. Table 18.4 presents a brief summary of the kinds of platyhelminths infecting herptiles and using four of those five categories.

Parasitic platyhelminths infecting herptiles may be classed into three groups according to their potential significance as agents of disease. Those groups comprise 1) platyhelminths occurring as adults, 2) platyhelminths occurring as larval or juvenile forms and potentially affecting the health of the host in which they occur,

PLATYHELMINTHS

Table 18.4. Comparative Transmission Modes of Platyhelminths Infecting Amphibians and Reptiles.

Transmission Class	Example	Transmission Agent
Direct-wholly aquatic	Monogeneans	Oncomiracidium
	Spirorchiid digeneans	Cercaria
	Nematotaeniid cestodes	Oncosphere
	Aspidogastreans	Cotylocidium
Indirect-wholly aquatic[a]	Adult cestodes	Plerocercoid Cysticercoid
	Larval cestodes	Procercoid Plerocercoid
	Adult digeneans	Metacercaria
	Larval digeneans	Cercaria
	Aspidogastreans	Juvenile
Indirect-partially terrestrial[b]	Adult cestodes	Plerocercoid Cysticercoid
	Larval cestodes	Procercoid
	Adult digeneans	Metacercaria
	Larval digeneans	Cercaria
Indirect-wholly terrestrial	Adult cestodes	Cysticercoid
	Adult digeneans	Metacercaria

[a]Infect aquatic amphibians or reptiles.
[b]Infect semi-terrestrial or terrestrial vertebrates, aquatic intermediate hosts, or aquatic amphibians or reptiles.

and 3) platyhelminths occurring as larval or juvenile forms which represent potential health hazards to human beings.

Reichenbach-Klinke and Elkan (1965) listed a number of digenean metacercariae which occur encysted in various organs, including the brain, of amphibians and may adversely affect their health, making them easier prey for the larger vertebrates which serve as definitive hosts. Freeman et al. (1976) reported a human death resulting from ingestion of poorly cooked frogs' legs infected with mesocercariae of the digenean *Alaria americana*. However, the vast majority of platyhelminths, larval, juvenile or adult, apparently pose no threat in natural situations to their amphibian or reptile hosts.

PATHOLOGY

There are sparse data implicating platyhelminths as etiologic agents of disease syndromes in amphibians and reptiles (Reichenbach-Klinke and Elkan, 1965; Marcus, 1977). Pathological syndromes associated with platyhelminth infections are characterized by 1) occlusion of organ ducts or tubular openings, 2) secondary bacterial infections resulting from lesions caused by attachment organs, or 3) pathological alterations of organ tissues in which larval or adult platyhelminths reside or through which they migrate.

Kazacos and Fisher (1977) reported finding specimens of the digenean Styphlodora sp. occluding renal tubules of a boa constrictor, Boa constrictor, and associated with mineralized debris, tubular epithelial hyperplasia and chronic interstitial nephritis. Myers (1971) reported a similar occurrence. Pathological changes most commonly associated with platyhelminths occluding ductal organs include hyperplasia of the epithelium lining of the duct, chronic inflammation and decreased release of the glandular product. Under natural conditions, amphibians and reptiles infected with such massive numbers would not survive long. Encapsulation of the platyhelminth or its eggs, as in the case of spirorchiid digeneans, in various organ tissues with resulting fibrocytic response and possible decreased organ function characterizes pathological changes associated with tissue-dwelling platyhelminths (Greiner et al., 1980; Kiel, 1975; Toft and Schmidt, 1975).

TREATMENT

Most platyhelminth infections are asymptomatic and most drugs effective against them are fairly toxic. Treatment besides surgical excision of some larval forms is not generally indicated (Marcus, 1977). Larval forms producing visible nodules, such as metacercariae of Clinostomum spp. in frogs, may be excised surgically. Monogeneans occurring on the skin of larval or perennibranch amphibians may be removed by bathing amphibians in the narcotizing agent MS-222 or in 0.5 to 1.0% formalin. For intestinal forms, Marcus (1977) recommended treating cestodes with dichlorophen and leaving digeneans untreated. Kiel (1975) also noted that there was no effective chemotherapeutic agent for digeneans, but recommended administrations of aqueous solutions of nicosamide (157 mg/kg body weight) or bunamide (50 mg/kg) in two doses given two to four weeks apart for cestodes. Frye (1973) provided a fuller account of possible chemotherapeutic agents for use in captive reptiles' infections.

REFERENCES

Brandt, B.B., 1936, Parasites of certain North Carolina salientia, Ecol. Monogr., 6:491-532.

Brooks, D.R., 1976, Parasites of amphibians of the Great Plains, II. Platyhelminths of amphibians in Nebraska, Bull. Univ. Nebraska State Museum, 10:65-92.

Brooks, D.R., 1977, Evolutionary history of some plagiorchioid trematodes of anurans, Syst. Zool., 26: 277-289.

Brooks, D.R., 1978a, Systematic status of proteocephaliid cestodes from reptiles and amphibians in North America with descriptions of three new species, Proc. Helm. Soc. Washington, 45:1-28.

Brooks, D.R., 1978b, Evolutionary history of the cestode order Proteocephalidea, Syst. Zool., 27:312-323.

Brooks, D.R., 1979, Testing hypotheses of evolutionary relationships among parasitic helminths: The digeneans of crocodilians, Amer. Zool., 19: 1225-1238.

Brooks, D.R., and Overstreet, R.M., 1978, The family Liolopidae (Digenea), including a new genus and two new species from crocodilians, Int. J. Parasitol., 8:267-273.

Carter, O.S., and Etges, F.G., 1973, Extraintestinal adult cestodes from Anolis carolinensis, J. Parasitol., 59:1140-1141.

Combes, C., 1972, Influence of the behaviour of amphibians on helminth life cycles, Zool. J. Linn. Soc., 51 (Suppl. No. 1):151-170.

Freeman, R.S., Stuart, P.F., Cullen, J.B., Ritchie, A.C., Mildon, A., Fernandes, B.J., and Bonin, R., 1976, Fatal human infection with mesocercariae of the trematode Alaria americana, Amer. J. Trop. Med. Hyg., 25:803-807.

Frye, F.L., 1973, "Husbandry, medicine and surgery in captive reptiles," V.M. Publ. Co., Bonner Springs.

Greiner, E.C., Forrester, D.J., and Jacobson, E.R., 1980, Helminths of mariculture-reared green turtles from Grand Cayman, BWI, Proc. Helm. Soc. Washington, 47:142-144.

Kazacos, K.R., and Fisher, L.F., 1977, Renal stypthlodoriasis in a boa constrictor, J. Amer. Vet. Med. Ass., 171:876-878.

Kiel, J.L., 1975, A review of parasites from snakes, Southwest Vet., 28:209-220.
Marcus, L.C., 1977, Parasitic diseases in captive reptiles, in: "Current veterinary therapy," 6th ed., R. Kirk, ed., W.B. Saunders Co., Philadelphia.
Prokopic, J., and Krivanec, K., 1975, Helminths of amphibians, their interaction and host-parasite relationships, Acta Sci. Nar. Brno., 9:1-48.
Reichenbach-Klinke, H., and Elkan, E., 1965, "The principl diseases of lower vertebrates," Academic Press, New York.
Schroeder, P.J., and Ulmer, M.J., 1959, Host-parasite relationships of Spirorchis elegans Stunkard (Trematoda: Spirorchiidae), Proc. Iowa Acad. Sci., 66:443-454.
Shoop, W.L., and Janovy, J., Jr., 1978, Adult cestodes from the coelomic cavity of the teiid lizard, Cnemidophorus sexlineatus, J. Parasitol., 64: 561-562.
Toft, J.D., II, and Schmidt, R.E., 1975, Pseudophyllidean tapeworms in green tree pythons (Chondropython viridis), J. Zoo Anim. Med., 6:25-26.
Tuff, D.W., and Huffman, D.G., 1977, An index to the gener of hosts in Yamaguti's Systema Helminthum, Texas J. Sci., 28:161-191.
Yamaguti, S., 1959-1963, "Systema helminthum," Vol. 1-5, Interscience Publishing, New York.
Yamaguti, S., 1971, "Synopsis of digenetic trematodes of vertebrates," Keigaku Publ. Co., Tokyo.

NON-HEMOPARASITIC PROTOZOANS

Werner Frank

Department of Parasitology

University of Hohenheim

INTRODUCTION

Only a limited number of the numerous protozoan parasites described from reptiles and amphibians cause pathogenic processes or are the cause of death of poikilothermic animals. Few investigations exist dealing with such problems, while on the other hand, the majority of publications are descriptions of new species or reports of new hosts having been found for certain species. Detailed research was done until two decades back concerning only the morphology of the parasites and sometimes their life cycles, but relatively few publications can be found in which the host response was investigated and that only on the cellular level. Nothing is mentioned in these earlier publications concerning the humoral reactions. Since the late 1950s, more and more observations have been published in which the pathogenic capacity of parasites against cold-blooded vertebrates is taken into consideration.

In this chapter only such protozoans are mentioned which are not blood-inhabiting species. It is not always easy to separate blood protozoans from intestinal or tissue forms. A number of genera can be found in the tissues as vegetative forms like Saurocytozoon or the primary stages of Plasmodium, while on the other hand, the sexually differentiated stages, the gametocytes or gamonts, can be found only in blood corpuscles. Even in these cases where the parasites are normally exclusively to be found in the muscular system, there are known

Table 19.1. Classification of Protozoa Associated with Amphibians and Reptiles.

Classification	Name	Characteristics[a]
PHYLUM	Sarcomastigophora	With flagella, and/or pseudopodia; typically asexual propagation
Subphylum	Mastigophora	One or more flagella
Class	Zoomastigophorea	Heterotrophic, one to many flagella
Order	Kinetoplastida	One to two flagella, one mitochondrion, typically with kinetoplast
Family	Trypanosom(at)idae	One flagellum, many species with undulating membrane
Genus	Leptomonas	
Order	Proteromonadida	One or two pairs of flagella, one mitochondrion, cysts exist
Family	Proteromonadidae	
Genus	Proteromonas	
	Karotomorpha	
Order	Retortamonadida	Two to four flagella; mitochondrion and Golgi apparatus absent; all species are parasitic, cysts present
Family	Retortamonadidae	
Genus	Retortamonas	
	Chilomastix	
Order	Diplomonadida	Two nuclei and eight flagella in two symmetrically arranged groups in genera with two "karyomastigonts"; mitochondria and Golgi apparatus absent
Suborder	Enteromonadina	Only one "karyomastigont"
Family	Enteromonadidae	

NON-HEMOPARASITIC PROTOZOANS

Genus	Enteromonas		
	Trimitus		
Suborder	Diplomonadina		Two "karyomastigonts"
Family	Hexamitidae (syn. Octomitidae)		
Genus	Hexamita		
	Spironucleus		
	Giardia (syn. Lamblia)		
	Octomitus		
Order	Oxymonadida		One or more "karyomastigonts", each containing four flagella in two pairs, axostyle, mitochondrion, and Golgi apparatus absent; cysts in some species
Family	Polymastigidae		
Genus	Monocercomonoides		
Order	Trichomonadida		Four to six flagella, one recurrent flagellum forming typically an undulating membrane or the proximal part of the recurrent flagellum adherent to the body surface; parabasal apparatus and axostyle present; mitochondrion absent; sexual reproduction and cyst formation not known
Family	Monocercomonadidae		Three to five anterior flagella; recurrent flagellum free or in the proximal part in many species adherent to the surface of the body; some species with low undulating membrane; parabasal apparatus with variously shaped structure
Genus	Monocercomonas		

Table 19.1. Classification of Protozoa Associated with Amphibians and Reptiles. (Continued)

Classification	Name	Characteristics
Family	Hexamastix Hypotrichomonas Trichomonadidae	Four to six flagella; one recurrent flagellum forming an undulating membrane along the surface of the body
Genus	Trichomitus Tetratrichomonas Tritrichomonas	
Subphylum Class Order	Opalinata Opalinatea Opalinida	Numerous short flagella (cilia); two or many nuclei
Family Genus	Opalinidae Protoopalina Opalina Zelleriella Cepedea	
Subphylum	Sarcodina	With pseudopodia; flagella when present are temporary
Superclass	Rhizopoda	With pseudopodia of various organization
Class Order Suborder	Lobosea Amoebida Tubulina	Pseudopodia often as lobopodia No flagellate stage

Family	Endamoebidae	Parasitic in invertebrates and vertebrates; delicate endosome; cysts are typical
Genus	Entamoeba	
Family	Hartmannellidae	Lobopodia; cysts are formed; large endosome; free-living and parasitic
Genus	Hartmannella	
Suborder	Acanthopodina	With filipodia; cysts are formed; large endosome
Family	Acanthamoebidae	
Genus	Acanthamoeba	
Order	Schizopyrenida	Typically with temporary flagellate stages; large endosome
Family	Vahlkampfiidae	With lobopodia; cysts are formed
Genus	Naegleria	With temporary flagellate stage (two flagella)
	Vahlkampfia	Without flagellate stage
PHYLUM	Apicomplexa	With apical complex (polar ring(s), rhoptries, conoid, micronemes); vegetative and sexual multiplication
Class	Sporozoea	Infective stages are sporozoites; monoxenous (homoxenous) or heteroxenous
Subclass	Coccidia	Life cycle typically consisting of merogony, gametogony and sporogony; intracellular development
Order	Eucoccidiida	
Suborder	Adeleina	Macrogametocyte and microgametocyte form syzygy; one to four microgametes
Family	Klossiellidae	Parasitic in invertebrates and vertebrates

Table 19.1. Classification of Protozoa Associated with Amphibians and Reptiles. (Continued)

Classification	Name	Characteristics
Genus	Klossiella	
	Klossiab	
Suborder	Eimeriina	Macrogamete and microgamete developing independently; many microgametes; sporozoites typically enclosed in sporocyst within oocyst, rarely outside sporocyst; monoxenous (homoxenous) and/or heteroxenous
Family	Toxoplasm(at)idae	Life cycle heteroxenous (vertebrates as intermediate and definitive hosts); "tissue-cyst forming isosporoid coccidia"
Genus	Toxoplasma	Species from poikilothermic animals are of uncertain status
	Besnoitia	Reptiles function as intermediate host (and definitive host?)
Family	Sarcocystidae	Life cycle heteroxenous, similar to Toxoplasm(at)idae; reptiles function as intermediate and definitive host
Genus	Sarcocystis	
	Frenkelia	It is doubtful that reptiles are hosts
Family	Eimeriidae	Monoxenous; oocysts with solid walls; number of sporocysts and sporozoites are characteristic for each genus

	Genus	Eimeria	
		Isospora	
		Caryospora	
		Cyclospora	
		Hoarella	
		Octosporella	
		Pythonella	
		Wenyonella	
		Dorisiella	
		Tyzzeria	
		Globidium	
	Family	Cryptosporidiidae	
	Genus	Cryptosporidium	
PHYLUM		Myxospora (syn. Myxozoa)	Spores with one or more polar-capsules and coiled pole-filaments; spores of multicellular origin; all species are parasitic
	Class	Myxosporea	Spores with one to six (typically two) polar-capsules; coelozoic and histozoic species in poikilothermic vertebrates
	Order	Bivalvulida	Spore wall with two valves
	Suborder	Platysporina	Spores with two pole-capsules at one pole
	Genus	Myxobolus	
		Henneguya	
	Suborder	Bipolarina	Spores with two polar-capsules, one at each pole
	Genus	Myxidium	

Table 19.1. Classification of Protozoa Associated with Amphibians and Reptiles. (Continued)

Classification	Name	Characteristics
PHYLUM	Microspora	Unicellular, spores with polar tube and polar cap; without polar-capsule; mitochondria absent
Class Order Suborder Genus Suborder Genus	Microsporea Microsporida Pansporoblastina Pleistophora Apansporoblastina "Microsporidium"	Collecting group of species insufficiently known (Glugea, Nosema, Pleistophora-pro parte)
PHYLUM	Ciliophora	Two types of nuclei (macro- and micro-); numerous cilia or ciliary organelles typically in at least one stage of the life cycle; binary fission transverse, sexual conjugation; cysts formed in many species; for classification of the members found in or on amphibians and reptiles see text

[a] Characteristics of the parasitic members only.
[b] The report of Klossia pachyleparon from Varanus nebulosus (Colley and Else, 1975) is the first species of this genus found in a vertebrate host, although it may be a spurious finding.

examples where trophozoites are transitory in the peripheral blood, e.g. Sarcocystis chamaeleonis (Frank, 1966a). In spite of these facts the chapter will deal with the protozoan groups and species listed in Table 19.1. Many new findings during the last few years show that the systematic grouping of organisms is not a steady one (Baker, 1977; Honigberg et al., 1964; Levine, 1970; Levine et al., 1980; Tadros and Laarman, 1976, 1982).

The life cycles of the various protozoan groups are different. The more primitive ones like the Mastigophora and the Sarcodina show only vegetative cell divisions either as binary fission (Flagellates) or sometimes multiple division (Entamoeba). In the Apicomplexa vegetative multiplication (merogony) happens as well as sexual propagation (gamogony). Many protozoans are monoxenous (homoxenous) while others are heteroxenous using vectors as intermediate hosts or they transport the infective stages to a new host. It is possible also that the intermediate host belongs to the food chain of the definitive host. Species passing into the environment often form resistant cysts or "spores".

PHYLUM SARCOMASTIGOPHORA
SUBPHYLUM MASTIGOPHORA

Members of the Zoomastigophorea belong to various orders: Kinetoplastida (mainly blood-inhabiting forms), Proteromonadida, Retortamonadida, Diplomonadida, Oxymonadida, Trichomonadida (Table 19.2). Many of these species are parasites as inhabitants of the intestinal tract of warm-blooded hosts as well as of poikilothermic animals, but the majority are parasites of invertebrates. With few exceptions, the flagellates of vertebrates live more or less as commensals in particular parts of the intestine while they prefer the cloacal ampulla in amphibians and reptiles. In reptiles they are common inhabitants of the intestinal tract and can be detected easily during postmortem examination. They have been mentioned always when such studies have been conducted. Jones (1980) reported that large numbers of flagellates are always found in the intestines of reptiles but none are found associated with mucosal lesions in the specimens examined. Up to a few years ago it was generally believed that flagellates caused no disease in amphibians and reptiles, and Telford (1971) mentioned the apathogenicity of these organisms found in reptiles. But at least one species, Hexamita parva, causes a disease, hexamitiasis, in chelonians (Zwart and Truyens, 1975).

Table 19.2. Distinguishing Criteria of the Various Flage.

Genus	Total number of flagella; recurrent flagella ( )	Number of nuclei	Undulating membrane
Leptomonas	1	1	-
Proteromonas	2 (1)	1 Anterior 1/4	-
Karotomorpha	4	1 Anterior 1/3	-
Chilomastix	4 (1) Short	1 Anterior	-
Retortamonas	2 (1)	1 Anterior	-
Enteromonas	4 (1) Longer than body	1 Anterior	-
Trimitus	3 (1) Longer than body	1 Anterior	-
Hexamita	8 (2)	2 Anterior	-
Spironucleus	8 (2)	2 Anterior	-
Giardia	8 (2)	2 Anterior	-
Octomitus	8 (2)	2 Anterior	-
Monocercomonoides	4 in 2 sep. pairs (1 or more)	1	-
Monocercomonas	4 (1)	1	-
Hexamastix	6 (1)	1	-
Hypotrichomonas	4 (1)	1	+ Shallow, shorter than body
Trichomitus	4 (1)	1	+
Tetratrichomonas	5 (1)	1	+ As long as body
Tritrichomonas	4 (1)	1	+

late Protozoan Genera from Amphibia and Reptilia.

Number of mitochondria	Cyst nuclei ( )	Axostyle	Golgi apparatus
1	-	-	-
1 Around nucleus	+ (1)	-	+ Ant. of nucleus
1	+ (1)	-	+ Ant. of nucleus
-	+	-	-
-	+	-	-
-	+	-	-
-	?	-	-
-	+	-	-
-	+ (4)	-	-
-	+	-	-
-	+	-	-
-	+ (1)	+	-
-	-	+	+
-	-	+	+
-	-	+	+
-	-	+	+
-	-	+	+
-	-	+	+

Table 19.2. Distinguishing Criteria of the Various Flagel (Continued)

Genus	Parabasal apparatus	Kinetosomes (basal bodies)
Leptomonas	-	1
Proteromonas	-	2 Orthogonally arranged
Karotomorpha	-	2 Pairs
Chilomastix	-	4
Retortamonas	-	4
Enteromonas	-	2 Pairs
Trimitus	-	3
Hexamita	-	2 Pairs opposed in each mastigont
Spironucleus	-	2 Pairs opposed in each mastigont
Giardia	-	2 Pairs in association between nuclei
Octomitus	-	2 Pairs opposed in each mastigont

late Protozoan Genera from Amphibia and Reptilia.

Body form	Cytostome	Remarks
Slender	-	With kinetoplast, a DNA containing part of the single mitochondrion
Elongated, pointed posteriorly	-	Food obtained by pinocytosis
Carrot shaped	-	Food obtained by pinocytosis
Pyriform, ant. rounded	1 Conspicuous ant. part	All kinetosomes equipped with flagella; recurrent flagellum associated with cytostome
Pyriform, ant. rounded	1 Conspicuous ant. part	Four kinetosomes are present, only two possess flagella, the others are barren
Pyriform	1 Shallow	Recurrent flagellum protrudes through cytostomal groove
Pyriform	1 Shallow	Probably similar to Enteromonas
Pyriform or ovoid	2	Axially symmetrical diplomonads with double set of organelles; each recurrent flagellum traverses one cytostome, emerges posteriorly as free-trailing flagellum, with 8 flagella altogether
Elongated, tapered posteriorly	2 Narrow	
Pear-shaped	-	With adhesive disk ventrally; 2 flagella emerge ventrally, 2 antero-laterally, 2 postero-laterally and 2 caudally
Broadly ovoid, caudally protruding in short spike	-	Axially symmetrical diplomonads with 8 flagella, 2 nuclei and double set of organelles

Table 19.2. Distinguishing Criteria of the Various Flage
(Continued)

Genus	Parabasal apparatus	Kinetosomes (basal bodies)
Monocercomonoides	--	2 Separate groups
Monocercomonas	+	--[a]
Hexamastix	+ Janicki type	--
Hypotrichomonas	+	--
Trichomitus	+	--
Tetratrichomonas	+	--
Tritrichomonas	+	--

[a]Possess kinetosomal complexes, individual kinetosomes cannot be seen by light microscopy.

The flagellates are acquired by a new host via food or water contaminated with infectious stages. The life cycles are simple and sexual processes are lacking. The multiplication is a typical binary fission of the trophozoites parallel to the longer axis of the cell. Cysts or resting stages are present in certain groups.

On the other hand, the diet of the host probably influences the establishment of infection (Kulda and Nohynkova, 1978). But this is only the result of proper physico-chemical conditions depending on the associated bacterial flora. It seems that in poikilothermic animals, as well as in mammals, a carbohydrate diet is more favorable than the uptake of much protein by feeding on insects or other prey. As mentioned above, the effect is only an indirect one of changes in the bacterial flora induced by the different resources. Peterson (1960) postulated that the density of intestinal bacteria is the most important factor influencing the reproduction of intestinal flagellates. A derangement of the equilibrium between

late Protozoan Genera from Amphibia and Reptilia.

Body form	Cytostome	Remarks
Ovoid	-	Recurrent flagellum accompanied by funis and adhered with its anterior part to the body surface
Ovoid	-	Recurrent flagellum free or adherent with proximal part to body surface; without costa
Ovoid	-	Recurrent flagellum not adhered to the body surface; without costa
Ovoid	-	Without costa
Ovoid	-	With costa
Ovoid	-	With costa
Ovoid	-	With costa

the number of bacteria and flagellates can cause an unchecked multiplication of the protozoans and the preferences for particular regions of the intestine may be lost.

In such cases, the otherwise harmless commensals may change into forms with pathogenicity in parts of the midintestine. The result is damage to the mucosa. In the feces blood coagulums or digested blood can be found. It is scarcely understood whether the flagellates are really pathogenic or only secondary invaders to a pathological condition of another etiology. The significance of such reports, as for example Frank (1976a,b), is of minor value since experimental evidence is lacking.

The sporadic reports of pathological destructions due to certain flagellates normally not known as pathogens probably are the result of particular conditions in a certain host caused by various factors. The often extreme conditions of captivity may be the reason for such findings in exhibited amphibians and reptiles. It would be urgent to investigate the flagellate infections of poikilothermic animals to find out either the facts leading to the change in the behavior of these organisms or whether there are a number of typical pathogenic species. For the many species described see Walton (1964, 1966, 1967).

Order Kinetoplastida
Family Trypanosomatidae

Members of the order Kinetoplastida are characterized by possession of a kinetoplast, a DNA-containing structure in the single mitochondrion close to the basal bodies of the flagella. All species have one or two flagella, pseudopodia are absent. The single vesicular nucleus shows a prominent endosome. Most of the species are parasites of invertebrates as well as vertebrates. A number of them are free-living under more or less anaerobic conditions. Species of the Trypanosomatidae are known to cause serious diseases of domestic animals and of man (genera Trypanosoma and Leishmania).

Leptomonas. Species of this genus are parasitic in invertebrates, mainly arthropods; the vast majority in insects. Wallace (1966, 1979) published a comprehensive study of these forms. Leptomonads have only two stages in their life cycle, the promastigote and the amastigote, often misinterpreted as a cyst. They are monogenetic. There exists some taxonomic confusion between Leptomonas and Herpetomonas (Wallace, 1966). The flagellates are usually found in the gut content of their invertebrate hosts and more rarely in the hemocoel or the salivary glands.

Leptomonas spp. from vertebrates are a group of organisms difficult to be discussed, since up to now they have been insufficiently characterized. It seems doubtful that stages found in the hindgut of lizards can be classified as true stages of Leptomonas. Vickerman (1976) called them "Leptomonas-like flagellates". Such flagellates can be found not rarely in the hindgut of chameleons kept in terraria where they may cause a colitis (Frank, 1976a), but unfortunately, nothing is known concerning the circumstances which change the behavior of these flagellates in captive reptiles from a commensalic to a parasitic and facultatively pathogenic way of life. In such animals the flagellates have extended to the midgut and the gut contents consist only of a clean culture of leptomonads mixed with a mass of the intestinal mucosa is the typical finding in these chameleons.

Leptomonads are common in the intestinal tract of chameleons (Brygoo, 1963; Vickerman, 1965). Pathological destructions have not been mentioned in chameleons from the wild. It is questionable in what respect the finding of a Leptomonas sp. in the gut and blood of a New World iguanid, Anolis carolinensis, can be accepted (Leger, 1918). The pathogenicity of Leptomonas spp. in chameleons observed in captivity is of interest for keepers (to cure the lizards), but possibly it is only the result of the changed environment in which the lizards live (humidity, temperature, etc.) and food. These most primitive trypanosomatids come from insects fed on by the lizards. Until further information is available the leptomonads are to be characterized as secondary invaders with facultative pathogenicity probably only for caged chameleons. Dollahon and Janovy (1971) investigated the gut contents of several Basiliscus, Ameiva, Cnemidophorus and Anolis and showed clearly that insect flagellates, Leptomonas and/or Herpetomonas, do persist in the lizard intestine for several days. To classify the relationship between Leptomonas spp. from reptiles it would be necessary to establish clone cultures and experimental infections in insects and chameleons. It is questionable if the species mentioned by Reichenbach-Klinke and Elkan (1965), particularly from Reichenow (1953), are all valid leptomonads.

If still in good health, chameleons may be cured of leptomonad infection with metronidazole drugs. These compounds are useful also against other flagellate infections of the intestinal tract as well as against amoebae.

Order Proteromonadida
Family Proteromonadidae

The former classification of the proteromonadids together with the trypanosomatids and bodonids in the one order Kinetoplastida cannot be accepted any longer. The wrongly termed "parabasal body", sometimes identified with a kinetoplast, is a large mitochondrion. But despite its basophilic properties it does not possess a morphologically differentiated area rich in DNA like the typical mitochondrial structure of the Kinetoplastida. A newly published classification of the Protozoa (Levine et al., 1980) accommodated these facts. The proteromonadids are now grouped in a separate order of their own with the single family Proteromonadidae. For detailed characterization see Kulda and Nohynkova (1978).

Only two genera of this family may be valid ones. They are parasites of amphibians and reptiles and of a few mammals. Karotomorpha is restricted to Amphibia while Proteromonas is also found in Reptilia. The species of both genera are flagellates inhabiting the intestine

Table 19.3. Species of Proteromonas.[a]

Species	Host	Geographic distribution
P. lacertae-viridis (syn. Schizobodo tarentolae, P. hemidactyli, P. ophisauri, P. uromastixi, P. chameleoni)	Snakes and many lizard genera, e.g., Iguana, Phrynosoma, Sceloporus, Xantusia, Chamaeleo, Tarentola, Hemidactylus, Ophisaurus, Uromastix	North, Central and South America; Europe; Africa
P. longifila	Urodelan and anuran amphibians, e.g., Ambystoma jeffersonianum, A. maculatum, A. opacum, A. mexicanum, Desmognathus fuscus, Triturus spp., Salamandra spp., Rana pipiens	North America; Europe
P. regnardi	Emys orbicularis	Europe
P. kakatiyae	Hemidactylus sp.	India
P. warangalensis	Mabuya carinata	India

[a]Sources: Flynn, 1973; Kulda and Nohynkova, 1978; Rao et al., 1978a.

of their hosts. They can be found preferably in the cloacal ampulla where they live as commensals. Up to now no pathological destructions are described.

It seems that similar to other intestinal flagellates the number of proteromonadids found in a host depends on the physico-chemical condition of the gut content. It is not uncommon during post-mortem examination to observe nearly pure cultures of these flagellates not only in the hindgut but also extended to the end of the midgut. This suggests that the mass reproduction of these flagellates has its origin in other disturbances of the intestinal tract, perhaps in a bacterial infection. Based on this reflection, the proteromonadids are only secondary invaders of other parts of the intestine than the cloacal region, but possibly they make worse the primary alterations.

<u>Proteromonas</u>. The species are biflagellate with the origin of both flagella in the anterior part of the cell. One flagellum is recurrent. The trophozoit is an elongated cell more or less pointed posteriorly. Multiplication occurs by longitudinal binary fission. Uninucleate spherical or oval cysts with thickened walls are formed.

Species of <u>Proteromonas</u> can be found in lizards, snakes, tortoises and urodelan amphibians (Table 19.3). If Anura can be infected has to be verified. Differentiating features among species are body size, location of the nucleus, location, size and shape of the large mitochondrion and of the Golgi apparatus. The relative length of the flagella is a further criterion. The size of the species differs from only a few microns up to about 25 microns. It seems possible that the size of the cells may be influenced by the environmental gut contents.

In reptiles, <u>P</u>. <u>lacertae-viridis</u> has a wide host range and geographic distribution. Up to now it is doubtful whether other species in reptiles exist and whether <u>P</u>. <u>longifila</u> from mainly urodelan amphibians is a separate species or only a synonym for <u>P</u>. <u>lacertae-viridis</u> (Kulda and Nohynkova, 1978). Despite these arguments new species have been described from Indian lizards (Rao et al., 1978a). The four other species from reptiles, now synonymized with <u>P</u>. <u>lacertae-viridis</u>, were accepted by these authors as valid species. While <u>P</u>. kakatiyae looks similar to other proteromonadids, <u>P</u>. <u>warangalensis</u> has a different appearance. These latter organisms are more or less ball-like, only few of the pictured specimens show a somewhat pointed posterior end. Flynn (1973) listed a further species, <u>P</u>. <u>regnardi</u> from the European pond turtle, <u>Emys</u>

Table 19.4. Species of Karotomorpha.[a]

Species	Host	Geographic distribution
K. bufonis (syn. K. swezyi, K. ambystomae)	Anura and Urodela, e.g., Rana pipiens, Bufo americanus, B. bufo, Ambystoma tigrinum, A. mexicanum, Desmognathus fuscus, Triturus helveticus, T. torosus, T. viridescens	North America; Europe

[a]Sources: Flynn, 1973; Kulda and Nohynkova, 1978.

orbicularis not mentioned in the comprehensive review given by Kulda and Nohynkova (1978). Further investigation is necessary to clear-up whether the differences between the species are stable ones or whether they are influenced by external factors.

Karotomorpha. Synonyms for this genus include Monocercomonas, Tetramitus, Tetramastix and Polymastix. The few species described possess four flagella in two groups. All arise from the anterior part of the cell. One flagellum is recurrent. The body of the trophozoite is carrot-shaped and posteriorly pointed. The organisms are about 12 to 16 microns long and 2 to 6 microns wide. Multiplication is by longitudinal binary fission. Uninucleate spherical or oval, thick-walled cysts are formed. The karotomorphs are non-pathogenic parasites (commensals) in the hindgut and cloacal ampulla of various amphibians from America and Europe. It is to be expected that these flagellates may be found also in amphibians from other zoogeographical areas. It seems that all species described are synonymous to the one K. bufonis with possibly worldwide distribution (Table 19.4). The differences between the supposed species were misinterpretations of certain structures.

Order Retortamonadida
Family Retortamonadidae

The single family Retortamonadidae represents the order which includes only two genera: Retortamonas and Chilomastix. None of the species are really pathogenic to their hosts, in which they live as commensals of the digestive tract. Retortamonas is restricted to a few mammals including man, as well as amphibians, reptiles and insects. Chilomastix may be found in all five classes of vertebrates and in a few invertebrates (termites and leeches, Aulastomum). Some authors suggest that two species have a potential pathogenicity: C. mesnili for man and C. gallinarum for poultry.

The trophozoite of these flagellates is an uninucleate, mobile, pyriform cell, anteriorly rounded and posteriorly elongated. Two (Retortamonas) or four (Chilomastix) flagella are present, one of which is always recurrent. Four kinetosomes (basal bodies) exist in both genera, but in Retortamonas only two are associated with flagella. A conspicuous cytostome united with the recurrent flagellum is typical for these organisms. In Chilomastix it is shorter than the three free ones. The free flagella are inserted anteriorly. The trophozoites multiply by longitudinal binary fission. A pyriform or ovoid cyst with a thick wall is the second stage in the life cycle. Cysts are passed with the feces and are the infectious stages.

Differentiating features of the species are the relative length and thickness of the flagella, the size of the cell and the cytostome. Revision of the family would doubtless reveal several synonyms among the species since they have a wide host range and possibly a wide geographical distribution (Tables 19.5 and 19.6).

Order Diplomonadida
Suborder Enteromonadina
Family Enteromonadidae

This family was established by Kulda and Nohynkova (1978) and was accepted by Levine et al. (1980) in the newly revised classification of Protozoa. The family includes tiny flagellates of three genera, two of them, Enteromonas and Trimitus (Table 19.7), are harmless commensals in the digestive tract of amphibians and reptiles. The pyriform flagellates are very small, frequently less than 5 microns in length and only 2 to 3 microns in width. The number of flagella is four for Enteromonas and three for Trimitus, in both genera one longer flagellum is recurrent, adherent to the body in the beginning but free-trailing at the end. A delicate cytostome is present. Up to now oval-shaped cysts only have been found in Enteromonas, but surely they also exist in Trimitus. The cysts possess four nuclei if they are fully developed. Some similarities to the Hexamitidae seen by electron microscopic investigations show the close relationship between the Enteromonadidae and the Hexamitidae, but they only possess one karyomastigont instead of the two in the Hexamitidae.

Order Diplomonadida
Suborder Diplomonadina
Family Hexamitidae

Much taxonomic confusion existed in this family as indicated by several names of the various genera, now listed as synonyms. Recently published investigations with the electron microscope, together with light microscopic studies, revealed the possibility to differentiate the genera exactly (Kulda and Nohynkova, 1978). The family consists of six genera, two of them are free-living or saprozoic (Trepomonas, Trigonomonas), members of Hexamita are free-living as well as parasitic, and species of the other three genera are exclusively parasitic (Spironucleus,

Table 19.5. Species of Retortamonas (syn. Embadomonas).[a]

Species	Host	Geographic distribution
R. boae	Boa constrictor	Central and South America
R. dobelli (syn. R. saurarum)	Rana pipiens, R. clamitans, R. catesbeiana, R. temporaria, Acris gryllus, Bufo bufo, Salamandra spp., newts, Natrix spp., Pituophis melanoleucus, Thamnophis spp., Heloderma suspectum	North America; Europe
R. cheloni	Testudo elegans	India
R. testudae	Tortoises	Asia
R. viperae	Vipera russellii	India
Retortamonas sp.	Tortoises	South America

[a]Source: Flynn, 1973; Krishnamurthy and Madre, 1976; Kulda and Nohynkova, 1978.

Table 19.6. Species of Chilomastix.[a]

Species	Host	Geographic distribution
C. bursa (syn. C. wenyoni)	Calotes nemoricola, Phrynosoma spp., Sceloporus spp., Xantusia spp.	Asia; Mexico; United States of America
C. caulleryi	Anuran and urodelan amphibians, e.g., Rana pipiens, Bufo bufo, Ambystoma maculata, A. mexicanum, A. tigrinum, Salamandra spp., Triturus spp.	United States of America; Europe
C. gigantea (syn. C. caulleryi?)	Salamandra spp., Pseudotriton sp.	Europe
C. quadrii (similar to C. bursa)	R. tigrina, R. cyanophlyctis	India
Chilomastix sp.	Tortoises and turtles	United States of America
Chilomastix sp.	Lacertidae	North Africa
C. hemidactyli	Hemidactylus giganteus	India

[a]Source: Flynn, 1973; Kulda and Nohynkova, 1978; Madre, 1979; Rao et al., 1976a.

Table 19.7. Species of Enteromonadidae.[a]

Species	Host	Geographic distribution
Enteromonas (syn. Tricercomonas) Enteromonas sp.	Triturus vulgaris	Europe
Trimitus (syn. Alexeiefella) T. ranae (syn. T. parvus?)	Urodelan and anuran amphibians, Rana pipiens, R. temporaria, Bufo bufo, Triturus viridescens, Thamnophis radix	North America; Europe
T. trionici (syn. T. corralesi, A. cheloni)	Tortoises, Kinosternon scorpioides	North America; India

[a]Source: Kulda and Nohynkova, 1978.

Giardia syn. Lamblia, Octomitus). In amphibians and reptiles species of all four parasitic genera may be found in part potentially pathogenic.

All members of this family are axially symmetrical diplomonads which possess two karyomastigonts with a total of eight flagella, two nuclei and a double set of accessor organelles. The eight flagella are arranged anteriorly in two complexes. Two of the flagella are recurrent through the body of the organism but emerge posteriorly to become free-trailing. The shape of the trophozoites is pyriform or ovoid. Cytostomes exist only in members of the subfamily Hexamitinae while they are absent in the Giardiinae. The life cycle of the Hexamitidae include two stages, the trophozoite and the cyst, both of which are able to divide by longitudinal binary fission. Fully developed cysts always contain four nuclei and the corresponding accessory organelles.

The hexamitids are mainly parasites of the digestive tract of all five classes of vertebrates where they live purely extracellular, multiplying solely by binary fission Reports of intracellular multiplication are misinterpretations of artifacts or stages of other parasites, etc.

Hexamita. Synonyms for this genus include Diceromonas, Hexamitus, Octomastix, Octomitus and Urophagus. The trophozoites possess six flagella at the anterior end and two recurrent flagella which protrude caudally and continue as long trailing flagella. The body is ovoid or pyriform; two nuclei and two tube-like cytostomes are present. The trophozoites vary in size from species to species, but rarely reach more than 10 microns in the long axis. H. intestinalis measures 5 to 10 microns by 3 to 7 microns, while H. parva only 4 to 9 microns by 1 to 3 microns. A detailed description of the morphology including the ultrastructure of these flagellates is given by Kulda and Nohynkova (1978).

Species of this genus are both free-living and parasitic in various vertebrates as well as in invertebrates (Table 19.8). The incidence of infected amphibians may be as high as approximately 40% (Flynn, 1973). Non-pathogenic H. intestinalis often inundates not only the intestinal fluid, but also the gall of healthy Rana esculenta (Reichenbach-Klinke and Elkan, 1965). Pathogenicity has been reported only for a few species. In amphibians and reptiles only one species, H. parva, may be pathogenic to various speices of chelonians (Zwart and Truyens, 1975), but as Kulda and Nohynkova pointed out H. parva (syn. H.

Table 19.8. Species of the Subfamily Hexamitinae.[a]

Species	Host	Geographic distribution
Hexamita intestinalis (syn. Octomitus dujardini, H. ovatus)	Anuran and urodelan amphibians, e.g., Rana pipiens, R. temporaria, R. catesbeiana, R. esculenta, Bufo bufo, Hyla crucifer, Ambystoma maculatum, A. opacum, A. mexicanum, Desmognathus fuscus, Triturus torosus, T. viridescens, T. cristatus	United States of America; Asia; Europe
H. parva	Amphibians and chelonians, e.g., Cuora spp., Emys spp., Terrapene spp., Geoemyda spp., Clemmys spp., R. pipiens, B. americanus, A. tigrinum, A. maculatum, D. fuscus, T. torosus, T. viridescens	World-wide?
Spironucleus elegans (syn. O. dujardini, H. ovatus)	Anuran and urodelan amphibians	World-wide?

[a]Source: Flynn, 1973; Kulda and Nohynkova, 1978.

parvus, H. batrachorum, Octomitus dujardini, Octomastix parvus, O. decipiens) may be found in quite healthy amphibians and possibly in healthy chelonians. It seems that suitable conditions for the flagellates in the hosts and unsuitable environmental conditions for the hosts are necessary prerequisites for the infection to take a turn for the worse.

Grasse (1924) observed that H. parva, living as a commensal in many amphibians and particulary in aquatic chelonians, may cause marked epithelial desquamation in the urinary bladder of infected European tortoises, and suggested that these flagellates might be pathogenic to their hosts. The organisms found by Grasse were mainly in the intestinal tract but also occurred frequently in the urinary bladder of aquatic chelonians where they were numerous in the mucus excreted from the bladder wall. Similar observations did not come into account until Zwart and Truyens (1975) and Zwart et al. (1975) published detailed descriptions of the pathological changes observed in infected chelonians. They reported hexamitiasis caused by H. parva in nine chelonians belonging to eight different species: Testudo horsfieldii, T. marginata, Geochelone elegans, G. carbonaria, Cuora amboinensis, Terrapene ornata, Rhinoclemys p. punctularia and Mauremys caspica leprosa. All specimens had been kept in captivity for a long period of time.

The flagellates can be found in various organs, e.g., intestinal tract, biliary ducts of the liver, gall bladder urinary ducts of the kidneys and urinary bladder. It seems that the disease affects all organs which have an open connection with the intestinal tract. The urinary system appears to be particularly affected. The kidneys are in most cases markedly enlarged and flagellates can be seen in collecting ducts as well as in tubules, but normally they are absent in such regions which show signs of regeneration. The infection of the animals takes place after uptake of cysts from the contaminated environment and lasts for weeks or months.

Clinical signs of hexamitiasis are not characteristic with diseased chelonians being apathetic and experiencing weight loss.

Pathological alterations can be seen in the affected organs, but they are particularly pronounced in the kidneys. These organs are enlarged and they look pale. The renal tubules are dilated and may be seen with the naked eye. The tubules are filled up with innumerable parasites, cell debris and inflammatory cells. Acute, subacute and chronic changes can be observed in the epithelial cells as well as in the surrounding tissue, which is edematous and infiltrated by granulocytes (pseudoeosinophilic) and lymphocytes. The glomeruli always show damaged structures with cellular infiltration. Vascularization in the liver and periductal fibrosis in the parenchyma result after the invasion of flagellates into the bilary ducts. The epithelium of the ducts shows proliferation.

The disease follows an infection apparently originating from the intestinal tract, the primary site for these and related flagellates. It affects adjacent organs with direct tubular connection with the gut system. Destructions in the intestinal epithelium are rarely found. Only small, isolated ulcerations in the midgut and solitary desquamations and hypertrophic proliferations in the colon epithelium are described.

The process of disease is slowly progressing and death occurs mainly due to nephritis. Experimental evidence of the disease is lacking. It has been suggested that environmental conditions are necessary prerequisites but these are difficult to reproduce. Possibly a certain bacterial flora in the intestinal tract is fundamental to establish pathogenicity of these flagellates as are other factors. Debilitated animals harbor more of these flagellates than do healthy animals. Ronidazole is an effective d

Spironucleus. These flagellates represent the features of the family. The trophozoites are elongate, pear-shaped and more or less pointed posteriorly. The organisms measure between 5 and 12 microns by 2 to 5 microns. All species are parasitic and several of them are potentially pathogenic to their hosts, however, none of the species are known to cause disease in amphibians or reptiles (Table 19.8).

Giardia. Synonyms for this genus include Lamblia, Cercomonas, Dicercomonas, Hexamita and Megastoma. Flagellates of this genus differ from other genera in having an adhesive disk on the ventral surface of their body. With the help of this organelle they are able to suck at the epithelial cells of the digestive tract. It is believed that these organisms are the most evolved group of the Hexamitidae. All species are parasitic in vertebrates and are potentially pathogenic at least in some species. The disease they may cause is a type of diarrhea. For amphibians and reptiles pathological effects are unknown.

The trophozoites of Giardia look pear-shaped with a rounded anterior and pointed posterior end, but they represent only half of such a fruit. The ventral surface is more or less flattened and consists of the already mentioned adhesive disk. The dorsal side is convex as opposed to the concave ventral surface. The other characteristics are those of the family; cytostomes are absent (Kulda and Nohynkova, 1978). The swimming movements of these flagellates are typical and look staggering like a continuously turning cup.

The life cycle of Giardia includes two stages, the trophozoite and the ovoid cyst. Multiplication takes place in both stages by binary fission. Despite the fact descriptions of about 40 species are available, only a few seem to be valid. Up to now much taxonomic confusion existed. While certain authors postulate a rigid host specificity and believe that Giardia spp. of each host are independent species, other workers distinguish only three species. Both concepts appear to be incorrect. It can be supposed that the genus Giardia by analogy to other flagellates may include host-specific species as well as -ipecies without or with only low host-specificity. Most members of the genus Giardia live in the upper part of the small intestine attached to the epithelial cells. The size of the trophozoites varies from species to species. The most common G. agilis, from anuran tadpoles, has a probable world-wide distribution and represents a very slender form being about 18 to 22 microns long and only 5 microns wide. The few species accepted as valid by Kulda an Nohynkova (1978) from amphibians and reptiles are listed together with Octomitus species in Table 19.9.

Octomitus. The species of this genus also are improperly named as Hexamita and its synonyms. The main differences between members of this genus and Giardia are their broadly pear-shaped body and the short spike-like structure protruding the cell caudally. This intensively stainable structure is the posterior part of an axial rod, the columna. Cytostomes are absent like in Giardia. All species are harmless commensals of vertebrates. Probably all described species belong to O. neglectus with a suggested world-wide distribution.

Table 19.9. Species of the Subfamily Giardiinae.[a]

Species	Host	Geographic distribution
Giardia agilis	Tadpoles of anuran and urodele amphibians, e.g., Rana temporaria, R. esculenta, Xenopus laevis	World-wide?
G. serpentis	Causus rhombeatus, Lampropeltis spp.	Africa; United States of America
G. varani	Varanus niloticus, V. bengalensis	Africa; Asia
Octomitus neglectus (syn. O. dujardini, Hexamitus hoarei)	Anuran and urodele amphibians	World-wide?

[a]Source: Kulda and Nohynkova, 1978.

Order Oxymonadida
Family Polymastigidae (syn.: Monocercomonoididae)

The members of this flagellate family have been found predominantly in insects. Only several species of the genus Monocercomonoides inhabit the intestinal tract of certain vertebrates (amphibians, reptiles and mammals). The organisms live as harmless parasites in the intestinal contents. Pathogenic species are not known.

The oxymonads possess in the trophozoite stage only one karyomastigont with four flagella arranged in two pairs. At least one flagellum is recurrent accompanied by a funis and adhered with its anterior part to the body of the cell. Only one round nucleus with a large endosome is present. Cysts may be formed but are not described for all species.

Monocercomonoides. The life cycle of members of this genus is simple. Multiplication takes place only in the trophozoite stage by binary fission. The uninucleated cysts do not multiply. Infection occurs mainly by uptake of infectious cysts. Only a few species are reported from poikilothermic animals (Table 19.10). None of them are pathogenic. These flagellates have a more or less ball-like body, and they resemble somewhat some species of trichomonad flagellates without an undulating membrane. The size of the organisms vary from species to species but is between 5 to 15 microns by 5 to 15 microns.

Order Trichomonadida

Two families, Monocercomonadidae and Trichomonadidae, are parasitic in amphibians and reptiles. A comprehensive study dealing with the systematic relationships in this flagellate order was published by Honigberg (1963).

Characteristics for these flagellates are more or less elongated pyriform or broadly pyriform bodies, some of them look ball-like. One of the typical features of these uninucleated organisms is the undulating membrane occurring in all more evolved species. It is formed by one recurrent flagellum of the four to six anterior flagella. The number of anterior flagella together with other structures, i.e., the recurrent flagellum and its adherence to the cell, the axostyle, the parabasal apparatus (Golgi complex), the undulating membrane (when present), and the costa have to be taken into account to differentiate the genera of Trichomonadida. Mitochondria and cytostome are absent.

Table 19.10. Species of Monocercomonoides.[a]

Species	Host	Geographic distribution
M. lacertae (possible syn. M. filamentum, M. mehdii, M. singhi)	Lizards, snakes and tortoises, e.g., Xantusia spp., Phrynosoma spp., Sceloporus spp., Calotes spp., C. versicolor, Chamaeleo zeylanicus, iguanas, Pituophis catenifer, Testudo elegans	Asia; India; North America
M. viperae	Vipera russellii	India
M. rotunda	Anuran and urodelan amphibians, e.g., Bufo bufo, Salamandra spp.	Europe
M. dobelli	B. melanostictus	India

[a]Source: Flynn, 1973; Krishnamurthy and Madre, 1976; Kulda and Nohynkova, 1978; Madre and Krishnamurthy, 1976.

All species are parasitic in invertebrates and vertebrates, and inhabit mainly the intestinal tract of their hosts. So far as is known, these organisms live as commensals. Only a few species live in the urogenital system of certain mammals (cattle) as well as man, and the mouth cavity or esophageal region of columbiform and galliform birds. These parasites have been found by the present author in small cage birds as well.

The life cycle of trichomonadids is simple, mainly involving monomorphic flagellate stages multiplying normally only by binary fission. Multiple division stages are possibly caused by changed environmental conditions. As far as it is known, cysts surrounded by a thickened wall are not to be found among members of this order. Rounded motionless forms, often misinterpreted as cysts, are degenerating stages.

The pathogenic capacity of trichomonadids is proved only for a few species, none of them living in poikilothermic animals. Despite the commensalic way of life of the members of the order Trichomonadida, these flagellates often have been observed in moribund snakes kept in captivitiy and killed for diagnostic purposes as well as during post-mortem examination of the midgut of spontaneously died hosts (Flynn, 1973; Frank, unpubl.; Honigberg, 1963).

The trichomonadids always could be found in regions of the digestive tract (duodenum and anterior part of the midgut) in such animals in which these regions were heavily affected by bacterial infections, particularly by species belonging to the Pseudomonas/Aeromonas group. The mucosa in these areas was completely destroyed and caseously changed. The wall of the gut was very thickened and the lumen was filled up with a caseous core. These alterations also could be seen easily on the outside of the gut, looking like parallel ring-like structures.

It is suggested that the presence of trichomonadids in regions of the intestinal tract normally not inhabited by these flagellates is the result of a completely changed milieu of the content. Bacterial infection can lead to changed conditions which enable the flagellates to live in gut areas usually unsuitable for them. It is not possible to answer the question whether these flagellates are really pathogenic or not. Despite the secondary character of such an invasion (infection?), the flagellates are doubtless responsible for making the primary disease worse.

Hilgenfild (1968) observed trichomonadids in pathologically altered lungs of Crotalus atrox from Mexico, only a short time in captivity. This suggests that invasions by these flagellates may happen by chance in organs outside of the intestine. The transfer of these trichomonadids to a healthy Natrix natrix demonstrated, on the other hand, the commensalic way of life in otherwise healthy hosts. Walton (1964) mentioned liver lesions in Rana pipiens associated with Tritrichomonas augusta. But in this case the true pathogenicity could not be proved experimentally. Further studies concerning the possible (facultative?) pathogenicity of certain flagellates to their poikilothermic hosts seem to be needed.

Order Trichomonadida
Family Monocercomonadidae

Monocercomonas. Flagellates of this genus possess three anterior flagella and one recurrent flagellum which is equal to or longer (not over 2X longer) than the anterior flagella. The recurrent flagellum is free over its entire length or is adherent with its proximal part to the body surface.

The systematic confusion about valid species from amphibians and reptiles, as well as from other hosts, was discussed in detail by Honigberg (1963). He suggested that between 20 to 30 species may be valid ones, but the uncertainty partly results from the original descriptions of species being mainly not instructive enough to distinguish them all exactly. Honigberg (1963) suggested that the genus, despite its world-wide distribution, is rather infrequently found in North American amphibians. He reported only two species, M. colubrorum, and a second one found in an arboreal salamander, Aneides lugubris, from Northern California, which was rather similar to M. mabuiae or M. colubrorum.

The monocercomonadids of amphibians and reptiles are harmless commensals mainly in the large intestine and the cloaca of their hosts. Wallach (1969) mentioned that the Monocercomonas spp. are common intestinal parasites of lizards and snakes. In terminal infections, he found that these organisms may enter the bloodstream and be readily detected in blood smears, being easily identified by the typical fragile trichomonad motility. Despite these findings, the present author believes that these reports represent only sporadic incidents since no similar observations were personally made among thousands of post-mortem investigations.

Table 19.11. Common Monocercomonadids from Amphibia and Reptilia.[a]

Species	Host	Geographic distribution
Monocercomonas colubrorum (syn. M. mabuiae, Trichomastix lacertae, T. viperae, T. serpentis, T. mabuiae, Eutrichomastix serpentis)	Lizards and snakes, e.g., Coluber spp., Heterodon spp., Lampropeltis spp., Natrix spp., Pituophis spp., Thamnophis spp., Scincidae, Gekkonidae	World-wide?
M. moskowitzi (syn. M. mabuiae, M. vital-brasili)	Crotalus viridis, Coluber spp., Sceloporus spp., Gekko vittatus, Gehyra spp.	World-wide?
M. batrachorum (syn. Eutrichomastix batrachorum)	Frogs, toads, salamanders, newts, e.g., Ambystoma opacum, Desmognathus spp., Triturus viridescens, Rana temporaria	World-wide?
M. cyanophlycti	R. cyanophlyctis	India
M. melanosticti	Bufo melanostictus	India
M. aurangabadensis	B. melanostictus	India
M. neosepsorum	Neoseps reynoldsi	United States of America
M. tantillorum	Tantilla coronatum	United States of America
Hexamastix batrachorum (syn. Polymastix batrachorum)	Urodelan amphibians	World-wide?
H. kirbyi	Lizards, e.g., Sceloporus spp., Phrynosoma spp.	Mexico; United States of America

H. crassus	Lizards, e.g., _Phrynosoma_ spp., _Sauromalus obesus_	Mexico; United States of America
Hypotrichomonas acosta (syn. _Trichomonas acosta_)	Snakes and lizards, e.g., _Boa constrictor_, _Drymarchon corais_, _Coluber_ spp., _Heterodon_ spp., _Elaphe_ spp., _Lampropeltis_ spp., _Natrix_ spp., _Thamnophis_ spp., _Pituophis_ spp., _Heloderma horridum_, _H. suspectum_	North, Central and South America; North Africa
H. osmaniae	_Varanus_ sp.	India
H. hemidactyli	_Hemidactylus_ sp.	India
H. venkataramiahii	_Varanus_ sp.	India

aSource: Bovee and Telford, 1962a,b; Daykar et al., 1977; Flynn, 1973; Honigberg, 1963; Krishnamurthy, 1967; Krishnamurthy and Madre, 1979a,b; Moskowitz, 1951; Rao et al., 1976b.

Table 19.12. Common Trichomonadids from Amphibia and Reptilia.[a]

Species	Host	Geographic distribution
Trichomitus batrachorum (syn. Tritrichomonas batrachorum, Trichomonas batrachorum, T. natricis)	Rana pipiens, R. catesbeiana, R. esculenta, Hyla spp.; Bufo americanus, B. terrestris, B. bufo, Xenopus laevis, Ambystoma maculatum, A. jeffersonianum, A. mexicanum, A. tigrinum, Salamandra spp.; Triturus alpestris, Natrix spp.; Pituophis spp.; Thamnophis spp.; Phrynosoma spp.; Lacerta spp.	World-wide
Tetratrichomonas prowazeki (syn. Trichomonas prowazeki)	Amphibia and Squamata, e.g., R. catesbeiana, R. temporaria, B. bufo, B. terrestris, Triturus cristatus, T. torosus, T. viridescens, Salamandra spp.; Amphiuma spp.; Natrix spp.; Thamnophis spp.	North and South America; Europe
Tritrichomonas augusta (syn. Trichomonas augusta, T. batrachorum, T. lacertae, Monocercomonas batrachorum)	R. pipiens, R. esculenta, R. temporaria, R. sylvatica, R. clamitans, R. palustris, Acris gryllus, Hyla cinerea, H. crucifer,	World-wide

T. simhii	B. americanus, B. bufo, B. terrestris, A. jeffersonianum, A. maculatum, A. opacum, A. tigrinum, Desmognathus spp., T. viridescens, T. torosus, Xantusia spp.	
	R. pipensi	India

aSource: Flynn, 1973; Honigberg, 1963; Moskowitz, 1951; Rao et al., 1978b.

Krishnamurthy (1968) made a detailed comparison of all species of the genus Monocercomonas from reptiles accepted by him as valid. The species of Monocercomonas are listed together with members of Hexamita and Hypotrichomonas in Table 19.11. A few newly described species are included also, but whether or not they are really valid species remains to be proven.

Hexamastix. The genus is characterized by five anterior flagella and one recurrent flagellum of equal length and diameter to the anterior flagella. The best known species described from the large intestine of urodelan amphibians is H. batrachorum. Members of this genus are found not only in vertebrates but also in arthropods.

Hypotrichomonas. The characteristics of members of this genus are three anterior flagella and one recurrent flagellum, posteriorly free. The undulating membrane is shallow and shorter than the body. Species of Hypotrichomonas seem to inhabit the large intestine of squamate reptiles as well as of land tortoises. Their geographical distribution is assumed to be world-wide.

Order Trichomonadida
Family Trichomonadidae

Members of three genera can be found as parasites mainly of the intestinal tract of poikilothermic hosts, Trichomitus, Tetratrichomonas, and Tritrichomonas. Only a few reports exist in which trichomonadids are mentioned in other organs and are always associated with pathological destructions. Whether these flagellates are responsible for the alterations in the organs was discussed above. Members of the Trichomonadidae are listed in Table 19.12.

Trichomitus. The members are characterized by three anterior flagella and one recurrent flagellum forming an undulating membrane of varying length. The recurrent flagellum is posteriorly free. The synonymity of the various species mentioned in the literature was discussed by Honigberg (1963).

Tetratrichomonas. Members of this genus possess four anterior flagella and one recurrent flagellum associated with a well developed undulating membrane, extending for about the entire length of the cell with a free posterior part. Tetratrichomonas is widely distributed among amphibians, snakes and lizards, inhabiting the large intestine.

Tritrichomonas. Species of the genus Tritrichomonas typically possess three anterior flagella. The recurrent flagellum forms a well developed undulating membrane and is free posteriorly. Only one species, T. augusta, possibly divided into several groups, seems to be valid. This trichomonad is widely distributed among amphibians and reptiles.

PHYLUM SARCOMASTIGOPHORA
SUBPHYLUM OPALINATA

Order Opalinida
Family Opalinidae

Opalines are uniformly covered with longitudinally arranged, parallel rows of short flagella, the so-called cilia. They are mouthless and possess two to many similar nuclei (Fig. 19.1). Their size differs up to about 1 mm. All species are commensals of cold-blooded vertebrates. It is doubtful whether the two species described from termites are valid species (Sandon, 1976). The vast majority are found in anuran amphibians. Only a few are reported from reptiles and four species are from fish (Foissner et al., 1979). Sandon (1976) mentioned that there were about 11 species from fresh-water fish, two from marine

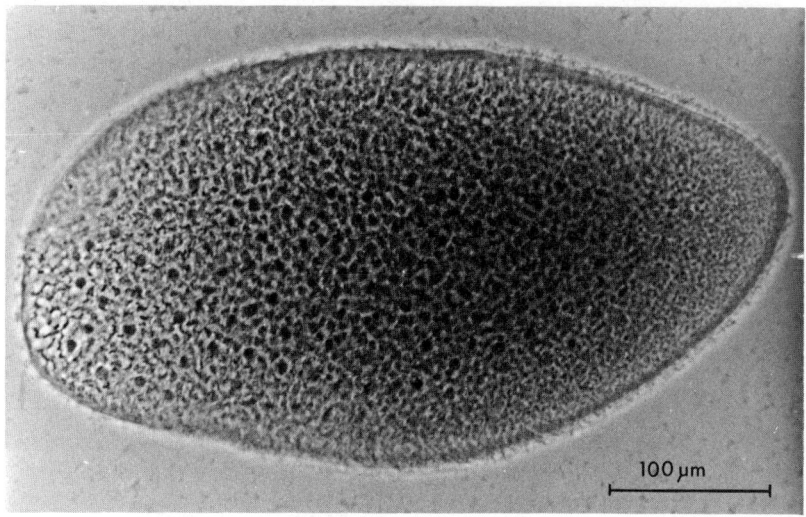

Fig. 19.1. Opalina ranarum, phase-contrast photography, showing the many nuclei and the ciliated border.

Table 19.13. Genera of the Family Opalinidae.

Genus	Characteristics
Protoopalina	Two nuclei; shape of the opalinid in transverse section is subcircular or circular; widest geographical distribution of the four genera; Metcalf (1923, 1940) suggested that it is the most primitive genus which may be found in fish, amphibians and reptiles; Sandon (1976), on the contrary, pointed out "that the opalinids may be a relict fauna much older than their usual hosts, the anurans, and that the genus Protoopalina may not represent the ancestral form of the group"
Opalina	Many nuclei; shape of the opalinid in transverse section is flattened (Fig. 19.1)
Zelleriella	Two nuclei; shape of the opalinid in transverse section is flattened
Cepedea	Many nuclei; shape of the opalinid in transverse section is subcircular or circular

fish and one from a fresh-water mollusc. The confusion whether the Opalinata belong to the Mastigophora or to the Ciliophora as a subclass Protociliata is no longer a subject of discussion. The new classification proposed by a group of specialists of the Society of Protozoologists classifies these protozoans as a separate subphylum in the phylum Sarcomastigophora (Levine et al., 1980).

Only four genera are distinguished (Table 19.13). They are characterized by the number of nuclei (two or many) and the shape of the organism in transverse section (circular or flattened). The characterization of the genera based only on the number of nuclei is not absolute as species of Zelleriella and Protoopalina have been described possessing more nuclei (four, eight and even more). The species described by Foissner et al. (1979) shows as a characteristic, a bridge-like structure of the nucleus membrane between the two nuclei. This structure has been observed in a few other opalinids as well (Sandon, 1976). The genus Hegeriella was created for an

Table 19.14. Zoogeographic Distribution of Opalinids and Main Groups of Hosts Parasitized.[a]

Genus	Palearctic	Ethiopian	Oriental	Neotropical	Nearctic	Australian
Protoopalina	10[b]	34[c]	17	7	5	12[d]
Opalina	18	9	38	13	62[e]	0
Cepedea[f]	5	12	42	14	5	0
Zelleriella[g]	2	1	5	47[h]	11	1

[a]Source: Wessenberg, 1978.
[b]Number of host species.
[c]Chiefly ranids, bufonids and leptodactylids.
[d]Chiefly hylids, ranids, bufonids and leptodactylids.
[e]Chiefly hylids, but also ranids and bufonids.
[f]Mainly associated with ranids, bufonids and hylids.
[g]Largely restricted to the Western hemisphere with its main distribution in South America.
[h]Chiefly leptodactylids in the Neotropical region, but also ranids, hylids and bufonids in the Neotropical and Nearctic regions.

Table 19.15. Some Opalinidae from Amphibia and Reptilia Inhabiting Common Hosts in the Americas, Europe, Africa, Asia and Australia.[a]

Species	Host	Geographic distribution
AMPHIBIA		
Protoopalina intestinalis	Rana temporaria, R. esculenta, Hyla arborea, Bufo spp., Bombina spp., Pelobates fuscus?, Triturus vulgaris, T. helveticus	Africa; Europe
P. caudata	Bombina bombina, B. variegata	Europe
P. xenopodos	Xenopus laevis	Africa
P. mitotica	Ambystoma mexicanum, A. tigrinum	North America
P. bibronii	Pseudophryne bibronii	Australia
Opalina obtrigona	H. arborea	Europe
O. cincta	Bufo bufo	Europe
O. obtrigonoidea	R. pipiens, R. sylvatica, R. palustris, H. crucifer, H. cinerea, Acris gryllus, B. americanus	North America
O. virguloidea	R. sylvatica, H. crucifer	North America
O. carolinensis	R. pipiens	North America
O. chlorophili	H. crucifer	North America
O. hylaxena	H. crucifer	North America

O. ranarum	R. temporaria, R. escu-lenta, H. arborea, B. bufo, T. alpestrin	Europe; Africa; Asia
O. discophrya	B. americanus	North America
O. triangularis	B. terrestris, B. melano-stictus	North America; Asia
O. larvarum	R. clamitans, R. pipiens, R. catesbeiana	North America
O. chattoni	B. melanostictus	Asia
O. sudafricana	B. regularis	Africa
Cepedea dimidiata	R. esculenta, B. bufo	Asia; Europe
C. scalpriformis	B. melanostictus	Asia
C. saharana	R. ridibunda	Asia; Africa
C. rubra	Leptodactylus ocellatus	South America
Zelleriella antunesi	L. ocellatus	South America
Z. corniola	L. ocellatus	South America
Z. cornucopia	L. ocellatus	South America
Z. artigasi	B. marinus	Central and North America

REPTILIA

Z. boipevae	Ophis meremmii	Brazil
Z. jaegeri	Liophis jaegeri	Brazil
P. nyanza	Varanus niloticus	Africa
Opalinidae gen. spec.	Testudo sp.	In captivity

[a]Source: Flynn, 1973; Metcalf, 1923, 1940.

opalinid species, H. dobelli, from Bufo valliceps, but Since it possesses only one nucleus (Earl, 1971) it seems not to be a valid species (Wessenberg, 1978).

The number of species described seems to be less than 400. According to Sandon (1976), only a number of species live in other hosts than anurans. Three species are found in Urodela, two in Varanidae and seven in Ophidia. Wessenberg (1978) gave some information about the geographical distribution of the opalinids (Table 19.14) which is limited, of course, by the distribution of their hosts (Table 19.15). A number of species can be found in several hosts, and on the other hand, a number of host species are known to harbor several species, even of different genera of opalinids. It can be suggested that many more species of opalinids exist as there have been described up to this time. The most comprehensive publications are the ones of Metcalf (1923, 1940), but a revision of the Opalinata under modern aspects of taxonomy may lead to a somewhat variant conception (Earl, 1973; Sandon, 1976).

The life history is complex and closely associated with the breeding season of amphibians. Nothing is known that regulates or stimulates the adequate processes in reptilian species. The opalinids live in the large intestine of their hosts where they are situated in the anterior most portion as trophonts, the full grown organisms. They are able to divide at any time by simple binary fission with each part growing to the usual size and form. These divisions restore the number of individuals lost by occasional passage of trophonts with the host feces.

During the breeding season of the host a certain number of trophonts undergo successive divisions, but these daughter cells (tomonts) do not grow to their normal size. They also have smaller numbers of nuclei. Several of these tomonts continue to divide and the result is many individuals with less than 12 nuclei. Such stages round off and secrete a cyst wall. In O. ranarum most cysts possess 4 to 8 nuclei and in O. virguloidea, 3 to 6. These cysts pass with the feces into the surrounding water where the amphibians mate. They are infectious for about 3 to 4 weeks. The percentage of the already mentioned stages varies characteristically during the egg-laying period of the hosts. A short time after the end of egg-laying about 40% of all stages are cysts.

The hatched tadpoles feed after a few days, among other things, on the detritus on the ground of the pools and ingest particles of feces containing opalinid cysts. In the intestine each cyst gives rise to a gamont. These rapid swimming individuals are collected in the hindgut of the tadpoles where they divide several times until they form uninucleate gametes of different sizes; one gamont forms a macrogamete, another a microgamete. When macrogametes and microgametes meet, they fuse and form a zygote which surrounds itself with a solid wall. The encysted zygote or zygocyst passes with the feces of the young tadpole. Possibly the cycle can be repeated if young tadpoles take these stages up again.

Zygocysts ingested passively by tadpoles approaching metamorphosis show a distinct way of further development. At first, the zygote looks like a miniature trophont, but repeated nuclei divisions without cell division and growth of the individual leads to a fully grown trophont. Before the end of metamorphosis, a number of such young trophonts undergo tomont formation and produce cysts in the same way described above. Possibly they act again as infectious cysts. During the metamorphosis, before the host gut shortens, the opalinids are found mainly in the small intestine, but after the completed metamorphosis they are all in the large intestine of the young frogs or toads.

The triggers for inducing all these complicated processes are the hormones of the host. El-Mofty (1974) induced sexual reproduction in O. sudafricana by injecting gibberellic acid into its host, B. regularis. El-Mofty and Sadek (1975a) induced encystation of the same opalinid by using fresh toad bile.

Opalinids possibly may be used in certain biological tests. El-Mofty and Sadek (1975b) used O. sudafricana for diagnosing disordered tryptophan metabolism in man. For further details the reader is referred to Wessenberg (1978).

As far as is known opalinids are not pathogenic, not even when they compete in the consumption of food. No records exist describing any damage to their amphibian hosts. This may be in respect to their localization in the large intestine where the only material present is not useful any more for the host, but a suitable nutrient for bacteria which produce substances taken up by the opalinids. The feeding process of these mouthless creatures is called endocytosis. Mass invasion of young tadpoles, where the opalinids are localized in the small intestine has not been studied.

The opalinids are commensals and not uncommonly hundreds and even thousands of individuals can be found in perfectly healthy hosts. They feed only on nutrients which would be otherwise passed with the feces. They never attack the mucosa of the intestine, but swim slowly amongst the gut contents. In a recently published investigation dealing with a new species, Protoopalina symphysodonis from a fresh-water fish, these problems also have been discussed (Foissner et al., 1979). It seems that a mass population of this opalinid may cause death of the hosts although nothing could be found in histological sections to correspond with the fatality of the infections However, fish possibly are not the original hosts of this species.

PHYLUM SARCOMASTIGOPHORA
SUBPHYLUM RHIZOPODA

Order Amoebida

The morphology of the pathogenic species for amphibians, Entamoeba ranarum, and for reptiles, E. invadens, corresponds well with that of E. histolytica of man as described by Albach and Booden (1978). Minor differences demonstrate the validity of the three species. Marked physiological and biochemical differences exist, e.g., the optimal temperature for the species from poikilotherms is only 25 to 28 C instead of 37 C for E. histolytica (except for the Laredo and similar strains growing at room temperature). Similar to E. histolytica, E. invadens has no mitochondria. Carosi (1974) proposed that amoebae of the Laredo type are the ancestors of E. invadens and E. histolytica. The locomotion of the members of the Amoebida is by pseudopodia, broad protrusions of the cytoplasm (lobopodia). Motility is sluggish, but some species show explosively extended pseudopodia formation, e.g., E. histolytica and often also E. invadens strains. Cultivation of amoebae is relatively easy. Monoxenic and axenic cultivation of many strains of various species has been successfully maintained.

Order Amoebida
Family Endamoebidae

From the several species of amoebae described from amphibians and reptiles, living as parasites in the intestinal tract, only two seem to be really pathogenic to their hosts, namely E. ranarum and E. invadens. The interpretation of pathogenicity among amoebae of cold-blooded verte-

brates is as difficult as that of E. histolytica of man
and certain other warm-blooded hosts. It depends surely
on certain environmental conditions and possibly also on
nutritional factors (Meerovitch, 1958). But as far as is
known, no exact data exist as to which conditions induce
pathological alterations after the uptake of infectious
stages of a distinct species and which prevent the disease.
A detailed study dealing with the problem of pathogenicity
of parasitic Entamoeba was published by Bos (1973).

Similar to the more or less symptomless carriers of
E. histolytica it seems that such possibilities also are
presented by E. invadens infections. Fresh-water terrapins
are proposed to act in this manner (Frank, unpubl.). It
is interesting to note that apparently healthy chelonians
are able to carry the amoebae in nature without any signs
of disease. Mishra and Gonzalez (1978) published a study
dealing with wild caught Mauremys caspica leprosa in
Tunisia. They found three out of 20 specimens examined
to be infected with E. invadens, but did not mention any
pathological changes. It seems that this is the first
true report of E. invadens found in free-ranging animals.
A very comprehensive study by Telford (1970) revealed a
high percentage of Entamoeba carriers among the more than
1000 California reptiles examined, belonging to various
families (Gekkonidae, Xantusiidae, Iguanidae, Teiidae,
Scincidae, Anguidae, Anniellidae), but he did not try to
determine the species of the amoebae so it is unclear if
E. invadens was present among them.

Suggestions that chelonians are carriers of these
amoebae in nature, but without pathological alterations,
have existed for a long time. About 15 years ago a German
hobbyist caught about 200 mud terrapins, Claudius angustatus, in Mexico and wanted to bring them to Europe. The
conditions during the transport lasting several weeks were
extremely bad, as he told the present author after his
arrival in Germany. During the voyage the first terrapins
died and after their arrival more died. All together more
than 50 terrapins perished. The author was able to examine
many of them and all showed the typical signs characteristic for reptilian amoebiasis. Despite the fact that all
other terrapins examined by cloacal swab and culture technique were positive, further deaths did not occur after
several weeks and improved conditions. Several of these
terrapins were kept for a long time in the laboratory of
the author with full success and one specimen for many
years. Although the animals were always shedding trophozoites and cysts with the feces, they never showed any
signs of disease. This description underlines the opinion

Table 19.16. Species of *Entamoeba* from Amphibia and Reptilia.

Species	Remarks
E. ranarum[a]	First described from Rana temporaria by Grassi (1879); life cycle studies by Sanders (1931); isolated from liver abscess of Ambystoma mexicanum (Frank, unpubl.); Ghosh (1977) reported this species from 10 amphibian genera and 22 host species from India, but did not mention pathogenicity to the hosts; cysts survive 25 weeks at 4 C (Neal, 1974)
E. curens[a]	Described from R. esculenta and Bufo bufo (Flynn, 1973); Ghosh (1977) found this species in the intestine of three amphibian genera and three host species in India
E. pyrrhogaster[a]	Described from Triturus viridescens (Flynn, 1973); Ghosh (1977) mentioned this species from R. temporaria and Cynops pyrrhogaster
E. invadens	Described from Python sebae by Rodhain (1934) from pathologically altered intestinal tissue; cysts survive seven weeks at 4 C (Neal, 1974)
E. insolita	Described by Geiman and Wichterman (1937) from Geochelone elephantopus
E. ilowaiskii[a]	Ghosh (1977) reported this species from R. temporaria; it is pathogenic to its hosts
E. serpentis	Described from a Brazilian snake, Drymobius bifossatus by Cunha and Fonseca (1917, 1918); proposed to be synonymous to E. invadens (Flynn, 1973; Ghosh, 1968)
E. terrapinae	Described from Chrysemys scripta elegans (Sanders and Cleveland, 1930); cysts survive 24 weeks at 4 C (Neal, 1974)
E. testudinis	Described from Testudo graeca by Hartman (1910); found also in T. chilensis and Geochelone sulcata (Wenyon, 1926) and Chrysemys picta (Sanders and Cleveland, 1930)

Table 19.16. Species of Entamoeba from Amphibia and Reptilia. (Continued)

Species	Remarks
E. barreti	Described from Chelydra serpentina by Taliaferro and Holmes (1924)
E. varani	Described from Varanus niloticus by Lavier (1928); identical with E. invadens?
E. knowlesi	Described by Rodhain and van Hoof (1947) from Terrapene carolina and Platysternon megacephalum; cysts survive 24 weeks at 4 C (Neal, 1974)
Entamoeba sp.	Described from Trionyx gangeticus by Knowles and Das Gupta (1930)
Entamoeba sp.	Described from Thamnophis spp. by Fantham and Porter (1953)
E. ctenosaurae	Described from Ctenosaura acanthura by Hegner and Hewitt (1940)[b]; coli-like amoeba
E. cuautla	Described from Ctenosaura acanthura by Hegner and Hewitt (1940)[b]

[a]E. ranarum, E. pyrrhogaster and E. ilowaiskii have quadrinucleated cysts; so far cysts from E. curens are not known.

[b]These authors described an amoeba from Ctenosaura acanthura which they proposed to belong to a new genus Martinezia. The simple descriptions and drawings given for all species make evident that M. baezi and a second unnamed species from Sceloporus clarkii probably belong to the order Schizopyrenida as they possess large spherical endosomes.

that amoebiasis of reptiles is a disease especially of exhibited specimens living, on the one hand, under unnatural conditions and, on the other hand, being exposed to continous infections in their cage environments.

A study of the Entamoeba spp. from amphibians by Ghosh (1977) revealed that these hosts harbor a number of species (Table 19.16), and that at least one of these species, E. ilowaiskii seems to be pathogenic to its hosts. With the exception of E. curens, all the other species investigated, E. ranarum, E. ilowaiskii and E. pyrrhogaster, form quadrinucleated cysts. So far a cyst from E. curens has not been recorded.

Entamoeba. Several species of amoebae are grouped in the genus Entamoeba. Only one, E. invadens, is known pathogenic to reptiles and Ghosh (1977) pointed out another one, E. ilowaiskii, to be pathogenic for amphibians. The validity of a number of species is questionable, they are listed in Table 19.16. The investigations of Albach and Shaffer (1965), Bosch and Deichsel (1972), Frank et al. (1976a,b) and Gelderman et al. (1971a,b) showed that E. invadens consists either of various strains of different characteristics or incorporates several forms up to now reported as one species.

A careful study and reexamination of intestinal amoebae from the hosts mentioned above and whenever possible the consideration of the original slides (when available) together with culture methods, infection experiments, etc., would be necessary to clear up the synonymy of species or their validity. First attempts have been made by Charoenlarp et al. (1971) to differentiate various species or strains of Entamoeba by serologic characteristics of glucokinases. They took into consideration E. invadens and E. terrapinae, but they concluded that not enough information was available for definite evidence of the systematic relationship of these species. But the investigations of Gelderman et al. (1971a,b) demonstrated that there are striking differences in the DNA base ratio content between various parasitic amoebae and that there also are differences in the genome size. They found that there already exist two distinct genospecies in the single species E. invadens. If strains of different origin would be taken into consideration, the results might differ (Bosch and Deichsel, 1972; Deichsel and Bosch, 1973).

Entamoeba invadens. In 1934 Rodhain isolated a parasitic amoeba from necrotic areas of the intestinal tract of a Python sebae in the Antwerp Zoo, which he named E. invadens. The name was selected because of the invasive capability of the vegetative stages, the trophozoites, into the intestinal tissues. The first detailed study of this amoeba dealing with the morphology and the life cycle was published by Geiman and Ratcliffe (1936). Morphologically and in the host-parasite relation there is a remarkable resemblance between E. histolytica of man and E. invadens of reptiles (Fig. 19.2). The stages in the life cycle are the trophozoite (with a size normally between about 10 and 35 microns, but with exceptions up to about

100 microns), the quadrinucleated fully developed cyst (with a size between 10 and 20 microns and which is the infective stage) and the precyst, a rounded-off trophozoite which starts the cyst formation. The precyst contains diffuse glykogen which is condensed in the mature cyst. Chromatoid bodies are characteristic for the cyst (Barker and Deutsch, 1958). A detailed electron microscopic study by Bidier (1977) took into consideration not only the fine structure of the amoeba, as did Siddiqui and Rudzinska (1965), but also the change of the surrounding tissues by the invasive trophozoites. The immunochemical composition of the surface and cytoplasmic membranes have been studied by McClaughin and Meerovitch (1975). The single nucleus of the trophozoite measures between 3.5 and about 10 microns (Frank et al., 1976a,b). Each nucleus contains a small centrally located granular endosome, the chromatin lies scattered inside the delicate nucleus membrane and is Feulgen stain positive.

Reproduction is by simple binary fission of the trophozoites (sexual processes are unknown), but multiplication also occurs in the cyst stage. The nucleus of the uninucleated trophozoite divides twice during the cyst formation and each cyst gives rise to four small uninucleated amoebulae, the young trophozoites, if they excyst in a new host (Bosch and Deichsel, 1972; Frank et al., 1976a,b; Geiman and Ratcliffe, 1936; Steck, 1963). Distribution

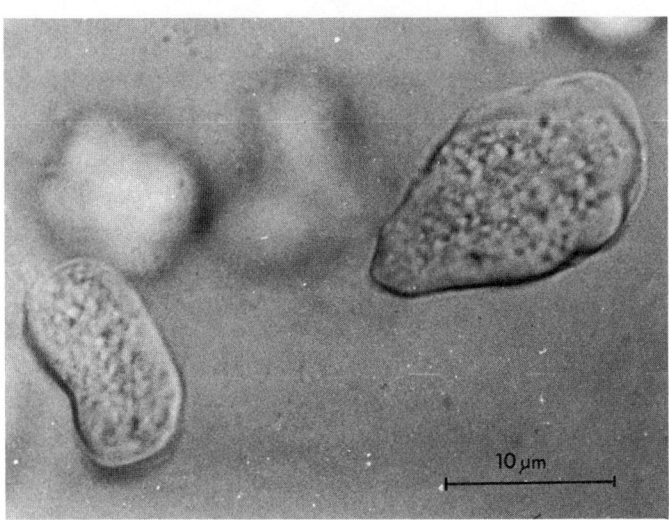

Fig. 19.2. Trophozoites of Entamoeba invadens, culture form.

of cysts is by certain insects, e.g., flies, ants, cockroaches and crickets (Frank, unpubl.).

The gross differences between E. histolytica and E. invadens are mainly the optimal temperature of about 25 to 28 C for E. invadens versus 37 C for E. histolytica. Morphologically the minuta and magna forms observed with E. histolytica have not been found for E. invadens. The missing distinct demarcation between the hyalin ectoplasm and the granular endoplasm, mentioned as a characteristic of E. invadens by Albach and Booden (1978) seems not to be a feature of all strains.

E. invadens seems to have a world-wide distribution among reptiles in captivity. Many publications dealing with enzootic disease outbreaks in zoological gardens show the danger particularly for exhibited snakes and certain lizards (Varanidae). The percentage of diseased animals, and finally the loss of these creatures, varies markedly, possibly depending upon the hygienic conditions in the exhibition and also on the exactness of the diagnosis. Also to be taken into account are the origin of the carcasses studied and the methods used. Frank (1976a,b), for example, mentioned only about 5% amoebiasis out of 4000 dissected reptiles. These results were based on dissections of carcasses of various origins and were determined either by microscopic examination of gut conten and detection of moving trophozoites or by culture technique for living trophozoites. Dolensek et al. (1976) reported a 30% loss of reptiles due to amoebiasis, but these results were based only on reptiles kept in exhibition by the New York Zoological Society. The loss of reptiles due to amoebiasis may be near 100% in a certain collection if the conditions are extremely bad, but altogether less than 5% loss seems to be an average among reptiles in captivity. It has been suggested that new drugs and better care have reduced the mortality in the last few years. Comprehensive reviews have been published (Borst et al., 1972; Donaldson et al., 1975; Fiennes, 1961 Frank and Loos-Frank, 1977; Hill and Neal, 1953; Ippen, 1971; Ippen and Schroeder, 1977; Steck, 1963). Infections of reptiles in nature are rarely observed.

As far as is known, all species of reptiles can be infected. Fatal disease is particularly observed among snakes and certain lizards (Hill and Neal, 1953; Ippen, 1959), but also may be found in very rare reptiles like the Komodo dragon, Varanus komodoensis (Gray et al., 1966). Amoebiasis also was observed in reptiles kept continuously at lower temperatures like the tuatara, Sphenodon punctatus

(Frank et al., 1976a). Extremely rare cases have been seen in animals normally living in sea water but kept under unnatural conditions. Frank et al. (1976b) described such cases found in Chelonia mydas kept for a short time in fresh water, and in Caretta caretta. Ippen (1959) diagnosed amoebiasis in a crocodile, Crocodylus porosus. Chelonians may be symptomless carriers as mentioned above. Altogether it can be assumed that all species may be infected and that under certain circumstances all can develop amoebiasis. Herbivorous reptiles are diseased rather rarely, but if they are fed a diet rich in protein amoebiasis may be caused. The common iguana, Iguana iguana, is a good example (Frank, 1966b).

The life history of E. invadens is direct without intermediate hosts. Fully developed cysts with four nuclei are the infective stages which are taken up mainly with contaminated water and more rarely with food. The cysts may be actively transported by various insects, common pests in zoological exhibitions. Mentioned in the literature are cockroaches, ants, flies and crickets. The cysts fed upon by these insects pass their digestive tract and are still infectious in the feces. Cysts of E. invadens may be transported from one cage to another by the keeper's contaminated hands, brushes or other utensils. In a new host the cysts pass the stomach and start to excyst in the posterior midgut/colon area. It is assumed that most nuclei of the cysts divide again before the young amoebulae escape through the softened cyst wall. The amoebulae grow to fully developed trophozoites in the gut content and start, after repeated cell divisions, either to penetrate the mucosa or to encyst. Infected animals shed with their feces numerous cysts as well as trophozoites. Invading trophozoites first destroy the tissues of the mucosa and submucosa, similar to E. histolytica in man. The lytic processes induced by the amoebae have been studied by electron microscopy (Bidier, 1977). In deeper layers the amoebae invade all kinds of tissue and penetrate the blood vessels. They are then transported by the circulatory system to all organs, primarily the liver. This hematogenous spreading goes hand in hand with the invasion of organs being in direct contact with already infected organs. Amoebic abscesses can be found in practically all organs (Frank, 1975).

The invasion of trophozoites into the tissues starts in the anterior part of the colon, but may spread in reptiles to the posterior part of the midgut and rarely up to the stomach. Lesions in the stomach wall are known. The duration of the disease depends on the vitality and the size of the infected reptile. Small snakes die after experimental infections within about three weeks, but the infection may last for several weeks in half or full-grown giant snakes.

As in man infected with E. histolytica, it has to be distinguished among reptiles between those only infected and without signs of disease and those showing signs of acute amoebiasis. In reptile collections the latent or unobtrusive carriers of the amoebae are more dangerous because they continuously shed cysts and function as reservoirs. In this respect it seems that chelonians, particularly fresh water terrapins and mud terrapins, are the most important carriers of amoebae beside crocodiles and water snakes. But in the author's opinion, infected reptiles which show no obvious signs of disease and do not develop any pathological changes in their organs, may belong to many other groups of reptiles. Nothing is known to explain the situation why one specimen shows amoebiasis in the strongest sense of the word while another stays healthy despite shedding cysts. Little is known about the prevalence of unobtrusive reservoir hosts in captivity and nothing of those hosts living in nature. It seems that in the course of pathobiology many similarities exist between E. histolytica and E. invadens infections.

The acute phase of the infection is uncharacteristic and is different between the various groups of hosts. It may be supposed that the disease may be best diagnosed in snakes. These creatures show some signs which are believed to be more or less characteristic. Ill snakes refuse to feed but drink much water. The feces shed at the beginning of the disease are mixed with blood and mucus which contain cell debris. Depending upon the size of the snake and varying between a few centimeters in small specimens and about 30 cm in giant snakes, a hard core in the intestine is palpable ventrally, anterior to the cloaca. This core is the area of the primary lesions and shows during post-mortem studies a hard caseous content and a thickened wall of the colon. This situation is already a progressive stage of the disease. Snakes show convulsions and try to press out feces with little success, however often drops of bloody mucus pass the cloaca. Often such specimens lie stretched out in a completely unphysiological position. The diagnosis among other reptiles is much more complicated because it is impossible to palpate the thickened and hardened colon area because of the pelvic girdle. The other signs can be observed particularly in lizards, i.e., refusal to eat, much drinking and lethargic behavior. In very advanced cases an enlarged and hardened liver may be palpable, but not in chelonians.

The duration of an acute amoebiasis, depending upon size and constitution of a certain specimen, lasts only one to two weeks in smaller lizards, about three weeks in smaller snakes and several weeks in larger snakes. It is interesting to note that the author has very often seen that well nourished snakes with a well developed fat body and in otherwise best condition suffered from fatal amoebiasis.

The primary processes in the course of amoebiasis are alterations in the anterior part of the colon, the area where a short caecum can be seen in boid snakes and other reptiles. First lesions are very small necrotic foci, the entrances of trophozoites. Very soon these foci join into bigger ulcerative processes which extend over the whole area. After a short time the mucosa is completely destroyed and the underlaying layers react by thickening the wall. The picture is that of an ulcerative colitis (Figs. 19.3 and 19.4). Trophozoites in the tissue are always present at the border to the unchanged tissue, never in the necrotic cell debris. The regeneration activity of the intestinal wall leads in some cases to a curious picture. Cross sectioned colons show concentric rings of membranes, one laying over the other (Fig. 19.5). In other specimens the intestinal content consists of a caseous material completely blocking the passage. The wall of the intestine is thickened and hyperemic. The picture seen during postmortem examination is very impressive and clear. The gut content has a yellowish/white color and looks crumbling to caseous in more or less chronic processes of a longer duration. Acute amoebiasis often observed in the posterior part of the mid-gut shows a bloody to brownish semi-liquid content, mainly consisting of innumerable amoebae. In such areas, and spread anteriorly, mass populations of flagellates, i.e., trichomonadids, are frequently seen. It is interesting to note that the author has never seen nematodes or cestodes in advanced amoebiasis and it seems that the physiological milieu caused by amoebae is unsuitable for helminths.

In affected visceral organs, particularly the liver, abscesses are characteristic. They are often only small foci with a diameter of a few millimeters, but in large lizards, can be the size of an orange (Fig. 19.6). A diffuse infiltration may occur and was observed by the author in snakes and lizards. The liver parenchyma was cracked (Fig. 19.7). Frank (1966b) described a very interesting type of generalized amoebiasis without any pathological changes in the intestine but with amoebic abscesses in the brain.

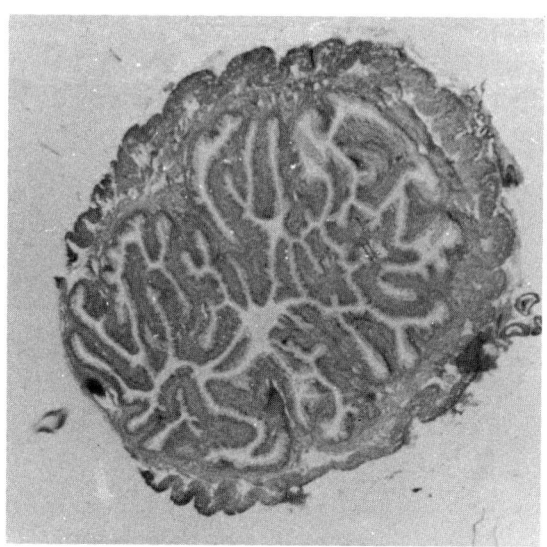

Fig. 19.3. Cross section of the mid-intestine of a healthy snake, Coluber gemonensis.

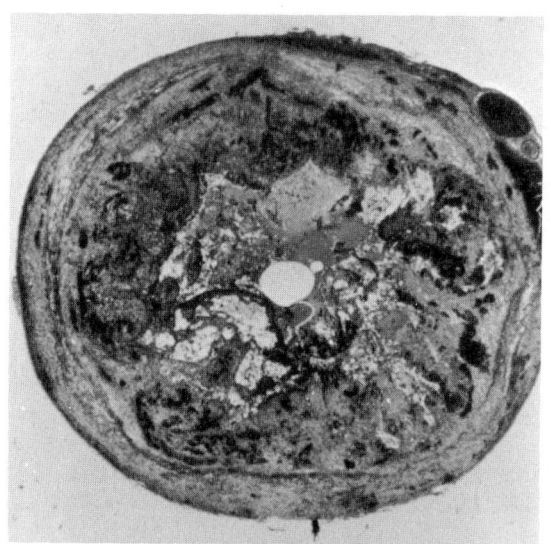

Fig. 19.4. Cross section of the mid-intestine (same region as in Fig. 19.3) with severe destruction caused by Entamoeba invadens. Experimental infection three weeks post-infection.

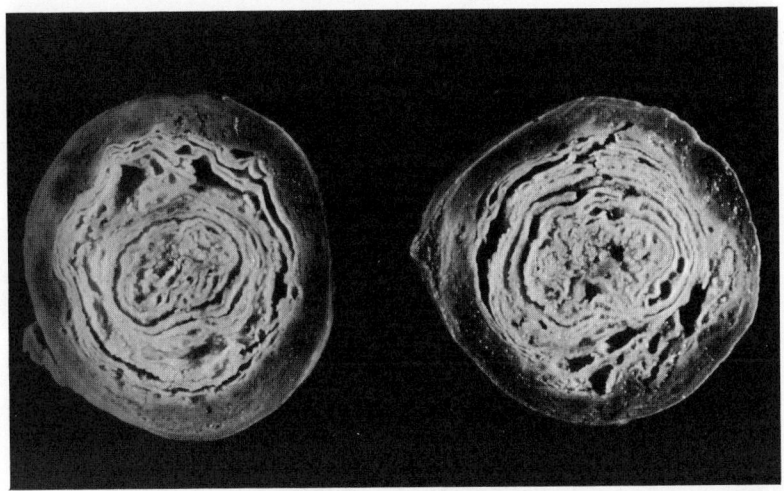

Fig. 19.5. Cross section of the colon region of a Heloderma horridum with the typical picture of "membraneous enteritis" caused by Entamoeba invadens.

Together with the invasion of trophozoites into intestinal tissue, the way is open for the invasion of bacteria which are transported via the blood stream to other organs. Such bacterial infections make the disease worse. Isolations from organs show the same species which are known to cause inflammations in the intestinal tract, e.g., Pseudomonas spp., Aeromonas spp. and Arizona spp. Detailed and comprehensive descriptions of the disease and the pathological alterations have been published (Bidier, 1972, 1977; Frank, 1966b; Frank et al., 1972, 1976a,b; Gabrisch, 1976; Ippen, 1959; Kramer, 1972; Meerovitch, 1961; Ratcliffe and Geiman, 1938; Reichenbach-Klinke, 1977; Soifer, 1978; Steck, 1962, 1963; Zwart, 1964).

Several methods have been proven to diagnose an infection with E. invadens in an early stage in the living reptile. Positive results should open a possibility for therapy to prevent amoebiasis but the examination is not always satisfactory. The best evidence is given when the moving trophozoites can be seen in a fresh preparation of feces, but this classical proof is rarely successful. A few techniques are described below:
a) Preparations of fresh feces
   A small piece of feces freshly taken from the cloaca or better from the colon by a cotton swab is diluted

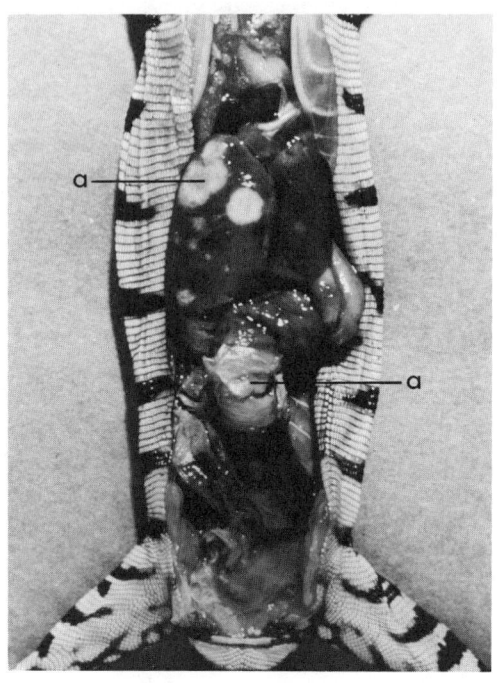

Fig. 19.6. Liver abscesses and severe destruction of the upper colon in a Varanus salvator caused by Entamoeba invadens. a=amoebic abscess in liver and intestine

with physiological saline or Locke solution and directly examined on a slide covered with a cover slip and a magnification of about 300X. The living trophozoite are easily seen. They move actively by pseudopodia formation. Cysts may be seen but are difficult to detect. At least two or three samples should be checked and the procedure repeated one to two days later.

b) Culture technique
Negative results give the possibility of taking a sample of feces in culture. Many methods are mentione in the literature mainly the so-called diphasic media used for E. histolytica. A solid phase medium consisting of special agar preparations or coagulated egg yolk or serum is overlayed by the liquid phase. The amoebae live on the surface of the solid phase. All media modified for E. invadens (Frank, 1966b; Steck, 1963) are based on the media described by Boeck and Drbohlav (1925) and Dobell and Laidlow (1926). If monophasic media are preferred then the bases are the

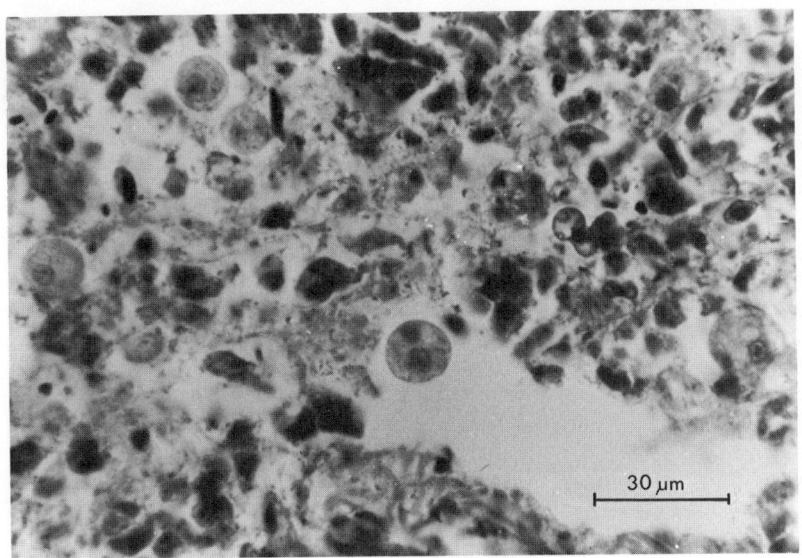

Fig. 19.7. Trophozoites of Entamoeba invadens (rounded off by fixation) free in the necrotic liver parenchyma of a snake, Coluber gemonensis. Note the tiny endosomes in the center of the nuclei.

preparations of Balamuth (1946) or Nelson (1947). For special purposes axenic or monoxenic cultures may be necessary (McConnachie, 1970; Stoll, 1957a,b; Thepsuparungsikul et al., 1971). The cultures have to be checked for amoebae after two to three days and again after a week. It is recommended that negative cultures be subcultured twice in the medium. Mass populations can be found within a few days.

c) Method with Lugol's solution
A small piece of feces, if possible freshly taken from the cloaca, is mixed on a slide with a few drops of Lugol's solution and covered with a cover slip. Mainly cysts can be detected with this technique being brown in color. The nuclei can easily be distinguished. Several samples must be checked to verify the infection.

d) MIF technique
Particularly if no laboratory equipment is at hand or other reasons prevent an immediate examination of feces, the fixation with MIF (merthiolate-iodine-formalin) is recommended. Cysts of amoebae and of other parasites can be recognized after weeks or months of fixation.

e) Immunofluorescence
For certain investigations, but not routine diagnosis, it is possible to label serum of reptiles with FITC for direct immunofluorescence (Frank and Sigmund, 1976). This method is useful to clear up histologically whether tissue fixed years ago is positive for amoebiasis or not. A titer from 1:16 seems to be positive. The indirect immunofluorescence technique also may be conducted.
f) Seropherogramme
For laboratory investigations the serum electrophoresi technique can be useful. Typical changes can be observed if the liver is affected (Frank et al., 1972)
g) Histological method
Trophozoites and precystic stages can be detected in fixed tissue on histological slides stained by various techniques. Some experience is necessary to differentiate the amoebae from the surrounding tissue.

Several authors have recommended various therapeutics to cure amoebiasis of reptiles. Two of these drugs seem to be most effective. Metronidazole often is used in various dosages from 62.5 mg/kg body weight daily (seven times) with a repetition after two weeks (Jes, 1975), up to a single dose of 275 mg/kg (Donaldson et al., 1975). Particularly in North America, emetine-hydrochlorid is recommended (Frye, 1973; Soifer, 1978) but it is difficult to secure in Europe. Various publications deal with the therapy of reptilian amoebiasis (Frank, 1975, 1976a; Frye, 1973; Gabrisch, 1976; Marcus, 1977; Schweinfurt, 1970; Soifer, 1978; Zwart, 1974).

Summarizing all facts dealing with amoebae and the disease they cause, amoebiasis is still the most serious parasitic infection of captive reptiles throughout the world. Therefore, prophylactic measures are the most important prior condition to prevent the disease among captive reptiles. One to the best methods is to keep the reptiles as long as possible, but at least six to eight weeks, in quarantine cages completely separated from the exhibition terraria. During this time it is necessary to examine fresh samples of feces a few times in accordance with the methods described above. Infected reptiles must be isolated. Disinfection of cages and utensils is as necessary as the removal of feces and the rest of the food. Bathing and drinking water has to be renewed as often as possible.

Some authors recommend the administration of certain drugs as a prophylactic measure. Conant (1971) gave 1 g aureomycin/month/40 to 50 kg body weight. Donaldson et al. (1975) used 275 mg/kg metronidazole to cure diseased reptiles in an exhibition diorama, as well as to prevent infection of snakes and lizards. The author's own use of therapeutics has been to cure diseased reptiles and not to give them chemical compounds with more or less unknown metabolic pathways for these species. Reptiles are stressed enough in captivity and care should be taken to ease the keeping away of all things which may disturb these sensitive creatures.

Pathogenic free-living amoebae. Free-living limax-amoebae are known to cause fatal disease in humans (Butt, 1966; Cerva and Nowak, 1968; Fowler and Carter, 1965). A rather comprehensive paper by Griffin (1978) summarized all data dealing with these specialized amoebae. The reader also is referred to the papers of an international colloquium on pathogenic free-living amoebae held in 1973 in Antwerp and published as the Proceedings of the Prince Leopold Institute of Tropical Medicine, 14:1-227 and in Ann. Soc. Belge Med. Trop., 54:227-450, 1974.

These amoebae are of interest in connection with amphibians and reptiles because they are free-living in water and muddy surrounding and can be isolated from these vertebrates as well as from invertebrates (Bosch and Deichsel, 1972; Frank, 1974; Frank and Bosch, 1972; Kasprzak et al., 1974). Independent of the systematic problems caused by these amoebae it can be assumed that some free-living amoebae play a part as pathogens at least in reptiles and that amphibians as well as reptiles may harbor these protozoans without any signs of disease, possibly functioning as carriers.

Frank (1974) showed that while such amoebae may be isolated from brains of reptiles showing pathological processes, e.g., Boa constrictor, Coluber hippocrepis and Iguana iguana, amphibians (European frogs) could be infected with these amoebae without producing any signs. Amoebae could be reisolated from experimentally infected frogs after six weeks. In addition, the author has found free-living limax-amoebae in brain lesions of a snake, Morelia sp., a lizard, Ophiosaurus apodus, and a terrapin, Kinosternon leucostomum. In the same reptiles pathological alterations could be observed caused by E. invadens. Many isolates of "free-living amoebae" have been established from the feces of quite healthy amphibians and reptiles and several records of these amoebae exist in the literature (Dolensek et al., 1976; Telford, 1970), but the classification of all these protozoans is still problematical. The systematic confusion where these amoebae have to be grouped seems still unresolved. The author follows the recommendations of Page (1976a,b), Griffin (1978) and Levine et al. (1980).

Order Amoebida
Suborder Tubulina
Family Hartmannellidae

Only one genus, Hartmannella, has been reported to be able to live not only free in water but also as a parasite. As far as is known this genus contains no species proven to be pathogenic. Earlier references refer possibly to amoebae now considered to be Acanthamoeba or even Naegleria (Griffin, 1978). If the so-called "interzonal bodies" appearing during mitosis are taken into account, Hartmannella is a synonym of Acanthamoeba (Das, 1974). One of the main characteristics to distinguish these amoebae, together with the other "pathogenic free-living amoebae", from other members of the class is the large central spherical endosome (karyosome) in the one nucleus present in the trophozoite (Fig. 19.8). Hartmannella may form cysts, but is unable to produce flagella in water. Members of this genus can be isolated from feces of amphibians and reptiles and possibly from pathologically altered tissue (Bosch and Deichsel, 1972; Frank and Bosch, 1972). Telford (1970) mentioned in his comprehensive investigation of California lizards that Hartmannella amoebae were very common among these lizards, but he never took into consideration pathological changes in

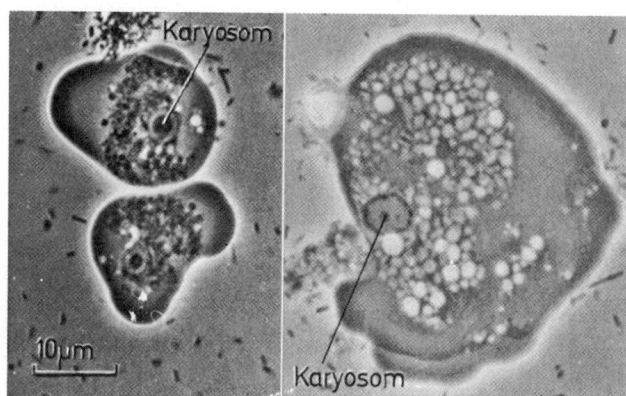

Fig. 19.8. Two amoebae of the "Hartmannella"-type from reptiles with a large endosome in the nucleus (left); compare the tiny endosome of Entamoeba invadens (right).

the reptiles harboring these protozoans. If the statements given above are considered, then the amoebae mentioned in these publications possibly may belong to one of the other genera.

Order Amoebida
Suborder Acanthopodina
Family Acanthamoebidae

Members of the genus Acanthamoeba, now known as facultatively pathogenic to man, are able to live as parasites in amphibians and reptiles (Griffin, 1978). Their characteristics are filiform pseudopodia and a large endosome in the nucleus. Cysts can be formed but as far as is known flagellate stages have never been observed. Because of the confusion in the nomenclature, the species isolated from lesions of reptiles may belong to either this genus or to Naegleria (Bosch and Deichsel, 1972; Frank, 1974; Frank and Bosch, 1972). The author has received personal communications from Balamuth and Das who considered these isolates as Naegleria and Tetramitus, respectively. It is hoped that these problems may be clarified in the near future.

Order Schizopyrenida
Family Vahlkampfiidae

Two genera, Vahlkampfia and Naegleria, are known to live as parasites in the intestine of amphibians and reptiles. Possibly a third genus, Tetramitus, can be found in these poikilothermic animals.

Vahlkampfia is a well known parasite often found in various amphibians and reptiles. The amoebae form broad pseudopodia and show a large spherical endosome in the nucleus. In water these protozoans are unable to produce flagella. As far as is known, Vahlkampfia spp. have no capability to cause pathological destructions in the intestine or in other organs and appear to be harmless commensals. Flynn (1973) mentioned five species from Europe and the United States, which were found in frogs, newts and lizards (Iguanidae-USA, Lacertidae-Europe). The species were V. ranarum (frogs-Europe), V. froschi (frogs-Europe), V. salamandrae (newts-USA), V. reynoldsi (Sceloporus undulatus-USA) and V. dobelli (Lacerta muralis-Europe).

Naegleria spp. are wide-spread in nature. They can be found in water and muddy surroundings particularly when there is a temperature of about 25 C. One of the characteristics differentiating them from other genera is the ability of these amoebae to form two flagella very quickly when contacting water. <u>Naegleria</u> spp. possess a large spherical endosome in the nucleus. The flagellate stages are supposed to be the principal infective stages for vertebrates as well as invertebrates, but possibly the amoebic trophozoites possess this capability. Species of this genus have been known since 1965 as dangerous pathogens in man. Possibly only one species, <u>N. fowleri</u>, is responsible for the disease called primary amoebic meningo encephalitis. Retrospective studies revealed that this disease was a cause of death in humans as early as 1909. Symmers (1969) demonstrated these amoebae in a lesion of a brain preserved in a museum. Since the investigations of Frank (1974) and Frank and Bosch (1972), it has been known that amoebae of the <u>Naegleria</u> type can cause lesions in the brains of poikilothermic animals. Such destruction had been observed in several reptiles but the same strains caused no lesions in <u>Rana temporaria</u> when experimentally transferred to these animals. Interesting to note is the hematogenous transport of these amoebae in amphibians. If amoebae were injected intraperitoneally they could be reisolated from the brain and vice versa. Griffin (1978) reviewed the literature of these free-living but facultatively pathogenic amoebae and mentioned a number of cases where these protozoans could be isolated from various vertebrates. It is suggested that the pathological alterations associated with limax-amoebae have been observed several times but always in reptiles kept in captivity. Whether similar relations exist in nature is unknown. Amphibians and reptiles (if they live in continuous contact with water) may act as carriers of these amoebae and potentially are able to spread these organisms in the environment. It would be necessary to investigate all types of free-living amoebae found as commensals or parasites in poikilothermic animals and to find a simple way of determination to distinguish the various strains exactly.

PHYLUM APICOMPLEXA

<u>Order Eucoccidiida</u>
<u>Suborder Adeleina</u>
<u>Family Klossiellidae</u>

Members of the family are sporadically found in rodents; only one species is known from reptiles. This species, <u>Klosiella boae</u>, has been recovered from the kidneys of a <u>Boa constrictor</u> (Zwart, 1963). The few species of the genus have been summarized by Taylor et

al. (1979). The Klossiellidae belong to the Adeleina;
their characteristics are that already at the beginning
of the gamogony the gametocytes come in contact with each
other and that the gametes are formed afterwards. The
zygote develops into an oocyst which is passed via feces.
In each oocyst several sporocysts, each with many sporozoites, come into existence. The accidental oral uptake
of sporulated oocysts is followed by new infections. The
oocysts of K. boae have a size of 36 to 53 by 14 to 22
microns. The vegetative stages develop in epithelial
cells of the renal tubules of B. constrictor. The host
response is mild. In spite of the supposed rarity of
these parasites, Zwart (1979) investigated several recently
imported B. constrictor and found about 0.5% of the snakes
infected.

Suborder Eimeriina
Families Toxoplasm(at)idae and Sarcocystidae

Species of these exclusively parasitic families are
known from many birds and mammals but they are rarely
found in poikilothermic vertebrates. Up to now only
species of the genera Besnoitia (Toxoplasmidae) and Sarcocystis (Sarcocystidae) are known to infect reptiles as
intermediate and/or definitive hosts. Munday et al. (1979)
mentioned for the first time that oocysts/sporocysts which
may belong to either Sarcocystis or Frenkelia were found
in the intestinal tract of three Australian reptiles
(Table 19.17). From amphibians, Levine (1976) and Levine
and Nye (1976, 1977) recorded three species of the genus
Toxoplasma from anurans, but Dubey (1977) termed them as
"sporozoans of unknown taxonomic position". The investigations by Munday et al. (1979) could not reveal these
apicomplexan families in 90 Australian amphibians belonging
to nine species in two families.

The investigations of Heydorn and Rommel (1972a,b),
Rommel and Heydorn (1972) and Rommel et al. (1972) first
confirmed the membership of these protozoans to the "cyst-forming isosporoid coccidia" (Frenkel, 1977) for which
two vertebrate hosts characteristically are obligatory
(Sarcocystis); the life cycle of the other genus seems to
be only facultatively heterogenous since it is possible
to maintain some species in mice indefinitely. Definitive
hosts of Besnoitia from reptiles have not been found up
to now (Smith and Frenkel, 1977). The intermediate host
with the vegetative multiplication stages (one or two
schizogonies and cyst formation in the muscles, Sarcocystis; or cyst formation in various organs, Besnoitia)
is for both genera a herbivorous or omnivorous animal.

Table 19.17. Reptiles as Intermediate and Definitive Hosts

Species	Host (Family)	Geographic distribution
INTERMEDIATE HOSTS		
S. platydactyli	Tarentola mauritanica (Geckonidae)	Minorca; Algeria; Tunisia
S. gongyli	Chalcides ocellatus (Scincidae)	Sicily
S. lacertae	Lacerta muralis (Lacertidae)	Italy
S. pythonis	Morelia argus (Pythonidae)	Australia
S. utae	Uta stansburiana (Iguanidae)	United States of America
S. scelopori	Sceloporus occidentalis (Iguanidae)	United States of America
S. chamaeleonis	Chamaeleo fischeri multituberculatus (Chamaeleonidae)	Tanzania
S. kinosterni (syn. S. gracilis)	Kinosteron scorpioides (Kinosternidae)	Brazil
Sarcocystis sp.	Eremias oliveri (Lacertidae)	South Africa
Sarcocystis sp.	Tortoises (Testudinidae)	Bulgaria
Sarcocystis sp.	Leiolopisma metallica (Scincidae) Varanus gouldii, V. varius (Varanidae)	Australia
S. atractaspidis[a]	Atractaspis leucomeles (Viperidae)	Kenya

of Sarcocystis.

Size of cysts (microns)	Size of trophozoites (microns)	References
2000 X 400	3.4 X 1.0	Bertram, 1892;
2000 X 400	4.0	Chatton and
2000 X 400	5.0-6.0 X 1.5-2.0	Avel, 1923; Dupouy and Kechemir, 1973; Weber, 1909a,b, 1910
200-800 X 30-60	3.0-4.0 X 1.0	Trinci, 1910
1800-2000 X 1000	6.5-7.3 X 1.5-2.0	Babudieri, 1931; Senaud and DePuytorac, 1964/1965
1100	4.0-7.0	Tiegs, 1931
950 X 120	5.5-7.0 X 1.5-2.0	Ball, 1944
600 X 180	5.2-6.0 X 1.5-2.0	Ball, 1944
1500 X 500-1000	10.0-13.0 X 2.0 (muscles) 10.0-14.0 X 3.0-3.8 (blood)	Frank, 1966a
8000 X 170-230	18.4 X 1.7	Lainson and Shaw, 1971
NA[b]	NA	Reichenbach-Klinke, 1977
NA	NA	Meshkov, 1975
NA	NA	Munday et al., 1979
NA	NA	Parenzan, 1947

(contd.)

Table 19.17. Reptiles as Intermediate and Definitive Host

Species	Intermediate host	Size of cysts (trophozoites) (microns)
DEFINITIVIE HOSTS		
S. singaporensis	Rattus norvegicus, R. tiomanicus, Rattus sp. (all experimental); R. rattus from Thailand had natural infection	1125 X 184 (6.9-8.6 X 2.0-2.9)
S. idahoensis	Peromyscus maniculatus	1600-9400 X 200-800 (6.0-7.0 X 2.0)
Sarcocystis sp.	R. fuscipes	2500 X 500
Sarcocystis sp. or Frenkelia sp.	Not known	Not known

aDoubtful validity; probably does not belong to Sarcocystis (Lainson and Shaw, 1971).
bNA=not available.

of Sarcocystis. (Continued)

Definitive host (Family)	Size of oocyst (sporocysts) (microns)	Geographic distribution	References
Python reticulatus (Pythonidae)	8.8-16.8 X 6.9-10.8 (7.2-12.0 X 6.9-9.1)	Malaysia; Thailand	Brehm, 1979; Brehm and Frank, 1980; Frank and Hafner, 1981; Zaman, 1975; Zaman and Colley, 1975
Pituophis melanoleucus deserticola (natural) P. m. catenifer P. m. annectans (experimental) (Colubridae)	13.0-14.0 X 22.0-23.0) (11.0-12.0 X 13.0-14.0)	North America	Bledsoe, 1979, 1980
Morelia spilotes variegata (Pythonidae)	9.6 X 13.8 (9.6 X 6.6)	Australia	Rzepczyk, 1974; Rzepczyk, and Scholtyseck, 1976
Austrelaps superba Notechis ater (Elapidae)	?	Australia	Munday et al., 1979

The definitive host is always an animal which preys upon other vertebrates. In the definitive host the gamogony and sporogony (Sarcocystis) or only the gamogony (Besnoitia) take place. Up to now a great number of studies considering the distribution, life cycles and cytology, including reptile infecting species, have been published and were summarized by Dubey (1977), Kalyakin and Zasukhin (1975), Mehlhorn and Heydorn (1978) and Tadros and Laarman (1976, 1982). In a comprehensive study, Rommel (1978) compared the life cycles of tissue cyst-forming coccidia and Frenkel et al. (1979), Melville (1980) and Tardos and Laarman (1982) discussed the taxonomic problems of these species which have arisen in relation to the international rules of zoological nomenclature.

Reptiles as intermediate hosts. Only a few publications deal with the existence of cysts in muscles or visceral organs of reptiles. If they do so, the cysts belong to either the genus Sarcocystis (Table 19.17) or Besnoitia. Reichenbach-Klinke (1977) mentioned that Elkan had found Toxoplasma gondii, but this unique finding could not be verified by other authors. The picture given is not instructive enough to identify Toxoplasma. On the other hand, experimental transmission of T. gondii from mice to reptiles failed under normal temperatures (Frank, unpubl.). However, Stone and Manwell (1969) have shown that Toxoplasma may be successfully transferred to reptile and even to amphibians especially when these animals were kept at higher temperatures. The parasites persisted at least 6 days or longer in some individuals, but more often when the animals were kept at 37 C rather than room temperature. Levit (1976) was able to infect reptiles with the low virulence Toxoplasma strain FCL if the reptiles were maintained at higher temperatures (31 to 35 C). A variation in susceptibility was observed with Agama and Vipera being most susceptible and Testudo and Natrix most resistant. Moreover, Levine (1977) grouped some species of protozoans from cold-blooded vertebrates under the genus Toxoplasma. The species are: 1) T. alencari (de Costa and Pereira, 1971) Levine and Nye, 1976, from the brain of the Brazilian frog Leptodactylus ocellatus; 2) T. ranae Levine and Nye, 1976, from brain pseudocysts of North American Rana pipiens; 3) T. serpai Scorza, Dagert and Itturriza Arocha, 1956, from the erythrocytes, liver, spleen, kidneys and brain of Venezuelan Bufo marinus; 4) T. brumpti Coutelen, 1932, from mononuclear leucocytes of Iguana tuberculata from Trinidad; and, 5) T. colubri Tibaldi, 1921, from white blood corpuscles of Coluber viridiflavus from Sardinia.

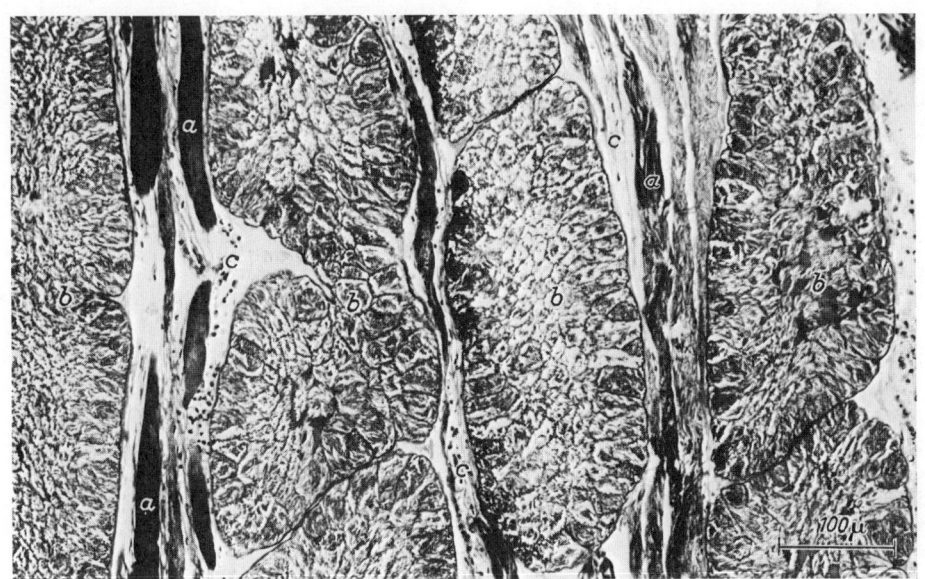

Fig. 19.9. Longitudinal section through muscle fibers of a Chamaeleo fischeri infected with vegetative stages (cysts) of Sarcocystis chamaeleonis. The so-called "Miescher's tubes" are chambered, most of them are empty, a sign of old, degenerating cysts. a=muscle fibers; b=Sarcocystis cysts; c=fibroblast cells, from Frank (1966a)

In his discussion, Levine (1977) wrote that "the only species of Toxoplasma whose complete life cycles are known are T. gondii and T. hammondi. It is not impossible that, when more becomes known about the other species, some of them may be transferred to other genera and other names may be found to be synonyms. In the meantime, the present position seems best." Dubey (1977) doubted these classifications since nothing is known concerning the life cycles and very little of the structure.

Apart from older descriptions, only a few findings of Sarcocystis cysts (Miescher's tubes) have been published in recent years. Frank (1966a) described S. chamaeleonis from Chamaeleo fischeri (Fig. 19.9) and Lainson and Shaw (1971, 1972) found S. kinosterni in the muscles of a Brazilian tortoise, K. scorpioides. The investigations of Meshkov (1975) and Munday et al. (1979) show that Sarcocystis cysts in the muscles of reptiles are more common than would be assumed from the few publications which exist in the widespread literature. All known species are given in Table 19.17.

Only a few details are known concerning the significance of these parasites for their intermediate hosts. Frank (1966a) mentioned marked muscle destructions with edematous swellings and gelatinous lysis of the masseter muscle of a C. fischeri. The walls of the cysts were destroyed and many trophozoites (cystozoites) were free not only in the tissue but also in the peripheral blood where their size differed from that of the trophozoites in cysts. Lainson and Shaw (1971, 1972) described the lesions caused by S. kinosterni in the skeletal muscles of K. scorpioides, all other muscles (cardiac and involuntary) were free of cysts. The lesions observed were usually associated with ruptured cysts. Remnants of the cysts were surrounded by intense round-cell infiltration. Heavily infected tortoises showed pale, soft and pulpy flesh. The fact that most of the tortoises that died in captivity proved to be very heavily infected suggests that infection may sometimes be fatal (Lainson and Shaw, 1971). The characterization of the lesions in tortoises corresponds well with the destructions described from the masseter muscle of C. fischeri (Frank, 1966a).

Besnoitia are tissue cyst-forming parasites in the intermediate host. The number of valid species from cold-blooded vertebrates seems to be doubtful. While Garnham (1964, 1966) mentioned that his B. sauriana from British Honduras must be a valid species since the cysts found in various organs of Basiliscus vittatus were different from those described by Schneider (1965) as B. panamensis from Ameiva ameiva, A. festiva, A. leptophrys, A. quadrilineata B. basiliscus, B. plumifrons, B. vittatus, Cnemidophorus lemniscatus and Sceloporun malachiticus, and contrary to the ones reported by Schneider (1967a) could not be transferred to mice. Schneider, nevertheless, synonymized the following species from the New World with B. darlingi: Sarcocystis sp. Darling, 1913; S. darlingi Brumpt, 1913; Fibrocystis darlingi Babudieri, 1932; B. panamensis Schneider, 1965; and, B. sauriana Garnham, 1966. In a further investigation, Schneider (1967c) studied B. darlingi from mammals and B. panamensis demonstrating cross-immunity between the two species. Smith and Frenkel (1977) accepted the synonym of the mammalian and lizard species and found cats to be the definitive hosts of the cysts. The cysts of B. darlingi from Panamanian lizards have a size of 200 to 500 microns and were found in the heart, lungs, spleen, kidneys, mesenteries and on occasion in the liver and lamina propria of the testis. The lizard parasites could be transferred to mice with initially initially low virulence, but the virulence increased with successive mouse passages (Schneider, 1965, 1967a,b).

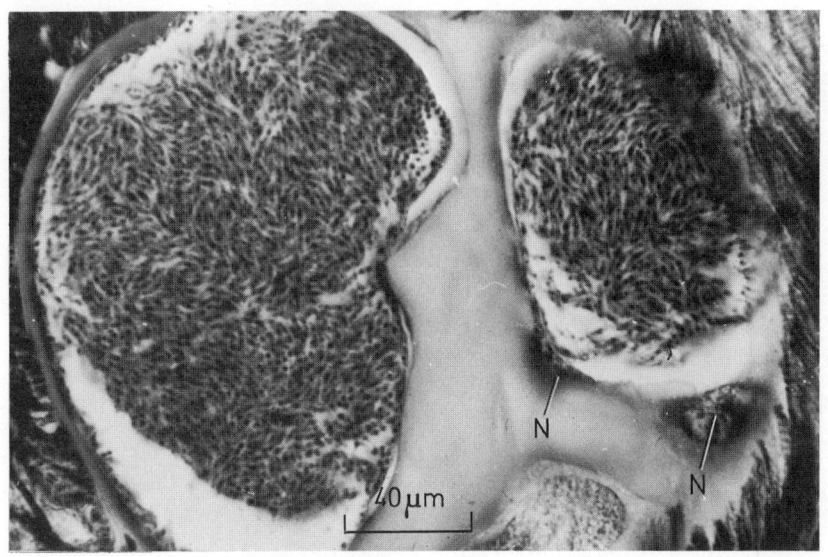

Fig. 19.10. Besnoitia cysts in the heart muscle of a Lacerta dugesii from Madeira Islands. n= nucleus

Pathological destructions caused by Besnoitia cysts depend on the degree of infection and the virulence of the strain.

Whether lizards are the natural intermediate hosts of B. darlingi or only one group of several intermediaries is just as unknown as the definitive host(s) of this species. Life cycle studies on other Besnoitia spp. included carnivores (cats) as definitive hosts. Frank and Frenkel (1981) briefly reported having found Besnoitia cysts in the heart muscle of a lizard, Lacerta dugesii, from the Madeira Islands (Fig. 19.10). It is the first record of these parasites in poikilothermic animals in the Old World. It is not known if Besnoitia cysts were present in other organs since no studies were done. It is interesting to note that in their natural environment the lizards are in close contact to cats and that many of them are caught by cats.

Reptiles as definitive hosts of Sarcocystis. Oocysts or sporocysts of the isosporoid type, probably belonging to species of the families Sarcocystidae or Toxoplasm(at)- idae, could be found repeatedly in the intestines or the feces of snakes from South America and East Asia during post-mortem examination (Fig. 19.11) (Frank and Loos-Frank, 1977). It can be assumed that a number of descriptions

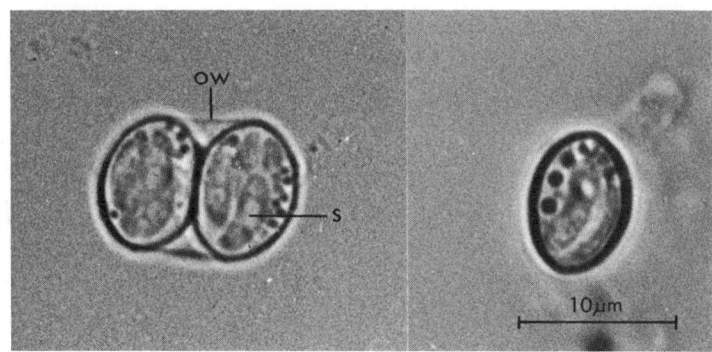

Fig. 19.11. Oocysts with two sporulated sporocysts (left) and a freed sporulated sporocyst (right) of Sarcocystis singaporensis from Python reticulatus. ow=oocyst wall; s=sporozoit, from Brehm and Frank (1980)

of Isospora spp. based on oocysts/sporocysts alone belong to the "tissue cyst-forming isosporoid coccidia". Life cycle studies of such isosporoid oocysts/sporocysts from three species of snakes established all three as members of the genus Sarcocystis, but comparing the descriptions of these stages given by Pellerdy (1974) and the characterization of Dubey (1977) for Besnoitia oocysts "...shed unsporulated - sporulation is completed within 2-4 days ...", the author suggests that some of the species listed by Pellerdy (1974) may also belong to the genus Besnoitia or even Frenkelia (Munday et al., 1979). Rzepczyk (1974) Reported oocysts/sporocysts of an anonymous Sarcocystis sp. from Morelia spilotes variegata. She found a suitable intermediate host in the endemic Australian rat, Rattus fuscipes, which was infected naturally. Although only transferring muscle cysts to snakes and not vice versa, she seems to have found in R. fuscipes the natural intermediate host of the above mentioned Sarcocystis sp. which develops in M. spilotes variegata as its definitive host. Other investigations confirmed that R. fuscipes and M. spilotes variegata are naturally associated in a food chain (Sprent, 1963).

The only species in which the complete life cycles could be studied experimentally, transferring muscle cysts to definitive hosts and the oocysts/sporocysts to the intermediate hosts several times, are S. singaporensis (Beaver and Maleckar (1981) separated this species into three distinguishable species, S. singaporensis, S. zamani and S. villivillosi; the complete life cycles of all

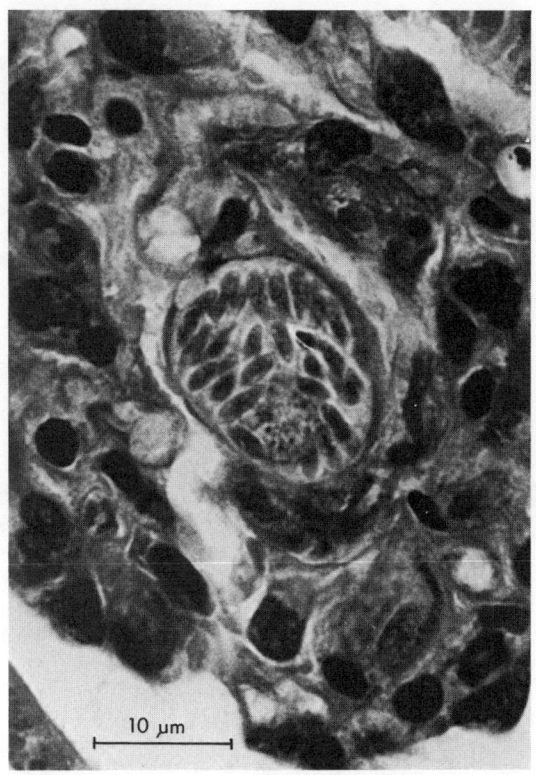

Fig. 19.12. Early developmental stage (meront) of <u>Sarcocystis singaporensis</u> in the kidney of an experimentally infected laboratory rat 10 days after feeding of about 150 oocysts/sporocysts.

these species are now known) and <u>S</u>. <u>idahoensis</u> (Figs. 19.12 to 19.14). Zaman and Colley (1975) published observations concerning the life cycle of <u>S</u>. <u>singaporensis</u> between oocysts/sporocysts shed via feces from the reticulated python, <u>Python reticulatus</u>, and the development of the vegetative stages in the rat, <u>R</u>. <u>norvegicus</u>. Further investigations of this species were made by Brehm (1979) and Brehm and Frank (1980). Recent publications by Bledsoe (1979, 1980) show that probably life cycles of <u>Sarcocystis</u> spp. between rodents as intermediate hosts and reptiles (snakes) as definitive hosts are more common as could be assumed a few years ago. Bledsoe reported the life cycle of <u>S</u>. <u>idahoensis</u> between deer mice, <u>Peromyscus maniculatus</u>, and the gopher snake, <u>Pituophis melanoleucus</u> (Matuschka (1981) reported for the first time

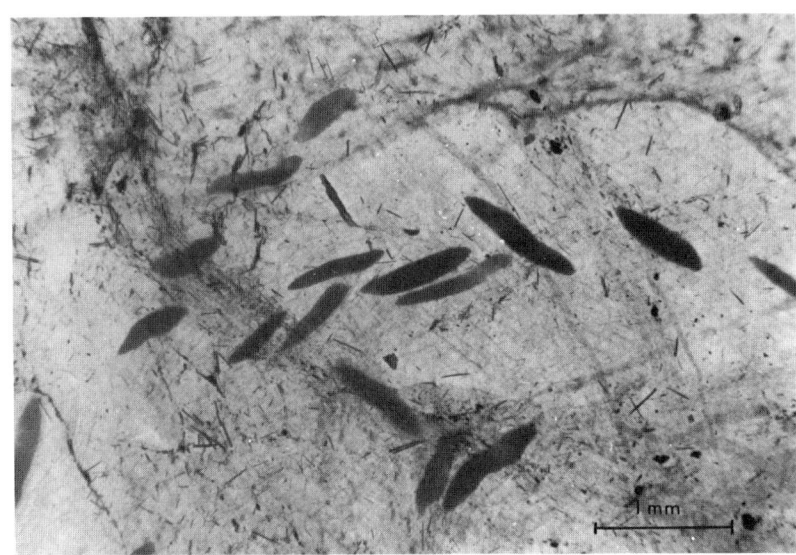

Fig. 19.13. Many cysts of <u>Sarcocystis</u> <u>singaporensis</u> in the muscles of an experimentally infected laboratory rat about two months post-infection, fresh preparation.

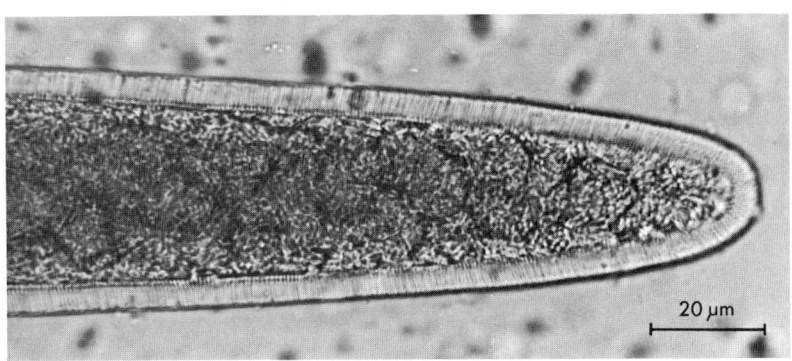

Fig. 19.14. Higher magnification of Fig. 19.13 to show details of the organization of a cyst.

a life cycle of a newly described <u>Sarcocystis</u> species, S. <u>podarcicolubris</u>, between two poikilothermic hosts. The lizards, <u>Podacris</u> (syn. <u>Lacerta</u>) <u>sicula</u> and <u>P</u>. (syn. <u>Lacerta</u>) <u>tiliquerta</u>, function as intermediate hosts and the snake, <u>Coluber</u> <u>viridiflavus</u>, as the definitive host).

<u>Pathogenesis in the intermediate host</u>. Brehm (1979) and Brehm and Frank (1980) showed that <u>S</u>. <u>singaporensis</u>

is highly pathogenic to rats. Even low numbers of sporocysts (150 to 300) given orally caused severe clinical signs with fever, diarrhea, bloody secretion from the eyes and nose. These signs correspond with the first and second schizogony in the visceral organs of the rat at the 9th and 16th day post-infection. Muscle cysts showed trophozoites (cystozoites) from the 40th day post-infection onward. Muscle cysts onwards the 60th day post-infection from the rats were infectious for snakes, P. reticulatus. The dissection of the rats showed hyperplastic spleen, swollen Peyer's patches and lymph nodes, and an orange-colored intestine which appeared to be hyalin. The animals were anemic.

The development in the definitive host could be completely investigated on tissue surgically taken from the midgut. Forty-five hours post-infection all cystozoites were in the epithelial cells and 90 hours post-infection the gamogony was performed. The sporogony occurred at the base of the epithelial cells and occasionally in the lamina propria. Four days post-infection the first oocysts were found in the tissue. In the feces from the 8th day post-infection onward fully sporulated oocysts and a high percentage of freed sporocysts were shed. The shedding of sporocysts lasted for at least 73 days.

Pathogenesis in the definitive host. Tissue reactions against the developmental stages in the intestinal cells could not be observed during any of the aforementioned studies. They may be dependent upon the degree of infection. Young P. reticulatus which had died after their arrival, often have many necrotic foci in the intestinal epithelium comparable with the early lesions of an E. invadens infection (Frank, unpubl.).

Host specificity. The most interesting result was strong host specificity of S. singaporensis. Brehm and Frank (1980) were not able to infect intermediate hosts other than Norwegian rats. These results correspond with the findings of Zaman (1976) which showed a very limited host range. The host specificity existed not only for intermediate hosts but also for the definitive host. It was not possible to infect other species of snakes, not even related species like P. molurus, from the same geographical area. It was postulated that S. singaporensis, and probably other Sarcocystis spp. as well, is species-specific for the definitive host, but the host range for intermediate hosts is possibly genus-specific. A number of species of the genus Rattus were tested and R. tiomanicus (Malaysia) is a suitable intermediate host as well as

Table 19.18. Distribution of the Eimeriidae.

	$Eimeria^a$ $(O=4\times2)$	$Isospora^b$ $(O=2\times4)$	$Caryospora$ $(O=1\times8)$	$Cyclospora$ $(O=2\times2)$	$Hoarella$ $(O=16\times2)$
AMPHIBIA					
Urodela	15	1	-	-	-
Anura	11	10	-	-	-
REPTILIA					
Lacertilia	35	18[c]	1	2	1
Chamaeleonidae	2	1	-	-	-
Ophidia	29	16[d]	11[e]	5	-
Crocodilia	3	2	-	-	-
Chelonia	18	-	-	-	-

[a] $O=4\times2$ means the oocyst contains four sporocysts, each with two sporozoites; $O=-\times8$ means the oocyst contains no sporocyst, but 8 naked sporozoites.
[b] Isospora species from reptiles probably belong in the majority to the "tissue cyst forming isosporoid coccidia", which should be included into the families Toxoplasmidae or Sarcocystidae with at least a facultative or obligatory two-vertebrate host life cycle. A number of species must possibly be included into the new genera Levineia or Cystoisospora (Dubey, 1977; Rommel, 1978).
[c] One species (I. varani) surely belongs to the Toxoplasmidae/Sarcocystidae "...the oocysts have yet to be observed" - a classical characterization of species of Sarcocystis since typically freed sporulated sporocysts pass with the feces in this genus. The host of I. varani is Varanus griseus. The other species may be true Isospora species since their hosts are herbivorous or are feeding on invertebrates.

Table 19.18. Distribution of the Eimeriidae.^{f} (Continued)

	Octosporella (O=8x2)	Pythonella (O=16x4)	Wenyonella (O=4x4)	Dorisiella (O=2x8)	Tyzzeria (O=-x8)
AMPHIBIA					
Urodela	–	–	–	–	–
Anura	–	–	–	–	–
REPTILIA					
Lacertilia	1	1	–	–	–
Chamaeleonidae	–	–	–	–	–
Ophidia	–	1	1	1	1
Crocodilia	–	–	–	–	–
Chelonia	–	–	–	–	–

^{d}Most of these species probably belong to Toxoplasmidae/Sarcocystidae. The given characterization is in accordance with the sporogonic stages of these genera. Snakes, on the other hand, are vertebrate preying reptiles and the chance that snakes are definitive hosts for tissue cyst-forming coccidia exists.

^{e}Altogether 12 species are known. C. dendrelaphis, the second ophidian Caryospora from Australia, was described by Cannon and Rzepczyk (1974) from the colubrid snake, Dendrelaphis punctulatus.

^{f}The genus Globidium represented by G. navillei (Host: Natrix natrix and N. viperinus) is a species with doubtful systematic position (Pellerdy, 1974).

other species of this genus from Thailand and Australia (Frank and Hafner, 1981).

The high infection rate of free-ranging snakes, P. reticulatus, is possibly the result of a high incidence of infected rats in the biotype of the snakes, and the spreading of sporocysts by invertebrates. Arthropods, for example coprophagous flies, can take up innumberable sporocysts from snake feces and easily transport them to food material of rats. Experiments have shown that even a few sporocysts fed orally to a rat were sufficient to cause severe infection. Hafner (1980) supposed that this system functioned in nature as well as in the laboratory. Nothing was known so far about definitive hosts of Sarcocystis spp. which can be found in the muscles of reptiles (Frank, 1976b), until the recent investigation of Matuschka (1981).

Suborder Eimeriina
Family Eimeriidae

Most of the numerous species of the Eimeriidae described from amphibians and reptiles are members of the genus Eimeria. A number of other genera can be found, but they are less common, the only exception being Isospora which will be discussed separately. The distribution of the various genera and their characterization is summarized in Table 19.18. The biology of only a few species from amphibians and reptiles is known. The pathogenicity of these coccidia for poikilothermic animals rarely has been investigated, but may be similar to that for warm-blooded vertebrates. New descriptions of species underline the frequency of these parasites in cold-blooded hosts (Colley and Else, 1975; Duszynski et al., 1977; Leibovitz et al., 1978; Mandal, 1976; Pluto and Rothenbacher, 1976; Wacha and Christiansen, 1977).

The descriptions of most species of the Eimeriidae are based exclusively on the oocyst stage which is passed from the host via feces. This stage is very easily detectable either in routine examinations of feces or during post-mortem studies. The observation of Seidel (1977) that in a post-mortem investigation of 173 snakes, 9% had a severe coccidian infection which was not detected during life, is a surprising statement and may not be generalized.

While the description of a species based only on the morphology of the oocysts is sufficient for Eimeria and probably for most other genera as well, problems of classification have arisen from new findings suggesting that members of the genus Isospora may belong to quite different coccidian groups. The majority of Isospora spp. from snakes, for example, probably have to be included in the "tissue cyst-forming isosporoid coccidia" (Dubey, 1977; Frenkel, 1977). The original descriptions of the oocysts of Isospora spp., as well as the drawings of oocysts and/or sporocysts of many species, show pecularities of the corresponding stages of the Toxoplasma(at)idae or Sarcocystidae. The delicate walls of the oocysts are shaped by closely underlying sporocysts. In some species the occurrence of freed sporocysts only in the feces is an unequivocal sign that these species have to be included in the already mentioned families (Hoare, 1933). Pellerdy (1974) summarized all known facts with parts of the original descriptions.

A revision of the genus Isospora of amphibians and reptiles is urgently needed. Further investigations concerning the life cycles of these coccidia may lead to a new classification of a certain number of species. The latest findings should be taken into account when new species are described.

The classification of members of the Eimeriidae is mainly based upon the morphology of the sporulated oocyst (Levine, 1973). The characteristics of the various genera are dealt with by Frank (1976b) and Todd and Ernst (1977). Problems have arisen in the genus Isospora during the past 10 years. Isospora contains two distinct groups of organisms which are structurally and biologically different. They can be characterized as follows.

Isospora Schneider, 1881, 1st group. The oocyst contains two sporocysts, each with four sporozoites. The wall of the oocyst is more or less thick and sturdy and sporulation typically occurs outside the host. Direct (monoxenous) fecal-oral transmission occurs without the involvement of intermediate hosts. The developmental stages are found mainly in epithelial or subepithelial cells. Various species may be found in herbivorous or invertebrate-feeding reptiles and amphibians. Examples include I. calotesi Bhatia, 1938 (host: Calotes versicolor) and I. hemidactyli Carini, 1936 (host: Hemidactylus mabuya).

Isospora Schneider, 1881, 2nd group. The oocyst, when present in the feces, contains two sporocysts, each with four sporozoites. A certain percentage of freed sporocysts can be seen. The oocysts have a delicate, unilayered, colorless wall which takes its shape from the closely adpressed sporocysts. Typically sporulation has occurred by the time of fecal passage, or it may take place within a few hours or days. The life cycle is heteroxenous with a facultative or obligatory two-vertebrate host intermediary. In the intermediate host, tissue cysts are formed, which can be seen macroscopically or microscopically. The intermediate hosts are herbivorous, omnivorous or invertebrate-feeders while the definitive hosts are always, at least in part, vertebrate preying or carcass feeding species. In accordance with the descriptions given by Pellerdy (1974) it can be supposed that I. crotali (Triffit, 1925), Hoare, 1925 (host: Crotalus confluens) and I. dirumpens Hoare, 1933, (host: Bitis arietans) are two examples of this group.

Biology of the Eimeriidae. Macrogametocytes and microgametocytes develop independently. The microgametocytes typically produce many microgametes with two or three flagella. The oocysts have 0, 1, 2, 4 or many sporocysts, each with one or more sporozoites (typically the sporozoites are enclosed in the sporocyst). Development (merogony or schizogony) is in the host cell proper while sporogony occurs typically outside the host. Endodyogeny and syzygy formation are absent and the zygote is not motile. The life cycle is monoxenous (Levine, 1973; Todd and Ernst 1977).

While the oocyst is the typical stage which can be found in the feces with ease (Fig. 19.15), it is more difficult to detect the vegetative stages in the tissues. Only histological slides show the meronts (schizonts), merozoites, gametocytes, gametes or zygotes. Knowledge about the life histories of coccidians from amphibians and reptiles is insufficient. Merogony (schizogony) and gamogony take place, according to the species, in various organs mainly the intestine, gall bladder, biliary ducts and very rarely, in the kidney tubules. The sites of development are always epithelial cells or underlying tissue layers. Despite the small number of investigations about the biology of coccidians of Amphibia and Reptilia, it can be assumed that the development of these species is identical with those species infecting warm-blooded vertebrates (Dubey, 1977).

The infection follows oral up-take of sporulated oocysts by feeding. In the intestine the sporozoites are freed and penetrate the intestinal mucosa. They come to their preference organs via the blood stream and develop into meronts intracellularly or the development takes place directly in the intestinal epithelial cells. The merogony

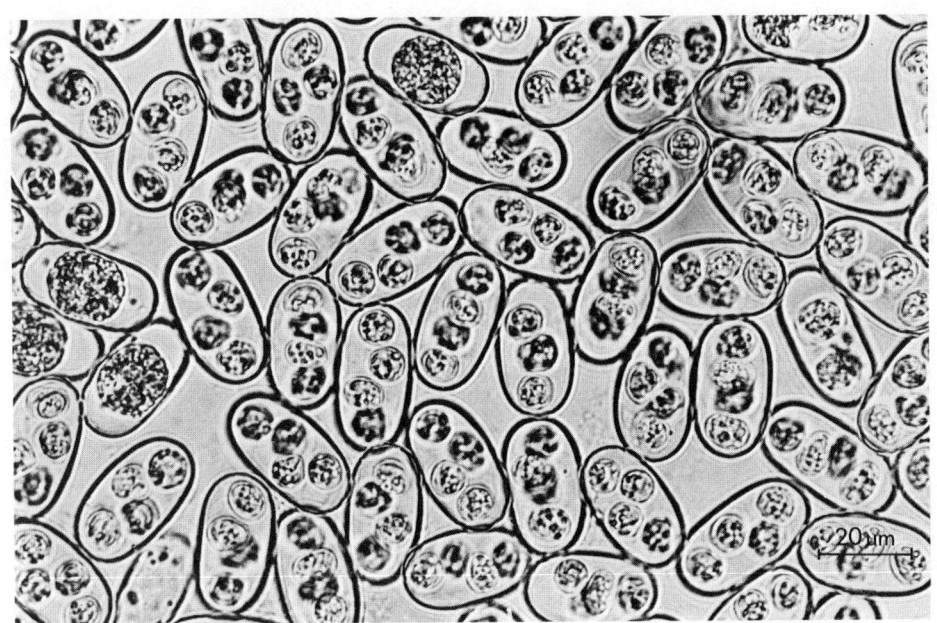

Fig. 19.15. Oocysts of an undetermined Eimeria sp. from a snake.

(schizogony) happens at least once; most species have two or more merogonies. The many merozoites penetrate cells in the neighborhood and repeat the merogony or develop into macro- or microgametocytes. Each macrogametocyte grows into one macrogamete, but several microgametes are formed from each microgametocyte. Fertilization between a microgamete and a macrogamete produces the zygote which is the oocyst after the walls have thickened. The young oocysts pass with the feces or urine. Sporulation mainly occurs outside the host. First sporoblasts are formed and in each sporoblast the sporozoites are differentiated and the sporoblasts become sporocysts. Very soon, often only one to few days, the oocysts are again infectious for new hosts. The length of the whole life cycle depends on the particular species, but normally is completed within several days.

Characteristic clinical signs are not correlated with coccidian infection. The disease, coccidiosis, is rarely observed (Frank, 1975; Gabrisch, 1976). Incidental diseases caused by Eimeriidae may occur. Sindermann (1977) described a coccidiosis of Chelonia mydas which probably was caused by Caryospora sp. Leibovitz et al. (1978) verified these observations and described the first species

of this genus from chelonians as C. cheloniae. This
coccidium is of economic importance for mariculture-reared
green sea turtles. Affected turtles ranged from 4 to 8
weeks old. The pathologic alterations in many young
turtles were most pronounced in the posterior third of the
intestine. The lumen of the gut was greatly dilated and
filled with blood, oocysts and tissue debris. All stages
of development could be found histologically. Cannon
(1967) reported C. demansiae from Australian elapid snake
Demansia psammophis. The snakes showed no congestion of
the intestine, but the lumen was full of a thick, pasty
material rich in oocysts. No histology was done.

Massive infection with Eimeria grobbeni caused cutaneous discoloration in Salamandra atra in Europe. Infected
salamanders were recognized by a conspicuous depigmentation
of their skin, particularly in the head, cervical and
abdominal regions. In the intestine, the site of development, desquamation of the epithelium and infiltration of
inflammatory cellular elements in the mucosa and submucosa
were characteristic.

In reptiles the pathological destructions of only two
Eimeria spp. were investigated. Fantham and Porter (1953)
studied E. bitis in a number of North American snakes,
namely, Thamnophis sirtalis, T. sauritus and Opheodrys
vernalis. The epithelium of the gall bladder was stripped
and ample connective tissue was present in the bladder
wall and biliary ducts. The bile was markedly viscid and
its color also had changed, varying from light green to
yellowish shades. They proposed that this species may be
identical with the species found by Fantham (1932) in a
puffadder, B. lachesis, in South Africa. This postulation
seems questionable.

A second Eimeria sp., E. cascabeli from rattlesnakes,
C. viridis viridis and C. v. helleri, was studied by
Vetterling and Widmer (1968). The different stages of
development occurred in the epithelial cells of the gall
bladder and extrahepatic ducts. The hosts responded to
these infections by a proliferation of the connective
tissue, erosions and liver enlargement. The species showed
a strong host specificity; attempts to infect C. cerastes
and T. sauritus with sporulated oocysts failed.

Only one other species, Cyclospora niniae from the
snake Ninia sebae sebae, has been investigated. Massive
infection of the intestine by these parasites provoked an
inflammatory cellular reaction which resulted in the detachment of the intestinal epithelium (Lainson, 1965).

An unpublished observation by Kutzer was that of a coccidiosis during the post-mortem examination of two pythons. Taking into account the explanations given in the section on Toxoplasm(at)idae and Sarcocystidae, it might have been an infection with a Sarcocystis sp. (S. singaporensis?). Similar remarks could be made about I. naiae infections mentioned by Frye (1973). The description of this species given by Pellerdy (1974) characterized it as a typical "tissue cyst-forming isosporoid coccidian". That this species should occur in Naja flava from South Africa, as well as in C. horridus from the New World, seems improbable.

Pathological destructions during the vegetative development can be seen according to the species of coccidians and the site and number of merogonies. As with warm-blooded vertebrates, young specimens of reptiles are especially subject to attack (Gabrisch, 1976), while on the other hand, adults or half grown specimens show either no or a mild response. They are the specimens which shed the oocysts for a long time and in captivity cause continuous infections if several animals of the same species are kept together. The author observed a high mortality rate among young Chamaeleo jacksonii bred in captivity due to an Eimeria infection of the gall bladder in spite of the good health of the mother. Examination of the feces of the mother, however, showed a continuous shedding of oocysts. Only a few young chameleons could be cured.

In spite of relatively high infection rates in some cases, pathological destructions have seldom been observed. E. ranae, for example, occurred in about 15% of the R. temporaria examined, but nothing is mentioned concerning their pathogenicity (Pellerdy, 1974). On the other hand, Seidel (1977) mentioned that 9% of 173 dissected snakes were infected with coccidia and that the coccidiosis was fatal in each case. A similar interpretation was published by Kiel (1975). The author's experience, based upon several thousand dissections, shows quite another picture. In amphibians and reptiles pathological alterations due to coccidia infections were very rare, with the exception of very young specimens. If alterations could be noticed, they belonged mainly to the "isosporoid coccidia". Oocysts of Eimeria spp. were commonly present in the feces and sporadically oocysts from Caryospora and also from "Isospora" could be seen. Stages of other genera were a rarity.

The same therapeutics which are used for birds and mammals can be attempted to cure coccidiosis in poikilothermic animals. Anticoccidial compounds are sulfonamide drugs in various preparations. The dosage administered varies from 40 mg/kg body weight up to 500 mg, depending upon the therapeutic used. As a rule the dosage has to be twice or three times the amount of the manufacturer's directions recommended for birds. It is advisable to administer the compound for several days (Frank, 1976a; Frye, 1973; Kiel, 1975; Lehmann, 1973; Wallach, 1969).

Suborder Eimeriina
Family Cryptosporidiidae

The members of the family are separated from the Eimeriidae by having microgametes without flagella and by their development in the host taking place just under the surface membranes of the host cells or within its striated border and not in the cell proper (Todd and Ernst 1977). All species are grouped in the only genus, Cryptosporidium. The oocysts are characterized by having no sporocyst, but instead, four naked sporozoites. Only a few species from reptiles are known; no record exists for amphibians. Pellerdy (1974) mentioned one species from Lacertilia and one from Ophidia. The records by Anderson et al. (1968), Duszynski (1969) and Triffit (1925) were not accepted by Vetterling et al. (1971) because no tissue stages were known up to that time. A new situation occurred since Brownstein et al. (1977) published a detailed study of an anonymous Cryptosporidium sp. from snakes with a full description of the tissue stages and the oocysts. The authors investigated 14 snakes of four species kept in captivity for a long period.

The species are characterized as follows. The oocyst are ball-like or ovoid with a size of 2.8 to 3.6 microns. During sporulation a residual body is formed. The schizonts in the tissue measure 2.5 to 3.0 microns and the four to eight filiform merozoites (trophozoites) are 1.6 to 2.0 microns in size. The development seems to be monoxenous. Infection experiments with mice as possible intermediate hosts failed. The infection of the hosts (snakes) occurred by taking up sporulated oocysts through feeding or drinking. It is possible that arthropods may transport the minute oocysts and so spread the infectious stages comparable to the carrier function of insects with Sarcocystis sporocysts (Hafner, 1980).

The development of the vegetative stages occurs exclusively in the mucosa of the stomach of snakes and causes a massive thickening of the wall (hypertrophic gastritis). The lumen becomes narrow. This situation leads to typical clinical signs with regurgitation of food and loss of weight. A swelling of the stomach region can sometimes be observed. McKenzie et al. (1978) reported identical signs from an Australian elapid snake, Pseudechis porphyriacus, housed for two years in a zoo in Queensland. The snake regurgitated fed mice within 30 to 60 minutes of ingestion. Autopsy revealed that the longitudinal rugae of the stomach were thickened. This is the first report of cryptosporidiosis in an Australian reptile and in elapid snakes.

The signs of cryptosporidiosis (regurgitation of prey) are similar to those caused by certain bacterial infections of the intestinal tract with necrotic decay of the mucosa and submucosa and thickening of the wall. In such cases the food passage may be blocked which then results in an identical reaction (Frank, 1976a).

The developmental stages of Cryptosporidium spp. occur in the mucosal cells just beneath the microvilli and cause a thickening of the mucosa which is edematous and rich in mucus. Necrotic areas often can be seen in histological slides. Lamina propria and submucosa also show edematous destruction with round-cell infiltration. Numerous plasma cells and lymphocytes can be distinguished. McKenzie et al. (1978) found all developmental stages of a Cryptosporidium sp., but not oocysts, histologically. This fact may be the reason why the other snakes of the same species kept together with the infected one showed no signs of disease. Bacteria of the genera Citrobacter, Proteus and Streptococcus may be isolated from infected snakes and McKenzie et al. (1978) mentioned two species of Salmonella. These findings must not be necessarily associated with a Cryptosporidium infection since these genera are common in reptiles (Mayer and Frank, 1974). In connection with the disease, other organs may be implicated. The liver appears pale yellow-brown and shows fatty degeneration. While the infection can be diagnosed by finding the minute oocysts in feces, up to now it is not known how to cure diseased snakes.

Organisms of uncertain status

Some genera mentioned by Reichenbach-Klinke and Elkan (1965) as parasites of amphibians and grouped together with the "Sporozoa" have still an unknown systematic position: Dermocystidium, Dermosporidium and Dermomycoides.

Flynn (1973) quoted them as stages possibly belonging to a fungus. The photographs of the "spores" given by

Reichenbach-Klinke and Elkan (1965) look quite similar to the so-called "spherules" (Frank et al., 1974), which cou be identified as an unusual and, up to that time, unknown stage in the development of a Mucor species. Similar to the genera mentioned above, this Mucor fungus causes derm lesions which look sometimes like a cyst, but they also produce skin tumors and severe destructions in practicall all visceral organs, particularly the liver and kidneys. The alterations can be seen microscopically. The spherule can easily be transferred to healthy amphibians by inject- ing homogenates of diseased organs. Within a few weeks post-inoculation an identical disease results. On agar plates a number of daughter organisms come free from each "spherule" and by budding each of them produces a typical Mucor mycelium. Conidiospores are produced and if they are inoculated into amphibians the result is the growth of the peculiar "spherules".

A further confusion has arisen since Levine (1978) erected a new class in the Apicomplexa, Perkinsea, with the single order Perkinsida, the single family Perkinsidae with the single species Perkinsus (syn. Dermocystidium) marinus, not identical with the species described from amphibians. This classification was accepted in the newly revised classification of the protozoa (Levine et al., 1980). Up to now it seems best to omit these three genera from the Apicomplexa until more information is available.

PHYLUM MICROSPORA

Order Microsporida

Microspora are a distinct group of protozoans which show some similarities to the Myxospora in having a polar filament, but not enclosed in a polar capsule, and an infective agent, the sporoplasm. The extreme smallness of the microsporidians with spores belonging to the small- est eucaryotic cells and the well adapted organization allowing them to live exclusively as intracellular para- sites of invertebrates and vertebrates characterize these organisms as a group of their own. Furthermore, it is suggested that there is no relationship between both phyla As a peculiarity, but also known from other protozoans, th microsporidians possess no mitochondria (Canning, 1977; Mitchell, 1977; Vavra, 1976).

The most fascinating process occurs when the unicell- ular spores come in contact with the tissues of a suitable host after ingestion of contaminated diet or water. The polar filament gets everted and comes in close contact with a host cell. The sporoplasm is then squeezed through the narrow, hollow tube of the filament and is injected into the host cell. This way of penetrating a host cell is unique but ensures that the delicate sporoplasm never reaches extracellular conditions.

Up to now, about 700 species of microsporidians infecting invertebrates as well as all five classes of vertebrates have been described (Canning, 1967, 1975, 1976; Hazard and Oldacre, 1975). The majority of species can be found in invertebrates with preference for arthropods. Fish are the most often infected vertebrates. Only a few species are known from amphibians and reptiles, belonging to the genera Pleistophora (suborder: Pansporoblastina) and Microsporidium. The last mentioned genus is a "collecting group" of unclassified Microsporida. All species insufficiently described are included in this genus until more information is available. Species now grouped into the genus Microsporidium have previously been described as species of Nosema, Glugea or Pl(e)istophora (Sprague, 1976, 1977) (Table 19.19). It would be desirable to get more information concerning the life cycle of microsporidians of both host groups in question, including their importance to the hosts.

Most species of microsporidians infecting amphibians and reptiles were discovered by post-mortem examination and/or histological examination. The whitish elongate cysts like Pleistophora myotrophica in the toad, B. bufo, or P. danilewskyi in its reptilian host can be easily seen during dissection. Signs of species parasiting the skin of the host are rarely found. Only Weiser (1950) reported a small white cyst of Microsporidium (syn. Nosema) tritoni on a tadpole, Triturus vulgaris. P. myotrophica infections in B. bufo were first observed in England by Canning and Elkan (1963, 1964). The disease normally lasts for a long period (about two years) but always ends fatally. This microsporidian infection could be found in Germany also (Frank, unpubl.) The white long cysts of P. myotrophica are macroscopically similar to several species of Sarcocystis and run parallel to the muscle fibers. Microscopically extensive destructions can be seen. Macrophages invade the masses of parasites and phagocytose spores, but they are without success in stopping the further development of the parasite. Long standing infections cause emaciation and subsequently the death of the toads. Further information about pathological alterations in the tissues infected by "Plistophora sp." are given for Sphenodon punctatus kept in captivity for about four months

Table 19.19. Microsporidian Species from Amphibia and

Host species	Microsporidian species	Type of reproduction
AMPHIBIA		
Bufo lentiginosus, B. bufo (syn. B. vulgaris)	Pleistophora bufonis (syn. Betramia, Plistophora)	Repeated binary fission (vegetative); 30 sporoblasts in a cyst, each develops into one spore
B. bufo	P. myotrophica (syn. Plistophora)	Binary fission, multiple fission and plasmotomy; sporonts give rise to large number of spores
Rana temporaria	Microsporidium danilewskyi[a]	Vegetative stages rarely seen; intracellular stages show early dissociation of the sporoblasts which results in isolated spores
Triturus vulgaris	M. tritoni (syn. Nosema)	Only a few vegetative stages could be found, they were uni- or binucleate; "sporont" round to egg-shaped, 5 X 3 microns; sporoblast elongated

Reptilia.

Spore (microns)	Site of development	Pathogenicity	Geographic distribution
Ends oval, the middle region with a slight constriction; 3.0 X 1.5; macrospores 4.0 X 4.5	"ova" of Bidder's organ	None reported	North America; Switzerland
Oval, 3.5-6.7 X 2.3 (when fresh); 3.2-4.5 X 1.9-2.6 (in section)	Striated muscle	Toads become emaciated; high mortality rates; lysis of myofibrils leads to the formation of fusiform spaces which are packed with spores; atrophy of the muscles occurs	England
Ovoid, 3.0-3.5 with a clear vacuole in either end	Muscles	None reported	Poland; Italy; Belgium; Switzerland
Not reported	Only seen in larva; infection occurred as white swelling anterior to the anus; the developing stages can be found	The lenticular cyst measured about 2 mm and was subcutaneous with thin and inconspicuous wall	Czechoslovakia

(contd.)

Table 19.19. Microsporidian Species from Amphibia and

Host species	Microsporidian species	Type of reproduction
REPTILIA		
Coluber gemonensis (syn. C. carbonaria)	P. heteroica (syn. Plistophora, Nosema)	Vegetative stages, no data; spherical vesicles with 8, 16, 64 or more spores
Sphenodon punctatus	Plistophora sp.[b]	Various stages from fusiform bodies 18.0-21.0 X 7.0-11.0 microns to schizogony containing numerous spherical uninucleate individuals to mature spores derived from a group of sporoblasts were observed in the muscle fibers
Chalcides tridactylus, Emys orbicularis, Natrix natrix, Lacerta sp.	M. danilewskyi[a] (syn. Plistophora, Nosema, Pleistophora, Glugea)	Compare text by Rana temporaria
N. natrix	M. ghigii[c] (syn. Glugea, Plistophora, Nosema)	Vegetative stages not seen; a few plasmodia and a few groups of spores apparently enclosed in membranes were seen; the great majority of the spores were isolated

Reptilia. (Continued)

Spore (microns)	Site of development	Pathogenicity	Geographic distribution
	in the connective tissue		
Ovoid, 6.0-7.0 X 2.0-3.0, with a clear terminal vacuole	No data	None reported	Italy
Pyriform, 3.9 X 2.2 with anterior and posterior vacuoles (stained)	Tongue and skeletal muscles	Muscle tissue white, fragile with "extensive destruction and myositis"	Stephens Islands, New Zealand; observed after 4 months in captivity in North America
Ovoid, 3.0 X 3.5 with a clear vacuole in either end	Muscles	None reported	Poland; Italy; Belgium; Switzerland
2.0 X 2.5	Intestinal tissue, surrounding the infected cestodes		Italy

(contd.)

Table 19.19. Microsporidian Species from Amphibia and

Host species	Microsporidian species	Type of reproduction
Lacerta muralis	Microsporidium[d] sp.	The occurrence of free spores in the foci rather than tight packed or membrane bound groups suggest that the species belongs to Nosema or Glugea

[a]The same species infects trematodes, Encylometra bolognensis and Telorchis ercolanii, parasitic in the intestinal tract of reptiles. The general state of confusion surrounding this species and the various synonymous names makes it convenient to group it provisionally in the "collective genus" Microsporidium.
[b]It is not clear if this is a species of Pleistophora, since no pansporoblastic membrane was seen.
[c]In spite of systematic confusion, this species is provisionally grouped in the "collective genus" Microsporidium. The same species is found in cestodes parasitic in the intestinal tract of the snake.
[d]Canning and Landau, 1971.

(Liu and King, 1971). The invaded tongue and skeletal muscles looked white and were fragile. They showed "extensive destruction and myositis". Unfortunately, the description is insufficient to group the species.

PHYLUM MYXOSPORA (SYN. MYXOZOA)

Up to recent times, the systematic position of the Myxospora was questionable. The multicellularity of both spores and trophozoites makes the classification difficult

Reptilia. (Continued)

Spore (microns)	Site of development	Pathogenicity	Geographic distribution
No data	Gut epithelium	The microsporidians were seen as foci of spores lying in a vacuole in the host cell; the spores were positioned close to the host cell nucleus between it and the mucus goblet	France

and some authors did not agree with the Myxosporea being true protozoans (Lom, 1973). The polar capsules (cnidocysts) of the myxosporidians show a close relationship to the nematocysts of the metazoan Cnidaria (Coelenterata) (Lom, 1969a,b, 1973). Despite these facts the Myxosporea are now included into the subkingdom Protozoa (Levine et al., 1980). Hundreds of species have been described from cold-blooded vertebrates, the majority of them from fish. Only a limited number of species (Table 19.20) are to be found in amphibians and very rarely in reptiles (chelonians). Although nothing is known about the life cycles of these species, it has been suggested that they are similar to or identical with species from fish (Mitchell, 1977).

Most of the myxosporidians show a tissue specificity but not a well developed host specificity. They can be distinguished as coelozoic species inhabiting the lumen of hollow organs such as the gall bladder and the urinary tract. The cytozoic species usually form cysts in the intercellular spaces of the muscles or other organs. The characterization of the genera is based mainly on spore morphology and the validity remains questionable for many species. The relationship of the Myxosporea to the Microsporea is not accepted by all authors.

Table 19.20. Species of Myxosporea in Amphibians and Reptiles.

Species	Host	Geographic distribution	Location in host
Leptotheca ohlmacheri	Various frog and toad species	North America; Europe	Kidneys
Myxosoma ranae	Rana temporaria, tree frogs	Australia; Europe	Various tissues
Myxobolus conspicuus	Notophthalmus v. viridescens	North America	Muscles
Myxidium serotinum	Various frog species; common toad	North America	Gallbladder
M. immersum	Various toad species; frogs	South America	Gallbladder
M. chelonarum	Various turtle species	North America	Bile duct; gallbladder
M. americanum	Soft-shelled turtles	North America	Kidneys

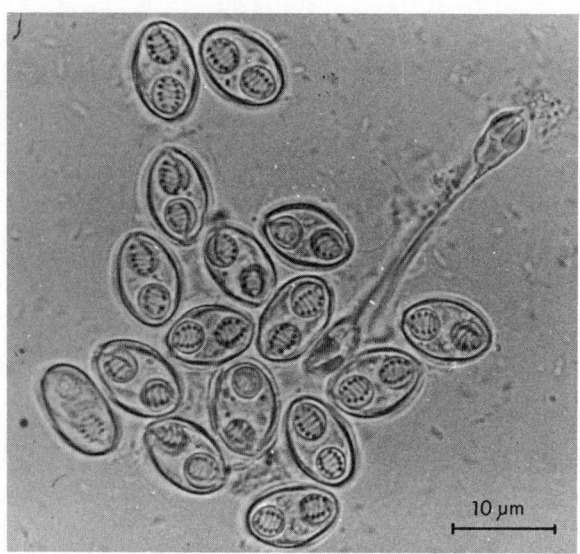

Fig. 19.16. Spores of Myxidium sp. and Henneguya sp. from the gall bladder of Pipa sp.

The class Myxosporea is subdivided into the order Bivalvulida with three suborders (Bipolarina, Eurysporina and Platysporina) and the order Multivalvulida. All myxosporidians have a spore which is the infectious stage. A new host can only be infected by accidental uptake of contaminated water. The members of the Platysporina possess two (one) pole-capsules (cnidocysts) situated at one end of the ovoid or ball-like spores, while on the other hand, the Bipolarina have two pole-capsules each at one end of the ovoid or banana-shaped spores. The size of the spores varies between a few microns up to about 16 microns. The spores are shaped by several cells.

The Myxosporea are represented in amphibians and reptiles by the genera Leptotheca, Myxobolus, Myxosoma, Henneguya and Myxidium. The few species recorded from amphibians are discussed by Walton (1964, 1966, 1967) and are listed in part by Flynn (1973). Dual infections in one host are possible. The author found two undetermined species belonging to two different genera (Myxidium and Henneguya) in the gall bladder of an adult female Pipa sp. kept in captivity for only a few months. The gall was gelatinous, possibly an effect due to the myxosporidian infection (Fig. 19.16).

The resistant spores require a certain time outside the host for aging before they become infectious. It is generally believed that only a single host is involved in the life cycle of the myxosporidians. Invertebrates and possibly birds preying on infected vertebrates can act as transport hosts. In such cases, spores may pass without morphological change through the intestinal tract. Oral uptake of infective spores is the usual way of infection. The life cycle starts if spores come into contact with the intestinal mucosa of suitable hosts. The spirally coiled filaments of the polar-capsules become everted and the sporoplasm(s) comes forth, penetrates the epithelium and finally reaches the organs preferred by certain species. The sporoplasms show an ameboid locomotion and subsequently grow as trophozoites to a large, frequently macroscopic stage, which is reached after repeated nuclear divisions. In cytozoic species the cellular host response forms a solid connective tissue capsule around the parasite, the so-called myxosporidian cyst. Coelozoic species may eventually float freely in the contents of the lumen organ.

The sporogonic phase starts when certain nuclei become surrounded by cytoplasm of high viscosity. These cells are generative ones which are able to divide again to form multicellular sporonts. One, several or many sporonts, depending upon the species, are formed in each trophozoit and one or two sporoblasts are differentiated in each sporont. The fully developed spores with the characteristics of the certain species usually can be found first in the center of the trophozoit. Only if these spores reach the environment of the host (water) can the maturation be completed. The spores are then infectious.

The pathogenicity of the myxosporidians depends on their group membership. Coelozoic species are less harmful to their hosts than cytozoic forms. The significance of the species parasitizing amphibians and reptiles is not known, not even in cases where the incidence is as high as 3% like in Notophthalmus v. viridescens with Myxobolus conspicuus. Unusual localizations (testes and ovaria) are reported for M. hylae, a parasite of the Australian golden tree frog, Hyla aurea (Reichenbach-Klinke and Elkan, 1965). For none of the five species of myxosporidians of amphibians and two species of reptiles (Flynn, 1973) have pathological effects been described.

It seems that the gall bladder is possibly the oldest site of a myxosporidian infection. The species parasitizing the gall generally are not found elsewhere in their hosts. Interesting aspects are postulated by Clark and

Shoemaker (1973). They suggested that the sporogony of
M. serotinum, specific to the gall bladder of certain
amphibians, is stimulated by metamorphic hormones of the
hosts. In spite of a general low pathogenicity of the
coelozoic species living in the gall bladder, Sindermann
(1970) pointed out that the higher the incidence of infection, the more pathological destructions can be found.

PHYLUM CILIOPHORA

Ciliophora are characterized by simple cilia or
ciliary organelles in at least one stage of the life cycle.
The main criteria separating them from other protozoans
are the two nuclei (macronucleus and micronucleus).
Vegetative division occurs by transverse binary fission,
sexuality by conjugation, autogamy and cytogamy. Most
species are free-living, but many are symbiotes, others
are commensals and only a few are true parasites in various hosts. Many ciliates, including the parasitic ones
are able to form cysts which normally are the infective
stage.

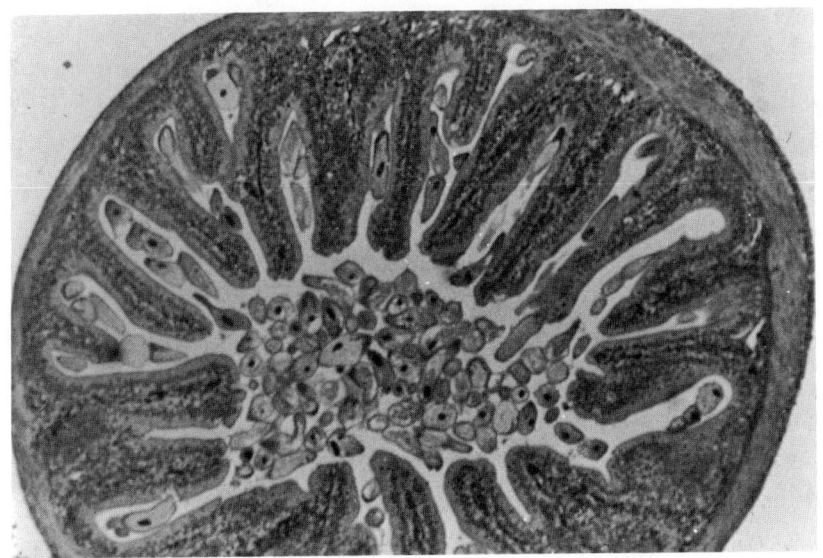

Fig. 19.17. Cross-section of the rectum of a Rana sp.
with many ciliates between the intestinal
crypts.

Table 19.21. Species of Balantidium, Nyctotherus, Cepedietta and Trichodina from Amphibia and Reptilia.[a]

Species	Hosts	Geographic distribution
Balantidium entozoon	Rana temporaria, R. esculenta, Bufo bufo, Triturus vulgaris, T. cristatus	Europe
B. elongatum	R. temporaria, R. esculenta, T. vulgaris, T. cristatus, T. alpestris	Asia; Europe
B. duodeni	R. temporaria, R. esculenta	Asia; Europe
B. helenae	R. temporaria, R. esculenta	Asia; Europe
B. nucleus	R. temporaria, R. esculenta	Europe
B. giganteum	R. esculenta	Asia; Europe
B. falciformis	R. palustris	North America
B. bacteriophorus	Chelonia mydas	Carribean Sea off the coast of Nicaragua
B. amblystomatis	Ambystoma tigrinum	North America
B. testudinis	Testudo spp.	Asia; Africa; South America
Balantidium sp.	B. americanus, Hyla cinerea, R. sylvatica	North America
Balantidium sp.	Xenopus laevis	Africa
Balantidium sp.	Newts	North America
Balantidium sp.	Iguanas	West Indies
Nyctotherus cordiformis	R. pipiens, R. clamitans, R. catesbeiana, R. sylvatica, R. palustris, R. esculenta, H. cinerea, H. crucifer, H.	World-wide

NON-HEMOPARASITIC PROTOZOANS

N. kyphodes	arborea, Acris sp., B. americanus, B. bufo, T. viridescens, T. torosus	
N. teleascus	Tortoises	Asia
N. beltrani	Tortoises	Asia
N. woodi	Ctenosaura acanthura	Mexico
N. hardwickii	Xantusia sp.	North America
N. trachysauri	Uromastix hardwickii	India
Nyctotherus sp.	Trachysaurus rugosus	Australia
Cepedietta michiganensis (syn. Haptophrya)	Iguanas	West Indies
	R. pipiens, R. sylvatica, B. americanus, A. opacum, A. jeffersonianum, Desmognathus sp.	North America
C. gigantea	R. esculenta, Eurycea lucifuga, salamanders	North America; Europe; Africa
C. virginiensis	R. palustris	North America
C. tritonis	T. alpestris	Europe
Trichodina urinicola	R. esculenta, T. vulgaris, T. cristatus, T. helveticus, toads	Africa; Europe; North America
T. pediculus	R. esculenta	Asia; Europe; North America
T. fultoni	Necturus sp.	North America

aSource: Amrein, 1952; Corliss, 1979; Dyer and Peck, 1975; Flynn, 1973; Hegner, 1940; Janakidevi, 1961; Johnston, 1932.

In amphibian and reptilian hosts the Ciliophora are mainly represented by two genera, Balantidium and Nyctotherus (Gurski et al., 1967). None of the reported species of these genera are known to be pathogenic to its host (Table 19.21). According to Corliss (1979), members of the Ciliophora may be found either as inhabitants of the intestinal tract (Fig. 19.17) (Fenchel, 1980) or, like members of the genus Trichodina, as parasites of the urinary bladder, skin or gills (Lom, 1959). Other members of the same order (Peritrichida) may be part of the aufwuchs of semi-aquatic or semi-terrestrial hosts belonging exclusively to the chelonians (Goodrich and Jahn, 1943). As far as the author knows, aufwuchs containing ciliophora protozoans are not described from crocodilians, but it is supposed that these reptiles also may have such epibionts. It seems that the epibionts despite being sessile on various substrates also have preferences (Bovee, 1976). In addition to the above mentioned genera, Corliss (1979) mentioned several other genera belonging to various families in his comprehensive treatise of the Ciliophora; they are listed in Table 19.22.

Table 19.22. Classification of the Phylum Ciliophora from Amphibia and Reptilia.

Classification	Name	Remarks
Class	Kinetofragminophorea	
Order	Trichostomatida	
Family	Balantidiidae	Many species are described from the intestines of various amphibian and reptilian hosts, but whether if all are valid species is doubtful
Genus	Balantidium	Single genus
Order	Colpodida	
Family	Colpodidae	
Genus	Colpoda	Only one species found in a skink
Order	Suctorida	Occur as symphorionts (aufwuchs) on semi-aquatic reptiles such as turtles (Goodrich and Jahn, 1943)
Class	Oligohymenophorea	
Order	Hymenostomatida a	
Family	Tetrahymenidae	
Genus	Tetrahymena	Intestine of tadpoles
Order	Astomatida	
Family	Haptophryidae	Intestine of anuran and especially urodelan amphibians
Genus	Cepedietta (syn. Haptophrya)	Several species, all in amphibians
Order	Peritrichida	
Family	Vorticellidae	Aufwuchs (epibionts) on turtles
Family	Trichodinidae	
Genus	Trichodina	Several species are described from amphibians, particularly larvae and members living permanently in water

Table 19.22. Classification of the Phylum Ciliophora from Amphibia and Reptilia. (Continued)

Classification	Name	Remarks
Family	Epistylididae	Only a few species are described as epizoic forms (aufwuchs) on chelonians
Genus	Epistylis finleyi	Trionyx muticus
	E. bishopi	T. muticus
	E. plummeri	T. muticus
	E. chrysemydis	Chrysemys marginata belli
Family	Operculariidae	
Genus	Opercularia jahni	T. muticus
Class	Polymenophorea	
Order	Heterotrichida	
Family	Nyctotheridae	Found in the intestines of amphibians and reptiles
Genus	Nyctotherus	Janakidevi (1961) mentioned that at that time 13 species were recorded from reptiles, 4 from snakes, 3 from chelonians and 6 from Lacertilia
	Nyctositum	Affa'a (1979) created a new genus Nyctositum for a heterotrich ciliate he found in tadpoles of Acenthixalus spinosus from Cameroon. The new species, N. amieti, is similar to Nyctotheroides, but clearly distinguished
Family	Sicuophorida	Found in the intestines of amphibians, particularly Anura, and reptiles
Genus	Sicuophora	

| Geimania | Found exclusively in reptiles |

a Walton (1964), Reichenbach-Klinke and Elkan (1965) and Flynn (1973) mentioned one ciliophoran, Glaucoma sp., which was found in the brain and spinal cord of an axolotl, Ambystoma mexicanum, but with unknown pathological effects. As this genus belongs to the family Glaucomidae, it is doubtful whether the determination of the organisms found was correct, because all members of this family (Order Hymenostomatida) are characterized as free-living by Corliss (1979). But possibly it was only an invasion into the otherwise affected organs from the surrounding water.

b It seems that despite the capacious possibilities to function as aufwuchs or epibionts "those peritrichs associated with turtles are mostly found only with them" (Bovee, 1976).

REFERENCES

Affa'a, F.M., 1979, Nyctositum amieti, n. gen., n. sp. cilie endocommensal du tetard d'Acanthixalus spinosus (Amphibien, Anoure), Protistologica, 15:333-336.

Albach, R.A., and Booden, T., 1978, Amoebae, in: "Parasit. protozoa," Vol. 2, J.P. Kreier, ed., Academic Press, New York.

Albach, R.A., and Shaffer, J.G., 1965, Free amino acid analyses of four strains of Entamoeba histolytic and of Entamoeba invadens in CLG medium, Protozoology, 12:659-665.

Amrein, Y.U., 1952, A new species of Nyctotherus (N. wood: from Southern California lizards, J. Parasitol. 38:266-270.

Anderson, D.R., Duszynski, D.W., and Marquardt, W.C., 196 Three new coccidia (Protozoa: Telosporea) from kingsnakes, Lampropeltis spp., in Illinois, with a redescription of Eimeria zamenis Phisalix, 1921, J. Parasitol., 54:577-581.

Babudieri, B., 1932, I Sarcosporidi e le Sarcosporidiosi, Arch. Protistenk., 76:421-580.

Baker, J.R., 1977, Systematics of parasitic protozoa, in: "Parasitic protozoa," Vol. 1, J.P. Kreier, ed., Academic Press, New York.

Balamuth, W., 1946, Improved egg yolk infusion for cultivation of Entamoeba histolytica and other intestinal protozoa, Amer. J. Clin. Pathol., 16:380.

Ball, G., 1944, Sarcosporidia in Southern California lizards, Trans. Amer. Microscop. Soc., 63:144-148.

Barker, D.G., and Deutsch, K., 1958, The chromatoid body of Entamoeba invadens, Exper. Cell Res., 15:604-610.

Beaver, P.C., and Maleckar, J.R., 1981, Sarcocystis singaporensis Zaman and Colley (1975), 1976, S. villi villosi sp. n. and S. zamani sp. n.: Development morphology and persistence in the laboratory rat, Rattus norvegicus, J. Parasitol., 67:241-256.

Bertram, A., 1892, Beitrage zur Kenntnis der Sarcosporidie nebst einem Anhange uber parasitische Schlauche in der Leibeshohle von Rotatorien, Zool. Jahrb. Abt. Anat. Ontog., 5:581-604.

Bhatia, B.L., 1938, Protozoa, Sporozoa, in: "The fauna of British India," London.

Bidier, I., 1972, Elektronenmikroskopische Untersuchungen an der reptilpathogenen Amoebe, Entamoeba invadens Rodhain, 1934 (Protozoa, Amoebozoa), Dipl. Arb. Univ. Hohenheim (Parasitologie).

Bidier, I., 1977, Licht- und Elektronenmikroskopische Untersuchungen an Entamoeba invadens Rodhain, 1934, als Beispiel einer gewebezerstorenden Entamoeba-Art (Protozoa, Amoebida), Diss. rer. nat. Univ. Hohenheim.

Bishop, E.L., Jr., and Jahn, T.L., 1941, Observations on colonial peritrichs (Ciliata; Protozoa) of the Okoboji region, Proc. Iowa Acad. Sci., 48:417-421.

Bledsoe, B., 1979, Sporogony of Sarcocystis idahoensis in the gopher snake, Pituophis melanoleucus (Daudin), J. Parasitol., 65:875-879.

Bledsoe, B., 1980, Sarcocystis idahoensis sp.n. in deer mice, Peromyscus maniculatus (Wagner), and gopher snakes, Pituophis melanoleucus (Daudin), Protozool., 27:93-107.

Boeck, W., and Drbohlav, J., 1925, The cultivation of Endamoeba histolytica, Amer. J. Hyg., 5:371-407.

Borst, G.H.A., Vroege, C., Poelma, F.G., Zwart, P., Strik, W.J., and Peters, J.C., 1972, Pathological findings on aminals in the Royal Zoological Gardens of the Rotterdam Zoo during the years 1963, 1964 and 1965, Acta Zool. Pathol. Antwerp, 56:3-20.

Bos, H.J., 1973, The problem of pathogenicity in parasitic Entamoeba, Acta Leiden., 40:1-112.

Bosch, I., and Deichsel, G., 1972, Morphologische Untersuchungen an pathogenen und potentiell pathogenen Amoeben der Typen "Entamoeba" und "Hartmanella-Acanthamoeba" aus Reptilien, Z. Parasitenk., 40: 107-129.

Bovee, E.C., 1976, New epizootic peritrichs of the soft shelled turtle, Trionyx muticus, Trans. Amer. Microscop. Soc., 95:682-687.

Bovee, E.C., and Telford, S.R., 1962a, Protozoan inquilines from reptiles. I. Monocercomonas neosepsorum n. sp., from the sand skink, Neoseps reynoldsi Stejneger, Quart. J. Florida Acad. Sci., 25:96-103.

Bovee, E.C., and Telford, S.R., 1962b, Protozoan inquilines from reptiles. II. Monocercomonas tantillorum n. sp., from the Florida crowned snake, Tantilla coronata Baird and Girard, Quart. J. Florida Acad. Sci., 25:104-108.

Brehm, H., 1979, Untersuchungen uber die Entwicklung von Sarcocystis singaporensis Zaman und Colley, 1976 in der Ratte (Rattus norvegicus Berkenhout, 1769) und in dem Netzpython (Python reticulatus Schneider, 1801), Vet-med. Diss., Univ. Munchen.

Brehm, H., and Frank, W., 1980, Der Entwicklungskreislauf von Sarcocystis singaporensis Zaman und Colley,

1976 im End- und Zwischenwirt, Z. Parasitenk., 62:15-30.
Brownstein, D.G., Standberg, J.D., Montali, R.J., Bush, M. and Fortner, J., 1977, Cryptosporidium in snakes with hypertrophic gastritis, Vet. Pathol., 14: 606-617.
Brygoo, E.R., 1963, Contribution a la connaissance de la parasitologie des cameleons malgaches, Ann. Parasitol. Hum. Comp., 38:526-739.
Butt, C.G., 1966, Primary amebic meningoencephalitis, New England J. Med., 274:1473-1476.
Canning, E.U., 1967, Vertebrates as hosts to Microsporidia with special refernce to rats infected with Nosema cuniculi, J. Helminthol. Suppl. 2 (Protozool.), :197-205.
Canning, E.U., 1975, The medical importance of Microssporida, Folia Parasitol. (Praha), 2:10.
Canning, E.U., 1976, Microsporidia in vertebrates: Hostparasite relations at the organismal level, in: "Comparative pathobiology," Vol. 1, L.A. Bulla and T.C. Cheng, eds., Plenum Press, New York.
Canning, E.U., 1977, Microsporida, in: "Parasitic protozoa," Vol. 4, J.P. Kreier, ed., Academic Press, New York.
Canning, E.U., and Elkan, E., 1963, Microsporidiosis in Bufo bufo, Parasitology, 53:11-12.
Canning, E.U., and Elkan, E., 1964, Plistophora myotrophic spec. nov., causing high mortality in the common toad, Bufo bufo L., with notes on the maintenanc of Bufo and Xenopus in the laboratory, J. Protozool., 11:157-166.
Canning, E.U., and Landau, I., 1971, A microsporidian infection of Lacerta muralis, Trans. Royal Soc. Trop. Med. Hyg., 65:431.
Cannon, L.R.G., 1967, Caryospora demansiae sp. nov. (Sporozoa: Eimeriidae) from the Australian snake, Demansia psammophis (Elapidae), Parasitology, 57:221-226.
Cannon, L.R.G., and Rzepczyk, C.M., 1974, A new species of Caryospora Leger, 1904 (Sporozoa:Eimeriidae) from an Australian snake, Parasitology, 69:197-200.
Carini, A., 1936, Sur une Isospora de l'intestine de l'Hemidactylus mabuyae, Ann. Parasit. Hum. Comp., 14:444-446.
Carosi, G., 1974, Etude comparative de l'ultrastructure d'Entamoeba moshkovskii, des amibes parasites du genre Entamoeba et des amibes "free-living" du groupe "Hartmannella-Naegleria," Ann. Soc. Belge Med. Trop., 54:41-53.

Cerva, L., and Nowak, K., 1968, Amoebic meningoencephalitis: Sixteen fatalities, Science, 160:92.
Charoenlarp, P., Warren, L.G., and Reeves, R.B., 1971, Serologic characteristics of glucokinases from Entamoeba histolytica and related species, Protozoology, 20:365-366.
Chatton, E., and Avel, M., 1923, Sur la Sarcosporidie du Gecko et ses cytophaneres, C.R. Soc. Biol. (Paris), 89:181-185.
Clark, J.G., and Shoemaker, J.P., 1973, Eurycea bislineata (Green), the two-lined salamander, a new host of Myxidium serotinum Kudo and Sprague, 1940 (Myxosporida, Myxidiidae), J. Protozool., 20: 365-366.
Colley, F.C., and Else, J.G., 1975, Eimeria nebulosa n. sp. and Klossia pachyleparon n. sp. from the monitor lizard, Varanus nebulosus, in Malaysia, Ann. Parasitol. Hum. Comp., 50:669-673.
Conant, R., 1971, Reptile and amphibian management practices at Philadelphia Zoo, Int. Zoo Yearbook, 11:224-230.
Corliss, J.O., 1979, "The ciliated Protozoa: Characterization, classification and guide to the literature," Pergamon Press, New York.
Coutelen, F., 1932, Existence des toxoplasms chez les lacertiliens. Un toxoplasme nouveau chez un iguane de la Trinite, C.R. Soc. Biol. (Paris), 110:85-87.
Cunha, A.M., and Fonseca, O., 1917, Sobre uma nova entameba, Entamoeba serpentis n. sp. (Nota previa), Brazil-Med., 31:279.
Cunha, A.M., and Fonseca, O., 1918, Sobre a Entamoeba serpentis, Mem. Inst. Osw. Cruz, 10:95-98.
Das, S.R., 1974, Importance of appropriate techniques for various studies on small free-living amoebae and their bearing on the taxonomy of the order Amoebida, Proc. Int. Coll. Antwerp, Prince Leopold Inst. Trop. Med. No., 14:11-23.
Daykar, P., Devi, A.T., Rao, S.B., and Rao, T.B., 1977, New flagellate Hypotrichomonas venkataramiahii sp. n. from the gut of Varanus sp. from Warangal, A.P., India, Acta Protozool. (Warszawa), 16:225-229.
Deichsel, G., and Bosch, I., 1973, Automatische Klassifikation von Amoben durch zwei grafentheoretische Verfahren, EDV in Medizin und Biologie, 3:69-73.
Dobell, C., and Laidlow, P.P., 1926, On the cultivation of Entamoeba histolytica and some other entozoic amoebae, Parasitology, 18:283-318.

Dolensek, E.P., Bihn, J.P., and Napolitano, R.L., 1976, Intestinal protozoan inhabitants in exhibited reptiles, J. Protozool., 23:Abstract 19A.

Dollahon, N.D., and Janovy, J., 1971, Insect flagellates from feces and gut contents of four genera of lizards, J. Parasitol., 57:1130-1132.

Donaldson, M., Heyneman, D., Dempster, R., and Garzia, L. 1975, Epizootic of fatal amebiasis among exhibited snakes: Epidemiologic, pathologic and chemotherapeutic considerations, Amer. J. Vet. Res., 36:807-817.

Dubey, J.P., 1977, Toxoplasma, Hammondia, Besnoitia, Sarcocystis and other tissue cyst-forming coccidia in: "Parasitic protozoa," Vol. 3, J.P. Kreier, ed., Academic Press, New York.

Dupouy, J., and Kechemir, N., 1973, Les Cestodes de Reptiles en Algerie Essai de revision du genre Oochoristica Luhe (Cestoda, Anoplocephalidae), Bull. Soc. Hist. Nat. Afr. Nord. Alger, 64:47-9

Duszynski, D.W., 1969, Two new coccidia (Protozoa: Eimeriidae) from Costa Rican lizards with a review of the Eimeria from lizards, J. Protozool., 16:581-585.

Duszynski, D.W., Altenbach, M.J., Marchiondo, A.A., and Speer, C.A., 1977, Eimeria crotalviridis sp. n. from prairie rattlesnakes, Crotalus viridis viridis, in New Mexico with data on excystation of sporozoites and ultrastructure of the oocyst wall, J. Protozool., 24:359-361.

Dyer, W.G., and Peck, S.B., 1975, Gastrointestinal parasites of the cave salamander, Eurycea lucifuga Rafinesque, from the southeastern United States, Can. J. Zool., 53:52-54.

Earl, P.R., 1971, Hegneriella dobelli gen. n., sp. n. (Opalinidae) from Bufo valliceps and some remarks on the systematic position of the Opalinidae, Acta Protozool., 9:41-47.

Earl, P.R., 1973, Suppressions and other taxonomic changes in the protozoan subphylum Opalinida, Publ. Biol. Inst. Inv. Cient, UANL, Mexico, 1:25-33.

El-Mofty, M.M., 1974, Induction of sexual reproduction in Opalina sudafricana by injecting its host, Bufo regularis with gibberellic acid, Int. J. Parasitol., 4:203-206.

El-Mofty, M.M., and Sadek, I.A., 1975a, The effect of fresh toad bile on the induction of encystation in Opalina sudafricana parasitic in Bufo regularis, Int. J. Parasitol., 5:219-224.

El-Mofty, M.M., and Sadek, I.A., 1975b, The use of Opalina sudafricana in a biological test for diagnosing

disordered metabolism of tryptophan in human
subjects, Int. J. Parasitol., 5:225-229.
Fantham, H.B., 1932, Some parasitic protozoa found in South
Africa, South Afr. J. Sci., 29:627-640.
Fantham, H.B., and Porter, A., 1953/54, The endoparasites
of some North American snakes and their effects
on the Ophidia, Proc. Zool. Soc. London, 123:
867-898.
Fenchel, T.M., 1980, The protozoan fauna from the gut of
the green turtle, Chelonia mydas L. with a
description of Balantidium bacteriophorus sp.
nov., Arch Protistenk., 123:22-26.
Fiennes, R.N., 1961, Diseases of snakes caused by internal
parasites, III Internationales Symposiums uber
die Erkrankungen der Zootiere, Akademie der
Wissenschaften der DDR, Berlin.
Flynn, R.J., 1973, "Parasites of laboratory animals,"
Iowa State Univ. Press, Ames.
Foissner, W., Schubert, G., and Wilbert, N., 1979, Morphology, in fraciliature, and silverline system
of Protoopalina symphysodonis nov. spec. (Protozoa: Opalinata), an Opalinidae from the intestine
of Symphysodon aequifasciata Pellegrin (Perco-
idei: Cichlidae), Zool. Anz. (Jena), 202:71-85.
Fowler, M., and Carter, R.F., 1965, Acute pyogenic
meningitis probably due to Acanthamoeba sp.:
A preliminary report, British Med. J., 2:740-742.
Frank, W., 1966a, Eine Sarcocystis-Infektion mit patho-
logischen Veranderungen bei einem Chamaeleo
fischeri durch Sarcocystis chamaeleonis n. spec.
(Protozoa, Sporozoa), Z. Parasitenk., 27:317-335.
Frank, W., 1966b, Generalisierte Amobiasis ohne Darmsymp-
tome bei einem Leguan (Iguana iguana) (Reptilia,
Iguanidae), hervorgerufen durch Entamoeba
invadens (Protozoa, Amoebozoa), Z. Trop. Med.
Parasitol., 17:285-293.
Frank, W., 1974, Limax-amoebae from cold-blooded verte-
brates, Proc. Int. Coll. Antwerp Prince Leopold
Inst. Trop. Med. No., 14:119-125.
Frank, W., 1975, Haltungsprobleme und Krankheiten der
Reptilien. Diagnose und Behandlung, Tierarztl.
Praxis, 3:343-364.
Frank, W., 1976a, Amphibien-Reptilien, in: "Zootierkrank-
heiten," H.G. Klos and E.M. Lang, eds., Parey
Verlag, Berlin.
Frank, W., 1976b, "Parasitologie," E. Ulmer Verlag, Stutt-
gart.
Frank, W., and Bosch, I., 1972, Isolierung von Amoeben
des Typs "Hartmannella-Acanthamoeba" und Naeg-
leria aus Kaltblutern, Z. Parasitenk., 40:139-
150.

Frank, W., and Frenkel, J.K., 1981, Besnoitia in a palaearctic lizard (Lacerta dugesii) from Madeira, Z. Parasitenk., 64:203-206.

Frank, W., and Hafner, U., 1981, Host range and host specificity of Sarcocystis, Zentralbl. Bakterio Parasitenkd. Hyg. Abt. I Orig. A, 250:355-360.

Frank, W., and Loos-Frank, B., 1977, Interessante Krankheitsbilder bei Amphibien und Reptilien, die durch Bakterien, Pilze und Parasiten bedingt sind- eine Ubersicht nach 15-jahriger Erfahrung XIX Internationales Symposiums uber die Erkrankungen der Zootiere, Akademie Verlag, Berlin.

Frank, W., and Sigmund, U., 1976, Nachweis einer Entamoeba invadens-Infektion mit Hilfe der Immunofluoreszentechnik bei Reptilien, Kleintierpraxis, 21:173-212.

Frank, W., Bachmann, U., and Braun, R., 1976a, Aubssergewohnliche Todesfalle durch Amobiasis bei einer Bruckenechse (Sphenodon punctatus), bei jungen Suppenschildkroten (Chelonia mydas) und bei einer unechten Karettschildkrote (Caretta caretta). I. Amobiasis bei Sphenodon punctatus, Salamandra, 12:94-102.

Frank, W., Roester, U., and Scholer, H.J., 1974, Sphaerulen-Bildung bei einer Mucor Species in inneren Organen von Amphibien, Zentralbl. Bakteriol. Parasitenkd. Hyg. Abt. I Orig. A, 226:405-417.

Frank, W., Sachsse, W., and Winkelstrater, K.H., 1976b, Aubssergewohnliche Todesfalle durch Amobiasis bei einer Bruckenechse (Sphenodon punctatus), bei jungen Suppenschildkroten (Chelonia mydas) und bei einer unechten Karettschildkrote (Caretta caretta). II. Amobiasis bei Chelonia mydas und Caretta caretta, Salamandra, 12:120-126.

Frank, W., Will, R., and Zwart, P., 1972, Leberamoebiasis bei Reptilien und die Serumeiweiz-Elektropherogramme, Z. Parasitenk., 39:63-64.

Frenkel, J.K., 1977, Besnoitia wallacei of cats and rodents; with a reclassification of other cystforming isosporoid coccidia, J. Parasitol., 63:611-628.

Frenkel, J.K., Heydorn, A.O., Mehlhorn, H., and Rommel, M., 1979, Sarcocystinae: Nomina dubia and available names, Z. Parasitenk., 58:115-139.

Frye, F.L., 1973, "Husbandry, medicine and surgery in captive reptiles," V.M. Publ. Co., Bonner Springs.

Gabrisch, K., 1976, Diagnose und Therapie von Parasitosen bei Reptilien, Prakt. Tierarzt "Coll. Veterinarium (1975)", 57:37-40.

Garnham, P.C.C., 1964, Discovery of Besnoitia in the basilisk lizard, Trans. Royal Soc. Trop. Med. Hyg., 58:286.

Garnham, P.C.C., 1966, Besnoitia (Protozoa: Toxoplasmea) in lizards, Parasitology, 56:329-334.

Geiman, Q.M., and Ratcliffe, H.L., 1936, Morphology and life-cycle of an amoeba producing amoebiasis in reptiles, Parasitology, 28:208-228.

Geiman, Q.M., and Wichterman, R., 1937, Intestinal protozoa from Galapagos tortoises (with descriptions of three new species), J. Parasitol., 23:331-347.

Gelderman, A.H., Bartgis, I.L., Keister, D.B., and Diamond, L.S., 1971a, A comparison of genome sizes and thermal denaturation-derived base composition of DNA from several members of Entamoeba (histolytica group), J. Parasitol., 57:912-916.

Gelderman, A.H., Keister, D.B., Bartgis, I.L., and Diamond, L.S., 1971b, Characterization of the deoxyribonucleic acid of representative strains of Entamoeba histolytica, Entamoeba histolytica-like amebae, and Entamoeba moshkovskii, J. Parasitol., 57:906-911.

Ghosh, T.N., 1968, Observations on the type specimen of Entamoeba serpentis (Cunha and Fonseca, 1917), J. Protozool., 15:164-166.

Ghosh, T.N., 1977, Studies on the genus Entamoeba. III. Entamoeba from amphibians, J. Protozool., 24: (suppl. 2) Abstract 131.

Goodrich, J.P., and Jahn, T.L., 1943, Epizoic Suctoria (Protozoa) from turtles, Trans. Amer. Microscop. Soc., 62:245-253.

Grasse, P.P., 1924, Octomastix parvus Alex. Diplozoaire parasite de la cistude d'Europe, C.R. Seances Soc. Biol., Ses. Fil., 91:439-442.

Gray, C.W., Marcus, L.C., McCarten, W.C., and Sappington, T., 1966, Amoebiasis in the Komodo dragon, Varanus komodoensis, Int. Zoo Yearbook, 6:279-283.

Griffin, J.L., 1978, Pathogenic free-living amoebae, in: "Parasitic protozoa," Vol. 2, J.P. Kreier, ed., Academic Press, New York.

Gurski, D.R., John, J.L., and Pierce, S., 1961, Isolation of Balantidium sp. from the blue tongued skink (Tiliqua nigrolutea), J. Protozool., 8: Suppl. 11.

Hafner, U., 1980, Arthropods as vectors of Sarcocystis sporocysts, Zentralbl. Bakteriol. Parasitenkd. Hyg. Abt. I Ref., 267:296-297.

Hartmann, M., 1910, Uber eine neue Darmamobe, Entamoeba testudinis n. sp., Mem. Inst. Osw. Cruz, 2:3-10.

Hazard, E.J., and Oldacre, S.W., 1975, "Revision of the Microsporida (Protozoa) close to Thelohania, with descriptions of one new family, eight new genera and thirteen new species, U.S. Dept. Agriculture Research Service, Tech. Bull., No. 1530.

Hegner, R., 1940, Nyctotherus beltrani n. sp., a ciliate from an iguana, J. Parasitol., 26:315-317.

Hegner, R., and Hewitt, R., 1940, A new genus and new species of amoebae from Mexican lizards, Parasitology, 26:319-321.

Heydorn, A.O., and Rommel, M., 1972a, Beitrage zum Lebens zyklus der Sarkosporidien. II. Hund und Katze als Ubertrager der Sarkosporidien des Rindes, Berl. Munch. Tierarztl. Wochenschr., 85:121-123

Heydorn, A.O., and Rommel, M., 1972b, Beitrage zum Lebenszyklus der Sarkosporidien. IV. Entwicklungsstadien von S. fusiformis in der Dunndarmschleim haut der Katze, Berl. Munch. Tierarztl. Wochenschr., 85:333-336.

Hilgenfeld, M., 1968, Protozoare Infektionen bei Zootieren (Kaltblutler, Vogel, Saugetiere) unter besondere Berucksichtigung der Pathologie des Respirations traktes, X Internationales Symposiums uber die Erkrankungen der Zootiere, Akademie Verlag, Berlin.

Hill, W.C.O., and Neal, R.A., 1953, An epizootic due to Entamoeba invadens at the gardens of the Zoological Society of London, Proc. Zool. Soc. London, 123:731-737.

Hoare, C.A., 1933, Studies on some ophidian and avian coccidia from Uganda with a revision of the classification of the Eimeridae, Parasitology, 25:359-388.

Honigberg, B.M., 1963, Evolutionary and systematic relationships in the flagellate order Trichomonadida Kirby, J. Protozool., 10:20-63.

Honigberg, B.M., Balamuth, W., Bovee, E.C., Corliss, J.O., Gojdics, M. et al., 1964, A revised classification of the phylum Protozoa, J. Protozool., 11:7-20.

Ippen, R., 1959, Die Amobendysenterie der Reptilien, Kleintierpraxis, 4:131-137.

Ippen, R., 1971, Zur Problematik des Parasitenbefalls bei Reptilien, XIII Internationales Symposiums uber die Erkrankungen der Zootiere, Akademie Verlag, Berlin.

Ippen, R., and Schroder, H.D., 1977, Zu den Erkrankungen der Reptilien, XIX Internationales Symposiums uber die Erkrankungen der Zootiere, Akademie Verlag, Berlin.

Janakidevi, K., 1961, A new ciliate from the spiny-tailed lizard, Z. Parasitenk., 21:155-158.
Jes, H., 1975, Jahresbericht Aquarium 1974, Z. Kolner Zoo, 18:15-23.
Johnston, T.H., 1932, The parasites of the "stumpy tail" lizard, Trachysaurus rugosus, Trans. Royal Soc. Australia, 56:62-70.
Jones, D.M., 1980, The Zoological Society of London. Scientific report 1977-1979, Department of Veterinary Science, J. Zool. London, 190:483-512.
Kalyakin, V.N., and Zasukhin, D.N., 1975, Distribution of Sarcocystis (Protozoa, Sporozoa) in vertebrates, Fol. Parasitol. Praha, 22:289-307.
Kasprzak, W., Mazur, T., and Rucka, A., 1974, Studies on some pathogenic strains of free-living amoebae isolated from lakes in Poland, Proc. Int. Coll. Antwerp Prince Leopold Inst. Trop. Med. No., 14:127-133.
Kiel, J.L., 1975, A review of parasites in snakes, Southwestern Vet., 28:209-220.
Knowles, R., and Das Gupta, B.M., 1930, On two intestinal protozoa of an Indian turtle, Indian J. Med. Res., 18:97-104.
Kramer, M., 1972, Een overzicht van hetgeen bekend is over amoebiasis bij reptilien, Lacerta, 30:87-96.
Krishnamurthy, R., 1967, Hypotrichomonas osmaniae n. sp. from a varanid lizard, Curr. Sci., 21:583-584.
Krishnamurthy, R., 1968, Studies on the morphology of the monocercomonad flagellates from reptiles in India. III. A review, with a key to the species, Riv. Parassitol., 29:233-240.
Krishnamurthy, R. and Madre, V.E., 1976, Retortamonas viperae n. sp., a new flagellate from the rectum of a viper, Marathwada Univ. J. (Nat. Sci.), 15:129-131.
Krishnamurthy, R.f and Madre, V.E., 1979a, Studies on two flagellates of the genus Monocercomonoides Travis, 1932 (Mastigophora: Polymastigina) from amphibians and reptiles in India, Acta Protozool. Warszawa, 18:251-257.
Krishnamurhty, R., and Madre, V.E., 1979b, Studies on the morphology of three new species of moncercomonad flagellates from amphibians in India, Arch. Protistenk., 121:64-72.
Kulda, J., and Nohynkova, E., 1978, Flagellates of the human intestine and of the intestines of other species, in: "Parasitic protozoa," Vol. 2, J.P. Kreier, ed., Academic Press, New York.
Lainson, R., 1965, Parasitological studies in British Honduras. II. Cyclospora niniae sp. nov. (Eimeri-

idae, Cyclosporinae) from the snake, Ninia sebae sebae (Colubridae), Ann. Trop. Med. Parasitol., 59:159-163.

Lainson, R., and Shaw, J.J., 1971, Sarcocystis gracilis n. sp. from the Brazilian tortoise, Kinosternon scorpioides, J. Protozool., 18:365-372.

Lainson, R., and Shaw, J.J., 1972, Sarcocystis in tortoise A replacement name S. kinosterni for the homonym S. gracilis Lainson and Shaw 1971, J. Protozool. 19:212.

Lavier, G., 1928, Entamoeba varani n. sp. amibe parasite de reptile, Ann. Parasitol. Hum. Comp., 6:152.

Leger, L., 1918, Infection sanguine par Leptomonas chez un saurien, C.R. Seances Soc. Biol. Fil., 54: 354-356.

Lehmann, R., 1972, Zur Behandlung der Coccidiose bei Reptilien, Salamandra, 8:48-49.

Leibovitz, L., Rebell, G., and Boucher, G.C., 1978, Caryospora cheloniae sp. n.: A coccidial pathogen of mariculture-reared green sea turtles (Chelonia mydas mydas), J. Wildlife Dis., 14:269-275.

Levine, N.D., 1970, Taxonomy of the Sporozoa, J. Parasitol., 46:208-209.

Levine, N.D., 1973, Introduction, history and taxonomy, in: "The coccidia," D.M. Hammond and P.L. Long, eds., Univ. Park Press, Baltimore.

Levine, N.D., 1977, Taxonomy of Toxoplasma, J. Protozool., 24:36-41.

Levine, N.D., 1978, Perkinsus gen. n. and other new taxa in the protozoan phylum Apicomplexa, J. Parasitol., 64:549.

Levine, N.D., and Nye, R.R., 1976, Toxoplasma ranae n. sp. from the leopard frog, Rana pipiens L., Protozoology, 23:488-490.

Levine, N.D., and Nye, R.R., 1977, A survey of blood and other tissue parasites of leopard frogs, Rana pipiens, in the United States, J. Wildlife Dis., 13:17-23.

Levine, N.D., Corliss, J.O., Cox, F.E.G., Deroux, G., Grain, J., Honigberg, B.M., et al., 1980, A newly revised classification of the Protozoa, J. Protozool., 27:37-58.

Levit, A.V., 1976, Effect of temperature on the susceptibility of reptiles to Toxoplasma, Protozool. Abstr., 2:119-120 (1978).

Liu, S.K., and King, F.W., 1971, Microsporidiosis in the tuatara, J. Amer. Vet. Med. Ass., 159:1578-1582.

Lom, J., 1959, A contribution to the systematics and morphology of endoparasitic trichodinids from amphibians, with a proposal for uniform specific characteristics, J. Protozool., 5:251-263.

Lom, J., 1969a, On a new taxonomic character in Myxosporidia, as demonstrated in descriptions of two new species of Myxobolus, Fol. Parasitol. (Praha), 16:97-103.

Lom, J., 1969b, Notes on the ultrastructure and sporoblast development in fish parasitizing myxosporidians of the genus Sphaeromyxa, Z. Zellfschg. Mikrosk. Anat., 97:416-437.

Lom, J., 1973, Current status of Myxo- and Microsporidia, Prog. Protozool. Abstr. Pap. 4th Int. Congr. Protozool.

Madre, V.E., 1979, Two species of flagellates of the genus Chilomastix Alexeieff, 1912 (Mastigophora: Retortamonadida) from amphibians and reptiles in India, Acta Protozool., 18:243-250.

Madre, V.E., and Krishnamurthy, R., 1976, Studies on two flagellates from the rectum of the viper, Vipera russelli in Aurangabad, Marathwada Univ. J. (Natur. Sci.), 15:143-147.

Mandal, R., 1976, Caryospora bengalensis sp. n. and Eimeria fibrilosa sp. n. new coccidia (Protozoa: Eucoccida) from a freshwater snake, Enhydris enhydris (Schneider), Acta Protozool., 15:405-410.

Marcus, L.C., 1977, Parasitic diseases of captive reptiles, in: "Current veterinary therapy," P. Kirk, ed., W.B. Saunders Co., Philadelphia.

Matuschka, F.R., 1981, Life cycle of Sarcocystis between poikilothermic hosts. Lizards are intermediate hosts for S. podarcicolubris sp. nov., snakes function as definitive hosts. Z. Naturforschg., 36c:1093-1095.

Mayer, H., and Frank, W., 1974, Bakteriologische Untersuchungen bei Reptilien und Amphibien, Zentralbl. Bakteriol. Parasitenkd. Hyg. Abt. I Orig. A, 229:470-481.

McClaughin, J., and Meerovitch, E., 1975, Immunochemical studies of the surface and cytoplasmic membranes of Entamoeba invadens (Rodhain, 1934), Can. J. Microbiol., 31:1635-1646.

McConnachie, E.W., 1970, Encystation in axenic cultures of Entamoeba invadens, J. Protozool., 17:Suppl. 25.

McKenzie, R.A., Green, P.E., Hartley, W.J., and Pollitt, C.C., 1978, Cryptosporidium in a red-bellied black snake (Pseudechis porphyriacus), Australian Vet. J., 54:365-366.

Meerovitch, E., 1958, Some biological requirements and host-parasite relations of Entamoeba invadens, Can. J. Zool., 36:513-523.

Meerovitch, E., 1961, Infectivity and pathogenicity of polyxenic and monoxenic Entamoeba invadens to snakes kept at normal and high temperatures and the natural history of reptile amoebiasis, J. Parasitol., 47:791-794.

Mehlhorn, H., and Heydorn, A.O., 1978, The Sarcosporidia (Protozoa, Sporozoa): Life cycle and fine structure, Adv. Parasitol., 16:43-91.

Melville, R.V., 1980, Nomina dubia and available names, Z. Parasitenk., 62:105-109.

Meshkov, S., 1975, Sarcosporidia in tortoises from Bulgaria, C.R. Acad. Bulg. Sci., 28:1547-1548.

Metcalf, M.M., 1923, The opalinid ciliate infusorians, United States National Mus. Bull., 120:1-471.

Metcalf, M.M., 1940, Further studies on the opalinid ciliate infusorians and their hosts, Proc. United States National Mus., 87:465-634.

Mishra, G.S., and Gonzalez, J.P., 1978, Les parasites des tortue d'eau douce en Tunisie, Arch. Inst. Pasteur Tunis, 55:303-326.

Mitchell, L.G., 1977, Myxosporida, in: "Parasitic protozoa," Vol. 4, J.P. Kreier, ed., Academic Press, New York.

Moskowitz, N., 1951, Observations on some intestinal flagellates from reptilian hosts (Squamata), Morphology, 89:257-321.

Munday, R.L., Hartley, W.J., Harrigan, K.E., Presidente, P.J., and Obendorf, D.L., 1979, Sarcocystis and related organisms in Australian wildlife: II Survey findings in birds, reptiles, amphibians and fish, J. Wildlife Dis., 15:57-73.

Neal, R.A., 1974, Survival of Entamoeba and related amoebae at low temperature. I Viabilitiy of Entamoeba cysts at 4 C, Int. J. Parasitol., 4:227-229.

Nelson, E.C., 1947, Alcoholic extract medium for the diagnosis and cultivation of Entamoeba histolytica, Amer. J. Trop. Med. Hyg., 27:545-552.

Page, F.C., 1976a, A revised classification of the Gymnaamoebia (Protozoa, Sarcodina), Zool. J. Linn. Soc., 58:61-77.

Page, F.C., 1976b, "An illustrated key to freshwater and soil amoebae," Freshwater Biol. Ass. Sci. Publ. No. 34.

Parenzan, P., 1947, Sarcosporidiosi psorospermosi da nuova specie (Prot.: Sarcosystis atractaspidis n. sp.) in rettile (Atractaspis), Boll. Soc. Nat. Napoli, 55:117-119.

Pellerdy, L.P., 1974, "Coccidia and coccidiosis," 2nd ed., Parey Verlag, Berlin.

Peterson, W.J., 1960, Population changes in the cecal Protozoa of rats and some factors influencing them, Exp. Parasitol., 10:293-312.

Pluto, T.G., and Rothenbacher, H., 1976, Eimeria juniataensis sp. n. (Protozoa: Eimeriidae) from the map turtle, Graptemys geographica, in Pennsylvania, J. Parasitol., 62:207-208.

Rao, T.B., Rao, T.S.B., and Devi, A., 1976a, Chilomastix hemidactyli n. sp. from a lizard, Hemidactylus, of Warangal, A.P., India, Acta Protozool. (Warszawa), 15:289-292.

Rao, T.B., Rao, T.S.B., and Devi, A., 1976b, On a new species of the genus Hypotrichomonas Lee, 1960 (Subfamily: Hypotrichomonadinae) from Hemidactylus species, Current Sci., 45:263-264.

Rao, T.S.B., Devi, A., Dayakar, P., Reddy, M.D., and Rao, T.B., 1978a, New flagellates, Proteromonas kakatiyae sp. n. of Hemidactylus and Proteromonas warangalensis sp. n. of Mabuya carinata from Warangal, Andhra Pradesh, India, Acta Protozool. (Warszawa), 17:1-7.

Rao, T.S.B., Devi, A., Reddy, M.D., Dayakar, P., and Rao, T.B., 1978b, A new species of the genus Tritrichomonas (Kofoid, 1920) from Rana pipensi, Riv. Parassitol., 39:39-42.

Ratcliffe, H.L., and Geiman, Q.M., 1938, Spontaneous and experimental amebic infection in reptiles, Arch. Pathol., 25:160-184.

Reichenbach-Klinke, H.H., 1977, "Krankheiten der Reptilien," 2nd ed., Fischer Verlag, Stuttgart.

Reichenbach-Klinke, H.H., and Elkan, E., 1965, "The principal diseases of lower vertebrates," Academic Press, New York.

Reichenow, E., 1953, "Lehrbuch der Protozoenkunde," 6th ed., Fischer Verlag, Jena.

Rodhain, J., 1934, Entamoeba invadens n. sp. parasite de serpents, C.R. Soc. Belge Biol., 117:1195.

Rodhain, J., and Hoof, M.T., van, 1947, Entamoeba knowlesi n. sp. parasite de deux tortues: Terrapina cinosternoides et Platysternum megacephalum, Ann. Parasitol. Hum. Comp., 22:129-137.

Rommel, M., 1978, Vergleichende Darstellung der Entwicklungsbiologie der Gattungen Sarcocystis, Frenkelia, Isospora, Cystoisospora, Hammondia, Toxoplasma und Besnoitia, Z. Parasitenk., 57: 269-283.

Rommel, M., and Heydorn, A.O., 1972, Beitrage zum Lebenszyklus der Sarkosporidien. III. Isospora hominis (Railliet et Lucet, 1891) Wenyon, 1923, eine Dauerform der Sarkosporidien des Rindes und des

Schweins, Berl. Munch. Tierarztl. Wochenschr., 85:143-145.

Rommel, M., Heydorn, A.O., and Gruber, F., 1972, Beitrage zum Lebenszyklus der Sarkosporidien. I. Die Sporocyste von S. tenella in den Fazes der Katze Berl. Munch. Tierarztl. Wochenschr., 85:101-105.

Rzepczyk, C., 1974, Evidence of rat-snake cycle for Sarcocystis, Int. J. Parasitol., 4:447-449.

Rzepczyk, C., and Scholtyseck, E., 1976, Light and electro microscope studies on the Sarcocystis of Rattus, Z. Parasitenk., 50:137-150.

Sanders, E.P., 1931, The life-cycle of Entamoeba ranarum, Grassi (1879), Arch. Protistenk., 74:365-371.

Sanders, E.P., and Cleveland, L.R., 1930, The morphology and life-cycle of Entamoeba terrapinae spec. nov from the terrapin, Chrysemys elegans, Arch. Protistenk., 70:267-272.

Sandon, H., 1976, The species problem in the opalinids (Protozoa, Opalinata), with special reference to Protoopalina, Trans. Amer. Microscop. Soc., 95:357-366.

Schneider, C.R., 1965, Besnoitia panamensis sp. n. (Protozoa: Toxoplasmatidae) from Panamanian lizards, J. Parasitol., 51:340-344.

Schneider, C.R., 1967a, The distribution of lizard besnoitiosis in Panama, and its transfer to mice J. Protozool., 14:674-678.

Schneider, C.R., 1967b, Cross-immunity evidence of the identity of Besnoitia panamensis from lizards and B. darlingi from opossums, J. Parasitol., 53:886.

Schneider, C.R., 1967c, Besnoitia darlingi (Brumpt, 1913) in Panama, J. Protozool., 14:78-82.

Schweinfurt, W., 1970, Perorale Behandlung der Amoebiasis bei Schlangen, Salamandra, 6:44-45.

Scorza, J.V., Dagert, C., and Iturriza Arocha, L., 1956, Estudo sobre hemoparasitos de Bufo marinus L. da Venezuela. 1. Hemogregarinas. 2. Una nuova especie da Toxoplasma, Mem. Inst. Osw. Cruz., 54:373-392.

Seidel, B., 1977, Beobachtungen bei einigen Endoparasiten von Schlangen, XIX Internationales Symposiums uber die Erkrankungen der Zootiere, Akademie Verlag, Berlin.

Senaud, J., and DePuytorac, P., 1964/1965, Observation de la Sarcosporidie du lezard (Lacerta muralis), Arch. Zool. Exp. Gen., 104:182-184.

Siddiqui, W.A., and Rudzinska, M.A., 1965, The fine structure of axenically grown trophozoites of Entamoeba invadens with special reference to the nucleus and helical ribonucleoprotein bodies, J. Protozool., 12:448-458.

Sindermann, C.J., 1970, "Principal diseases of marine fish and shellfish," Academic Press, New York.

Sindermann, C.J., 1977, Coccidian diseases of green turtles, in: "Disease diagnosis and control in North American marine aquaculture," Vol. 6, C.J. Sindermann, ed., Elsevier Sci. Publ. Co., New York.

Smith, D.D., and Frenkel, J.K., 1977, Besnoitia darlingi (Protozoa: Toxoplasmatinae): Cyclic transmission by cats, J. Parasitol., 63:1066-1071.

Soifer, F., 1978, Parasitic diseases of reptiles, in: "Zoo and wild animal medicine," M.E. Fowler, ed., Saunders Co., Philadelphia.

Sprague, V., 1976, Classification and phylogeny of the Microsporidia, in: "Comparative pathobiology," Vol. 1, L.A. Bulla and T.C. Cheng, eds., Plenum Press, New York.

Sprague, V., 1977, Annotated list of species of Microsporidia, in: "Comparative pathobiology," Vol. 4, L.A. Bulla and T.C. Cheng, eds., Plenum Press, New York.

Sprent, J.F.A., 1963, The life history and development of Amplicaecum robertsi an ascaridoid nematode of the carpet python (Morelia spilotes variegatus). II. Growth and host specificity of larval stages in relation to the food chain, Parasitology, 53:321-337.

Steck, F., 1962, Pathogenese und klinisches Bild der Amoebaendysenterie der Reptilien, Acta Trop., 19:318-354.

Steck, F., 1963, Die Amoebendysenterie der Reptilien. Aetiologie, Epidemiologie, Diagnostik und Bekampfung, Acta Trop., 20:115-142.

Stoll, N.R., 1957a, Axenic culture of Entamoeba invadens in the absence of tissue, J. Protozool., 4: Suppl. 6.

Stoll, N.R., 1957b, Axenic serial culture in cell-free medium of Entamoeba invadens, a pathogenic amoeba of snakes, Science, 126:1236.

Stone, W.B., and Manwell, R.D., 1969, Toxoplasmosis in cold-blooded hosts, J. Protozool., 16:99-102.

Symmers, W.S.C.S., 1969, Primary amoebic meningoencephalitis in Britain, British Med. J., 4:449-454.

Taliaferro, W.H., and Holmes, F.O., 1924, Entamoeba barreti n. sp. from the turtle, Chelydra serpentina: A description of the amoeba from the vertebrate host and from Barret and Smith's cultures, Amer. J. Hyg., 4:160-168.

Tadros, W., and Laarman, J.J., 1976, Sarcocystis and related coccidian parasites: A brief, general review, together with a discussion on some biological aspects of their life cycles and a new proposal for their classification, Acta Leiden., 44:1-137.

Tadros, W., and Laarman, J.J., 1982, Current concepts on the biology, evolution and taxonomy of tissue cyst-forming eimeriid coccidia, Adv. Parasitol., 20:293-468.

Taylor, J.L., Wagner, J.E., Kusewitt, D.F., and Mann, P.C. 1979, Klossiella parasites of animals: A literature review, Vet. Parasitol., 5:137-144.

Telford, S.R., Jr., 1970, A comparative study of endoparasitism among some southern California lizard populations, Amer. Midland Natur., 83:516-554.

Telford, S.R., Jr., 1971, Parasitic diseases of reptiles, J. Amer. Vet. Med. Ass., 159:1644-1652.

Thepsuparungsikul, V., Seng, L., and Bailey, G.B., 1971, Differentiation of Entamoeba: Encystation of Entamoeba invadens in monoxenic and axenic cultures, J. Parasitol., 57:1288-1292.

Tibaldi, E., 1921, Una nuova specie di Toxoplasma, Riv. Biol., 3:612-616.

Tiegs, O.W., 1931, Note on the occurrence of Sarcocystis in muscle of Python, Parasitology, 23:412-414.

Todd, K.S., and Ernst, J.V., 1977, Coccidia of mammals except man, in: "Parasitic protozoa," Vol. 3, J.P. Kreier, ed., Academic Press, New York.

Triffit, M.J., 1925, Observations on two new species of coccidia parasitic in snakes, Protozoology, 1:19-26.

Trinci, G., 1911, Nota sopra una Sarcocystis parassita di Gongylus ocellatus Wagl. con considerazioni critiche sulla morfologia e sulla biologia dei Sarcosporidi, Monit. Zool. Ital., 22:309-326.

Vavra, J., 1976, Structure of the Microsporidia, in: "Comparative pathobiology," Vol. 1, L.A. Bulla and T.C. Cheng, eds., Plenum Press, New York.

Vetterling, J.M., and Widmer, E.H., 1968, Eimeria cascabeli sp. n. (Eimeriidae, Sporozoa) from rattlesnakes, with a review of the species of Eimeria from snakes, J. Parasitol., 54:569-576.

Vetterling, J.M., Jervis, H.R., Merrill, T.G., and Sprinz, H., 1971, Cryptosporidium wrairi sp. n. from the guinea pig, Cavia porcellus, with emendation of the genus, J. Protozool., 18:243-247.

Vickerman, K., 1965, The identity of Leishmania chamaeleonis Wenyon, 1921, Trans. Royal Soc. Trop. Med. Hyg., 59:372.

Vickerman, K., 1976, The diversity of the kinetoplastid flagellates, in: "Biology of the Kinetoplastida," Vol. 1, W.H.R. Lumsden and D.A. Evans, eds., Academic Press, New York.

Wacha, R.S., and Christiansen, J.L., 1977, Additional notes on the coccidian parasites of the soft-shelled turtle, Trionyx spinifera Le Sueur, in Iowa, with a description of Eimeria vesicostieda sp. n., J. Protozool., 24:357-359.

Wallace, F.G., 1966, The trypanosomatid parasites of insects and arachnids, Exp. Parasitol., 18:124-193.

Wallace, F.G., 1979, Biology of the Kinetoplastida of arthropods, in: "Biology of the Kinetoplastida," Vol. 2, W.H.R. Lumsden and D.A. Evans, eds., Academic Press, New York.

Wallach, J.D., 1969, Medical care of reptiles, J. Amer. Vet. Med. Ass., 155:1017-1034.

Walton, A.C., 1964, The parasites of Amphibia, Wildlife Dis., 40.

Walton, A.C., 1966, Supplemental catalog of the parasites of Amphibia, Wildlife Dis., 48.

Walton, A.C., 1967, Supplemental catalog of the parasites of Amphibia, Wildlife Dis., 50.

Weber, A., 1909a, Alteration des fibres musculaires striees sous l'influence des Sarcosporidies, C.R. Soc. Biol. (Paris), 66:566-568.

Weber, A., 1909b, Sur la morphologie de la Sarcosporidie du Gecko (Sarcocystis platydactyli Bertram), C.R. Soc. Biol. (Paris), 66:1061-1062.

Weber, A., 1910, Recerches sur la Sarcosporidie du Gecko (Sarcocystis platydactyli Bertram), Arch. Anat. Microbiol., 11:167-178.

Weiser, J., 1960, Zur Kenntnis der Krankheiten der Lurche, Vestn. Cesk. Spol. Zool., 24:232-233.

Wenyon, C.M., 1926, "Protozoology," Bailliere, Tindall and Cox, London.

Wessenberg, H.S., 1978, Opalinata, in: "Parasitic protozoa," Vol. 2, J.P. Kreier, ed., Academic Press, New York.

Zaman, V., 1975, Revision of S. orientalis Zaman and Colley, 1975, South East Asian J. Trop. Med. Public Health, 6:603.

Zaman, V., 1976, Host range of Sarcocystis orientalis, South East Asian J. Trop. Med. Public Health, 7:112.

Zaman, V., and Colley, F.C., 1975, Light and electron microscope observations of the life cycle of Sarcocystis orientalis sp. n. in the rat (Rattus norvegicus) and the Malaysian reticulated python (Python reticulatus), Z. Parasitenk., 47:169-185.

Zaman, V., and Colley, F.C., 1976, Replacement of Sarcocystis orientalis Zaman and Colley, 1975, by Sarcocystis singaporensis n. sp., Z. Parasitenk 51:137.
Zwart, P., 1964, Studies on renal pathology in reptiles, Pathol. Vet., 1:542-556.
Zwart, P., 1974, Maladies des reptiles, Zoo Anvers, 39: 152-158; 40:14-22; 40:63-67.
Zwart, P., and Truyens, E.H.A., 1975, Hexamitiasis in tortoises, Vet. Parasitol., 1:175-183.
Zwart, P., Borst, G.H.A., and Truyens, E.H.A., 1975, Hexamitiasis bei Schildkroten, XVII Internationales Symposiums uber die Erkrankungen der Zootiere, Akademie Verlag, Berlin.

HAEMOPARASITES OF REPTILES

Sam R. Telford, Jr.

Florida State Museum

Gainesville

INTRODUCTION

The haemoparasites of reptiles include representatives of all taxonomic groups which parasitize the other vertebrate classes: trypanosomatid flagellates, haemogregarines, haemosporidia and filariid nematodes, as well as a heterogeneous assemblage of organisms or inclusions which possibly contains viruses, bacteria, rickettsiae, piroplasmids and probably artifacts of staining as well.

The literature describing these organisms is widely scattered in frequently obscure regional or short-lived journals, and requires some multilingual competence to understand, as much of it has never been translated due to its lack of direct human or veterinary medical importance. Wenyon (1926) presented the most thorough review of reptilian haemoparasite groups, except for filariids, which today remains essential as a key to the earlier literature. Subsequent literature reviews have dealt with single taxonomic groups, except for Pienaar (1962) and Brygoo (1963a,b). Increased interest in recent years has led to a broadening of our knowledge of these parasites and their hosts, and recognition of a multiplicity of species in most groups. It is remarkable, however, how little more has been learned of reptilian trypanosomatids, haemogregarines, haemoproteids, and parasites of dubious nature since Wenyon. Particularly lacking are life-history studies, data which could help elucidate systematic relationships presently somewhat speculative or based upon analogy to better known mammalian (particularly human) and avian parasites.

Ecological/epizootiological data are rarely available for most of these parasites in turtle and crocodilian hosts, with only slightly more at hand for snakes. The haemoparasites of lizards are best known due to the large number examined to date, of which those surveys cited in this chapter represent only the most accessible in the literature. Regretably, it has been necessary for the author to refer endlessly to his personal research, much of which remains unpublished and is thus without the refinement given by expert reviewers.

SAURIAN LEISHMANIASIS

Leishmanias as parasites of reptiles are poorly known Although Leishmania species are important and common parasites of man and other animals, and can cause serious disease and often death, there is no evidence of deleterious effects upon survival of their reptilian hosts.

About a dozen species of saurian Leishmania have been described since the first isolation from a lizard was made by Sergent et al. (1915) (Table 20.1). The genus Leish-

Table 20.1. Leishmania Species Described from Lizards.

Species	Host spp.
agamae David, 1929	Agama stellio
nicollei Chodukin and Sofieff, 1940	A. sanguinolenta; Phrynocephalus sp.
sofieffi Markov et al., 1964	Phrynocephalus sp.
chameleonis Wenyon, 1921	Chameleo vulgaris
tarentolae Wenyon, 1921	Tarentola mauritanica
hemidactyli MacKie et al., 1923	Hemidactylus brooki
ceramodactyli Adler and Theodor, 1929	Ceramodactylus doriae
gymnodactyli Chodukin and Sofieff, 1947	Gymnodactylus caspius
hoogstraali McMillan, 1965	H. turcicus
henrici Leger, 1918	Anolis sp.
zmeevi Andrushko and Markov, 1955	Eremias sp.
adleri Heisch, 1958	Latastia longicauda

mania is related to trypanosomes, and is presently placed in the same family, the Trypanosomatidae. It is thought that leishmanias have evolved from insect flagellates possibly similar to Leptomonas, a parasite of modern insects (Garnham, 1971), and that reptiles probably were their first vertebrate hosts (Zuckerman and Lainson, 1977). During their life cycle leishmanias show morphological changes which have been given descriptive names that refer to the position of the flagellum. For practical purposes these will be referred to simply as the promastigote and amastigote forms. Promastigotes are motile, extracellular stages with a prominent flagellum. They are found within the gut of the vector insect and possibly in the bloodstream of the saurian host. This term is used also for the culture form of the parasite. Amastigote stages (Figs. 20.1 and 20.2) are intracellular, rounded and lack an external flagellum. In mammalian hosts they parasitize reticulo-endothelial cells in various organs and tissues, especially liver, spleen, bone marrow and the skin. In reptiles, however, amastigotes are known with certainty only from circulating blood cells, no visceral foci of infection have been demonstrated (Telford, 1979b) except for L. chameleonis found in the large intestine of chameleons. This species, however, may not belong to the genus Leishmania but rather to Herpetomonas (Gardner, 1977).

Distribution

With a single exception, all records of leishmanial infection in reptiles come from the Old World: Mediterranean Europe, North Africa, East Africa, Middle East and southern Russia through the Indian subcontinent into China. Leger (1918) described Leptomonas henrici from an Anolis species (Iguanidae) of Martinique. Intensive studies on haemoparasites of many Neotropical lizard species during

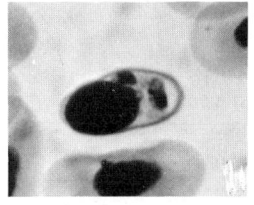
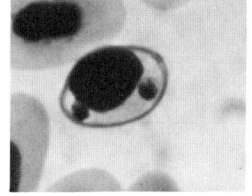

a b

Fig. 20.1a,b. Leishmania sp. amastigotes in thrombocytes of Agama agilis, Pakistan. X1480

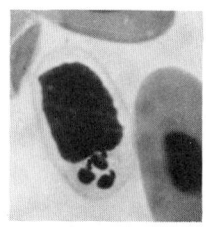 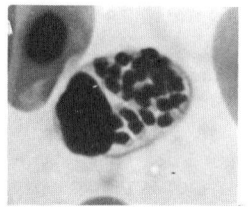

Fig. 20.2a,b. Leishmania sp. amastigotes in thrombocytes of Teratoscincus scincus, Pakistan. X1480

the last decade have not confirmed the presence of saurian leishmaniasis in the New World. Most infections have been reported from lizards in arid or semi-arid environments and among the families Gekkonidae, Agamidae, Chameleontidae, Lacertidae and Scincidae. Soviet scientists, who have done the most extensive surveys for saurian Leishmania, also found 8 of 207 Turkmenian snakes infected: one infection each in Coluber rhodorhachis, C. karelini, Psammophis schokari and in two Echis carinatus (Belova and Bogdanov, 1968).

The incidence of leishmanial infection among lizards is most accurately determined by surveys employing culture techniques, as parasitemia of circulating blood cells is usually very low and it is not known if cells infected by amastigotes are alway present in the circulation or if they may be sequestered in capillaries underlying skin or within organs during part of the life cycle. The most extensive survey was reported by Belova (1971), in which 3,818 lizards of six families and 21 species were collected in the Turkmenian SSR. Positive cultures were obtained from 223 lizards (5.8%) of 11 species, all gekkonids, agamids or lacertids which comprosed 99.3% of the sample. Varanids, anguids and scincids collected in very low numbers were negative. Nearly two-thirds of the Leishmania infections were found in gekkonids (62.8%), with proportionately fewer in agamids (26.5%) and lacertids (10.8%), despite the predominance of agamids in the total lizards sampled. Gekkonids and lacertids were represented in nearly equal numbers. Gymnodactylus caspius showed the highest overall infection rate (15.3%, N=907), and accounted for 62.3% of the total infections found, followed by Agama sanguinolenta (6.0%, N=683) infections which represented 18.4% of the total number of infections. Infection rates varied somewhat from locality to locality, with usually more than one species infected per locality.

Some prevalence data are provided by two surveys in which blood smears were examined. A survey in Lebanon by Edeson and Himo (1973) found 4% of 200 A. stellio with blood cells parasitized by amastigotes. Telford (1979) reported amastigote-parasitized thrombocytes in Teratoscincus scincus (18.8%, N=16) and A. agilis (9.7%, N=72), with an overall infection rate among 848 Pakistani lizards from 6 families and 37 species of 1.2%. Both the Lebanese and Pakistani surveys probably are significant underestimates of actual prevalence of leishmanial infection, as cryptic infections would not be revealed except by culture.

Etiology

Leishmaniasis results from the infection of the vertebrate host by flagellates of the genus Leishmania transmitted from probable vector insects, phlebotomine sandflies of the genus Sergentomyia, by ingestion of infected flies or by their bite, neither of which route has been demonstrated. Leishmania spp. enter circulating blood cells, usually thrombocytes, lymphocytes or monocytes, sometime following transmission where they evidently reproduce by binary fission. No visceral focus of infection is known and the amastigote seems to be the characteristic form present in the reptilian host (Telford, 1979b).

Transmission

Vector transmission of saurian Leishmania spp. has not been accomplished experimentally. Phlebotomine sandflies (Diptera: Psychodidae) are probable vectors. Serological studies of strains isolated from promastigotes found in S. sintoni in Iran (Nadim et al., 1968) and in S. arpaklensis in the Soviet Union (Saf'janova, 1966) proved them to be of saurian origin rather than mammalian. Promastigotes of saurian species appear to develop both anteriorly and posteriorly in sandflies, thus suggesting that infection could take place by more than one route, i.e., by bite or by ingestion of the vector.

Transmission of leishmaniasis is confined to that period of the year during which the presumed sandfly vectors are active, i.e., from late spring to early fall in southern Asia. The first generation of sandflies for the season probably becomes infected by feeding on chronically infected lizards newly emerged from hibernation. Belova (1966, 1971) reported an infection rate of 20% among G. caspius in early April in Serakhs, Turkmenia, before emergence of sandflies which pass the winter as uninfected larvae. Following the establishment of infection in this first generation of sandflies, transmission might occur to subadult and adult lizards not previously infected, with infection of subsequent generations of sandflies coming from either the new active infections or older, chronically infected lizards. As sandfly densities increase through the season to reach their maximum in late summer-early fall, so too would the prevalence of promastigote infections among them. Nadim et al. (1968) reported promastigote infections in 25% of S. sintoni in the Turkmenian Sahara of Iran, and demonstrated their saurian origin serologically. Coinciding with the peaks of sandfl density and promastigote incidence among them would be entry of large numbers of hatchlings into the lizard populations. The highest parasitemia by Leishmania amastigotes in thrombocytes of T. scincus on the Afghan border of Pakistan, 2.7 to 8.5%, was seen in hatchling lizards collected in mid-September (Telford, 1979b). Belova (1966 reported the gecko infection rate in Serakhs to be 26% at the height of the transmission period, with only a slight decline to 20% by the following spring.

Pathogenesis and pathology

No studies have been done on the pathogenesis of Leishmania in reptiles and there are no descriptions of pathological alterations due to the parasite in its natura: host species. Presumably infection of circulating blood cells by amastigotes will cause their eventual destruction, but in view of the very low parasitemias recorded thus far, 0.1 to 15.0% of thrombocytes (Telford, 1979b), it is unlikely that host survival is affected. Belova (1971) believed that saurian hosts remain infected for life, while epizootiological data suggest that infection must last for 5 to 6 months as a minimum. Belova observed natural infections to persist as long as 1.5 to 2 months in the laboratory, and Telford (1979b) found parasitemia of thrombocytes in T. scincus to remain relatively constant at 0.1 to 0.8% over an 82 day period.

Diagnosis

Leishmanial infections are usually detected by culture of heart or hepatic blood or pieces of tissues from heart, spleen, liver, lung or bone marrow in N.N.N. medium, or on slants of blood agar overlain by an enrichment medium containing antibiotics (Belova, 1971). Examination of impression smears from organs revealed infections in some endemic areas (Edeson and Himo, 1973; Telford, 1979b). Smears of peripheral blood stained by the Geimsa technique for at least one hour should be carefully examined at

X400 to X1,000, with special attention given to thrombocytes, lymphocytes and monocytes. As parasitemia may be no higher than 0.1% of thrombocytes, several hundred of these cells must be examined to exclude patent leishmanial infection. Culture techniques are the most efficient.

Immunity and prognosis

There is no evidence that leishmanial infections reduce the longevity of reptilian hosts. Infection probably continues for life and no studies have demonstrated whether or not immunity can develop in reptilian hosts to leishmania.

Control

Transmission of leishmaniasis among captive reptiles would require capable vectors to occur naturally in the area, and in view of a probably high degree of specificity at the invertebrate host level, is most unlikely. It might be possible for infection to develop should an infected lizard be eaten by another, but this is too speculative to require elaboration.

TRYPANOSOMIASIS

Trypanosomiasis in reptiles is caused by infection with flagellates of the genus Trypanosoma (Fig. 20.3). Infections by the various species in their natural hosts are apparently non-pathogenic but experimental transmission to different hosts can be fatal.

At least 58 species of Trypanosoma are known from crocodilians, turtles, lizards and snakes (Table 20.2). Additionally, there are more than 40 infections recorded in the literature as "Trypanosoma sp." (Brygoo, 1966), some of which represent distinct species, as well as several named species which are obvious synonyms. Very few life cycles are known and virtually no natural vectors have been proven, although several have been identified as probable because of their capacity to serve as laboratory vectors and their ecological association with the reptilian hosts. The species are distinguished by morphological differences among the trypomastigote forms which inhabit the reptilian blood stream. Very few descriptions contain enough quantitative data to permit estimates of intraspecific variations. Systematics of this group are confused due to the paucity of life history data and the absence of comparative biochemical studies which are proving valuable for mammalian trypanosome identifications.

Table 20.2. *Trypanosoma* Species Described from Reptiles, 1902-1980.

Geographic distribution	Reptilian family	*Trypanosoma* sp.
United States and Mexico	Emydidae	chrysemydis Roudabush and Coatney, 1937
	Chelydridae	chrysemydis Roudabush and Coatney, 1937
	Iguanidae	serveti Pelaez and Streber, 1955
		scelopori Ayala, 1970
Tropical America	Anguidae	gerrhonoti Ayala, 1971
	Testudinidae	testudinis Floch and Abonnenc, 1942
	Emydidae	platemysi Floch and Abonnenc, 1942
	Iguanidae	superciliosae Walliker, 1965
		plicae Lainson et al., 1975
	Scincidae	rudolphi Carini and Rudolph, 1912
	Gekkonidae	ocumarense Scorza and Dagert, 1955
		thecadactyli Christensen and Telford, 1972
		torrealbai Telford, 1980
	Sphaerodactylidae	gonatodi Telford, 1980
		torrealbai Telford, 1980
	Colubridae	brazili Brumpt, 1914[a]
		butantanense Arantes and da Fonseca, 1931[a]
		erythrolampri Wenyon, 1908
		mattogrossense Arantes, 1935
		merremii Arantes and da Fonseca, 1931[a]
		philodriasi Pessoa, 1968
		vitali Lavier, 1943[a]
	Boidae	hogei Pessoa, 1968
		constrictor Pessoa and Fleury, 1969
	Viperidae	salamantae Pessoa and Fleury, 1969
		cascavelli Pessoa and Biasi, 1972

Region	Family	Species
East Asia	Eublepharidae	ryukyuense Miyata, 1977
Southeast and	Emydidae	damoniae Laveran and Mesnil, 1902
Southern Asia		vittatae Robertson, 1908
	Gekkonidae	hemidactyli MacKie et al., 1923
		leschenaulti Robertson, 1908
		pertenue Robertson, 1908b
		phlebotomi Shortt and Swaminath, 1931
Australia and	Colubridae	primeti Mathis and Leger, 1909
Oceania	Chelydidae	chelodina Johnston, 1907
	Scincidae	egerniae Mackerras, 1961
	Gekkonidae	phylluri Mackerras, 1961
Africa	Testudinidae	leroyi Commes, 1919
	Pelomedusidae	mocambicum Pienaar, 1962
		neitzi Dias, 1952
		pontyi Bouet, 1909
		sheppardi Dias, 1952
	Crocodilidae	grayi MacKie, 1914c
	Varanidae	grayi MacKie, 1914c
		varani Wenyon, 1909c
	Chamaeleontidae	chamaeleonis Wenyon, 1909
		therezieni Brygoo, 1963
	Iguanidae	domerguei Brygoo, 1965
	Gerrhosauridae	betschi Brygoo, 1966
	Scincidae	boueti Martin, 1907
		mochli Berghe et al., 1957
	Gekkonidae	gallayi Bouet, 1909b
		loricatum Garnham and Duke, 1953b
		petteri Brygoo, 1966
	Colubridae	platydactyli Catouillard, 1909b
		clozeli Bouet, 1909
		haranti Brygoo, 1965
	Boidae	psammophis Fantham and Porter, 1950
		sebae Fantham and Porter, 1950

(contd.)

Table 20.2. Trypanosoma Species Described from Reptiles, 1902-1980. (Continued)

Geographic distribution	Reptilian family	Trypanosoma sp.
	Elapidae	najae Wenyon, 1909 voltariae MacKie, 1919

[a] possible synonyms (Brygoo, 1965).
[b] possible synonyms (Bray, 1964).
[c] possible synonyms (Bray, 1964).

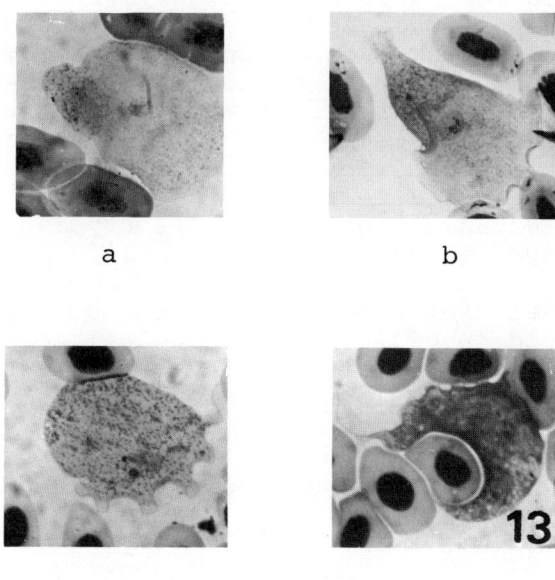

Fig. 20.3. Trypanosoma spp. from lizards.
   a. T. gonatodi from Gonatodes albogularis, Panama. X750
   b. T. torrealbai from Gonatodes taniae, Venezuela. X750
   c. T. serveti from Anolis poecilopus, Panama. X750
   d. Trypanosoma sp. from Gecko gecko, Thailand. X750

Distribution

Reptilian Trypanosoma spp. have been reported from North, Central and South America, Africa and Mediterranean Europe, the Indian subcontinent and southern Russia, Southeast Asia, southern Japan, Australasia and Oceania. Most of the described species (93%) are known from the tropics or subtropics. Throughout Africa, Mediterranean Europe and southern Asia, Trypanosoma in lizards is sympatric with Leishmania, related trypanosomatid saurian parasites which also utilize phlebotomine sandflies as vectors.

Because reptilian trypanosomes seldom show moderate to high parasitemias in infected hosts, it is difficult to assess the reliability of available survey data.

Reported infection rates are probably gross underestimates of true prevalence when based upon examination of single slides or samples taken on a single occasion, as very low parasitemias may easily fluctuate between positive and negative when slides are taken at daily intervals. The effect of low parasitemias on results obtained from initial versus second examinations of single slides was shown by Telford (1977), who detected on initial examination only 28.6% of the actual number of Anolis trypanosome infections found upon repeated examinations.

Survey data for crocodilians and turtles are inadequate to provide useful epizootiological conclusions. Studies by Hoare (1929, 1931b) indicated that a majority of adult Crocodylus niloticus in Uganda were infected by T. grayi. This may be typical over much of the range of C. niloticus which coincides with riverine tsetse fly distribution. Glossina spp. are often found infected with T. grayi during routine dissections in the course of medical and veterinary research on trypanosomiases (Wenyon 1926; Molyneux, 1977). No trypanosomes are known from American or Asian crocodilians, but this may represent lack of research only. Turtle trypanosomes have been reported more often and from many areas of the world, but no good data on prevalence or seasonality and age distribution of infected hosts are available. A survey of snakes based upon a large sample was presented by Pessoa et al. (1974), but conclusions are limited due to the broad geographical area and considerable time span over which the samples were collected. They found 18 Trypanosoma infections among 2113 snakes obtained by Instituto Butantan from south-central Brazil, a prevalence rate of only 0.9%. These comprised 3.8% of 474 haemoparasite infections found and came from 6 of the 45 snake species examined. Infection rates were highest in Rachidelus brazili (28.6%) and Boa constrictor (13.8%), and were much lower in others: Xenodon merremi (0.7%), X. neuwiedii (3.3%), Epicrates cenchris (2.7%) and Crotalus durissus (1.7%).

Trypanosome infections appear to be most common in continental areas which are temperate to subtropical, semi-arid grasslands or tropical to subtropical, humid and forested (Tables 20.3 and 20.4). Inasmuch as saurian trypanosomes appear to use phlebotomine sandflies as vectors, one might expect some prevalence of mixed infections of Leishmania spp. and Trypanosoma spp. in both Sergentomyia sandflies and various lizards in those areas of Africa, Mediterranean Europe and southern Asia where the two trypanosomatid genera are sympatric, but this has not yet been demonstrated.

Table 20.3. References for Saurian Haemoparasite Surveys.

Area	No. lizards examined	References
California, central	1367	Ayala, 1973; Telford, 1972, 1977 (unpubl.); Wood and Wood, 1936
California, southern	922	Telford, 1970a
Florida	1992	Telford, 1978b; Thompson and Huff, 1944b
Texas-Arizona	240	Telford, 1970b, 1972 (unpubl.); 1978a
Mexico	358	Telford, 1970 (unpubl.); Thompson and Huff, 1944b
Middle America	572	Telford, 1977
Panama	1905	Telford, 1977
Venezuela	851	Telford, 1978c, 1980
Caribbean	463	Telford, 1975, unpubl.
Africa, west	520	Baker, 1961; Bray, 1959; Schwetz, 1931a,b, 1934
Africa, east	1419	Ball, 1967; Telford, unpubl.
Madagascar	1099	Brygoo, 1963a,b
New Guinea	154	Ewers, 1968
Australia, east	294	Mackerras, 1961
Japan, Honshu	1855	Telford, 1965-1967 (unpubl.)
Japan, Ryukyus	166	Telford, 1965-1968 (unpubl.)
Thailand-Malaysia	384	Telford, 1976-1980 (unpubl.)
Pakistan	848	Telford, 1975-1977 (unpubl.)
Russia, southern	605	Andrushko and Markov, 1955a, b, 1956; Krasilnikov, 1965; Markov and Bogdanov, 1961; Markov et al., 1964, 1968

Approximately 70% of the described saurian trypanosome species are known from gekkonid, scincid, anguid and gerrhosaurid hosts which tend to be secretive in terrestrial or arboreal habitats, and 26% from chamaeleontids and iguanids which are markedly arboreal or saxicolous. A single species only, apparently, is known from varanids, which may share the parasite with crocodilians due to their predilection for riverine habitat. According to Bray (1964) *T. grayi* and *T. varani* are possibly synonymous. The crocodile trypanosome uses *Glossina* rather than phlebotomine sandflies as vectors. No agamid trypanosomes are

Table 20.4. Geographic Distribution of Saurian Trypano-

Physiographic/climatic characteristics	Area	No. lizard examined
Continental, temperate to subtropical, arid, desert or montane	California, southern Pakistan Russia, southern	922 848 605
Subtotal:		2375
Continental, temperate to subtropical, semi-arid, grasslands or montane	California, central Texas-Arizona Mexico Africa, east Australia, east	1367 240 358 1419 294
Subtotal:		3678
Continental, tropical to subtropical, humid, forest	Florida Middle America Panama Venezuela Africa, west Thailand-Malaysia	1992 572 1905 851 520 384
Subtotal:		6224
Insular, temperate, humid, forest	Japan, Honshu Japan, Ryukyus	1855 166
Insular, subtropical, humid, forest	Caribbean Madagascar	463 1099
Insular, tropical, humid, forest	New Guinea	154
Subtotal:		3737
Total:		16,014

[a]Saurian Leishmania present, but not detected by blood smears.

yet described, although some have been reported in the literature from these generally ecological equivalents of iguanids (Brygoo, 1966). Phlebotomine sandflies show greater abundance in the types of habitats in which burrow inhabitating, secretive or arboreal hosts live, and the correlation between host habitats and vector habitat with prevalence of trypanosomes is thus expected.

somatid Parasites from Survey Data given in Table 20.3.

No. haemoparasite infections	% Infections comprised by Trypanosoma	Leishmania
119	0.0	0.0
181	0.0	5.5
140	0.7	---a
440	0.7 x̄	5.5 x̄
377	1.9	0.0
48	6.2	0.0
74	0.0	0.0
312	25.0	---
113	10.4	0.0
924	8.7 x̄	0.0 x̄
261	0.0	0.0
120	2.5	0.0
759	4.5	0.0
338	0.8	0.0
156	4.5	0.0
164	28.7	0.0
1798	8.2 x̄	0.0 x̄
280	0.0	0.0
7	14.3	0.0
97	0.0	0.0
300	87.8	---
21	28.6	0.0
705	43.6 x̄	0.0 x̄
3867		

Within the range of single host species, trypanosome prevalence can vary widely as described by Ayala (1973) for T. scelopori in Sceloporus occidentalis where one host deme showed an infection rate of 5% in contrast to 0.4% overall from among 733 lizards from other areas. Telford (1977) reported an infection rate of 9% for T. gonatodi among 142 Gonatodes albogularis collected in Panama, but all infections found came from a single deme in San Blas Territory, where 31% of 45 lizards were infected compared to 97 negative G. albogularis from the Canal Zone. Differences in prevalence such as these are probably due to

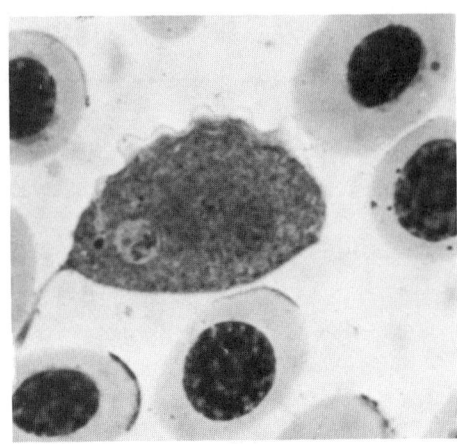

Fig. 20.4. <u>Trypanosoma</u> <u>thecadactyli</u> from <u>Thecadactylus</u> <u>rapicaudus</u>, Panama. X750

variation in some critical microhabitat requirement of the vector which does not influence distribution of the vertebrate host.

Few data are available which provide information on seasonality. Telford (1977) reported an infection rate of 72% for T. thecadactyli (Fig. 20.4) in its only host Thecadactylus rapicaudus. Infections were found in seven months of the year in Panama, with no significant difference seen between dry season (January-May, 57%) and wet season (June-December, 78%). This large gecko has an intimate, probably continuous association with the presume sandfly vector Lutzomyia trinidadensis in caves, outbuildings and tree buttresses (Christensen and Telford, 1972). The particular microhabitats used by both sandfly and geck are probably less influenced by monthly variation in rainfall than would be the arboreal canopy and forest floor. T. serveti was found in six species of Panamanian Anolis (Telford, 1977), but only in the dry season when the infec tion rate was 2.4% among 587 anoles examined. Another 366 anoles of the same species in the same localities were examined in the wet season and found to be negative. This significant difference in infection rate by season possibly reflects the effect of heavy rain on resting sites of the presumed sandfly vectors. Although too few G. albogularis were collected in the late wet season for good comparison, the infection rate by T. gonatodi in the dry season was still significantly greater (60.9%, N=37) than in the wet season when no infections were found.

Etiology

At present all reptilian trypanosomes are included within Trypanosoma. It is possible to separate those few species for which life history data are available into two groups based upon the developmental pattern within the invertebrate vectors, but the significance of certain variations reported remains unclear. Generally, those trypanosomes which parasitize aquatic reptiles are probably transmitted by leeches, and transform from the trypomastigotes ingested by the leech into epimastigotes which multiply by binary fission, then transform into metacyclic trypanosomes which are infective for the reptile where they become trypomastigotes. This pattern also is present in the tsetse fly transmitted crocodile trypanosomes. Where known, trypanosomes of non-aquatic reptiles utilize dipterans as vectors, of which only phlebotomine sandflies have been satisfactorily incriminated. Trypomastigotes from the reptile become amastigotes in the vector, then sphaeromastigotes and finally epimastigotes which appear to be the infective stage for the reptile. Multiplication can continue in all of the vector stages.

Trypanosomiasis results from the introduction of infectious metacyclic trypanosomes or epimastigote stages by the vector into the reptilian host. These stages enter the host's blood stream either directly by inoculation through the vector's bite or indirectly through the mucous membranes of the oral cavity or through the gut wall following ingestion of the vector by the reptile. In T. butantanense, which parasitizes Xenodon merremi, division of trypomastigotes by binary fission occurs in the blood stream (Arantes and da Fonseca, 1931), thus permitting heavy parasitemias to develop. Most reptilian trypanosome infections, however, show such low parasitemias both in natural and experimental infections (Woo, 1969) that it seems unlikely that division in the peripheral blood is usual in their life cycles. The level of parasitemia achieved is probably directly related to the number of infective stages introduced, with little reproduction occuring in the reptilian host. There is no evidence that reptilian trypanosomes aggregate in visceral foci or invade host tissue. Infection by some species possibly persists for the life of the host (Shortt and Swaminath, 1931). An individual T. rapicaudus, however, positive for T. thecadactyli at capture and for eight months following, became negative by xenodiagnosis thereafter (Christensen and Telford, 1972), thus indicating that infections can be lost by development of immunity or in absence of opportunity for reinfection.

Transmission

Reptilian trypanosomes demonstrate two basic life history patterns: that shown by leech transmitted species which parasitize aquatic reptiles, and one characteristic of dipteran transmitted trypanosomes infecting primarily lizards.

Trypomastigotes in the blood stream of aquatic turtl and snakes transform into epimastigotes in the crop or stomach of leeches and divide by binary fission in the multiplicative phase of the life cycle. Epimastigotes then turn into transitional forms which become metacyclic trypomastigotes, the infective stage for the turtle or snake. This development pattern was first indicated by Robertson (1909) for T. vittatae in Glossiphonia sp. and Limnatis granulosa fed on Emyda vittata of Ceylon. This was confirmed by Woo (1969) for T. chrysemydis parasitic in Chrysemys picta marginata in North America. Trypomast gotes of T. chrysemydis obtained in turtle blood by Placobdella parasitica and P. rugosa produced epimastigot by four days post-infection in leeches kept at 21 C to 23 C. Transitional stages were seen in 8 to 13 days and some metacyclic trypomastigotes by 22 days, with many of the latter present by the 34th day. When kept at 31 C, the developmental cycle was shortened: epimastigotes were present by day 2, transitional forms on day 4 and metacyclic trypomastigotes by days 14 to 16.

Although transmitted by dipterans, T. grayi, which parasitizes C. niloticus, follows the developmental patte characteristic of leech transmitted species. Trypomastigotes in the blood stream are taken by tsetse flies and transform into epimastigotes in the midgut where they divide. As their number increase, epimastigotes enter the hindgut and become metacyclic trypomastigotes (Hoare, 1972). In the first two to three days, the epimastigotes are contained within the peritrophic membrane which surrounds the blood meal in the midgut, but by four to five days many have migrated to the hindgut. These reach the open end of the peritrophic membrane and escape into the extraperitrophic space attaching to the epithelium (Hoare, 1931a). By six to eight days, all have escaped from within the peritrophic membrane and have migrated anteriorly, re-invading the midgut and anterior hindgut, but this time occupying the extraperitrophic space. As division continues along the midgut from days 9 to 34, transformation to infective metacyclic trypanosomes begins and these migrate posteriorly to complete development in the ileum of the hindgut. Eventually, the infection

becomes restricted to the ileum. When infected tsetse
flies enter the open mouths of basking crocodiles and
defecate while feeding, metacyclic trypanosomes enter the
crocodile's blood stream through the mucous membranes and
become trypomastigotes. Infection also probably occurs
by crushing of flies when crocodiles close their jaws.
The morphology of T. grayi and its life cycle in C. niloticus and G. fuscipes in Uganda was described by Hoare
(1929, 1931a,b), while Molyneux (1977) reported finding
T. grayi in G. tachinoides and G. palpalis of Upper Volta.

Some variation in life cycle pattern and modes of
transmission has been reported. Brumpt (1914) described
development of T. brazili from Helicops modestus in the
leeches, P. braziliensis and P. cantenifer. Epimastigotes
were seen in 4 days post-feeding, and metacyclic trypomastigotes in 19 days. Development occurred in the leech
stomach without invasion of the proboscis sheath, which
led Brumpt to suggest that infection occurred by ingestion
of the leech. Although Woo (1969) did not find metacyclic
forms of T. chrysemydis in the salivary glands or proboscis
of leeches, transmission to clean turtles was accomplished
only by bite of leeches, and not by their ingestion,
indicating the infective metacyclic trypomastigotes entered
the turtle blood stream either by migration or regurgitation from the crop while leeches fed. Pessoa and Fleury
(1969) found T. hogei from R. brazili to develop in the
leech Haementeria lutzi, with formation of promastigote
and epimastigote stages only, the latter presumably being
infective. Infection was thought to persist for the life
of the leech.

With the exception of tsetse fly-transmitted T. grayi,
the dipteran-transmitted trypanosomes of land reptiles
appear to develop to infective stages only in phlebotomine
sandflies, and usually progress from ingested trypomastigotes to amastigotes, then to sphaeromastigotes and ultimately form epimastigotes, the infective stage. Multiplication can occur, apparently, in all stages but trypomastigotes. The anuran parasite, T. rotatorium, was shown by
Desser et al. (1973) to develop in the mosquito, Culex
territans: amastigotes formed in 1 to 3 hours and divided
within the midgut for 3 to 70 hours. Sphaeromastigotes
were present in the hindgut by 83 hours and epimastigotes
were seen from 100 hours, with no conversion to metacyclic
trypomastigotes observed. DeBiasi et al. (1975) reported
some development of T. salamantae from E. cenchris crassus
in C. dolosus by 24 hours after feeding, but did not
describe progression to infective stages. They reported
infection per os of two laboratory-born Bothrops alter-

natus by culture forms of T. phylodriasi originally isolated from Philodryas nattereri. Prepatent time was five days. Other workers have been unable to infect mosquitoe with reptilian trypanosomes (Christensen and Telford, 197 Woo, 1969) with the exception of Brygoo (1963a). He fed C. pipiens fatigans on a chamaeleon infected by T. therezieni, and found epimastigotes present in the mosquito digestive tracts, undergoing division, in 18 to 24 hours, but between 48 to 60 hours all flagellates disappeared. Oddly, inoculation of engorged mosquitoes into chamaeleon within 6 hours after the blood meal produced infection, but such inoculations after more than 24 hours failed to induce infection.

Shortt and Swaminath (1931) described the developmen of T. phlebotomi from Hemidactylus frenatus in the sandfl S. babu shortii. In 3 to 5 hours following ingestion of infected blood, the trypanosomes are ovoid or nearly spherical; division begins in the amastigote form in the midgut, within hyaline cysts which contain 40 to 60 amast gotes each by 24 hours. Some flagellated forms appear in 36 to 40 hours, with most having flagella by 72 hours. Motile epimastigotes were found in the midgut and hindgut by 113 hours. Division within secondary cysts in the midgut continues to produce epimastigotes which enter the hindgut. Transmission to clean H. frenatus followed ingestion of infected flies with patent infection observec in 17 to 25 days. Adler and Theodor (1935) found development of T. platydactyli restricted to the esophagus and midgut of S. minuta fed on infected Tarentola mauretanica and possibly observed transmission per os to a clean geckc Ayala and McKay (1971) found a similar development patterr for T. sceleropi and T. gerrhonoti in the sandfly, L. vexator occidentis, with epimastigotes usually present in the cardia and occasionally in both stomach and esophagus. Christensen and Telford (1972), however, described the development of T. thecadacyli in L. trinidadensis as showing epimastigotes present 3 to 14 days post-feeding, primarily in the hindgut with some persisting in the midgu through day 7. Midgut and hindgut infections of T. boueti (Fig. 20.5) in S. bedfordi fed on Mabuya striata were described by Ashford et al. (1973) in Ethiopia. Amastigotes were first seen at 48 hours, they became sphaeromastigotes by 72 hours and continued division in the midgut. Shortly thereafter, transformation to epimastigotes occurred in the midgut and the hindgut was invaded. Voiding of the blood meal remnants at 4 to 5 days eliminated most flagellates from the midgut, but the hindgut retained tightly packed epimastigotes after evacuation of the bloodmeal. The presence of developed infections

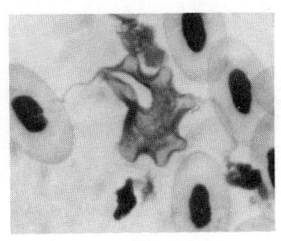 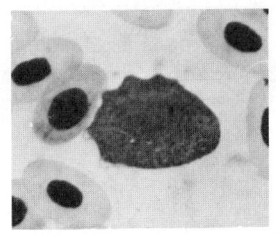

a   b

Fig. 20.5a,b. Trypanosoma boueti, a polymorphic parasite of Mabuya quinquetaeniata, Kenya. X750

in the esophagus, midgut and cardia (T. scelopori, T. gerrhonoti, T. platydactyli) as well as in the hindgut (T. phlebotomi, T. thecadactyli, T. boueti) suggests differing modes of transmission according to site of development in the vector. The former group is possibly transmitted by bite and the latter by ingestion.

Some variation in life cycle stages has been reported from in vitro studies. Grewal (1955) mentioned dividing promastigote forms of T. garnhami from H. brookii angulatus, and reported forms which looked like metacyclic trypomastigotes but which were not infective. Sergent et al. (1914) found promastigotes of T. platydactyli in vitro, but Chatton and Blanc (1918) reported culture forms to be epimastigotes. The former workers may have isolated L. tarentolae instead of T. platydactyli.

Successful experimental transmission of T. therezieni by parenteral inoculation of infected blood was accomplished by Brygoo (1963a), who also infected chamaeleons by feeding them the liver from a Chamaeleo lateralis previously itself infected parenterally with T. therezieni. Many attempts to transmit various Neotropical saurian trypanosome species by Telford (unpubl. data) have failed, in contrast to Brygoo's results.

Pathology

The only study to report pathogenicity by a reptilian trypanosome is that of Brygoo (1963a). Most natural infections show low parasitemias and it is difficult to imagine any pathologic consequences. Shortt and Swaminath (1931) commented that T. phlebotomi seems to be "quite innocuous" to its host, H. frenatus, and Brygoo (1963a) described T. therezieni as non-pathogenic to its natural host, C.

brevicornis. Parenteral inoculation of infected blood into four other Chamaeleo spp., none of which were natural hosts to T. therezieni, always produced fatal infections. C. parsoni and C. verrucosus, which weighed 100 to 300 g, died 25 to 35 days following infection, but the much smaller C. lateralis, rarely weighing more than 15 g, did not survive longer than 11 to 18 days. In C. lateralis no parasites were seen in peripheral blood for 4 to 5 days post-inoculation. After the sixth day, however, trypanosomes appeared and their numbers increased until the death of the animal, at which time the blood resembled a pure culture of trypanosomes accompanied by some blood cells. The blood stream trypanosomes seen in C. lateralis appear to be epimastigote forms capable of prolific division, while those seen in C. brevicornis were normal trypomastigotes which probably rarely, if ever, divide in the saurian blood stream. Examination of tissues from naturally infected C. brevicornis and experimentally infected C. lateralis found no divisional stages in the tissues. Dying hosts, however, showed varitable emboli of trypanosomes in the pulmonary capillaries. C. lateralis which showed 800 to 900,000 blood cells per mm^3 before infection died at 13 to 14 days following infection showing 200 to 300,000 erythrocytes per mm^3, but Brygoo was reluctant to consider this to be a parasite-induced anemia. No anemia was evident in naturally infected chamaeleons.

Diagnosis

The diagnosis of reptilian trypanosome infections may be made from either fresh or fixed and stained blood smears. A drop of fresh blood in reptilian Ringer's solution and covered with a coverslip can be examined under 10 to 40X magnification. Movement of trypanosomes is usually detected if the field is darkened slightly. Stained smears should be screened under the same magnifications with close attention given to the margins of the smears. Identification must be made under oil immersion at 1,000X when trypanosomes are located, and measurements should be made of at least 20 specimens using most or all of the characters employed by Telford (1979a).

Immunity and host specificity

There have been no studies on possible immunity by reptilian hosts towards trypanosome parasites.

Crocodilian and turtle trypanosomes seem to be slightly less host specific than are ophidian and saurian species, to judge from published records (Brygoo, 1966). If Bray (1964) is correct, T. grayi and T. varani are conspecific and infect both crocodilians and varanid lizards. Records listed by Brygoo (1966) for turtle trypanosome species indicate that 11 described forms parasitize 16 host speces. One species, T. chelodina, however, parasitizes five different hosts (Mackerras, 1961); the other 10 species average 1.1 hosts each. Woo (1969) has provided some experimental evidence bearing upon host specificity. C. serpentina, C. picta marginata and Graptemys geographica were infected with T. chrysemydis by inoculation with crop and caecal contents of infected leeches, but Clemmys guttata and Emydoidea blandingi were refractory to infection. From data of Pessoa et al. (1974a) and records listed by Brygoo (1966), 16 apparently valid species of snake trypanosomes infect 19 host species. Most saurian trypanosomes are known from single host species. T. serveti, however, parasitizes three iguanid genera, Sceloporus, Anolis and Corytophanes, and at least 10 species (Telford, 1979c), and the African skink parasite, T. boueti under its apparent synonyms T. perroteti, T. martini, T. macroscinci and T. mabuiae (Bray, 1964), parasitizes five Mabuya species. The remaining 25 apparently valid species parasitize 28 different hosts, without accepting Bray's synonymy of geckkonid trypanosomes. It appears, then, that each host group has one or two eurytopic Trypanosoma species and the remainder are highly host specific parasites, infecting only one or two host species. Vector data are inadequate for generalization, but high host specificity toward vectors has probably contributed to a limitation of potential vertebrate hosts among reptilian trypanosome species.

Treatment and control

No information is available on treatment of reptilian trypanosomiasis. In view of the usually low parasitemias found, prognosis would appear to be excellent without treatment.

Trypanosomiasis among captive reptiles can be prevented by eliminating potential vectors (leeches, tabanid and psychodid flies, perhaps mosquitoes) from enclosures. Transmission by ingestion of an infected animal by another is a possibility, in view of Brygoo's experiments (1963a), but seems unlikely. Control measures in nature are impractical in view of the relative scarcity of trypanosome infections in natural populations and the normally low parasitemias.

HAEMOGREGARINES

The most common group of intracellular sporozoan haemoparasites found in reptiles are the haemogregarines, some genera of which parasitize each vertebrate class. Although parasitemias may be intense and of long duration, there is little documented evidence that haemogregarines are pathogenic to their hosts.

The number of named haemogregarine species probably runs into the hundreds, most having been described from erythrocytic stages alone under the illusion that presence in a different host indicates specific identity. All are transmitted by arthropod or annelid vectors, but the mode of transmission may be mechanical only or show sporogonic development within the vector, which provides a useful basis for classification. Natural vectors are unknown for most species, but a number of capable laboratory vectors have been demonstrated.

Haemogregarines have been reported from crocodilians, turtles, the tuatara, Sphenodon punctatus, lizards and amphisbaenians, and are the dominant and characteristic haemoparasites of snakes. Classification to the generic level appears reasonably stable at present, but requires knowledge of development in the vector as well as the reptile. Without life cycle data, therefore, most described species have to be considered as "haemogregarine sensu lato".

Distribution

Haemogregarines are known from virtually every geographic area in which reptiles occur, but unfortunately too few systematic surveys have been published. References cited here are by no means the only ones available; these were chosen to illustrate the cosmopolitan distribution of haemogregarines. To avoid a ponderous citation, many listed by Wenyon (1926) will be so mentioned rather than giving the original source.

Among the Crocodilia, haemogregarines are known from Africa (Hoare, 1932), India, Ceylon, Sumatra, North and South America (Wenyon, 1926) and from the three families, Crocodilidae, Gavialidae and Alligatoridae. Laird (1950) reported Haemogregarina tuatarae from S. punctatus. Haemogregarines are known from all families of freshwater and terrestrial turtles on all continents (Acholonu, 1974; Mackerras, 1961; Wenyon, 1926), but not from the marine turtles. Table 20.5 shows the prevalence of both haemogregarines and haemococcidia among saurians worldwide. Haemococcidia such as Schellackia have apparently not yet been identified in the Australia-New Guinea area, but probably will be found there inasmuch as they occur everywhere else. All major snake families on all continents have been host to haemogregarines (Mackerras, 1961; Miyata, 1974; Mohiuddin et al., 1967; Moreno and Bolanos, 1977; Pessoa et al., 1974a; Wenyon, 1926), but not to haemococcidia which are apparently restricted to saurians among the Reptilia. A single amphisbaenid species, Amphisbaena alba, was found infected by haemogregarines in Brazil (Pessoa, 1968) and Venezuela (Telford, unpubl. data).

There have been so few published surveys on haemogregarine prevalence in the reptilian fauna of given areas, except for saurians, that it is difficult to form any valid conclusions on epizootiology. Such data are virtually lacking for crocodilians, although Hoare (1932) commented that all of the Nile crocodiles he examined, at all ages, were infected by Hepatozoon pettiti. No better data are available for turtles except for North America where four surveys from defined areas showed prevalence ranging from 42 to 100%, with a majority of host species examined in each area found positive (Table 20.6). There are no data on seasonality and age distribution, and in each survey too few turtles were examined to attempt correlation of prevalence with habits or habitat.

Survey data for snakes is considerably better (Table 20.6) as indicative of cosmopolitan prevalence, but still does not provide useful information on some epizootiological parameters. Prevalence is remarkably similar among snakes from Florida, Central America, South America, East Africa, Madagascar, Japan and Pakistan, surprisingly low in a large sample from the Congo, and highest in a small sample from New Guinea. This suggests that climatic factors may not influence haemogregarine prevalence greatly nor, perhaps, phylogenetic differences among hosts. No haemogregarines are known from the families Typhlopidae, Leptotyphlopidae and Uropeltidae, where fossorial habits probably reduce the probability of a vector relationship evolving. A haemogregarine infection was seen in the hydrophiid, Laticauda colubrina (Telford, unpubl. data), but this is not too surprising in view of the fact that a tick, Amblyomma nitidum, is known to parasitize this seasnake (Audy et al., 1960). It is also possible that the trombiculid lung mite, Vatacarus ipoides, which parasitizes Laticauda spp. (Audy et al., 1960; Telford, 1967) might play a vector role. Upon summarizing data from 2,471 Neotropical snakes furnished by Moreno and Bolanos

Table 20.5. Geographical Distribution of Saurian Haemo-

Physiographic/climatic characteristics	Area	No. lizard examined
Continental, temperate to subtropical, arid, desert or montane	California, southern	922
	Pakistan	848
	Russia, southern	605
Subtotal:		2375
Continental, temperate to subtropical, semi-arid, grasslands or montane	California, central	1367
	Texas-Arizona	240
	Mexico	358
	Africa, east	1419
	Australia, east	294
Subtotal:		3678
Continental, tropical to subtropical, humid, forest	Florida	1992
	Middle America	572
	Panama	1905
	Venezuela	851
	Africa, west	520
	Thailand-Malaysia	384
Subtotal:		6224
Insular, temperate, humid, forest	Japan, Honshu	1855
	Japan, Ryukyus	166
Insular, subtropical, humid, forest	Caribbean	463
	Madagascar	1099
Insular, tropical, humid, forest	New Guinea	154
Subtotal:		3737
Total:		16,014

(1977), Pessoa et al. (1974a) and Telford (unpubl. data) in Table 20.7, it would seem that host habitats (arboreal-semiarboreal, terrestrial, aquatic-semiaquatic) do not significantly affect haemogregarine prevalence, although possibly the aquatic snakes may be less often parasitized. Again, the host species distribution by habits show no real differences in prevalence of haemogregarines, in view of the very few aquatic species represented. Although arboreal snakes in south-central Brazil show approximately the same prevalence of haemogregarines as do the same

gregarine Parasites from Survey Data given in Table 20.3.

No. haemoparasite infections	% Infections comprised by Adeleiina	Eimeriina
119	5.9	94.1
181	28.2	48.6
140	10.6	65.8
440	14.9 $\bar{x}$	69.5 $\bar{x}$
377	2.1	26.8
48	18.8	35.4
74	13.5	25.7
312	11.0	4.0
113	37.4	0.0
924	16.6 $\bar{x}$	23.0 $\bar{x}$
261	7.7	6.1
120	11.7	10.8
759	6.6	16.4
338	47.9	9.8
156	3.8	0.0
164	7.9	7.3
1798	14.3 $\bar{x}$	10.1 $\bar{x}$
280	0.0	10.0
7	0.0	0.0
97	1.0	28.9
300	9.0	2.3
21	42.9	0.0
705	17.6 $\bar{x}$	13.7 $\bar{x}$
3867		

group from Venezuela north to Honduras there is a striking difference in prevalence among terrestrial host species, with those from south-central Brazil showing considerably lower prevalence than the northern Neotropical samples. Table 20.8 shows the prevalence of haemogregarines among four families of Neotropical snakes. There seems to be little difference between Colubridae and Viperidae, but Boidae clearly has the highest prevalence and Elapidae the lowest. No data on seasonal or age prevalence are available.

Table 20.6. Haemogregarine Prevalence among Turtles and

Host area	No. examined	No. positive	Percent positive
TURTLES			
North America			
Illinois	26	11	42
Texas	44	33	75
Louisiana	95	95	100
Florida	71	30	42
SNAKES			
North America			
Florida	33	11	33
Central America			
Costa Rica	216	72	33
Costa Rica	39	17	44
Honduras	32	3	9
Panama	33	21	64
South America			
Venezuela	31	18	58
Brazil	2113	406	19
Japan	275	95	35
Africa, west	356	23	6
Africa, east	29	6	21
Madagascar	76	17	22
New Guinea	25	17	68
Pakistan	36	9	25

Among saurians, adeleine haemogregarines are less common than among snakes, but haemococcidia form an important component of the haemoparasite spectrum. From data shown in Table 20.5 it is evident that adeleines are most common in continental areas which are temperate or subtropical, semiarid to arid grasslands or montane habitats, somewhat less common in lizards of the desert floor or foothills, and least common in tropical or subtropical, humid and forested continental areas. The prevalence shown for the Venezuela sample reflects its origin: the dry tropical forest of west-central Venezuela, rather than moist tropical forest. The haemococcidia, on the other hand, are the dominant component of the saurian haemoparasite community in desert regions, and are

Snakes from Various Areas.

No. species examined	No. species positive	Reference
6	4	Marquardt, 1966
11	8	Wang and Hopkins, 1965
8	8	Acholonu, 1974
9	6	Telford, unpubl.
19	5	Telford, unpubl.
16	9	Moreno and Bolanos, 1977
19	7	Telford, unpubl.
11	3	Telford, unpubl.
8	7	Telford, unpubl.
14	10	Telford, unpubl.
45	35	Pessoa et al., 1974a
6	4	Miyata, 1974
25	10	Schwetz, 1931
12	4	Ball, 1967
16	9	Brygoo, 1963
12	11	Ewers, 1968
10	6	Telford, unpubl.

comparable to adeleines in prevalence in temperate or subtropical, semiarid to arid grasslands or mountains, and least common in the wet tropics or subtropics, where again they are similar to adeleines. Their proportionate abundance in xeric regions probably reflects their use of geckobiid or other mites as vectors instead of dipterans. One factor which reduces the proportionate representation of haemogregarines in non-desert areas is the abundance of plasmodiid, trypanosomatid and microfilarid parasites in those areas, and their scarcity in deserts. Haemogregarines have been relatively successful in accompanying colonizing lizard species to islands such as in the Caribean (Telford, unpubl. data) and the Galapagos (Ayala and Hutchings, 1974), again probably because of

Table 20.7. Prevalence of Haemogregarine Infections among Neotropical Snakes by Mode of Life.[a]

Habits	No. examined	Positive No.	percent	No. species examined	Species positive No.	percent
Arboreal/semi-arboreal	298	81	27.2	26	16	61.5
Terrestrial	1952	490	25.1	56	38	67.9
Aquatic/semi-aquatic	221	32	14.5	7	6	85.7
Totals	2471	603	24.4	89	60	67.4

[a]Data from Moreno and Bolanos, 1977; Pessoa et al., 1974a; Telford, unpubl.

Table 20.8. Prevalence of Haemogregarine Infections among Neotropical Snakes by Host Family.

Family	Snakes examined No.	percent	Snakes positive No.	percent	No. species examined	Species positive No.	percent
Boidae	103	4.2	44	42.7	6	5	83.3
Colubridae	1276	51.6	290	22.7	58	41	70.7
Viperidae	1035	41.9	268	25.9	20	13	65.0
Elapidae	57	2.3	1	1.8	5	1	20.0

Table 20.9. Prevalence of Haemogregarines in Saurians at

Host species	Family	Locality
Sceloporus occidentalis and S. graciosus	Iguanidae	California, southern San Jacinto Mtns.
S. jarrovi	Iguanidae	Arizona, southeastern Pinaleno Mtns. Chiricahua Mtns.
Agama tuberculata	Agamidae	Pakistan Himalayas: Naran
Lygosoma himalayanum	Scincidae	Pakistan Himalayas: Lake Saif-ul-Maluk
Euspondylus brevifrontalis	Teiidae	Venezuela Andes: Apartaderos

[a]Data from Telford, 1970a,b, 1980 and unpubl.

the nature of their vectors. Mountains have not provided barriers to haemogregarine distribution, and particularly not for the haemococcidia. Data presented in Table 20.9 demostrate that prevalence of both adeleine and eimeriine haemogregarines can remain high in montane habitats as far as 3,800 m elevation, again, probably because acarine vectors are less affected by elevation and cold than are most dipterans. Karyolysus spp., transmitted by the mite Sauronyssus sauraram, have been found as far north as 58 N latitude in southern Sweden (Svahn, 1974).

Few data are available on age-group distribution of haemogregarines. Among southern California lizards, Telford (1970b) found haemococcidia to be present only in the older age groups of Sceloporus spp., but in Uta stansburiana infections were found in first, second and third year lizards with the infection rate increasing stepwise. Seasonality data on haemogregarine and haemococcidian infections in Panamanian anoles were presented by Telford (1977). Haemogregarine prevalence was very similar throughout the dry and early wet seasons, but rose slightly in the late wet season. Haemococcidian infections were at their lowest prevalence in the late dry season, then rose sharply in the early wet, peaking during the late wet season, and then declining in the early dry season.

Higher Elevations.[a]

Elevation (m)	No. examined	Percent positive for haemogregarines	haemococcidia
1950	63	0.0	8.0
1800-2000	57	0.0	42.0
2400-2700	35	0.0	17.0
2700-2970	36	0.0	28.0
3213	21	0.0	48.0
2375	64	13.0	70.0
3000	46	26.0	11.0
3800	15	0.0	47.0

In southern California lizards, Telford (1970b) reported spring to be the period of highest, demonstrable haemogregarine parasitemia, prior to the appearance of hatchlings. Sexual differences appeared in the onset of parasitemia: male U. stansburiana showed an increase in infection rate from 12 to 57% from pre-reproductive (September 29 to February 6) to reproductive (March 18 to April 29) periods, with no males found infected in the post-reproductive period (May 20 to September 14). Female rates did not increase significantly from pre-reproductive to reproductive periods, but reached 18% in a post-reproductive sample comparable to that for males. In Sceloporus magister collected at 915 m, 15 females were negative while 5 of 17 males were infected by haemogregarines.

Svahn (1974), studying populations of Karyolysus spp. (Fig. 20.6) in Lacerta agilis and L. vivipara of Denmark and southern Sweden, found initial infections present in August and September. Gametocytes persisted in erythrocytes through hibernation, providing the source of infection for the vector, S. saurarum, which was present in great numbers in early spring. As many as 250 nymphs of S. saurarum were found on a single lizard. Laboratory studies indicated that a period of about 65 days is required between ingestion of a first blood meal containing Karyolysus gametocytes by female mites, and the appearance of gametocytes in a second lizard following ingestion of

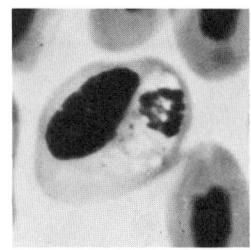 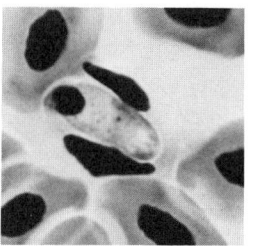

a   b

Fig. 20.6a,b. Karyolysus ca. lacertae in erythrocytes of Lacerta muralis, Switzerland. X1480

infected nymphal mites, which is consistent with appearance of infections in lizards by August-September in nature.

Etiology

Two primary divisions exist in the classification of haemogregarine Coccidiida, the Eimeriina and Adeleiina. The Eimeriine coccidia undergo both sporogony and gametogony in the reptile host, using vectors for mechanical transfer only. Two genera are found with certainty among the Reptilia: Schellackia (Figs. 20.7 to 20.9) and Lainsonia (Fig. 20.10), both of which belong to the Lankesterellidae. These are distinguished by differences in development within the reptile host, as described below. The genus Lankesterella (Fig. 20.11), although reported from reptiles, is probably confined to amphibian and avian hosts (Lainson et al., 1976). Although all haemogregarines are coccidian sporozoans, the eimeriine haemogregarines are often called haemococcidia, in reference to their development occurring solely within the reptile, as with intestinal coccidia of this host group.

Haemogregarines which have sporogonic development in invertebrate vectors belong to the Adeleiina. Gametogony occurs in the vertebrate host. Three genera of Haemogregarinidae are commonly seen in reptiles: Haemogregarina, Hepatozoon and Karyolysus. Klossiella (Klossiellidae) has been reported from an ophidian host (Zwart, 1964), but is rarely if ever seen in circulating blood, transmission perhaps relying upon ingestion of sporocytes in feces by the usual mammalian hosts or through predation upon infected mammals by other mammals and birds (Landau, 1973) or snakes. The genera Haemogregarina, Hepatozoon and Karyolysus CANNOT consistently be distinguished solely by either

HAEMOPARASITES OF REPTILES

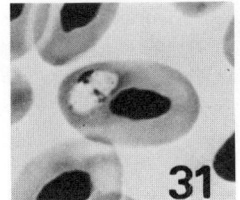

a

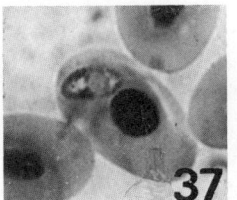

b

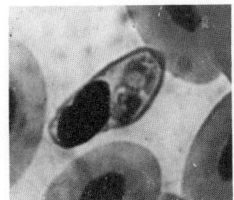

c

Fig. 20.7a,b,c. Schellackia spp. from lizards. X1480
- a. S. ca. bolivari from Lacerta muralis, Switzerland
- b. Schellackia sp. from Takydromus tachydromoides, Japan
- c. Same species as in b except the parasite is situated in a thrombocyte

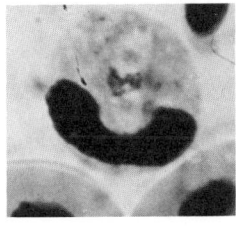

a

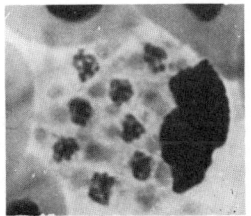

b

Fig. 20.8a,b. Leucocytes of Anolis cybotes, Haiti, infected with Schellackia ca. golvani. X1480

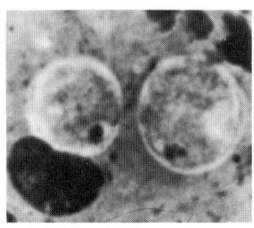
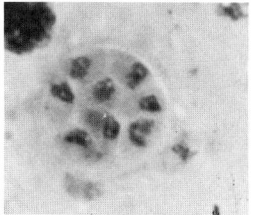

a   b

Fig. 20.9a,b. Developing oocysts of Schellackia ca.
               golvani in an impression smear from the
               small intestine of Anolis cybotes, Haiti.
               X1480
               a. Developing oocysts
               b. Mature oocysts

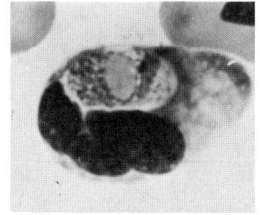
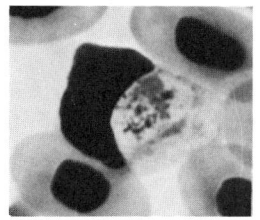

a   b

Fig. 20.10a,b. Lainsonia spp. in leucocytes of Venezuelan
               lizards. X1480
               a. L. legeri in Tupinambis teguixin
               b. L. iguanae in Iguana iguana

erythrocytic stages or characteristics of the schizonts
which occur in various host tissues. Generic designation
of the many described adeleiine haemogregarine species is
impossible without knowledge of the developmental pattern
in vectors. This is why taxonomic distinction of haemogregarines found in blood smears is discouraged unless there
is some obvious characteristic unique to that parasite
(Ball, 1967). Comparative development of the three genera,
described in detail below, shows that Haemogregarina produces sporocysts within the vector gut, Hepatozoon forms
oocysts containing sporocysts in the haemocoele, and
Karyolysus produces sporokinetes (and motile spores) within
oocysts in the gut wall which enter ova and form sporocysts in developing mite larvae, thus showing transovarian
transmission.

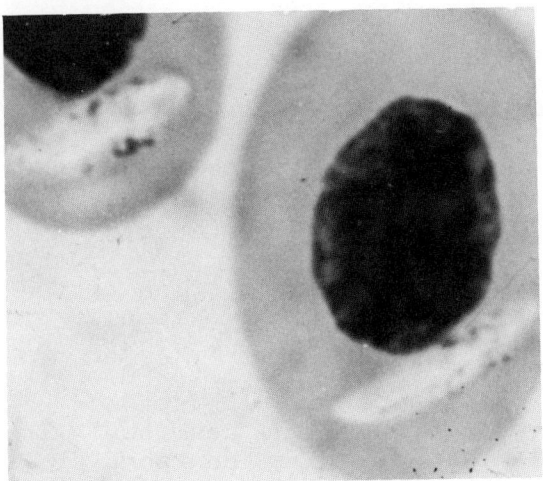

Fig. 20.11. Lankesterella sp. from the anuran, Atelopus varius, Panama. X1480

Transmission

Mites of the genera Sauronyssus (Liponyssus of Reichenow, 1920) and Geckobiella (Bororris and Ball, 1955) are demonstrated capable vectors for Schellackia and probably function as such in nature. Culex pipiens has proven to be a suitable laboratory vector (Lainson et al., 1976). No natural vector is known for Lainsonia; experimental infection was accomplished by both the oral route and parenterally, using infected blood (Landau et al., 1974). Schellackia also has been transmitted by intraperitoneal inoculation of infected blood (Bonorris and Ball, 1955; Telford, unpubl. data), but the prepatent period is considerably longer by the parenteral route. The natural mode of infection is probably by ingestion of the vector and presumably infection could result from ingestion of infected vertebrates as well. Vectors for the haemococcidia are purely mechanical. Intracellular sporozoites in saurian blood are ingested by the vector. As digestion proceeds or possibly by their own effort, sporozoites escape from blood cells and accumulate in epithelial cells lining the vector gut (Lainson et al., 1976). No development or multiplication occurs in the vector. When the vector is ingested by a new host, sporozoites initiate sexual and asexual cycles in the reptile.

Evolution of a complex vector relationship proceeds further with the adeleine haemogregarines. Ingestion of gametocytes in reptilian blood cells initiates the sexual cycle in the vector, the products of which are sporozoites infective for the vertebrate host. Sporogonic patterns differ among the genera Haemogregarina, Hepatozoon and Karyolysus forming the basis for generic differentiation.

According to Reichenow (1910) gametocytes of Haemogregarina stepanowi in turtle blood are ingested by a leech, Placobdella catenigera. Within the leech gut gametocytes associate in pairs (szygy), and are encased by formation of a cyst wall adhering to the lumenal epithelium. Macro- and microgametocytes are formed, fertilization occurs, and the resulting zygote begins division, producing sporozoites. Sporozoites developing within the oocyst are released when it ruptures, penetrate the gut wall and pass through the haemocoele into the dorsal blood sinus, accumulating in the leech proboscis. Transmission occurs when a new host is bitten. Robertson (1910) found a similar sporogonic pattern for H. nicoriae in the leech, Ozobranchus shipleyi. Apparently, the complete sporogony of other Haemogregarina spp. has not been observed, although partial success was achieved by Ball (1958). Many species, earlier described as Haemogregarina, Have been found to belong to Hepatozoon when sporogony Was obtained in experimental vectors (Ball et al., 1967; Hoare, 1932; Pessoa et al., 1974a) or when more carefully studied (Michel, 1973). Evidence was presented by Pessoa et al. (1971) which they thought demonstrated a species of Haemogregarina to develop in C. pipiens fatigans and C. dolosus because the oocyst developed on the stomach wall rather than in the haemocoele. However, they described, and their photographs confirmed, the presence of an oocyst containing sporocysts with sporozoites which is diagnostic for Hepatozoon (Fig. 20.12). The only proven Vectors, then, for Haemogregarina are leeches.

As originally described in the rodent mite, Laelaps echidninus, vector development of Hepatozoon differs from Haemogregarina in that male and female gametes fuse to form a zygote and then a motile ookinete develops which penetrates through the gut wall into the haemocoele (Miller, 1908). Robin (1936) also described for H. mesnili Of Gecko gecko, a pryriform zygote which penetrated the gut lining of mosquitoes to begin oocyst formation in the haemocoele. Ball and Oda (1971) found that association of H. rarefaciens gametocytes (Fig. 20.13) free from their host erythrocyte, takes place in the mosquito haemocoele, fertilization occurs and the zygote forms the young oocyst without, apparently, becoming a motile ookinete. This implies that vermicules (free, elongate gametocytes) migrate individually through the gut wall into the haemo-

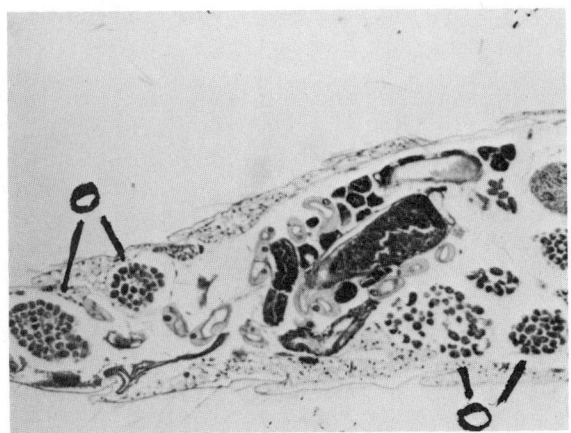

Fig. 20.12. Hepatozoon fusifex oocysts (o) in the haemocoele of Culex tarsalis. X25

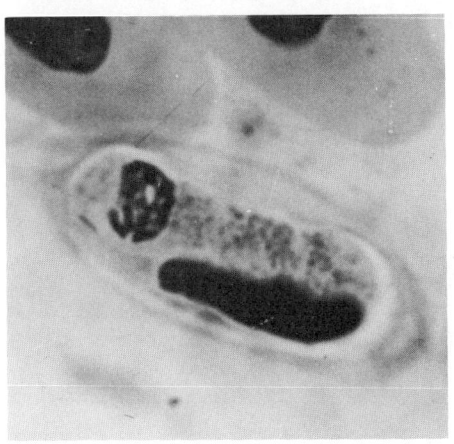

Fig. 20.13. Hepatozoon rarefaciens from Drymarchon corais. X825

coele, a substantial difference of probable significance to generic classification. Sporocysts containing sporozoites then form within the oocyst and transmission occurs when the vector is ingested. Hepatozoon spp. from reptiles can develop successfully in a variety of vectors: leeches (Pessoa and Cavalheiro, 1969a,b), triatomid bugs (da Rocha e Silva, 1975), tsetse flies (Hoare, 1932), ixodid ticks (Ball et al., 1969; Michel, 1973), mites (Lewis and Wagner, 1964), phlebotomine sandflies (Ayala, 1970a) and both culicine and anopheline mosquitoes (Ball et al., 1967,1969;

Landau et al., 1972; Mackerras 1962a; Pessoa and de Biasi 1973b; Robin, 1936).

In Karyolysus male and female gametocytes associate in pairs without fusing and enter epithelial cells of the vector mite gut where a cyst wall forms around them (Reichenow, 1921). Gametes form, fertilization occurs and the zygote becomes an oocyst with nuclear division producing sporokinetes within the oocyst. This ruptures and sporokinetes enter the haemocoele. Some reach the ovary, enter the ova and form sporocysts while the larval mite develops. As embryonic tissues take shape, sporocyst occupy cells which become gut epithelium and reach maturit by the time the nymphal mite has its first blood meal. Svahn (1975) found sporocysts to contain sporozoites 5 to 7 days after maternal mites had their second blood meal, and nymphs taking their first blood meal about 10 days after eggs were laid contained mature sporocysts. As digestion takes place, epithelial cells may be shed into the lumen and sporozoites leave the mite with feces which may be ingested by lizard hosts (Wenyon, 1926). More likely, the infected mites are ingested by lizards, as demonstrated by Svahn (1975). Vectors of Karyolysus are mites of the genus Sauronyssus (Reichenow, 1921; Svahn, 1974; 1975).

It is possible that non-vectorial transmission can occur either by predation or congenitally. Landau (1973) believed that resistant cysts in viscera, derived directly from Hepatozoon sporozoites, provided a mechanism for transmission from infected prey (lizard) to snake predators, and demonstrated that the tissue stage of Hepatozoon could survive passage through a lizard host, in which it could not produce gametocytes, to ultimately infect a snake which ingested the lizard. Predation also might transmit haemococcidian infections from infected prey lizards to uninfected predator lizards, inasmuch as sporozoites occur in blood cells and transmission by ingestion of infected blood has been shown to be possible (Landau et al., 1974). Congenital transmission of haemogregarines was reported by Biasi et al. (1971) who found several litters of young Bothrops moojeni and Crotalus durissus, born to parasitized females, themselves infected. Congenital transmission of Hepatozoon sp. was evident when several still-born Boa constrictor showed parasitized erythrocytes and the mother was infected by H. fusifex (Telford, unpubl. data).

Pathogenesis

Infection by haemogregarines results when the infective sporozoites enter the reptile host from the vector, either by ingestion or inoculation. Development in the reptile is similar for all with respect to schizogony and gametogony. A basic difference, however, distinguishes the haemococcidian genera Schellackia and Lainsonia from the adeleines: asexual reproduction, gametogony, sexual reproduction and sporogony occur in the reptile for the haemococcidians, but asexual reproduction and gametogony alone occur for the adeleines within reptiles. Ingested or inoculated sporozoites of Schellackia enter epithelial cells of the intestine and multiply by schizogony. Some schizonts then produce gametocytes, gametes form, fertilization yields a zygote, and this becomes an oocyst in which sporozoites are produced. Fertilization occurs in the gut epithelium or the lamina propria and zygotes form oocysts usually in the lamina propria. Sporozoites then enter blood cells in the intestinal capillaries 30 to 45 days post-infection (Bonorris and Ball, 1955; Lainson et al., 1976). Some sporozoites parasitize erythrocytic cells exclusively or only white blood cells, while others may use both types (Lainson et al., 1976). Sporozoites carried to the viscera may accumulate in reticuloendothelial cells of the liver, spleen and lung where in at least one species an extraintestinal asexual division may occur (Lainson et al., 1976).

In Lainsonia, by contrast, sporozoites entering the saurian host penetrate reticuloendothelial cells of internal organs where they undergo schizogony, gametogony and sexual reproduction, producing oocysts (Landau, 1973). Sporozoites then enter red or white blood cells and become available to the vector, or accumulate in the reticuloendothelial cells where they remain indefinitely in infective diapause (Lainson et al., 1976).

Ingested or inoculated sporozoites of adeleine haemogregarines enter the bloodstream and are carried to various organs, most commonly liver, spleen and lung, where those of Hepatozoon and Karyolysus occupy endothelial cells of capillaries or other cells in the liver. Sporozoites of Haemogregarina enter red blood cells which may tend to be sequestered within certain viscera. In Haemogregarina schizogony occurs within the erythrocytes (Acholunu, 1974; Reichenow, 1910; Robertson, 1910), giving rise to a generation of merozoites which then invade new red blood cells and undergo a second schizogony. Merozoites from this division can enter blood cells and produce gametocytes or possibly other generations of schizonts. The presence of haemogregarine schizogonic stages in circulating erythrocytes is suggestive, but not conclusive, evidence that the genus Haemogregarina is present.

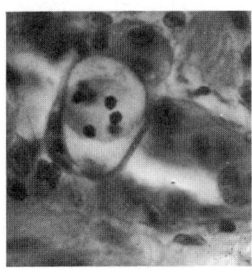 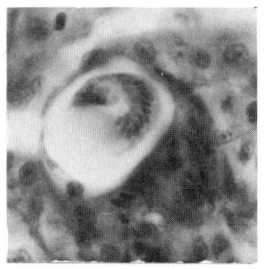

a b

Fig. 20.14. Schizonts of Hepatozoon fusifex in the lung of Boa constrictor. X375
a. Y-type schizont
b. X-type schizont

In Hepatozoon, and some Karyolysus infections, at least two generations of schizonts develop in their visceral site (Fig. 20.14) with one generation (Y-schizont producing markedly fewer and larger merozoites per schizon (macromerozoites), but there is disagreement upon which type of schizont develops first in sequence and on the fate of its merozoites (Ball et al., 1967; Furman, 1966; Mackerras, 1961, 1962a; Svahn, 1975). As suggested by Reichenow (1921), possibly macromerozoites result from Y-schizonts derived from sporozoites and give rise to X-schizonts which initiate the sexual phase by producing micromerozoites which become gametocytes when they enter blood cells 20 to 50 days following infection (Table 20.10). Furthermore, some of the forms seen in circulatin red or white blood cells are trophozoites rather than youn gametocytes, but there is no concensus on how to differentiate them (Ball et al., 1967). Landau (1973) has postulated that some Hepatozoon sporozoites entering the reptile do not enter the two schizogonic cycles giving rise to gametocytes, but instead produce resistant cysts in the tissues. Their product can then initiate a new infection in suitable predators which eat the infected animal. In Karyolysus spp. there is often extensive disorganization of the erythrocyte nucleus. This is suggestive of the presence of that genus, but not diagnostic, for some Hepatozoon spp. also alter the appearance of the host cell nucleus (Ball, 1967) and many produce dramatic hypertrophy of the erythrocyte itself (Ball et al., 1967, 1969).

As schizogony continues, haemogregarine infections may become intense and acute infections are commonly seen.

No one, apparently, has charted the course of initial infection and demonstrated the rate at which parasitemia can increase, although Hull and Camin (1960) showed variations in the level of parasitemia of developed infections over a 52 day period.

Pathology

Although heavy parasitemias of haemogregarines are commonly seen, and infected reptiles easily obtained for laboratory study, there has been virtually no work done on the pathology of infection. Occasional reference to mild anemia is made, as by Pienaar (1962), but apparently only three papers have provided precise data. Beyer and Selivanova (1969) reported on nuclear DNA content in haemogregarines parasitizing diploid and triploid Lacerta and found that the presence of haemogregarines within the erythrocyte caused no change in the nuclear DNA content of the host cells even though the nuclei of these were morphologically deformed and fragmented. This is a commonly seen effect of being parasitized by haemogregarines and is characteristic of, but by no means exclusive to Karyolysus. Beyer and Sidorenko (1972) found that hemoglobin disappeared progressively from erythrocytes infected with haemogregarines, but the total protein amount remained unchanged. They suggested that perhaps metabolic changes occur in the infected erythrocyte which produce additional proteins induced by the parasite, commenting that this may be related to the hypertrophy of host cell that is often seen. Many haemogregarine species do cause tremendous hypertrophy of host cells, the extremes of which may be seen in H. rarefaciens and H. fusifex (Ball et al., 1967, 1969).

In a later paper, Beyer and Sidorenko (1973) reported that an activated increase in erythrocyte dehydrogenases in parasitized cells is an initial erythrocyte response to parasitization. They postulated that such metabolic changes may contribute to maintaining suitable environmental conditions for the parasite and to stabilization of erythrocyte integrity. This could increase the life span of the erythrocyte and, therefore, that of the parasite.

Diagnosis

Diagnosis of haemogregrine infection is made by microscopic examination of thin blood smears stained, preferably, with the standard dilution of Giemsa for one hour or more. Very few species can be identified satisfactorily

Table 20.10. Prepatent Periods Observed Following Intro- and Non-homologous Hosts.

Haemogregarine species and original host species	Experimental host species and type: (H) homologous (N) non-homologous
Schellackia occidentalis; Sceloporus occidentalis (exp.)	Sceloporus undulatus (N)
S. landaue	Polychrus marmoratus (H)
Lainsonia legeri	Tupinambis teguixin (H)
Hepatozoon rarefaciens; Drymarchon corais (exp.)	Boa constrictor (N); Pituophis catenifer (N)
H. fusifex	Boa constrictor (H)
H. mesnili	Gecko verticillatus (H)
H. sauromali; Sauromalus spp. (exp.)	Sceloporus spp. (N)
Hepatozoon sp.; B. constrictor (exp.)	Anolis carolinensis (N)
Hepatozoon sp.; B. constrictor (exp.)	P. catenifer (N) S. occidentalis (N)
Hepatozoon sp.; B. constrictor via P. catenifer	S. occidentalis (N)
H. tupinambis; T. teguixin	Crotalus durissus terrificus (N)
H. domerguei; Madagascarophis colubrina	Madagascarophis colubrina (H) Lioheterodon modestus (N) Python sebae (N) Oplurus sebae (N)
Karyolysus latus; Lacerta agilis or vivipara	Lacerta agilis (H) L. vivipara (H)
K. lacazei or K. lacertae (mixed); L. agilis or vivipara	L. agilis (H)

duction of Haemogregarine Sporozoites into both Homologous

Experimental vector	Infection route	Prepatent period (days)	Reference
Geckobiella texana	Oral Parenteral	30-45 79-97	Bonorris and Ball, 1955
Culex pipiens fatigans	Oral	30-45	Lainson et al., 1976
Infected blood	Oral	36	Landau et al., 1974
C. tarsalis	Parenteral; oral	20-47	Ball et al., 1967; Chao and Ball, 1969
C. tarsalis; Aedes togoi; Amblyomma dissimile	Oral	38	Ball et al., 1969
C. pipiens fatigans; A. albopicta	Oral	20	Robin, 1936
Hirstiella sp.	Oral	30	Lewis and Wagner, 1964
C. tarsalis	Oral	42-50	Booden et al., 1970
C. tarsalis	Oral Oral	25 45	Oda et al., 1971
C. tarsalis	Oral	32	Oda et al., 1971
C. pipiens fatigans	Oral	42	Pessoa et al., 1974b
C. pipiens fatigans	Oral	40	Landau et al., 1974
Anopheles stephensi	Oral	40 23 40	
Sauronyssus saurarum	Oral	32-37 40	Svahn, 1975
S. saurarum	Oral	30-31	Svahn, 1975

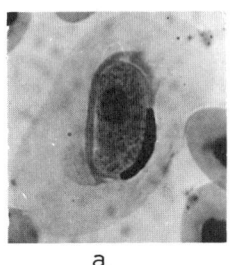 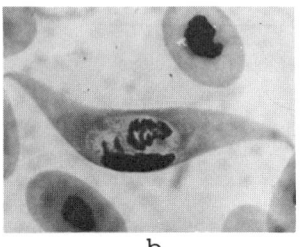

a b

Fig. 20.15a,b. Morphologically variable forms of Hepatozoon fusifex from Mexican snakes. X500

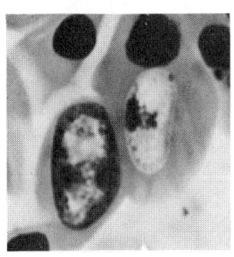 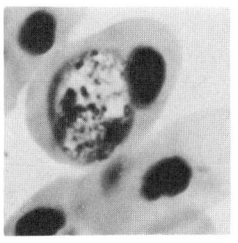

a b

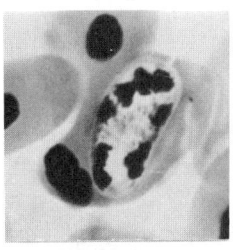 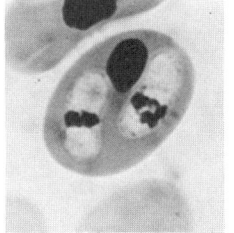

c d

Fig. 20.16a,b,c,d. Haemogregarina crocodilinorum in erythrocytes of Alligator mississippiensis, Florida. X1480

from blood smears (Figs. 20.15 and 20.16), though the presence of "haemogregarines sensu lato" is easily established (Fig. 20.17).

Immunity

There are apparently no precise data available on immune responses to haemogregarine infection. Svahn (1974) found that natural infection of Karyolysus spp. in L. agilis and L. vivipara disappeared 5 to 6 months later, but very heavy infections might persist as long as 8 months or more. Lizards which had recovered from low grade infections were not resistant to reinfection, but repeated reinfection and heavy infection appeared to cause some resistance to develop. No evidence was found of cross-resistance to infection by other Karyolysus spp. By repeated reinfections, parasitemia could be maintained at a low level for as long as 22 months, and Svahn suggested that this capacity for reinfection contributes to maintaining Karyolysus spp. in the lizard populations.

The degree of host specificity among haemogregarines is poorly known. Hull and Camin (1960), on the basis of parasite morphology in erythrocytes, thought all haemogregarine infections found in 13 snake genera, belonging to three families and housed by three zoos, to represent a single species. Other investigators (Marquardt, 1966; Roudabush and Coatney, 1937) have freely identified North American turtle haemogregarines (Fig. 20.18) as H. stepanowi, which is correctly applied only to parasites of European turtles in which the life cycle of that species was fully studied by Reichenow (1910). On the other extreme, many workers have not hesitated to name new species upon finding infections in different hosts. In a long series of papers, Pessoa named a number of species based upon differences in morphology of the erythrocytic, schizogonic and sporogonic stages, but finally admitted that the erythrocytic gametocytes are too variable and the schizonts and oocysts too similar to be of much value in distinguishing species (Pessoa and de Biasi, 1973a,b).

Experimental work has shown that some haemogregarines have very loose specificity with regard to both vector and vertebrate. Ball et al. (1967) have shown that H. rarefaciens of the colubrid snake, Drymarchon corais, can be transmitted to the boid, Boa constrictor, and ultimately to the colubrid, Pituophis catenifer (Chao and Ball, 1969), but not, apparently, to lizards of the genus Sceloporus (Oda et al., 1971), though they did produce a transitory infection in Anolis carolinensis. Mosquitoes of the

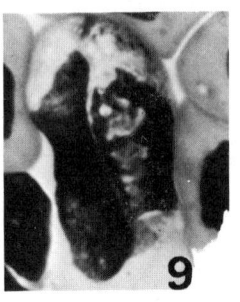

a

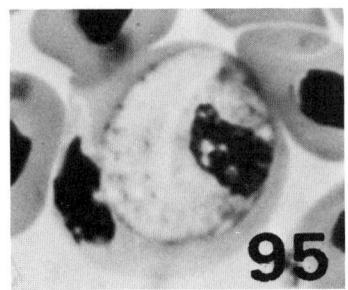

b

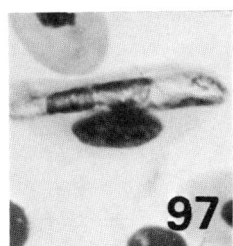

c

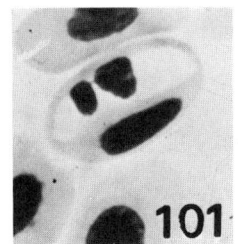

d

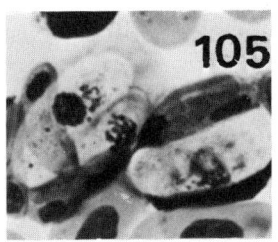

e

Fig. 20.17a,b,c,d,e. Morphological diversity of unidentified haemogregarines from various reptiles, all host cells are erythrocytes. X1480
  a. from Gecko gecko, Thailand
  b. from Cyrtodactylus scaber, Pakistan
  c. from Agama caucasica, Pakistan
  d. from Sceloporus poinsetti, United States of America (Texas)
  e. from Tupinambis teguixin, Venezuela

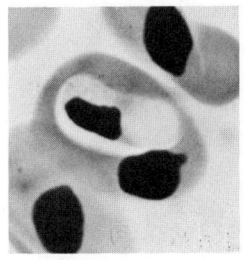
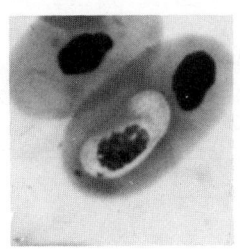

a b

Fig. 20.18a,b. Adeleid haemogregarine in turtles from Florida. X1480
a. from Chrysemys concinna
b. from Trionyx ferox

species C. tarsalis, Anopheles albimanus and Aedes sierrensis are all capable laboratory vectors for H. rarefaciens. Similarly, Ball et al. (1969) found that H. fusifex of B. constrictor will undergo sporogony in C. tarsalis, A. togoi and Amblyomma dissimile.

An Hepatozoon sp. (possibly H. fusifex) from B. constrictor can produce normal blood infections in A. carolinensis, though of only 3 to 4 months duration (Booden et al., 1970), in P. catenifer of at least 1.5 years duration and in S. occidentalis of one month duration (Oda et al., 1971). Similarly, Landau et al. (1972) transmitted H. domerguei of the colubrid, Madagascarophis colubrina, by the mosquitoes C. pipiens fatigans and A. stephensi to the colubrid, Lioheterodon modestus, the boid, Python sebae and the iguanid lizard, Oplurus sebae. They could not infect three Lacerta spp., but schizonts formed in tissues of L. muralis without gametocytes appearing in the blood. Pessoa et al. (1974b) were able to transfer H. tupinambis from the teiid lizard, T. teguixin, to the rattlesnake, C. durissus terrificus by C. pipiens fatigans. Pessoa et al. (1970) found the colubrid, Cyclagras gigas, parasitized by two species of Hepatozoon: H. migonei underwent sporogony in the leech, Haementeria lutzei, and H. cyclagrasi did so in the mosquito, C. quinquefasciatus.

The evidence on host specificity of haemogregarines is confusing at present and perhaps no real evaluation can be made until the newer biochemical tools are applied to species identification in this group of parasites. Certainly, many species of haemogregarines do exist, but probably not as many as have been named. Minchin (1907)

was correct when he said "In the present state of our knowledge, it is not new species of haemogregarines that are needed, but rather new facts about old species"
The dictum still holds.

Treatment and prognosis

No information is available on treatment of haemogregarine infections. Presumably some of the antimalarials or anticoccidials would be effective, but dosages need to established. Untreated haemogregarine infections seem to cause no discernible ill effects upon hosts, infected animals often surviving as well as uninfected individuals.

Control

As with all vector borne diseases among captive animals, transmission can be prevented by normal control measures against acarine, dipteran or leech pests. It might be well not to pen heavily infected small reptiles with larger ones to prevent transmission by predation. Control in nature is not practical.

MALARIA

Malaria in reptiles, common and widely distributed, is caused by three genera of related haemosporidian parasites: Plasmodium, Fallisia and Saurocytozoon. Infection by most species is of little apparent significance to survival of either the individual or population, but some species are at least potentially pathogenic, singly or synergistically in their effect.

At present there are 68 species and subspecies of malarial parasites described from lizards, most of which are Plasmodium (62), with few Fallisia (4) and Saurocytozoon (2) species reported (Table 20.11). Only three species are known from snakes, all Plasmodium. During their life cycle, all undergo sporogony in an insect vector, followed by schizogony and gametogony in the vertebrate host. Very few details of sporogony are known, no definitive proof of natural vector identity has been presented, and primary exoerythrocytic schizogony is yet undescribed. The species are distinguished by morphological differences in asexual and sexual stages found within circulating blood cells, and the extent of variatio to be expected in these stages is well known for less than half of the described forms. An acceptable scheme of classification has not been devised and that presented below lies between the current extreme positions.

Distribution

Saurian Plasmodium spp. have been described from North, Central and South America, Africa, Ceylon, Japan, Malaysia, Australia and Oceania. The preponderance of named forms from Tropical America is indicative only of the intensive effort in that region during the last decade. Species of Saurocytozoon are known from Brazil and Venezuela (Lainson and Shaw, 1969a; Lainson et al., 1974b; Telford, 1978a). Fallisia has been described thus far only from Brazil (Lainson et al., 1974a, 1975). Both genera occur in Southeast Asia as well (Telford, unpubl. data).

Three species of Plasmodium have been described from Neotropical snakes: Plasmodium wenyoni and P. tomodoni (Fig. 20.19) from Thamnodynastes pallidus and Tomodon dorsatus, two very similar Brazilian species (Garnham, 1965; Pessoa and Fleury, 1968), and P. pessoai (Ayala et al., 1978) from Lachesis muta and Spilotes pullatus of Costa Rica. Several records from Panamanian colubrids in adjacent Bocas del Toro (Gorgas Memorial Laboratory, 1964) probably refer to the latter species, while others from Brazil (Pessoa et al., 1974a) may represent undescribed species. All records of Plasmodium from African and Asian snakes appear to be haemoproteids instead. No plasmodiids are known from turtles or crocodilians.

In East and West Africa and Australia, where agamid, scincid and gekkonid lizards predominate in the saurian fauna, plasmodiid species are sympatric with haemoproteids. Elsewhere these haemosporidian families are allopatric, with haemoproteids known from agamids and gekkonids in Southern Asia, and plasmodiids parasitizing iguanids, teiids, scincids, anguids and gekkonids in the Western Hemisphere. Plasmodiids appear to have been more successful on islands, being found in lacertids of Japan and the Ryukyus, scincids of Oceania, chameleontids of Madagascar and iguanids of the Caribean, but both species and host diversity are reduced in insular situations. Haemoproteids occur in New Guinea and plasmodiids should be found there as well, given their sympatry as seen in Australian lizards. Saurian haemoproteids also are known from Ceylon where a plasmodiid parasitizes varanids, in contrast to the remainder of the Indian subcontinent where only haemoproteids have been found.

Although prevalence of saurian malaria often varies considerably among sites within relatively short distances, some broad ecological generalizations seem possible from

Table 20.11. Plasmodiid Species and Subspecies Described from Lizards, 1909-1980.

Geographic distribution	Reptilian family	Genus	Species
United States and Mexico	Iguanidae	Plasmodium	floridense Thompson and Huff, 1944
			mexicanum Thompson and Huff, 1944
			rhadinurum Thompson and Huff, 1944
			beltrani Pelaez and Perez-Reyes, 1952
			brumpti Pelaez and Perez-Reyes, 1952
			basilisci Pelaez and Perez-Reyes, 1959
Africa	Teiidae	Plasmodium	chirichuae Telford, 1970
	Agamidae	Plasmodium	josephinae Pelaez, 1967
			agamae Wenyon, 1909
			giganteum Theiler, 1930
	Chamaeleontidae	Plasmodium	acuminatum Pringle, 1960
			robinsoni Brygoo, 1962
			fischeri Ball and Pringle, 1965
	Scincidae	Plasmodium	mabuiae Wenyon, 1909
			maculilabre Schwetz, 1932
			pitmani Hoare, 1932
Asia, east	Cordylidae	Plasmodium	zonuriae Pienaar, 1962
Asia, south-east	Lacertidae	Plasmodium	sasai Telford and Ball, 1969
	Agamidae	Plasmodium	"minasense" Laird, 1960
			vastator Laird, 1960
Australia and Oceania	Varanidae	Plasmodium	clelandi Manawadu, 1972
	Agamidae	Plasmodium	giganteum australis Garnham, 1966
	Scincidae	Plasmodium	lacertiliae Thompson and Hart, 1946
			lygosomae lygosomae Laird, 1951

HAEMOPARASITES OF REPTILES 437

Tropical America	Gekkonidae	Plasmodium	lygosomae nucleoversans Garnham, 1966 egerniae Mackerras, 1961 mackerrasae Telford, 1979 aurulentum Telford, 1971 lainsoni Telford, 1978 scorzai Telford, 1978 gonatodi Telford, 1970 beebei Telford, 1978 tropiduri tropiduri Aragao and Neiva, 1909
	Sphaerodactyl-idae	Plasmodium	minasense carinii Leger and Mouzels, 1917 torrealbai Scorza and Dagert, 1957 balli Telford, 1969 utingensis Lainson et al., 1971 achiotense Telford, 1972 uncinatum Telford, 1973 vautieri Pessoa and Biassi, 1973 azurophilum Telford, 1975 multiformis Lainson et al., 1975 uranoscodoni Lainson et al., 1975 vacuolatum Lainson et al., 1975 colombiense Ayala and Spain, 1976 scelopori Telford, 1977
	Iguanidae	Plasmodium	guyannense Telford, 1979 marginatum Telford, 1979 minasense anolisi Telford, 1979 minasense capitoi Telford, 1979 minasense plicae Telford, 1979 tropiduri aquaticum Telford, 1979 tropiduri panamense Telford, 1979 iguanae Telford, 1980

(contd.)

Table 20.11. Plasmodiid Species and Subspecies Described from Lizards, 1909-1980. (Continued)

Geographic distribution	Reptilian family	Genus	Species
	Teiidae	Fallisia	modesta Lainson et al., 1974
			audaciosa Lainson et al., 1975
			simplex Lainson et al., 1975
		Plasmodium	cnemidophori Carini, 1941
			pifanoi Scorza and Dagert, 1956
			telfordi Lainson et al., 1971
			attenuatum Telford, 1973
			minasense diminutivum Telford, 1973
			minasense tegui Telford, 1979
	Scincidae	Fallisia	effusa Lainson et al., 1974
		Saurocytozoon	tubinambi Lainson and Shaw, 1969
		Plasmodium	diploglossi Aragao and Neiva, 1909
			minasense minasense Carini and Rudolph, 1912
			morulum Telford, 1970
			mabuyi Lainson et al., 1974
	Anguidae	Saurocytozoon	
		Plasmodium	diploglossi Aragao and Neiva, 1909

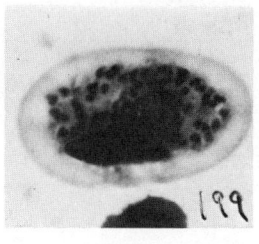
a

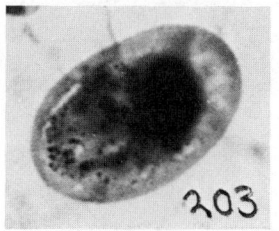
b

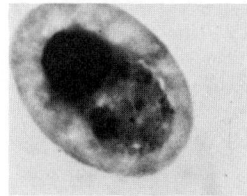
c

Fig. 20.19a,b,c. Plasmodium tomodoni from Tomodon dorsatus, Brazil. X1480
a. schizont
b. macrogametocyte
c. microgametocyte

comparison of published and unpublished survey data (Table 20.12). Plasmodiid infections are relatively most common in continental areas which are tropical or subtropical, humid and forested, showing greater species and host diversity there. Infections also are fairly common in continental areas which are subtropical or temperate, semi-arid to arid grasslands or montane habitats. There are no records from lizards of desert biomes, although malaria may be common in mountains bordered by desert, such as the Chiricahua, Huachuca and Pinaleno mountains of southeastern Arizona (Telford, 1970a). Only three species are known from hosts which must hibernate for at least four months of the year: P. mexicanum in Wyoming (Greiner and Daggett, 1973), P. chiricahuae in Arizona and Texas (Telford, 1970a, 1978b) and P. sasai in Honshu (Telford and Ball, 1969). The presence and abundance of lizard malaria on islands is probably more greatly influenced by phylogenetic relationships of potential hosts and vectors than by climatic and physiographic factors which seem to be important in continental areas. Saurian Plasmodium spp. appear to be more commonly found in hosts with semi-arboreal, cursorial or secretive habits (Table 20.13).

Table 20.12. Geographic Distribution of Saurian Haemo-

Physiographic/climatic characteristics	Area	No. lizar examined
Continental, temperate to subtropical, arid, desert or montane	California, southern Pakistan Russia, southern	922 848 605
Subtotal:		2375
Continental, temperate to subtropical, semi-arid, grasslands or montane	California, central Texas-Arizona Mexico Africa, east Australia, east	1367 240 358 1419 294
Subtotal:		3678
Continental, tropical to subtropical, humid, forest	Florida Middle America Panama Venezuela Africa, west Thailand-Malaysia	1992 572 1905 851 520 384
Subtotal:		6224
Insular, temperate, humid, forest	Japan, Honshu Japan, Ryukyus	1855 166
Insular, subtropical, humid, forest	Caribbean Madagascar	463 1099
Insular, tropical, humid, forest	New Guinea	154
Subtotal:		3737
Total:		16,014

There is some evidence that saurian malaria may be limited in its vertical distribution, perhaps due to altitudinal zonation of its vector (Telford, 1970a). P. chiricahuae (Fig. 20.20) was found to be most common between 1,800 to 2,000 m in the Pinaleno Mountains of Arizona (54%), declining in prevalence between 2,400 to 2,700 m (26%) and still less common from 2,700 to 2,800 m (6%). Comparable host samples from 2,850 and 3,242 m were negative. P. floridense is a common parasite in several Panamanian host species from sea level to 300 m (Telford,

sporidian Parasites from Survey Data given in Table 20.3.

No. haemoparasite infections	% Infections comprised by Plasmodiidae	Haemoproteiidae
119	0.0	0.0
181	0.0	14.9
140	0.0	2.9
440	0.0 $\bar{x}$	8.9 $\bar{x}$
377	60.0	0.0
48	39.6	0.0
74	55.4	0.0
312	47.4	3.2
113	5.2	20.0
924	41.5 $\bar{x}$	11.6 $\bar{x}$
261	81.7	0.0
120	73.3	0.0
759	64.7	0.0
338	36.1	0.0
156	71.8	2.6
164	36.6	0.0
1798	60.7 $\bar{x}$	2.6 $\bar{x}$
280	2.1	0.0
7	85.7	0.0
97	64.9	0.0
300	1.7	0.0
21	0.0	4.8
705	38.6 $\bar{x}$	4.8 $\bar{x}$
3867		

1974a, 1977). Huff and Marchbank (1953) found P. floridense parasitizing 5 to 6% of Sceloporus malachiticus in two localities at the base of El Volcan, Chirique Provence, Panama, but a large series of S. malachiticus taken at 1,650 m along the Rio Chiriqui Viejo on the slopes of El Volcan were negative for it (Telford, unpubl. data). There are no other records of saurian Plasmodium spp. from montane hosts except by Pelaez et al. (1948) who found P. mexicanum in S. torquatus from Chapultepec Park, Mexico City, which lies at an approximate elevation of 2,100 m.

Table 20.13. Distribution of Saurian Plasmodium Species

Geographic area	No. Plasmodium spp. described	cursorial	saxicolous
New World	42	25[a]	4
African	9	17	19
Asian/ Australian	10	30	10
All areas	61	24	7

[a]Percent of total Plasmodium spp. from each geographic area which parasitize hosts utilizing the niche. Hosts which can be classified in several categories are included in all with equal weight.

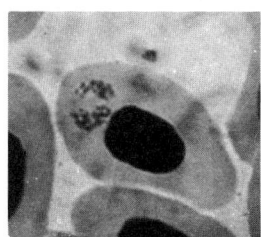

a

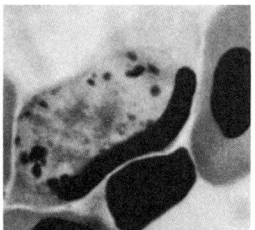

b

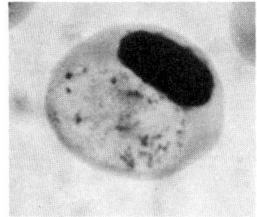

c

Fig. 20.20a,b,c. Plasmodium chiricahuae from Sceloporus jarrovi, Arizona. X1480
a. schizont
b. macrogametocyte
c. microgametocyte

among Host Species of Different Ecological Niches.

secretive	semi-aquatic or arboriparian	semi-arboreal	arbo-secretive	canopy dwelling
10	12	37	5	8
24	0	24	0	17
40	0	5	0	15
17	8	30	3	10

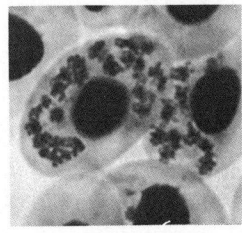

a

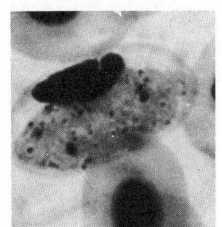

b

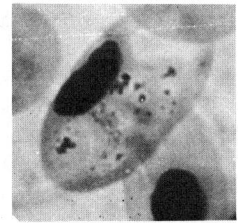

c

Fig. 20.21a,b,c. *Plasmodium mexicanum* from *Sceloporus occidentalis*, California. X1480
a. schizont
b. macrogametocyte
c. microgametocyte

The seasonal prevalence of saurian malaria is known to vary for both temperate and tropical species. Ayala (1970b) found new infections of P. mexicanum (Fig. 20.21) most commonly in spring and early summer, in adult and first year S. occidentalis prior to the appearance of hatchlings. Very few infections were seen in hatchlings in the fall in an area where nearly 60% of adult and yearling lizards were infected. A spring relapse among infected lizards apparently occurs (Ayala, 1970b), evidently in synchrony with emergence of the initial generation of phlebotomine sandflies and the appearance from hibernation of the susceptible lizard hatchlings from the previous fall. Ayala (1973) postulated that most malarial transmission may be accomplished by the first sandfly generation, even though maximum sandfly density occurs in late August with emergence of the third generation. Another temperate species, P. sasai, may follow a similar pattern in Honshu, where the few active infections found were in late April through June among adult and yearling Takydromus tachydromoides (Telford, unpubl. data). Although hatchlings can appear as early as mid-July, most hatch in September and October at a time when only chronic P. sasai infections, comprised primarily of gametocytes, were seen.

P. floridense also shows seasonality in transmission to its temperate host species, S. undulatus (Goodwin, 1951 and Anolis carolinensis (Jordan, 1964). Although infections were found in S. undulatus in all months in Georgia, hatchling lizards did not acquire infections until November, even though hatching occurs from mid-June through September. Acute infections were common during fall and winter, suggesting transmission in late summer and fall. Jordan (1964) found a similar pattern in A. carolinensis in Georgia, with infections predominantly new or acute and progressively increasing from August into November. This also is the period when the greatest variety and abundance of haematophagous arthropods appear in correlation with rainfall maxima. Unfortunately, vector studies by Jordan (1964) and D.G. Young (personal communication) have found oocyst development to occur in both culicine mosquitoes and phlebotomine sandflies respectively, withou production of sporozoites in either. P. floridense is the only species of saurian malaria for which annual fluctuations in prevalence have been demonstrated over a long period of time (Jordan and Friend, 1971).

The most thorough study to date of a tropical saurian malaria, P. colombiense, found transmission to be continuous throughout the year (Ayala and Spain, 1976), with fluctuations in prevalence related more to changes in host population structure than to variation in rainfall. Male A. auratus were more commonly infected (26%) than females (20%) and prevalence increased with host age and size. Most of the parasite population (81%) was found in mature lizards in the "middle age" group, which could result from high mortality among infected juveniles and acquisition of immunity by older lizards. Infections were rare prior to maturation, all four found were acute and two were overwhelming. No difference in parasitemia was found between reproductive and non-reproductive females. Two "epizootics" were observed in which over half the populations studied showed infection, mostly in acute stages. These ran their course in 6 to 8 months, with prevalence and parasitemia decreasing, the latter becoming chronic. After one year prevalence had dropped to 10% in both populations.

In the wet tropical forest of Panama, two subspecies of P. tropiduri (P. t. panamense in the arboreal A. biporcatus and P. t. aquaticum in the semi-aquatic A. lionatus and A. poecilopus) also apparently show continuous transmission. P. floridense in its tropical anole hosts also may be continuous in transmission, but the proportion of active infections appears to decline slightly in the late wet season (September to December). Data suggest, however, that other tropical saurian malaria species show seasonal transmission which is probably correlated with rainfall, influenced possibly by either vertebrate host or vector population dynamics. As described earlier (Telford, 1977), P. balli is apparently transmitted primarily in the late wet season. P. basilisci infection rate increases sharply in the early wet season (May to August) and the proportion of active infections found reaches its maximum in the late wet season, with both the infection rate and proportion of active infections dropping to minimum levels in the dry season (January to April). In the type population in San Blas Territory, eastern Panama, P. gonatodi was found during only the dry and early wet season, with active, acute infections seen in both March and June, but with greatest prevalence evident in March.

In the dry tropical forest of Venezuela, the three Plasmodium spp. parasitizing Ameiva ameiva may be transmitted primarily in the wet season (Telford, 1980). Only chronic infections of P. cnemidophori (Fig. 20.22) were found in the dry season, January to April, but from June to October (wet season), new and acute infections also were observed. P. attenuatum was most common in the dry season, but these infections were all of low parasitemia

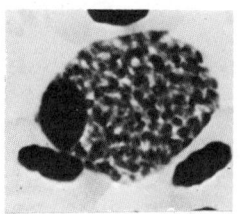
a

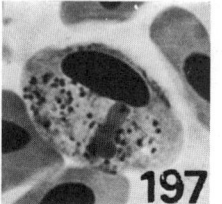
b

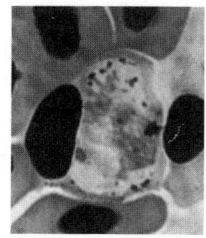
c

Fig. 20.22a,b,c. Plasmodium cnemidophori from Ameiva ameiva, Venezuela. X1480
a. schizont
b. macrogametocyte
c. microgametocyte

and showed asexual stages only, a characteristic of chroni infection by the P. minasense group of species. The heaviest infections, showing gametocytes, were in the wet season when the prevalence reached 10%. Although dry season samples of Tupinambis teguixin could not be obtained, transmission of P. minasense tegui apparently occurred in the late wet season as it was found only then and not during May to August. Saurocytozoon tupinambi was equally common in the early and late wet season with no apparent difference in the parasitemias.

Etiology

The classical approach to classification of the Haemosporidia divides the group into three families, Plasmodiidae, Haemoproteiidae and Leucocytozoidae (Garnham 1966), relying upon the presence or absence of malarial pigment (hemozoin), and an asexual cycle in circulating blood cells, along with the type of blood cell parasitized

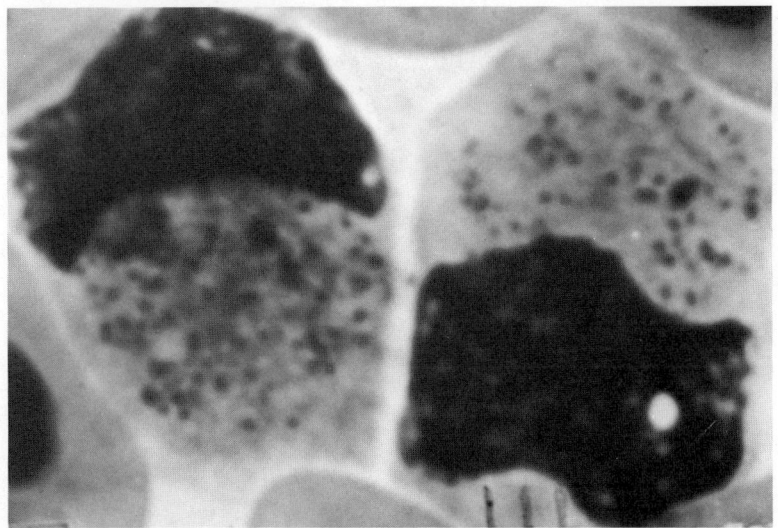

Fig. 20.23. Saurocytozoon tupinambi macrogametocyte (left) and microgametocyte (right). X1480

for definition of the families. Thus, sporozoan parasites of erythrocytes which have asexual cycles within them and show pigment are plasmodiids; erythrocytic parasites with pigment, but lacking the asexual cycle are haemoproteiids; and, parasites found in leucocytes, without pigment and asexual cycle are leucocytozoids. These distinctions hold for haemosporidia of mammals and birds, but with recently intensified studies on reptilian haemosporidia, species were found which did not fit the accepted classification. Two extreme viewpoints, therefore, have emerged in the literature. In strict adherence to the classical approach, an unpigmented parasite of leucocytes which may lack an asexual cycle in circulating blood cells, S. tupinambi (Fig. 20.23), was thought initially to be a leucocytozoid (Lainson and Shaw, 1969a). Later studies, however, showed that in most details its sporogonic pattern is essentially that of a plasmodiid (Landau et al., 1973), and there is some evidence suggesting that Saurocytozoon could have a schizogonic cycle of brief duration and low intensity which is completed before gametocytes appear (Telford, 1978a). Similarly, parasites with typical schizogonic and gametogonic cycles in erythrocytes, but which lacked visible pigment (Figs. 20.24 to 20.26), were placed in a separate family, Garniidae, and genus, Garnia (Lainson et al., 1971). Later, unpigmented parasites with both schizonony and gametogony in thrombocytes and leucocytes were designated Fallisia (Figs. 20.27 and 20.28) and placed in the Garniidae (Lainson et al., 1974a).

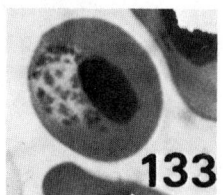 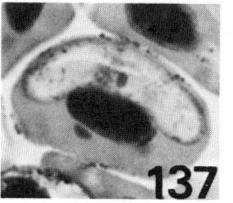

a   b

Fig. 20.24a,b. Plasmodium gonatodi from Gonatodes albogularis fuscus, Panama. X1480
a. schizont
b. macrogametocyte

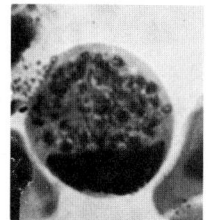 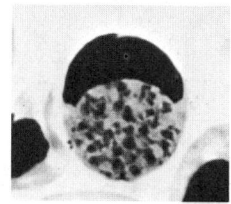

a   b

Fig. 20.25a,b. Plasmodium balli from Anolis lionatus and A. limifrons, Panama. X1480
a. schizont (from A. lionatus)
b. schizont (from A. limifrons)

    As an alternative to creation of new families and genera for parasites which differ only by the absence of pigment, Telford (1973) slightly broadened the definition of Plasmodiidae and Plasmodium, and synonymized Garniidae and Garnia with those taxa. Ayala (1977) went further and synonymized both Saurocytozoon and Fallisia with Plasmodium. This arrangement will probably not be supported as data gained from more sophisticated techniques become available. Accordingly, a classification is presented below which hopefully incorporates the significant concepts of both extremes, and which might serve until considerably more basic data on sporogony, exoerythrocytic schizogony and biochemistry are available.

    Plasmodiidae Mesnil, 1903. Parasites belonging to this family have a sexual phase in dipteran insects and

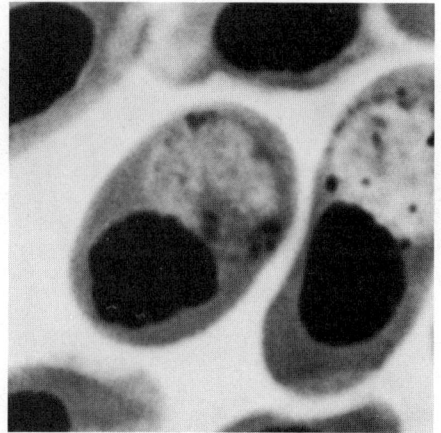

Fig. 20.26. <u>Plasmodium morulum</u> macrogametocyte (left) and microgametocyte (right). X1170

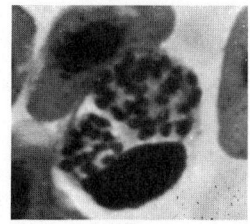

a

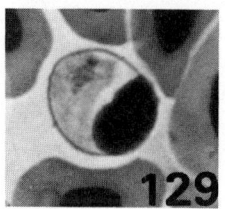

b

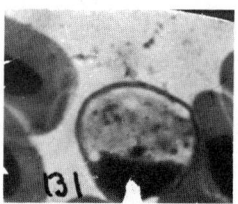

c

Fig. 20.27a,b,c. Fallisia sp. in thrombocytes from <u>Draco maculatus</u>, Thailand. X1480
a. schizont
b. macrogametocyte
c. microgametocyte

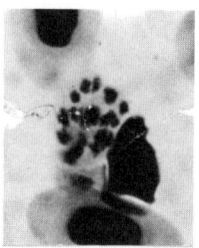
a

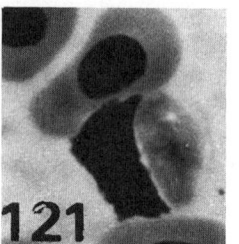
b

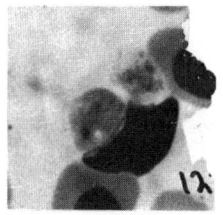
c

Fig. 20.28a,b,c. Fallisia simplex in lymphocytes from
Plica umbra, Guyana. X1480
  a. schizont
  b. macrogametocyte
  c. macrogametocyte (left) and micro-
     gametocyte (right) in double infection

asexual cycles in tissue and blood cells of the vertebrate
host. Gametocytes are produced and may occur in both
immature and mature erythrocytes and in certain white
blood cells. Production of malarial pigment is typical,
but constant only for those species parasitizing endothermic vertebrates. During sporogony, large expanding
oocysts form which produce several hundred sporozoites.

Genus Plasmodium Marchiafava and Celli, 1885. Plasmodiid parasites which have schizogonic and gametocytic
cycles in the erythrocytic series of cells, during which
malarial pigment may form.

Genus Saurocytozoon Lainson and Shaw, 1969. Unpigmented plamodiid parasites which have a gametocytic cycle
predominantly within lymphocytes and monocytes or their
near derivatives. Schizogonic cycle presumptive in circulating cells, transitory and not evident during gametogony.

Genus Fallisia Lainson, Landau and Shaw, 1974.
Unpigmented plasmodiid parasites with schizogonic and
gametocytic cycles within thrombocytes and leucocytes of
circulating blood. Schizogony relatively profuse and
continuing during gametogony.

Transmission

Male and female gametocytes of malarial parasites
are found in circulating blood cells of the vertebrate
host. When an appropriate dipteran vector takes a blood
meal from an infected mammal, bird or reptile, gametocytes
are ingested. Host cells lyse in the vector gut and macrogametocytes (females) round up in preparation for fertilization. After varying lengths of time during which intense
cytogenetic activity takes place, microgametocytes (males)
begin exflagellation which produces up to eight microgametes per mature microgametocyte. Their frenetic
activity results in contact with macrogametes and fertilization of the latter follows successful penetration by a
microgamete. The resulting zygote is termed an ookinete
and is a motile, elongate cell which soon penetrates the
vector gut wall to enter an epithelial cell. Oocyst formation, signifying the onset of sporogony, begins with
nuclear division. As oocysts increase in size, those of
Plasmodium spp. protrude into the vector haemocoele. In
S. tupinambi, as observed in an experimental host C.
pipiens, oocyst development occurs within the gut wall
(Landau, 1973), which appears to be the only significant
difference from sporogony of Plasmodium. P. mexicanum,
the only reptilian Plasmodium for which complete sporogony
has been described (Ayala, 1971), resembles avian and
mammalian species in forming oocysts which protrude into
the haemocoele of Lutzomyia vexatrix occidentalis and L.
stewarti. These phlebotomine sandfly species have an
intimate ecological relationship with S. occidentalis,
the primary vertebrate host of P. mexicanum in California
(Ayala, 1973), and are probably natural vectors. Nuclear
division continues and hundreds of elongate, thin sporozoites are produced as oocysts mature. As in avian and
mammalian species, sporozoites are released from ruptured
oocysts into the haemocoele. Some of these enter salivary
glands while others are found in the foregut (Ayala, 1971).
Transmission of P. mexicanum by bite of infected sandflies
has not been accomplished, but experimental infection of
laboratory-reared hatchling S. occidentalis by inoculation
of sporozoites from sandflies was successful (Ayala, 1971).
The mode of natural infection remains to be demonstrated;
it could occur by either bite or ingestion of the vector.
Although experimental transmission of S. tupinambi has not

been completed, sporozoites similar to those of Plasmodium spp. were produced by oocysts which developed in the gut wall of C. pipiens during a period of 16 days (Landau, 1973). Sporogony of Fallisia spp. has not been described.

No natural vectors have been demonstrated conclusively for reptilian malarial species. Experimental and ecological evidence strongly suggests that phlebotomine sandflies may serve as natural vectors of P. mexicanum in California (Ayala, 1971, 1973), but this does not preclude involvement of other haematophagous arthropods as vectors for some of the diverse species of Plasmodium, Fallisia and Saurocytozoon in their ecologically varied hosts. P. floridense can produce oocysts on the gut wall of Culex spp. (Jordan, 1964) and a sandfly, L. vexatrix orientalis (D.G. Young, personal communication), but the latter, at least, did not develop to maturity and produce sporozoites. Aedes aegypti has reportedly produced occasional oocysts of P. floridense (Jordan, 1964) and P. agamae (Bray, 1959). Attempts by other investigators to obtain sporogony of saurian malarial species have been negative with disappointing uniformity, despite the use of a variety of host-parasite-arthropod combinations. The single successful attempt to obtain infectious sporozoites suggests that specificity may be strict with respect to vector relationships for many species. Studies of sporogony are critical to obtaining a better understanding of reptilian malarias and should be encouraged despite the negative results obtained thus far by most investigators. The determination of geographical, seasonal and habitat concordance between the distribution of saurian malarias, their hosts and haematophagous dipterans with predilection toward reptilian blood can greatly assist the search for natural vectors (Ayala, 1977; Telford, 1974b, 1977).

Pathogenesis

Malaria results from the introduction of infectious sporozoites by the vector into the reptilian host. The prepatent phase is presumed to include primary exoerythrocytic schizogony, as in mammalian and avain malaria, but no proof of this is yet available. Experimentally induced infection by sporozoites has been successful only for P. mexicanum in S. occidentalis (Ayala, 1971); trophozoites were seen in erythrocytes following a prepatent period of 22 days. Infections induced by inoculation of infected blood apparently produce direct infection of erythrocytes; despite many attempts, no investigator has reported finding exoerythrocytic schizonts during the prepatent period of blood-induced infections. As in mammalian and avian

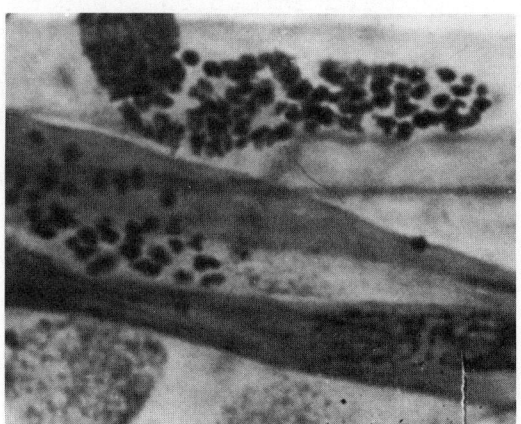

Fig. 20.29. Plasmodium mexicanum schizonts in the cerebral capillaries of Sceloporus undulatus. X760

malarias, trophozoites in blood cells develop into schizonts which undergo 2 to 8 nuclear divisions, depending upon the species, following which cytoplasm surrounding the nuclei divides to form merozoites during segmentation. Host cells then rupture and merozoites enter new host cells for additional schizogonic cycles, or develop into gametocytes. During active infection, and in some species chronic phase as well, secondary exoerythrocytic schizonts may be found in circulating leucocytes, usually lymphocytes or very commonly in thrombocytes. Phanerozoic schizonts of P. mexicanum have been reported from capillary endothelium of organs in several species of natural and experimental hosts (Thompson and Huff, 1944a) and may proliferate extensively in cerebral capillaries (Fig. 20.29) (Ayala, 1970b). This is the only Plasmodium species which is known to have schizogonic cycles in both fixed and circulating cells.

During active phase parasitemia increases more slowly than in mammalian and avian malaria, reaching its maximum level in 30 to 90 days in the several species studied (Goodwin and Stapleton, 1952; Scorza, 1970; Telford, 1972; Thompson and Huff, 1944a,b). If a high level of parasitemia is attained, a crisis stage may develop, with a relatively rapid decrease in parasitemia to very low levels or become apparently negative. Often, however, the drop in parasitemia may be gradual with an almost inperceptible shift into chronic phase and no evidence of crisis seen, especially in infections where no distinct peak of parasitemia occurs. Chronic infection apparently persists for the life of the host, during which parasitemia remains at low levels, with the parasite population often composed largely of gametocytes. Recrudescence may occur (Telford, 1972) during which renewed schizogony can significantly increase the level of parasitemia for brief periods, followed by a return to levels characteristic of chronic infection.

Pathology

The pathology of saurian malaria infections is poorly known. The course of experimental infections has been studied for only five species: P. azurophilum (Telford, 1975), P. floridense (Fig. 20.30) (Goodwin and Stapleton, 1952; Huff and Marchbank, 1953; Jordan, 1975; Thompson, 1944; Thompson and Huff, 1944b; Thompson and Winder, 1947) P. mexicanum (Ayala, 1971; Thompson, 1944; Thompson and Huff, 1944a), P. sasai (Telford, 1972; Telford and Ball, 1969) and, P. tropiduri (Fig. 20.31) (Scorza, 1970, 1971). Effect upon the hosts of P. floridense, however, is not described except for a casual comment by Goodwin and Stapleton (1952) that anemia was produced. Ayala (1977) has suggested that the degree of pathogenicity may be related to parasite size and proclivity to infect immature blood cells. Large species such as P. balli and P. cnemidophori, therefore, are assumed to be more pathogenic than are the small species related to P. minasense (Fig. 20.32) which almost exclusively parasitize mature erythrocytes. The species of medium size would then produce intermediate pathogenicity. There is insufficient information yet on the pathogenicity of saurian malaria to support this suggestion. By analogy to avian and mammalian malarias, however, one might expect host cells parasitized by large parasites to become more rigid than normal, thereby decreasing their ability to pass freely through capillary networks, blocking them and possibly producing emboli. Certainly mechanical effects alone are obvious in the distortion of both the host cell and its nucleus as recorded for many saurian Plasmodium spp. Two species, P. balli (Telford, 1969, 1974a) and an undescribed haemosporidian from geckoes (Telford, 1978c) produce particularly severe disorganization of the host cell nucleus resembling a lytic effect (Fig. 20.33).

For species other than P. mexicanum, pathology appears to be restricted to destruction of erythrocytic host cells which gives rise to varying degrees of anemia. Telford (1972) showed that infection by homologous strains of P. sasai in T. tachydromoides and T. smaragdinus resulted in

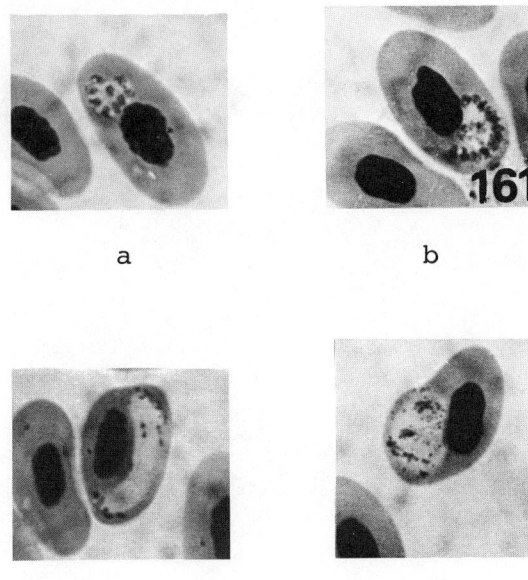

Fig. 20.30a,b,c,d. Plasmodium floridense from Sceloporus undulatus and Anolis carolinensis, Florida. X1480
   a. schizont (from S. undulatus)
   b. schizont (from A. carolinensis)
   c. microgametocyte (from S. undulatus)
   d. microgametocyte (from A. carolinensis)

a moderate erythropoietic response as indicated by increases of 24 to 31% in the proportion of immature erythrocytic cells present, in comparison to uninfected control lizards on the same sampling schedule. Scorza (1971) found that heavy experimental infections of P. tropiduri produced severe anemia in Tropidurus hispidus, characterized by a fall in hematocrit to as low as 12.0%, with hemoglobin values reaching minima of 0.2 to 0.4 g%. Normal values for these parameters in uninfected lizards subjected to similar sampling schedules were 21.0 to 45.9% and 6.9 to 11.3 g%, respectively. A mild, normocytic, normochromic anemia was produced without significant production of erythroblasts. Lizards with chronic natural infections did not differ significantly from the normal values.

In natural infections by P. colombiense in A. auratus, Ayala and Spain (1976) found significant anemia present,

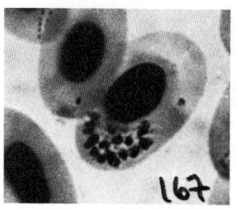
a

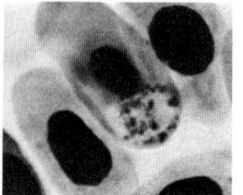
b

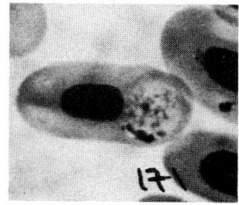
c

Fig. 20.31a,b,c. Plasmodium tropiduri from Tropidurus hispidus, Venezuela. X1480
a. schizont in procrythrocyte
b. macrogametocyte
c. microgametocyte

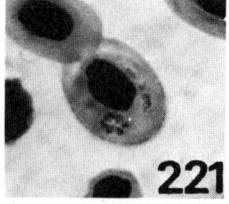
a

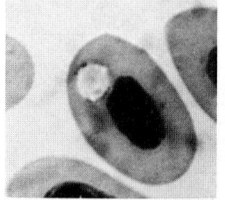
b

Fig. 20.32a,b. Plasmodium minasense anolisi from Anolis limifrons, Panama. X1170
a. schizont
b. microgametocyte

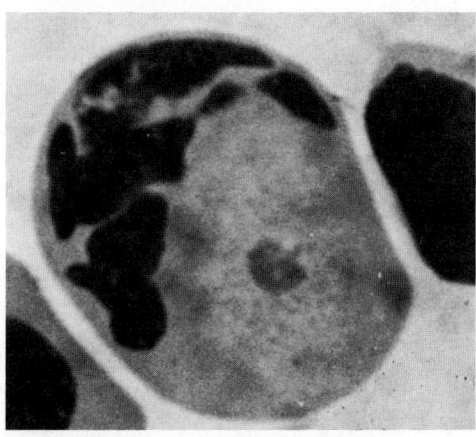

Fig. 20.33. Plasmodium balli microgametocytes from Anolis limifrons, Panama. X1480

with at least a suggestion that nearly complete replacement of the erythrocyte population can occur. Initial severe infections appear to be accomplished by a release of available, nearly mature polychromatophilic proerythrocytes, following which an acute erythropoietic response may occur or not, characterized by release of erythroblasts, mitosis and cell maturation in peripheral blood. In those infections showing a distinct peak of parasitemia, a crisis may occur, following which severe anemia results, accompanied by a deteriorated blood picture in which erythroblasts and early polychromatophilic proerythrocytes predominate. As infections become chronic, the blood picture returns to normal or nearly so. Pienaar (1962) found natural infections of P. zonuriae in Cordylus vittifer to produce hyperplastic compensating erythropoiesis when anemia was severe, with erythrocytes derived from both stem cells and lymphoid origins.

While P. mexicanum can produce severe, debilitating anemia in infected lizards (Ayala, 1970b; Thompson and Huff, 1944a) which probably is often fatal in juveniles (Ayala, 1970b), its most dramatic pathology is seen in the production of large exoerythrocytic schizonts in capillary endothelium of the brain (Ayala, 1970b), evoking similarity to human cerebral malaria as caused by P. falciparum. Thompson and Huff (1944a) described two patterns of exoerythrocytic schizogony for P. mexicanum: proliferation of asexual stages within circulating cells other than the erythrocytic series (elongatum-type) and schizogony within fixed cells of several kinds (gallinaceum-type), notably endothelium of the heart, liver, spleen, lung, meninges, lamina propria of the intestine and subcutaneous tissues. There is no evidence that the latter type of exoerythrocytic schizonts are always produced in infected natural hosts of P. mexicanum, although they have been found in fatal, fulminating infections in juvenile S. occidentalis (Ayala, 1970b). They were seen during infections produced in experimental, non-natural hosts by Thompson and Huff (1944a) and appear to be typical of fatal experimental (blood-induced) infections of S. woodi and S. undulatus from Florida (Telford, unpubl. data). It is possible that these large schizonts are purely pathologic, appearing only in severe infections which overwhelm the host's defense mechanisms and represent a deviation from the normal course of infection. Gallinaceum-type exoerythrocytic schizonts have not been described for other saurian Plasmodium spp., but the elongatum-type of exoerythrocytic schizogony seems characteristic of many

P. sasai infections are typically relatively innocuous to their hosts (Telford, 1972). Pirhemocyton infections, however, appeared to have exacerbated the course of malarial infections which became patent as Pirhemocyton disappeared from blood cells. Hosts died during ascending P. sasai parasitemias (Telford, 1972) possibly because their erythropoietic systems had been weaken by pirhemocytonosis. Neither infection was normally fatal to the host T. tachydromoides. Ayala (1973) has postulated that infections by the rickettsia Eperythrozoon may suppress P. mexicanum in nature.

The same strain of P. floridense has been shown to affect two natural host species differently (Jordan, 1975). Infections in S. undulatus have fewer nuclei in schizonts during the phase of acute rise (10.6) and decline (8.6), but produce higher peaks of parasitemia (up to 11,600/10,000 erythrocytes) and require more time to run their course (150 days) than in A. carolinensis. In A. carolinensis more nuclei are formed in schizonts (13.4 and 10.3, respectively), but peaks are lower (1,600/10,000 erythrocytes or less) and duration of active infection is shorter (71 days). Infection rates in these two hosts show differences which could be correlated with degree of pathogenicity. Jordan and Friend (1971) found infection rates of P. floridense in A. carolinensis to average 35% over a 15 year period, while they were far lower, 5% in S. undulatus during the same interval in Fargo, Georgia.

Diagnosis

The diagnosis of saurian malaria infections is made

by microscopic examination of thin smears from the peripheral or cardiac blood (Figs. 20.34 to 20.36). The simplest technique is to clip a toe and gently squeeze it until a drop of blood forms, touch it to the slide and smear it evenly along the surface with the edge of another slide. Toes on the forefeet usually bleed better than those on the hindfeet, and if care is given to the

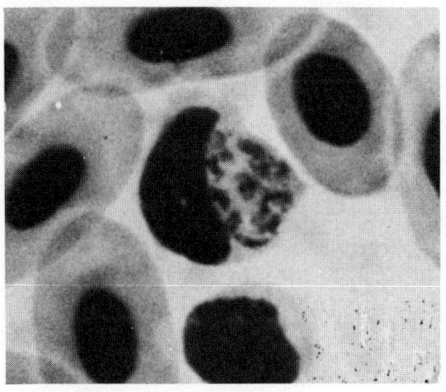

Fig. 20.34. Plasmodium pitmani schizont in a lymphocyte from Mabuya striata, Kenya. X1170

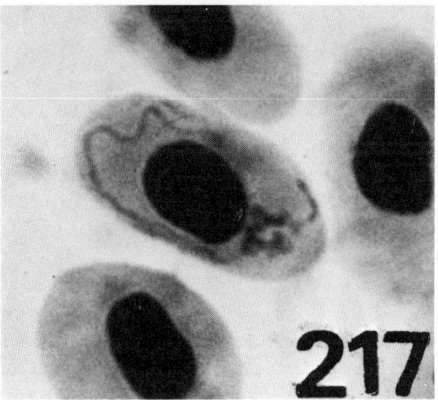

Fig. 20.35. Plasmodium rhadinurum from Iguana iguana, Mexico. X1480

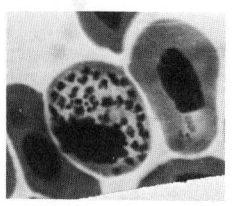
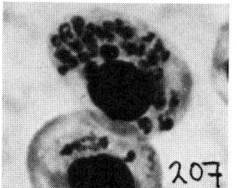

a   b

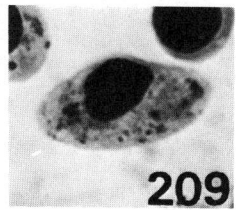

c

Fig. 20.36a,b,c. Plasmodium diploglossi from Mabuya mabouya, Panama. X1480
a. schizont
b. segmenting schizont
c. macrogametocyte

sequence of toe-clipping, a marking system can be utilized to distinguish individual lizards. Slides should be moved gently in the air or under an air jet until dry, then fixed in absolute methanol for 1 to 2 minutes. They are stood on end to dry and then stained, preferably immediately, by the Giemsa technique for 1 to 1.5 hours, with one part Giemsa stain diluted by 10 parts distilled water at a pH of 6.8 to 7.0. The stain should be washed off under running water from the tap and the slide again stood on end to dry. When dry it can be screened at 400 X to locate parasites which are then studied under oil immersion at 1,000 X. Identification should be based upon measured series of 20 to 25 each of mature schizonts and gametocytes, employing the criteria listed by Telford (1974a, 1979a). Slides collected in field surveys should always be accompanied by preserved voucher host specimens to provide positive identification.

Immunity

Only two papers have discussed immunity of saurian hosts to malarial parasites. Thompson (1944) studied the development of acquired immunity by several host species in experimental infections with P. floridense and P. mexicanum. Presence of a humoral response was indicated by morphological changes, degenerative in nature, in parasites during crisis in acute infections, while a cellular response was evident from increased phagocytosis. It was found that acquired immunity against P. floridense did not prevent infection by P. mexicanum. Comparative studies on the course of infection in lizards maintained at 20 C and 30 C found no effect on the development of the immune response, but demonstrated that the rate of progression of the infection increased as ambient temperatures rose (Thompson and Winder, 1947).

There is little experimental evidence which permits evaluation of natural immunity. Although limited success was obtained by Thompson and Huff (1944a,b) in inducing infections by P. mexicanum and P. floridense among several species of iguanid lizards, normal infections as indicated by good production of gametocytes were obtained only in lizards congeneric or conspecific with the natural hosts of both species. Gametocytes of P. mexicanum were produced in two Phrynosoma spp., but only in very low numbers and these hosts were refractory to infection by P. floridense. Infections of P. mexicanum produced in Crotaphytus collaris did not show gametocytes (Thompson and Huff, 1944a), but P. floridense infections in this host apparently did (Thompson, 1944). Repeated attempts to infect hosts of families different from those of the natural host species were unsuccessful for P. mexicanum and P. floridense (Thompson, 1944; Thompson and Huff, 1944a,b) and P. sasai (Telford, 1972). The experimental cross-familial infection of I. iguana and A. carolinensis with a supposed Plasmodium sp. from Lygosoma laterale by Herban (1971) needs confirmation. Despite inoculations of large numbers of parasites from four insular P. floridense strains (Haiti, Jamaica, Puerto Rico and Grand Cayman) into A. carolinensis from north Florida, only low levels of parasitemias by the Haiti strain resulted (Telford, unpubl. data).

Natural cross-familial infections have been reported for five saurian Plasmodium spp. (Table 20.14). The records for P. diploglossi and P. mexicanum appear to represent genuine infections of lizards belonging to different families. The parasites reported as P. tropiduri from Mabuya mabouya in Brazil (Lainson and Shaw, 1969b)

Table 20.14. *Plasmodium* Species Reported to Naturally Infect Lizards of Different Families.

Plasmodium spp.	Type host	Other reported hosts	References
diploglossi Aragao and Neiva, 1909	Diploglossus fasciatus (Anguidae)	Mabuya mabouya (Scincidae)	Ayala, 1978; Lainson and Shaw, 1969b; Telford, 1970b
tropiduri Aragao and Neiva, 1909	Tropidurus torquatus (Iguanidae)	Mabuya mabuya (Scincidae)	Lainson and Shaw, 1979b
aurulentum Telford, 1971	Thecadactylus rapicauda (Gekkonidae)	Anolis limifrons (Iguanidae)	Telford, 1977
mexicanum Thompson and Huff, 1944	Sceloporus ferrariperezi (Iguanidae)	Gerrhonotus multicarinatus (Anguidae)	Ayala, 1970b, 1973
minasense Carini and Rudolph, 1912	Mabuya mabuya (Scincidae)	Gonyocephalus borneensis (Agamidae)	Laird, 1960; Yap et al., 1967

and as P. minasense from Gonyocephalus spp. in Malaysia
(Laird, 1950; Yap et al., 1967) may instead represent
different, morphologically similar species. Asexual
stages only of P. aurulentum were found in A. limifrons
in a Panamanian locality at a time when transmission was
apparently occurring to its normal host, Thecadactylus
rapicaudus (Telford, 1977). Obviously little biological
significance attaches to cross infections which produce
only asexual stages, as with P. aurulentum in A. limifrons.
Adaptation of saurian malaria species to new hosts in
nature would happen occasionally, however, genetic exchange
and recombination occur in the dipteran vector thus
increasing the potential for finding acceptable hosts.

Host specificity between saurian and Plasmodium spp.
may be found to have a strong basis in natural resistance,
as many parasite and host species often coexist at high
prevalence levels in the tropical forest community, suggesting rather less importance for the role of ecological
non-overlap in maintaining host-parasite relationships.
Proper evaluation of natural resistance can be made only
after sporozoite transmission becomes possible in the
laboratory. Circumstantial evidence indicates that host
specificity for most saurian malarias is high, not low
as some investigators have intimated. The checklist of
Ayala (1978), with some unpublished data added, shows
that 61 Plasmodium spp. are known from 73 host genera
($\bar{x}$ 1.2) and 129 species ($\bar{x}$ 2.1). Three iguanid malarias
with multiple hosts have unduly influenced this calculation: P. floridense is known from 21 species, P. mexicanum
from seven and P. balli from eight species. With these
Eurytopic forms excluded, the remaining Plasmodium spp.
parasitize an average of 1.6 host species.

Treatment and control

The only information presented so far on treatment
of saurian malaria is that of Thompson (1946a,b) who
tested quinine against P. mexicanum and P. floridense,
and atabrine against the latter species alone. Quinine
was found to be toxic to lizards in daily doses exceeding
100 mg/kg of body weight. At doses of 75 mg/kg every two
days, quinine suppressed P. floridense infection in A.
carolinensis, with some morphological alterations of the
parasites seen within 48 hours and a discernible effect
against the level of parasitemia after 10 days. Cure
may not have been achieved inasmuch as parasites reappeared
in one lizard after 69 days of being microscopically negative. In P. mexicanum infections of S. undulatus consobrinus, quinine was effective only against parasites within

cells containing hemoglobin. Exoerythrocytic stages in blood and brain were not noticeably affected. This indicates that cure of P. mexicanum could not be achieved with quinine. Atabrine, given in varying doses of 19 to 100 mg/kg, suppressed P. floridense in a similar manner to quinine, with some damage to parasites evident within 24 hours. Both drugs, however, required several weeks to completely suppress the infections.

The severe anemia often produced in saurian malaria infections, which probably has the most serious effect on prognosis, can be treated successfully with administration of iron compounds. Scorza (1971) increased survival of infected lizards two-fold over untreated controls by intramuscular injection of 0.15 ml of an iron-dextran complex which contained 50 mg/ml of iron.

With the exception of P. mexicanum, infections by most saurian Plasmodium spp. seldom lead to death of the natural lizard hosts in captivity, if conditions of housing are satisfactory to meet the lizards' thermal and nutritional requirements under minimum stress. The severity of stress can affect the outcome of infection. The development of acquired immunity by infected lizards otherwise in good condition will normally control infections, maintaining them in a chronic state. A synergistic effect of malaria with concurrent infections by other haemoparasites may reduce survival, but experimental data are lacking. Certainly in tropical areas it is not unusual to find lizards infected simultaneously with three to five different haemoparasites: Plasmodium, haemogregarines, haemococcidia, Trypanosoma and microfilariae (Telford, 1977). Infections with two species of Plasmodium simultaneously are common and triple malarial infections have been seen (Telford, 1977, 1980). Very seldom is it possible to observe any physical or behavioural effect upon the hosts.

Control

Malaria in captive reptiles might possibly be transmitted if an uninfected reptile were to ingest another parasitized by asexual stages of Plasmodium, but such transmission has never been demonstrated. It is unlikely that natural transmission by haematophagous arthropods would occur, but this could be prevented by normal control measures effective against dipteran or acarine pests. There would be no point to applying control measures in the natural environment.

HAEMOPROTEIIDS

The haemosporidian family Haemoproteiidae is represented in turtles, lizards and snakes by 13 described species. Although pigmented and similar to plasmodiids in ultrastructure (Sterling and DeGiusti, 1972), haemoproteiids differ from them by absence of asexual reproduction in circulating blood cells, schizogony being confined to the internal organs. Only gametocytes in various stages of development are found in the blood. Garnham (1966) considered the turtle haemoproteiids to be of ancient origin and the family to be possibly ancestral to the saurian malarias. Details of sporogony and ultrastructure of the sporozoites tend to support this concept (Sterling and DeGiusti, 1974). Except for Haemoproteus metchnikovi in American turtles (DeGiusti et al., 1973), virtually nothing is known of the biology of reptilian haemoproteiids.

Distribution

Turtle haemoproteiids have been reported from the Indian subcontinent, Australia, Africa and North America. None are known from crocodilians. Saurian haemoproteiids are described from southern Asia, Africa, Australia, southern Europe and southern Russia (Andrushko and Markov, 1956; Ball, 1967; Bray, 1959) (Table 20.15). The only saurian haemoproteiid reported from the Western Hemisphere was probably described from a Plasmodium infection comprised of gametocytes only which is commonly seen in chronic malarial infections (Pessoa and Cavalheiro, 1970). Wenyon (1926) placed P. gonzalezi Iturbe and Gonzalez, 1921, in Haemoproteus despite clear mention of erythrocytic schizonts (Telford, 1978d) and this inappropiate allocation was accepted by others (Garnham, 1966). Snake haemoproteiids are known only from Africa. Gorgas Memorial Laboratory (1964) reported a haemoproteiid from snakes but this was probably a plasmodiid. With exception of the North American turtle haemoproteiids, distribution of the reptilian species strongly suggests a Gondwanaland origin for the group.

Saurian haemoproteiids are known with certainty from relatively dry to completely xeric areas in East Africa, Mediterranean Europe, southern Asia and Australia. Some occur in more lush, tropical areas in West Africa and Ceylon, but none appear to be parasites of rain forest lizards. Few data are available which provide epizootiological interpretations. A new, acute infection with H. kopki was found in a hatchling Teratoscincus scincus

Table 20.15. Haemoproteus Species Described from Reptiles, 1901-1980.

Haemoproteus sp.	Recorded host families	Geographic area
TURTLES		
H. metchnikovi Simond, 1901	Trionychidae Chelydridae, Emydidae	India, North America North America
H. testudinis Laveran, 1905	Testudinidae	Africa
H. roumei Bouet, 1909	Testudinidae	Africa
H. chelodina Johnston and Cleland, 1909	Chelydidae	Australia
H. cajali Pittaluga, 1912	Emydidae	Africa
H. balazuci Santos-Diaz, 1950	Testudinidae	Africa
H. caucasica Kraselnikov, 1965	Testudinidae	Southern Russia
SNAKES		
H. mesnili Bouet, 1909	Elapidae	Africa
LIZARDS		
H. simondi Castellani and Willey, 1904	Gekkonidae	Ceylon
H. kopki DeMello, 1916	Gekkonidae	India
H. phyllodactyli Shortt, 1922	Gekkonidae	Iran
H. grahami Shortt, 1922	Agamidae	Iran
H. tarentolae Parrot, 1927	Gekkonidae	Africa
H. catenatus Pessoa and Cavalheiro, 1970	Iguanidae	Brazil

on the Afghan border of Pakistan, concurrently infected by Leishmania in mid-September, while several chronic infections were present in nearby adult T. scincus collected in May (Telford, unpubl. data). No useful data are available for snake haemoproteiids.

Etiology

The classification of haemoproteiids in general is not satisfactory. The family is well-defined by the presence of pigment, absence of schizogony in blood cells and by sporogonic pattern, where known (Garnham, 1966). Without life history data from both vertebrate and vector, it is probably best to consider all reptilian haemoproteiids as Haemoproteus spp. Garnham (1966) proposed the generic name Simondia for turtle haemoproteiids and followed Mackerras (1961) in using Haemocystidium for the saurian species. As pointed out by Shortt (1922), no valid characteristics for generic differentiation of Haemocystidium from Haemoproteus are yet known. Mere presence in saurian or chelonian hosts is a poor basis for generic distinction. DeGiusti (1965, 1970) described megaloschizonts of H. metchnikovi as similar to those of H. columbae from avian hosts and to those of Hepatocystis kochi, the mammalian haemoproteiid. Ultrastructural studies of these exoerythrocytic schizonts (Sterling and DeGiusti, 1972) has confirmed this similarity. To date, the only exoerythrocytic schizonts found in saurian haemoproteiid infections are not similar to megaloschizonts (De Mello, 1934; Shortt, 1962) and if such a distinction is confirmed, this would provide a firm basis for recognizing Haemocystidium Castellani and Willey 1904, as a valid genus.

No generalizations about turtle haemoproteiids are appropriate in view of the fact that no real evidence exists which establishes a cosmopolitan distribution for H. metchnikovi described originally from Chitra indica of India. DeGiusti and Dobrzechowsky (1974) have demonstrated a narrow host specificity for the haemoproteiid they have studied and based on experimental sporozoite-induced infections have suggested that ecological speciation has occured. They justly criticized lumping of all turtle haemoproteiids as a single species, H. metchnikovi, as has been common practice (Garnham, 1966; Wenyon, 1926).

Transmission

A natural vector is known only for H. metchnikovi and no experimental vectors have been found for any reptilian haemoproteiid. DeGiusti et al. (1973) reported transmission of H. metchnikovi by the tabanid fly, Chrysops callidus. Tabanids were seen feeding on basking Chrysemys picta from June to August. Dissection of the flies revealed sporozoite infection rates of 8 to 11% in June, 28 to 38% in July and 45% in August. Salivary glands of the flies were heavily infected with over 1,000 sporozoites each from June to early August, but by mid-August the numbers of sporozoites found in flies diminished greatly, to as few as 1 to 5 per fly. Young oocysts were found beneath the basement membrane of the fly midgut and as they enlarged, bulged outward into the haemocoele from the midgut epithelium (Sterling and DeGiusti, 1974). At maturity oocysts measured about 20 microns and contained 100 to 200 sporozoites. Upon rupture of the oocyst, sporozoites evidently migrate forward and enter the salivary glands of the fly, where they await the next feeding upon a suitable turtle host. The duration of sporogony from ingestion of gametocytes in turtle blood, through fertilization and ookinete formation to infective sporozoites in the salivaries is unknown.

Vector identity is speculative for saurian haemoproteiids, but for H. kopki may prove to be phlebotomine sandflies in view of the fact that the T. scincus population studied had concurrent Leishmania infections and the harsh sand dune habitat on the Afghan border suggests absence of dipterans which require water to be present (Telford, 1979b). Mackerras (1961) fed Culex pipiens fatigans on Heteronota binoei infected with H. simondi with negative results, while Telford (unpubl. data) found nothing in ixodid ticks and geckobiid mites removed from Agama nupta fusca heavily infected by H. grahami. Dobell (1910) also found no developmental stages of H. simondi in geckobiid mites.

Pathogenesis

Only H. metchnikovi (Fig. 20.37) from North American turtles has been studied from sporozoite-induced experimental infections (DeGiusti and Dobrzechowski, 1974; DeGiusti et al., 1973). Following introduction by the vector, sporozoites enter cells in the turtle spleen. Here they develop into megaloschizonts which produce merozoites in 3 to 4 weeks. Cytoplasmic and nuclear divisions with the megaloschizonts produce multinucleate syncytia, the "pseudocytomeres" (Sterling and DeGiusti, 1972). Merozoites produced by budding from "pseudocytomeres" apparently can produce new megaloschizonts in spleen cells which provide for continuing infection of both spleen

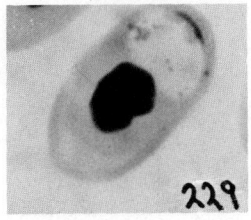 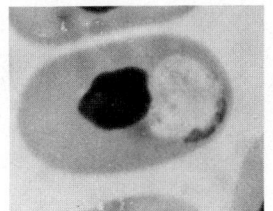

a   b

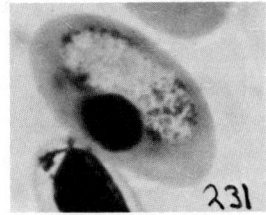

c

Fig. 20.37a,b,c. Haemoproteus metchnikovi from Chrysemys concinna, Florida. X1480
a. macrogametocyte
b. macrogametocyte
c. microgametocyte

cells and erythrocytes, or can enter erythrocytes directly, becoming gametocytic trophozoites and eventually gametocytes. Trophozoites are first visible in erythrocytes in 30 to 32 days (DeGiusti et al., 1973), producing a massive invasion of the erythrocytes which can contain up to 10 parasites each in multiple infections. Gametocytes develop slowly, becoming mature in about three months. Peak parasitemia occurs in 3 to 4 weeks following initial appearance of gametocytic trophozoites. By eight weeks the parasitemia drops to a level which remains relatively constant for up to nine months or longer (DeGiusti and Dobrezechowski, 1974).

Infections of two saurian haemoproteiids, H. grahami (Fig. 20.38) and H. kopki (Fig. 20.39) were studied by Telford (unpubl. data). In an initial natural infection of H. kopki, gametocytic trophozoites appeared in a hatchling T. scincus 23 days following capture, at which time it showed no parasites. As in H. metchnikovi infections, trophozoites appeared suddenly in a massive infection,

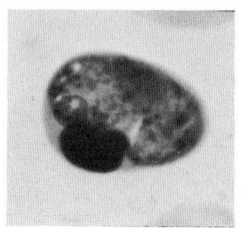
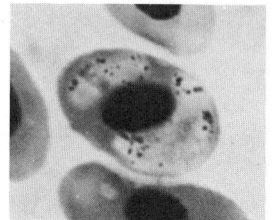

a b

Fig. 20.38a,b. Haemoproteus grahami from Agama nupta, Pakistan. X1480
a. macrogametocyte
b. day 18 of patency in experimentally inoculated lizards

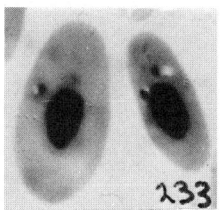
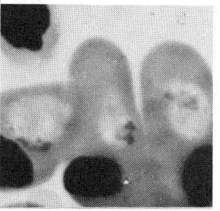

a b

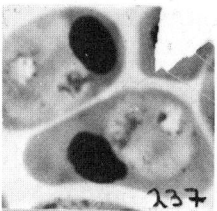
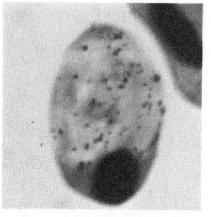

c d

Fig. 20.39a,b,c,d. Haemoproteus kopki from Teratoscincus scincus, Pakistan (initial infection). X1480
a. day 1 of patency: gametocytic trophozoites
b. day 7 of patency: young gametocytes
c. day 13 of patency: microgametocytes
d. day 22 of patency: macrogametocytes

with 34.9% of the erythrocytes parasitized. Peak parasitemia (53.8%) was reached three days later, then the infection declined as gametocytes grew, the first mature forms being seen in 12 days. An adult T. scincus showed a relapse infection 100 days following capture during which period only an occasional mature gametocyte was seen. Trophozoites appeared suddenly, but in a rather low parasitemia of 0.5%. They grew more slowly than in the initial infection, reaching mature size in 31 days, with peak parasitemia of 1.5% reached on day 10. New trophozoites were found only on day 1 of the initial infection, but continued to appear during a 13 day period in the relapse infection. A juvenile A. nupta fusca, negative at capture, was inoculated intraperitoneally with a suspension of spleen, liver and lung tissue from an adult lizard which showed a heavy parasitemia of young H. grahami gametocytes. Trophozoites were observed 14 days after inoculation in a parasitemia of 0.3%. These grew slowly, some reaching maturity in 21 days, with peak parasitemia seen on day 27. Trophozoites were present during a period of 27 days, similar to the relapse infection of H. kopki. Another juvenile lizard inoculated with infected blood from the same adult did not become infected.

Pathology

The few comments on the effect of Haemoproteus on reptilian hosts suggest that pathogenicity is low. DeGiusti and Dobrzechowski (1974) found profound changes to occur in the blood picture during the initial period of rising gametocytemia. During the third week following patency, the numbers of lymphocytes in the peripheral blood gradually dropped. Their numbers then increased sharply as the peripheral gametocyte population rapidly declined. By 8 weeks a stable low level of parasitemia was achieved which remained constant for many months. Riding (1930) commented that Tarentola annularis are apparently little disturbed by H. tarentolae infection despite parasitemias which may exceed 40%. De Mello (1934) described the effect of H. kopki on erythrocytes of Hemi-Dactylus brookii as a "dehemoglobinazation". This has been seen in infections by this species in T. scincus, but not in H. grahami infections in A. nupta fusca (Telford, unpubl. data). No significant parasite-induced anemia was found during infections of either H. kopki or H. grahami and it is unlikely that either parasite is pathogenic to its hosts. The continuing, often extensive destruction of red blood cells seen in saurian malaria infections does not occur in saurian haemoproteiid infections apparently because heavy production of new parasites is limited to an initial period, without successive asexual multiplication in the erythrocytes.

Diagnosis

Diagnosis is made from microscopic examination of stained thin blood films. The presence of pigmented gametocytes only in red blood cells is suggestive of haemoproteiid infection, but it must be remembered that chronic Plasmodium infections can show only gametocytes at very low parasitemias. If repeated examinations over a considerable period of time never indicate schizogonic forms to be present, then the parasite is probably Haemoproteus. This can be tested by experimental inoculation of infected blood into known clean lizards of the same species. A Plasmodium sp. will usually produce a new infection by blood transfer despite the apparent absence of stages other than gametocytes, and schizonts would be readily seen. Nothing should result if Haemoproteus is present (unless a mixed Plasmodium-Haemoproteus infection is at hand), unless merozoites are being released at the time blood samples are taken for inoculation. In a Haemoproteus infection induced in this manner, only gametocytes would appear in erythrocytes. Ball (1967) considered the complete absence of schizogonic stages, plus the resemblance of younger parasites present to gametocytes, as evidence that Haemoproteus was present. In Plasmodium infections schizogony always continues well into the gametogonic phase of active infection.

Immunity

DeGiusti and Dobrzechowsky (1974) found evidence that cell-mediated immunity against H. metchnikovi developed with controlled and stabilized gametocytemia in peripheral blood of C. picta. This was reflected during the third week of mounting gametocytemia following infection, when the lymphocyte population first declined gradually, then rose sharply accompanied by a rapid decrease in gametocytemia. They suggested that the immune mechanisms may destroy most of the early trophozoites, thus delaying the appearance of large populations of mature gametocytes, perhaps in correlation with approaching hibernation by the turtle host. The action of immune mechanisms also may be responsible for the early drop in parasitemia seen in infections of H. kopki and H. grahami (Telford, unpubl. data).

The Haemoproteus which infects C. picta is apparently highly host specific, as only C. scripta elegans could be

experimentally infected by sporozoites, and it produced
light peripheral blood parasitemias, in contrast to heavy
infections in the natural host. Neither Trionyx spinifer
nor Chelydra serpentina could be infected despite the fact
that both serve as haemoproteiid hosts elsewhere (DeGiusti,
1965; Wang and Hopkins, 1965). Although H. simondi was
reported from four genera and species of Australian geckos
by Mackerras (1961), she admitted that more than one
species might be present, but they agreed more closely
with H. simondi than with other described forms. Too few
detailed descriptions of reptilian Haemoproteus spp. have
been made to properly evaluate host specificity among those
known at present.

Treatment and control

There are no data available on treatment. Antimalarials might prove effective, but considerable experi-
mentation with dosages would be required. Prognosis should
be favorable as infected hosts seem competent to keep
gametocytemias low following the initial acute phase.

Separation of captive reptiles from possible invertebrate vectors is the most practical control measure. There
seems no justification for control in the wild.

PARASITES OF DUBIOUS NATURE

Parasites of dubious nature include those parasites
or inclusions described in reptilian blood cells for
which insufficient precise data are known to permit their
classification. Some are certainly protozoa, e.g., Dactylosoma, while others are of viral origin, e.g., Pirhemocyton. Frank (1974) suggested it is possible that artifacts of fixation or staining have been mistaken for parasitic organisms. Some of this group were reviewed by
Wenyon (1926), but unfortunately little more is known
about their exact nature now, and since then new "genera"
And "species" have been described. Only a description
and notes on pathogenicity, distribution and epizootiology,
where known, is given below. Generic designations in most
cases are those employed by the original authors. Johnston
(1975) has provided a host distribution list for several
of the infectious agents.

Dactylosoma Labbe, 1894

This genus is presently considered to be a piro-
plasmid; no substantial evidence supports this position,

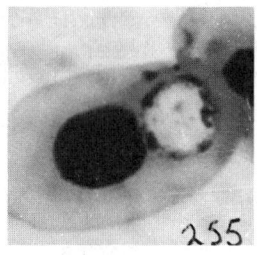
a

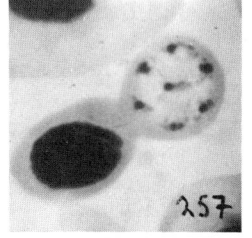
b

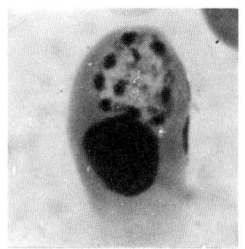
c

Fig. 20.40a,b,c. Dactylosoma sp. from Rana rugosa, Japan. X1480

but until the life cycle is known there seems to be no better classification available. Dactylosoma ranarum Kruse, 1890, was described from erythrocytes of European anurans (Fig. 20.40). Dactylosomids have since been reported from frogs and fish of North America (Fantham et al., 1942), Brazil (Pessoa and Cunha Neto, 1967), Japan (Miyata, 1976), Taiwan (Manwell, 1964), Indo-China (Mathis and Leger, 1911), West Africa (Dutton et al., 1907) and other areas (Wenyon, 1926). There are two records of Dactylosoma from reptiles. Awerinzew (1914) described Lankesterella amania from Chamaeleo fischeri, collected probably from northeastern Tanganyika (Pringle, 1960) rather than from "West Africa" as stated by Wenyon (1926). Wenyon placed L. amania in Dactylosoma, but others consider it to be a species incertae sedis (Brygoo, 1963c; Hoare, 1930). Kraselnikov (1965) described D. sauriae from Lacerta strigata, but his illustrations are not convincing; the parasite more closely resembles the genus Cytamoeba.

Dactylosoma undergoes schizogony in erythrocytes producing segmenters which bear a remarkable resemblance to those of Plasmodium spp. However, Dactylosoma is thought to be unpigmented, although Manwell (1964) described cytoplasmic granules which resembled pigment even under polarized light, presumably the diagnostic test for hemozoin. Elongate uninucleate parasites have been interpreted as gametocytes (Manwell, 1964; Wenyon, 1926); verification is still lacking. Species described from fish may represent a different genus (Jakowska and Nigrelli, 1956). Although leeches have been suggested as possible vectors, as has the the fish louse, Argulus (Manwell, 1964; Wenyon, 1926), it is more likely that a dipteran vector transmits anuran Dactylosoma, inasmuch as tadpoles and young frogs appear to be free of infection (Miyata, 1976). An ultrastructural and biochemical comparison of Dactylosoma with the unpigmented saurian plasmodiids might be worthwhile. No data suggest that Dactylosoma is pathogenic to its hosts.

Nuttallia Franca, 1910

This genus of babesiid piroplasms was reported from reptiles by Carpano (1939), who described Nuttallia guglielmi from the tortoise, Testudo campanulata. It is characterized as a small oval or pear-shaped organism which divides twice, producing four nuclei which are often arranged as a cross. Each nucleus is accompanied by a minute amount of cytoplasm and may be pyriform in shape; there are no rod-shaped forms present. Species of Nuttallia have been reported from various mammals, including horses, viverrids, rodents and bats, and appear to be transmitted by ticks (Wenyon, 1926). Although the type infection was described from a dead tortoise in the Cairo Zoological Garden, there was no evidence of pathogenicity. There have been no additional reports of the species.

Tunetella Brumpt and Lavier, 1935

Tunetella emydis from Mauremys leprosa was described by Brumpt and Lavier (1935) as being distinguished from Aegyptianella on the basis of much larger size and less intensely staining divisional stages. Large round or oval forms showed some evidence of binary fission, resembling babesiids. Some large forms showed prominent cytoplasmic projections which resembled pseudopods. Other minute bodies appeared, arranged in a "pseudo-schizogonic" pattern, suggesting that perhaps they had budded-off one of the larger forms. Carpano (1939) felt the resemblance of T. emydis to Aegyptianella was sufficient to include it in that genus. Carini (1937) described a similar parasite from Chelonia mydas as a second species, T. cheloniae. There have been no further reports of these organisms and their status remains unclear.

Aegyptianella carpani was described from Naja nigricollis by Battelli (1947). His figures show round to oval large stages with 1 to 4 chromatin dots which apparently give rise eventually to smaller, uninucleate, pyriform parasites that practically fill the cytoplasm of the erythrocyte. Another possibly related organism was reported from Testudo graeca by Peirce and Castleman (1974) who happily refrained from naming it. It resembled Nuttallia guglielimi more than other named forms, but did not produce the cruciform arrangement of chromatin characteristic of Nuttallia. If these odd parasites reported from reptiles are related to Aegyptianella, then perhaps they should be treated taxonomically as rickettsia-like organisms (Bird and Garnham, 1967) rather than as piroplasms.

Sauroplasma DuToit, 1937

These parasites are small, generally less than two microns in diameter and may appear as anaplasmoid bodies consisting of a granule of chromatin. They usually are associated with a vacuole or are ring-shaped. Both chromatin and cytoplasm are clearly differentiated when well stained with Giemsa. They apparently reproduce by both binary fission and budding (DuToit, 1937; Pienaar, 1962). Described originally from South American cordylid lizards, Sauroplasma also has been reported from Madagascan gekkonids (Uilenberg and Blanc, 1966), gerrhosaurids and chameleontids (Brygoo, 1963c). Frank (1974) examined the material described by Uilenberg and Blanc and considered their Sauroplasma to represent intraerythrocytic artifacts. Sauroplasma as described by DuToit (1937) and Pienaar (1962) resembles closely a parasite of Japanese lacertids (Telford, unpubl. data), and definitely appears to be an organism (Fig. 20.41). Ultra-structural studies are essential for elucidating the nature of this organism. Pienaar (1962) described a parasite of Naja nigricollis as a separate genus, Serpentoplasma, apparently because it was found in an ophidian host. Serpentoplasma is very similar to organisms seen in erythrocytes of a Mexican Trimorphodon biscutatus (Telford, unpubl. data) (Fig. 20.42); both should be regarded probably as Sauroplasma spp. They do not appear to be pathogenic (Pienaar, 1962). During a three year study, Sauroplasma infections in Japanese Takydromus tachydromoides appeared only from March to June (Table 20.16) and occurred almost entirely in first-year lizards (Telford, unpubl. data).

Table 20.16. Monthly Prevalence during Three Years (1965-1967) of Three Infective Agents in Correlation with Tick Infestation in a Population of Takydromus tachydromoides.

Infective agent	Prevalence (%)							
	March	April	May	June	July	August	September	October
Sauroplasma	2.5	1.2	4.6	0.7	0.0	0.0	0.0	0.0
Cytamoeba	3.4	6.8	2.8	7.1	14.0	9.1	3.6	5.2
Pirhemocyton	0.9	1.9	2.8	2.1	11.6	16.9	4.2	1.5
Ixodes nipponensis								
infestation rate	18.6	33.8	47.2	30.7	45.3	50.7	27.4	32.4
specific index[a]	1.3	1.6	2.2	2.1	5.2	3.1	2.3	3.1
No. lizards examined	118	162	176	140	86	77	165	136

[a]Mean number ticks per infested lizard.

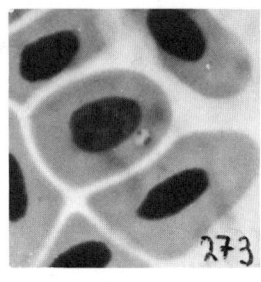 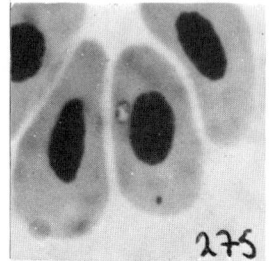

a b

Fig. 20.41a,b. Sauroplasma sp. from Takydromus tachydromoides, Japan. X1480

Sauromella Pienaar, 1962

A heavy infection of erythrocytes in the gecko, Pachydactylus capensis, was described under the name Sauromella haemolysus (Pienaar, 1962). The parasites were minute, basophilic, spherical or rod-like bodies which were seen singly or in groups in dehemoglobinized areas of the erythrocyte cytoplasm. They were frequently associated with vacuoles or albuminoid "bodies of a Piro-Hemocyton type"; multiplication appeared to be binary or multiple fission. Pienaar considered Sauromella to be of "acutely pathologic nature" due to dehemoglobinization of the red blood cells and their disorganization (nuclear pycnosis, karyoclasis and cytoplasmic disruption) which produced severe anemia and hyperactive erythropoiesis.

Bertariella Carini, 1930

This genus was proposed by Carini (1930) for parasites seen in erythrocytes of the anuran, Leptodactylus pentadactylus, which appeared to be related to Anaplasma, Aegyptianella, Grahamella, Bartonella and Eperythrozoon, all now thought to be rickettsial organisms. These were round or oval bodies of variable size, 1 to 2 microns, which stained blue with Giemsa; the small peripheral ring which defined the vacuole was sometimes absent. In better stained Geimsa preparations, it was possible to see an intensely staining granule. De Mello and Correa de Meyrelles (1937) found erythrocytic organisms in Calotes versicolor which resembled Carini's parasite and designated them Bertariella calotis. The saurian parasite appeared in variable form, from anaplasmoid to a small roundish body bounded by a distinctly staining membrane. A central granule (occasionally located peripherally) was surrounded

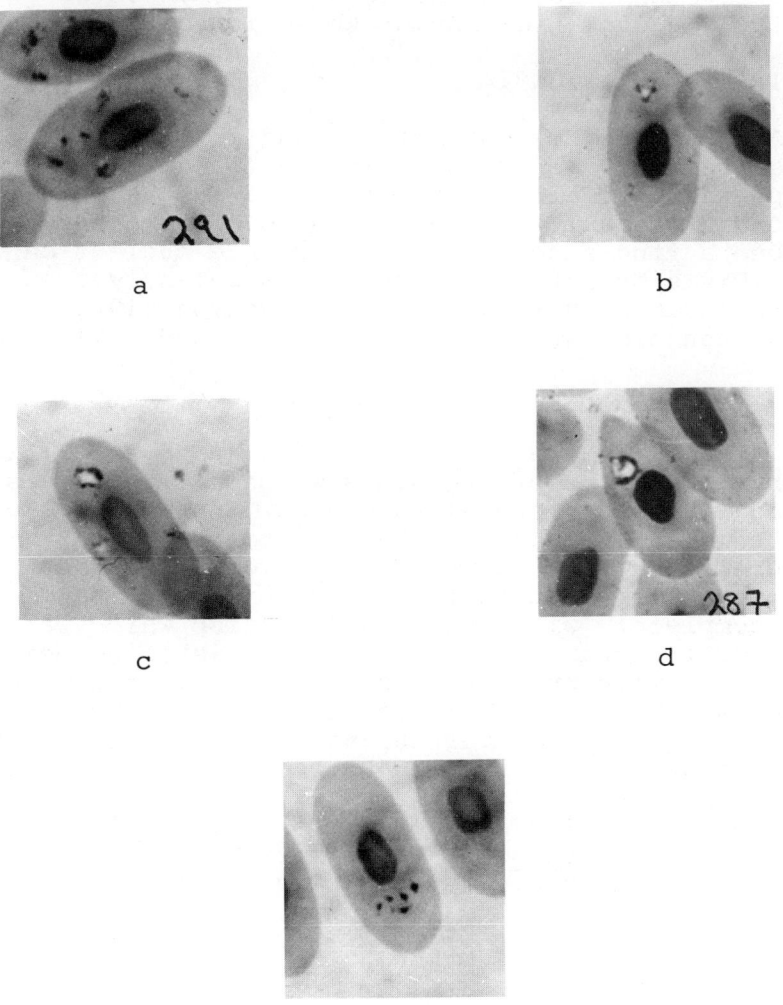

Fig. 20.42a,b,c,d,e.   Serpentoplasma? sp. from Trimorphodon biscutatus, Mexico.   X1480

usually by a colorless space, but this "protoplasm" sometimes stained blue or grayish blue. Correa de Meyrelles (1938) described B. carinii from the turtles, Lissemys punctata granosa, C. mydas and Caretta caretta. De Mello and Correa de Meyrelles (1937) had previously compared B. calotis with Grahamella talassochelys described by Cerruti (1931) from C. caretta and found the parasites very similar, but concluded that Grahamella was not an appropriate generic designation. No evidence of pathogenicity was shown for any of these infections.

Cingula Awerinzew, 1914

An erythrocytic infection found in Boodon lineatus by Awerinzew (1914) was described as Cingula boodontis. It appeared initially as a clear area in the cell which surrounded a small granule. A vacuole then formed which produced a ring-shaped structure with a nucleus on one side. Division into two organisms apparently occurred. Nothing further is known, although Wenyon (1926) reported having seen similar objects in snake blood cells.

Cytamoeba Labbe, 1894

Cytamoeba bacterifera (Figs. 20.43 to 20.45) is probably a complex of organisms which have been described from anurans and urodeles throughout the world. Fortunately, its investigators have been content to report it as C. bacterifera without naming additional species, although often remarking that their particular organisms did not agree completely with the type infection which was described from European frogs. There is no agreement upon its nature, with opinions ranging from piroplasm to virus, but perhaps Wenyon (1926) was close to the truth in providing gentle support for the view that the intraerythrocytic "parasites" are formed by the host cell in response to bacterial infection. The most recent opinion of De Sousa and Freire (1975), based upon cytochemical studies, suggested that Cytamoeba ia "an intracytoplasmic clump of modified organisms ... related with the bacteria, such as ... the Chlamydiae and Rickettsiae."

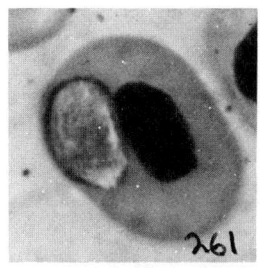

a

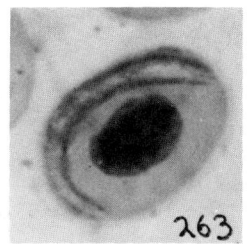

b

Fig. 20.43a,b. Cytamoeba sp. from Atelopus varius, Panama
X1480

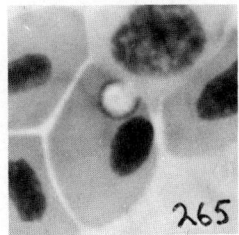
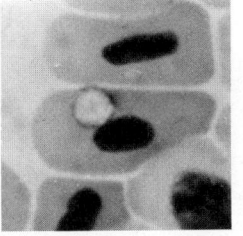

a   b

Fig. 20.44a,b. *Cytamoeba* sp. from *Takydromus tachydromoides*, Japan. X1480

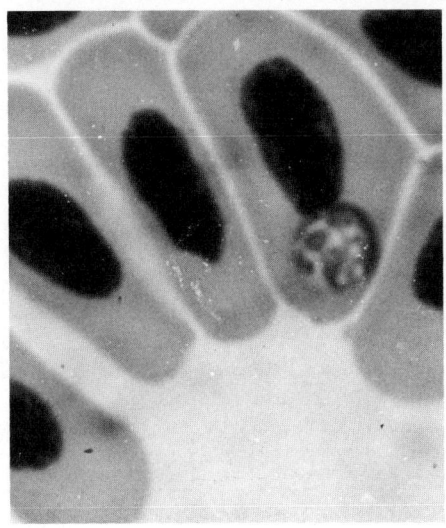

Fig. 20.45. *Cytamoeba* sp. from *Eumeces inexpectatus*, Florida. X1480

Cytamoeba appears as rounded to irregularly shaped structures 1 to 8 microns in diameter, which stain blue to reddish purple with Giemsa. No nucleus can be discerned, although dark granules are sometimes seen within the stained area. There may be a more deeply stained periphery, and sometimes a clear central area is present which lacks the definition of a vacuole. Rod-shaped bodies have been described within the organism, but are not present in all infections. Lehman (1961) has described reproduction as occurring by a constriction which produced, most commonly, two equal daughter cells.

Cytamoeba has not previously been reported from reptiles, although there would seem to be a strong probability that some of the odd organisms described under various names might be related. However, organisms which correspond to the various descriptions of Cytamoeba were common intraerythrocytic parasites in a population of the Japanese lacertid, T. tachydromoides, studied by Telford (unpubl. data). Their prevalence, overall, exceeded that of four other haemoparasites: Plasmodium, Schellackia, Sauroplasma and Pirhemocyton. Apparently, identical forms were common in the population of Rana japonica which was closely associated with the lizards. There can be little doubt that this was the source of infection, inasmuch as T. tachydromoides from other populations where aquatic anurans were absent were free from infection. Overall infection rates for three successive years varied annually: 1965-1.9%, 1966-6.7% and 1967-7.4%. The three year sample showed that upon emergence from hibernation in March, the infection rate was 3.4%, rising fairly evenly to a maximum 14.0% in July then declining to 5.2% by October as hatchling lizards entered the population (Table 20.16). First year lizards showed no infections before entering hibernation (September-October), 0.7% in the months following emergence (March-April), 2.5% in May-June and 6.5% by July-August. Older lizards, by contrast, showed no great differences before and after hibernation, 7.8% in September-October and 10.5% in March-April. The level of infection was 9.0% in May-June, but rose to a maximum of 21.8% in July-August. Although there was a correlation with the specific index of the only ectoparasite associated with the lizard population, Ixodes nipponensis (Table 20.16) was not found on the aquatic anurans present, which suggests that Cytamoemba is not tick-transmitted and the correlation was spurious. A dipteran vector, direct transmission by contact with infected animals or contaminated water or vegetation can be ruled out on the basis of available evidence. A similar organism has been seen in erythrocytes of the skink, Eumeces inexpectatus, in Florida (Telford, unpubl. data).

Pirhemocyton Chatton and Blanc, 1914

This group of organisms was first recognized by Chatton and Blanc (1914) in their description of Pirhemocyton tarentolae from the gecko, Tarentola mauritanica (Figs. 20.46 to 20.48). The parasite appeared initially as a red-staining dot about one micron in diameter within the host cell cytoplasm. As infection progressed, the size increased to 3 to 4 microns, with the shape usually circular and the central portion unstained, within which

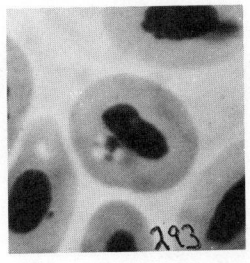 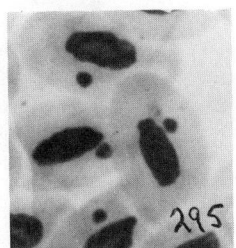

a   b

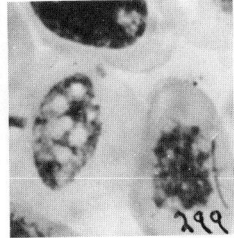

c

Fig. 20.46a,b,c. Pirhemocyton sp. from Takydromus tachydromoides, Japan. X1480

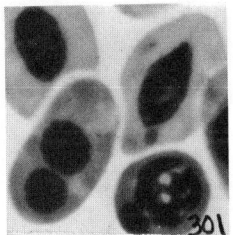 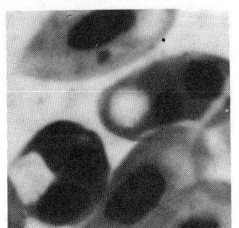

a   b

Fig. 20.47a,b. Pirhemocyton sp. from Calotes versicolor, Burma. X1480

a chromatin dot could be discerned. A globular albuminoid body was associated with the parasite, located elsewhere within the host cell. A second species, P. lacertae, was recognized by Brumpt and Lavier (1935) from Lacerta viridis, which corresponded closely to P. tarentolae except that the albuminoid bodies were not seen in the host cells.

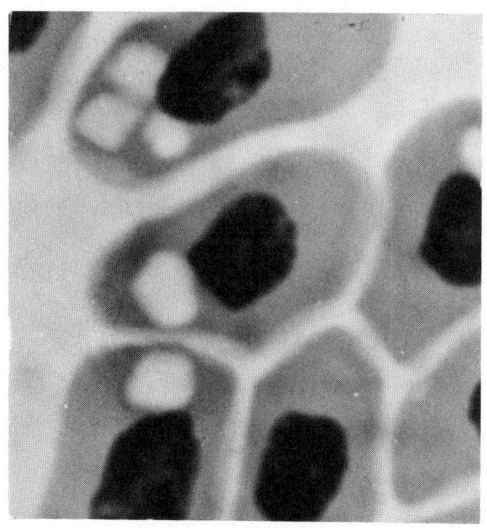

Fig. 20.48. Pirhemocyton sp. from Iguana iguana, Venezuela. X1480

Other "species" described since include P. zonuriae (Pienaar, 1962), P. granosa (Garnham, 1950), P. eremiasi (Blanc and Ascionc, 1958), P. chamaeleonis (Rousselot, 1953) and P. iguanae (Arcay de Peraza and de la Roca, 1971), all from lizards. Rousselot (1953) also had designated infections in six other saurian species by another six Pirhemocyton specific names. Mackerras (1961) reported a Pirhemocyton infection in a carpet python, Morelia spilotes variegata, while Pessoa and Pimenta de Campos (1966) described P. brazili from Brazilian snakes. The only record from turtles appears to be that of P. chelonarum by Acholonu (1974).

The taxonomic position of Pirhemocyton was unclear for many years; it was generally placed with the piroplasms. Blanc and Ascione (1958) suggested a possible viral nature of Pirhemocyton and this was confirmed by the ultrastructural study of Stehbens and Johnston (1966). They concluded that the visible "parasite" seen in erythrocytes represented the "assembly pool" of an icosohedral virus of DNA type, similar to Sericesthis iridescent virus and Tipula iridescent virus. Arcay de Peraza and de la Roca (1971) emphasized cytochemical studies of P. iguanae, which showed both RNA and DNA, as well as respiratory activity, to be present. They reverted to considering Pirhemocyton as similar to piroplasms, rather than accepting the ultrastructural evidence indicating a viral nature.

Some types of Pirhemocyton infection are evidently pathogenic to reptilian hosts. A severe anemia characterized by anisocytosis and poikilocytosis, gross cellular distortion and cytolysis were described by Pienaar (1962), Wood (1935) and Arcay de Peraza and de la Roca (1971). Nuclei of infected cells degenerated with marked pycnosis and karyorrhexis. Although he produced no mortality figures, Pienaar (1962) thought that heavy infections in cordylid lizards must be fatal because of the effects on haemopoiesis and production of severe anemia. Brygoo (1963), however, observed that although captive chamaeleons might die from pirhemocytonosis, it probably was not often fatal in nature. Pirhemocyton infections in T. tachydromoides appeared to be well tolerated by captive lizards, with spontaneous recovery observed in all cases after 1 to 3 months duration of infection (Telford, unpubl. data). Concurrent infection by Pirhemocyton and Plasmodium sasai, however, seemed to exacerbate the course of the malarial infection, causing very high parasitemias which terminated fatally, an otherwise unlikely conclusion to infection by P. sasai (Telford, 1972).

Pirhemocytonosis in snakes appears to be uncommon in comparison to lizards. De Sousa et al. (1973) examined 683 Brazilian snakes and found only 2.4% infected by either Pirhemocyton or Toddia. Only one infection seemed to be clearly due to Pirhemocyton, with many similarities noted between the two similar parasites. Pienaar (1962) found a 10% infection rate among 20 Cordylus vittifer, while Brygoo (1963) reported infection rates of 14, 1.9 and 1.8% among 250 Chamaeleo lateralis, 104 C. oustaleti and 57 C. pardalis, respectively. Mackerras (1961) found 26% of 70 Phyllurus platurus infected; 7.3% of 179 Agama agama examined by Baker (personal communication) were positive; and, a series of 22 T. sexlineatus from Thailand showed 82% infected with pirhemocytonosis (Telford, unpubl. data). In Japan, the Pirhemocyton infection rate varied from 1.5 to 22.6% in 1,885 T. tachydromoides from various localities in the Tokyo area (Telford, unpubl. data). The annual incidence in one population during three consecutive years was similar, 2.2 to 6.1%. Infection was acquired by hatchlings prior to hibernation, reaching 0.5 to 0.7% from emergence in March until July. The July-August infection rate in first year lizards increased dramatically to 15.1%. Older lizards showed a pattern of increasing infection from March-April (2.2%) through May-June (5.7%), with a sharp increase in July-August (14.6%) followed by a drop prior to hibernation in September-October (5.4%). Monthly population infection rates for the three year period are shown in Table 20.16, along with the infestation rate of

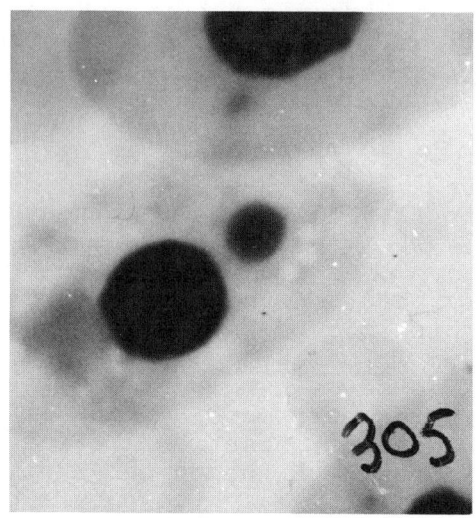

Fig. 20.49. Toddia sp. from Nerodia rhombifera, Mexico. X1480

Ixodes nipponensis and its specific index (mean number of ticks/infested lizard). Correlation appears to lie with the specific index rather than the infestation rate and suggests that pirhemocytonosis might be tick-transmitted to T. tachydromoides (Telford, unpubl. data).

Toddia Franca, 1911

This group of infectious agents was recognized by Franca (1911) for red-staining intraerythrocytic bodies found in anurans (Fig. 20.49). Associated with these bodies were crystalline rods. They have been seen in frogs from equatorial Africa and southeast Asia (Wenyon, 1926), the Ryukyu Islands (Miyata and Miyagi, 1977), Venezuela (Scorza and Dagert, 1956) and Brazil (Pereira et al., 1973). Marquardt and Yaeger (1967) described Toddia from Agkistrodon piscivorus in Louisiana and Pessoa (1967) reported it from the colubrid, Tomodon dorsatus, in Brazil. Arcay de Peraza et al. (1971) extended the host range of Toddia to lizards. Both Arcay de Peraza and de la Roca (1971) and De Sousa et al. (1973) have studied the affinity of Toddia to Pirhemocyton cytochemically. The latter group in particular feel there is little reason for generic distinction. Marquardt and Yaeger (1967) concluded that Toddia and Pirhemocyton were closely related and probably viruses of the DNA type. It is appropriate, therefore, to cease treating both of these infectious agents as genera and species under binomial zoological nomenclature.

Toddia infections are easily distinguished microscopically from Pirhemocyton by the crystalline nature of the cytoplasmic inclusions that accompany the red-staining bodies within the erythrocyte. The inclusions in Toddia infection may be rod-like, rectangular, square or hexagonal. Inclusions are not always seen in Pirhemocyton infection, but when present are opaque and non-crystalline in appearance, usually round but reported as rectangular in Iguana iguana (Arcay de Peraza and de la Roca, 1971). Effects on host cells do not differ significantly from those described above for Pirhemocyton. Virtually nothing is known on the epizootiological aspects of Toddia infection, but it appears to be much less common in reptiles than is Pirhemocyton infection. Marquardt and Yaeger (1967) found 2.4% of 163 A. piscivorus infected and De Sousa et al. (1973) found the same rate among 683 Brazilian snakes, some infections of which may have been Pirhemocyton.

FILARIASIS

Among the Reptilia, filariid nematodes are predominantly parasites of snakes and lizards. Fifteen genera and 50 species are known, one each from turtles and crocodilians, nine species of three genera from snakes and 39 species representing 14 genera from lizards (Table 20.17). Three species may be pathogenic to natural and accidental hosts, but others appear to be innocuous. Natural vectors remain unproven, but several species of four genera can develop to infective stages in mosquitoes

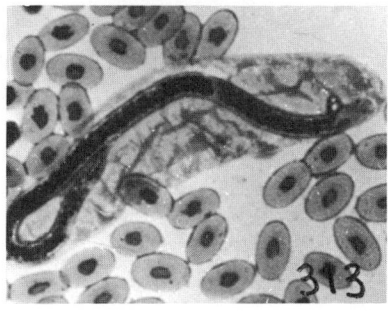

Fig. 20.50. Macdonaldius oschei from Boa constrictor. X250

Table 20.17. Filarial Species Described from Reptiles.

Geographic distribution	Reptilian family	Filarial species
North America	Emydidae	Cardianema cistudinis Leidy, 1856
	Boidae	Macdonaldius oschei Chabaud and Frank, 1961
		M. colimensis Telford, 1965
	Colubridae	M. oschei Chabaud and Frank, 1961
		M. seetae Khanna, 1933
		M. colimensis Telford, 1965
	Viperidae	M. oschei Chabaud and Frank, 1961
	Helodermatidae	M. andersoni Chabaud and Frank, 1961
		Splendidofilaria corophila Hannum, 1943
	Iguanidae	M. grassii Caballero, 1954
		Piratuba prolifica Pelaez and Perez-Pelaez, 1958
South America	Alligatoridae	P. lanceolata Pelaez and Perez-Pelaez, 1958
	Boidae	Oswaldofilaria bacillaris Molin, 1958
	Viperidae	Hastospiculum oncocercum Chitwood, 1932
	Colubridae	H. oncocercum Chitwood, 1932
		M. carinii Vaz and Pereira, 1935
		H. digiticaudatum Teixeira and Freitas, 1955
	Iguanidae	O. brevicaudata Rodhain and Vuylsteke, 1937
	Teiidae	O. petersi Bain and Sulahian, 1975
		O. belemensis Bain and Sulahian, 1975
	Scincidae	O. spinosa Bain and Sulahian, 1975
	Unidentified lizard	P. digiticaudata Lent and Freitas, 1941
Australia	Agamidae	O. chlamydosauri Breinl, 1913
		M. innisfailensis Mackerras, 1962
		M. pflugfelderi Frank, 1964

	Varanidae	Pseudothamugadia physignathi Johnston, 1912
		H. gouldi Yorke and Maplestone, 1926
		Piratuba queenslandensis Mackerras, 1962
		P. varanicola Mackerras, 1962
Africa	Gekkonidae	Thamugadia hyalina Seurat, 1917
	Agamidae	Foleyella candezei Fraipont, 1882
		F. agamae Rodhain, 1906
		F. rodhaini Tendeiro, 1953
		Saurositus agamae Macfie, 1924
		H. macrophallos Parona, 1889
		S. peyrierasi Prod'hon, 1970
		Befilaria urschi Chabaud et al., 1959
Madagascar	Varanidae	Madathamugadia opluri Chabaud et al., 1959
	Gekkonidae	F. brevicauda Chabaud and Brygoo, 1962
		F. furcata Linstow, 1899
	Iguanidae	Madathamugadia zonosauri Chabaud et al., 1959
	Chamaeleontidae	Solafilaria guibei Chabaud et al., 1959
	Gerrhosauridae	F. philistinae Schacher and Khalil, 1967
Middle East	Agamidae	Saurositus baal Sulahian and Schacher, 1969
		Brygoofilaria agama Sulahian and Schacher, 1968
Asia, southern	Colubridae	F. schikhobalovi Skarbilovitsch, 1947
		F. skrjabini Skarbilovitsch, 1947
	Boidae	H. setiferum Chitwood, 1932
		H. spinigerum Chandler, 1929
	Lacertidae	F. schikhobalovi Skarbilovitsch, 1947
	Agamidae	Conispiculum guindiensis Pandit et al., 1929
		Saurositus indicus Deshmukh and Mehdi-Ali, 1965
	Varanidae	H. bipinnatum Linstow, 1899
		H. macrophallos Parona, 1889
		H. indicum Mirza and Basir, 1939
		H. spinigerum Chandler, 1929
		H. varani Skrjabin, 1923

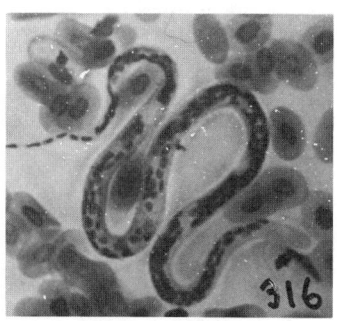

Fig. 20.51. Macdonaldius seetae from Pituophis melanoleucus, Mexico. X250

and an argasid tick has been used successfully as a laboratory vector for one species.

Distribution

Cardianema testudinis, the sole filariid known from turtles, was described from the eastern United States in 1856 and has not been rediscovered. Macdonaldius spp. (Figs. 20.50 and 20.51) are known from snakes and lizards of the southwestern United States and Mexico (Telford, 1965b), South America and Australia, as is Piratuba, a lizard parasite. Oswaldofilaria parasitizes caimans and lizards in South America and lizards in Australia. The single species of Splendidofilaria known from reptiles, S. corophila has not been seen again since its discovery in Heloderma suspectum of Arizona (Hannum, 1943). Hastospiculum seems most common in Asian varanid lizards, but also is known from Asian boids and South American boids and viperids. Pseudothamugadia is known to parasitize Australian agamid lizards and Thamugadia was found in a North African gekkonid. Foleyella has a broad distribution in temperate amphibians (Schacher and Crans, 1973), but also is known from African and Middle Eastern agamid lizards, Russian colubrid snakes and lacertids, and Madagascan chameleons. Saurositus parasitizes African, Middle Eastern and Asian agamids and Madagascan gekkonids, while Brygoofilaria is found in Middle Eastern agamids. Conispiculum, previously known only from Indian agamids (Pandi et al., 1929), has been found in an agamid, Japalura polygonota, in the Ryukyu archipelago (Miyata et al., 1978). Three genera appear to be endemic to Madagascar: Befilaria in gekkonids, Madathamugadia in iguanids and gerrhosaurids and Solafilaria in gerrhosaurids.

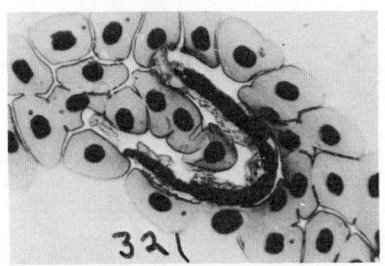

Fig. 20.52. Unidentified microfilaria from Cordylus cataphractus, South Africa. X250

The prevalence of filariasis among snakes and lizards is based upon finding microfilaria on blood smears. Often the adult worms are not found or not looked for, so identifications of species often are not made (Fig. 20.52). Field data on snake filariasis appear limited to one study from western Mexico (Telford, 1965b). A total of 119 snakes, belonging to 18 species, collected in Colima, Mexico were examined and 51 were found positive for Macdonaldius spp. Examination of approximately 100 additional snakes from other parts of Mexico resulted in negative findings. Seven species, all host to Macdonaldius, comprised 85% of the Colima snakes, with 53 infections among them: 46 M. oschei, 1 M. seetae, 2 M. colimensis and 2 mixed infections of M. oschei-M. colimensis. Infection rates among the three most common host species were 80.6% for Boa constrictor, 69.2% for Trimorphodon biscutatus and 39.3% for Drymarchon corais. M. oschei parasitized B. constrictor, T. biscutatus, D. corais, Lampropeltis doliata, Clelia clelia, Conophis vittatus and Crotalus basiliscus. M. seetae was found once in T. biscutatus and M. colimensis in T. biscutatus and B. constrictor. No explanation is at hand for the high prevalence of snake filariasis in Colima. The examination of 2,113 snakes from south-central Brazil by Pessoa et al. (1974a) found no microfilarial infections, nor were any seen by Telford (unpubl. data) or Moreno and Bolanos (1977) among 358 snakes from Venezuela, Panama, Costa Rica and Honduras.

Saurian survey data (Table 20.18) show filariasis infections to comprise 1.7 to 11.3% of haemoparasite infections in most areas in which they have been found. Among 300 haemoparasite infections studied by Brygoo (1963a) among Madagascan lizards, filariasis was represented by 65.3% of the total. Nearly two-thirds of the Madagascan sample was formed by chamaeleontids which showed exceptionally high infection rates of Foleyella furcata in three

Table 20.18. Geographic Distribution of Saurian Filari-

Physiographic/climatic characteristics	Area	No. lizard examined
Continental, temperate to subtropical, arid, desert or montane	California, southern Pakistan Russia, southern	922 848 605
Subtotal:		2375
Continental, temperate to subtropical, semi-arid, grasslands or montane	California, central Texas-Arizona Mexico Africa, east Australia, east	1367 240 358 1419 294
Subtotal:		3678
Continental, tropical to subtropical, humid, forest	Florida Middle America Panama Venezuela Africa, west Thailand-Malaysia	1992 572 1905 851 520 384
Subtotal:		6224
Insular, temperate, humid, forest Insular, subtropical, humid, forest Insular, tropical, humid, forest	Japan, Honshu Japan, Ryukyus Caribbean Madagascar New Guinea	1855 166 463 1099 154
Subtotal:		3737
Total:		16,014

host species: Chamaeleo pardalis (50.9%), C. oustaleti (59.2%) and C. verrucosus (48.8%). With their arboreal habits, chamaeleons are probably more easily and continuously accessible to the presumed mosquito vectors than are terrestrial or secretive hosts. Otherwise, the survey data show general similarity in the proportionate representation of filariasis among haemoparasite communities except in arid, continental areas where prevalence is apparently much lower. The Pakistani data (Telford, unpubl. data) are misleading inasmuch as microfilariae

asis from Survey Data given in Table 20.3.

No. haemoparasite infections	No. host species	Host species infected (%)	Microfilariae infection (%)
119	27	0.0	0.0
181	37	2.7	2.8
140			
440			2.8 $\bar{x}$
377	5	0.0	0.0
48	21	0.0	0.0
74	30	13.3	5.4
312	38	16.3	11.2
113	13	30.8	11.3
924			6.0 $\bar{x}$
261	16	6.3	4.2
120	41	4.9	1.7
759	34	32.4	7.8
338	21	19.1	4.4
156	8	37.5	9.0
164	17	11.8	1.2
1798			4.8 $\bar{x}$
280	3	0.0	0.0
7	7	0.0	0.0
97	29	3.5	5.2
300	42	23.8	65.3
21	17	5.9	9.5
705			26.7 $\bar{x}$
3867			

were seen only in one host species of 37 examined and that was Teratoscincus scincus. The infection rate was 31.3% in an apparent focus of intense haemoparasite transmission with Haemoproteus kopki (31.3%) and Leishmania sp. (25.0%) also present in the same host in one locality. Similarly, the East African data (Telford, unpubl. data) are distorted by the high prevalence of microfilariae among three Mabuya spp., where 20% of M. striata, M. quinquetaeniata and M. maculilabris were infected in one locality, in comparison to 5.8% in another area.

The only data available on seasonal prevalence of reptilian filarial infections were presented by Telford (1977). Panamanian anoles showed microfilarial infection rates varying from 4.8 to 5.7% from early dry season through the early wet season, with a minimum prevalence of 2.9% seen in the late wet season. There are no age or sex distribution data available at present.

Etiology

Under the scheme of classification proposed by Chabaud and Anderson (1959), the reptilian filarial worms (Nematoda: Filaroidea) were placed in two families. A single genus, Hastospiculum, represents the Diplotriaenidae in reptilian hosts. These are oviparous and produce embryonated eggs which presumably pass to the outside via the digestive tract where the arthropod intermediate host eats them and is in turn ingested by the definitive host. The remaining genera found in reptiles are viviparous and produce microfilarial larvae into the blood stream or subcutaneously, perhaps, where they are ingested by haematophagous arthropods, develop to the infective stage and are then reintroduced to a new host when the arthropod feeds again. The reptilian species belong to five subfamilies of the Onchocercidae: Onchocercinae (Macdonaldius, Befilaria), Dirofilariinae (Foleyella), Splendidofilariinae (Splendidofilaria, Cardianema, Thamugadia, Pseudothamugadia, Madathamugadia, Brygoofilaria), Oswaldofilariinae (Piratuba, Solafilaria, Oswaldofilaria, Conspiculum), and Eufilariinae (Saurositus).

Transmission

Microfilariae in the circulating blood are ingested by vector arthropods upon feeding on the infected reptile host. If the vector ingests too many microfilariae death can result, due apparently to the trauma caused by larval filariae penetrating the vector gut wall (Brygoo, 1960; Mackerras, 1962b; Pandit et al., 1930). Those microfilariae which are sheathed (enclosed within the egg membrane) quickly escape from their sheaths in the vector gut. Unsheathed larvae penetrate the gut wall and enter the vector haemocoele where they seek out particular sites for development. Foleyella spp. enter the adipose tissue of mosquito vectors (Bain, 1970; Schacher and Crans, 1973; Schacher and Khalil, 1968) as do Oswaldofilaria spp. (Bain and Chabaud, 1975; Mackerras, 1953; Prod'hon and Bain, 1972) and Conspiculum guindiensis (Pandit et al., 1930). Saurositus agamae, however, develops in mosquito wing muscles (Bain, 1969), while $\underline{M}$. oschei uses the lumen of the Malpighian tubules in the argasid tick, Ornithodoros talaje (Frank, 1964b,c). The first stage larvae moult, becoming second stage, which may be short and often stubby (termed "sausage-shaped"), in 3 to 4 days for Foleyella and Saurositus (Bain, 1969, 1970), 7 to 8 days for Oswaldofilari (Bain and Chabaud, 1975; Prod'hon and Bain, 1972) and 2 to 5 days for M. oschei (Frank, 1964b). Development continues for 2 to 20 days (Foleyella, 9 days; Saurositus, 2 days; Oswaldofilaria, 8 days; M. oschei, 14 to 20 days), and the second moult produces the third stage larvae which then become infective. These are now considerably elongated and slender. They may then leave the site of development, migrating into the vicinity of the vector's mouthparts. Duration of larval development in the vector requires varying lengths of time, depending upon vector and filarial species and the temperature at which the vector is maintained.

Natural vectors remain unknown. Both Culicine and Anopheline mosquitoes have proven capable as laboratory vectors for Saurositus, Oswaldofilaria, Foleyella and Conispiculum. Some of the species used probably are natural vectors where their ranges overlap those of the reptilian hosts. Macdonaldius probably uses an ixodid tick rather than argasids in nature, as argasids seldom are found on reptiles (Telford, 1965b). Unknown filarial larvae are often found during dissections of wild-caught mosquitoes and phlebotomine sandflies and some of these, perhaps, may represent reptilian filarial species.

Pathogenesis

Filariasis develops in the reptile host following introduction of the infective third stage larvae via the bite of the vector. Details of the migration made through the reptile's body by the larvae, if any, are unknown, but at some time following the infective bite the larvae reach the appropriate site for development. This site is often specific for filarial species (Table 20.19) and may be subcutaneous, in hepatic sinuses, the heart chambers, major blood vessels, the intestinal mesentery or simply the coelomic cavity. Either while enroute to this final site or upon reaching it, the third stage larva moults, changing into its fourth stage. The larva grows during the fourth stage and moults a final time into an adult female or male. The adults copulate and females produce living larvae or microfilariae in the Onchocercid nematodes. Apparently, no life cycle is known for the reptilian Diplotriaenid, Hastospiculum, which is oviparous. Microfilariae represent the first larval stage and must moult four times before maturing, twice in the vector and twice in the definitive host. Maturation may take several months. Pandit et al. (1930) found patent microfilaremia of C. quindiensis in Calotes versicolor after 68 days; Mackerras (1953) observed microfilariae of Oswaldofilaria chlamydosauri present in Amphibolurus barbatus 4.5 to 5 months following injection of third stage larvae. Once established, filarial infections may persist for long periods of time. Mackerras (1962) reported that the microfilaremia obtained in A. barbatus gradually increased during the first year of patency and microfilariae were still abundant in two lizards which died 34 months following infection. Telford (1965b), studying natural infections, observed little change in the level of microfilaremia of M. colimensis in T. biscutatus during 21 months, nor in M. oschei infection followed for 13 months in D. corais and 10 months in B. constrictor. As filarial worms die they may become calcified in the site of development and infections of Macdonaldius spp. commonly show mixtures of calcified, dead adult worms and living, reproductive individuals together in blood vessels. This possibly results from repeated infection with calcified worms representing earlier infections than the living. It was suggested that higher microfilaremias were correlated with the presence of calcified adults (Telford, 1965b) which implies that microfilarial life span might extend past that of adults.

Pathology

Pathogenicity has been described from three reptilian filaria: M. oschei, M. seetae and M. colimensis. Frank (1964a) found M. oschei infections in Python reticulatus and P. molurus from the Stuttgart Zoological Gardens associated with extensive dermal lesions in which the skin itself had eroded. Adult worms were present in large numbers in mesenteric and carotid arteries. Other boid species in the collection also showed microfilarial infections and a few adult worms were recovered from some of them, but they had no overt signs of disease. Telford (1965b) found filarial infections to be common in boids, colubrids and a viperid in the vicinity of Colima, Mexico. None of these showed dermal lesions despite evidence of long-standing infection and massive parasitemias by both adults and microfilariae. Both M. oschei and M. colimensis adults were found in the renal portal veins and post vena cavae in such numbers that bulbous swellings of the veins, resembling aneurysms were formed, which upon section showed the veins to be nearly occluded by tangled masses of adult worms. Sections of lung tissues usually showed large numbers of microfilariae in the capillaries. M. seetae

Table 20.19. Location of Adult Filarial Worms within the Infected Host.

Species	Site within body	Reference
Hastospiculum spp.	Serous membranes	Yamaguti, 1961
Macdonaldius spp.	Arteries and veins, heart	Frank, 1964a; Telford, 1965b
Oswaldofilaria chlamydosauri	Subcutaneous in thoracic region and throat	Mackerras, 1962
O. bacillaris	Thoracic muscles	Prod'hon and Bain, 1972
Conispiculum guindiensis	Coelomic mesenteries; pelvic region; along trachea	Pandit et al., 1929
Saurositus agamae	Coelomic mesenteries	Bain, 1969
S. peyrierasi	Subcutaneous; coelomic cavity	Prod'hon, 1970
Brygoofilaria agamae	Periesophageal and peritracheal connective tissue; pericardial cavity; intestinal mesentery	Sulahian and Schacher, 1968
Befilaria urschi	Subcutaneous; peritoneum	Brygoo, 1965b
Madathamugadia opluri	Coelomic cavity	Brygoo, 1965b
Foleyella furcata	Subcutaneous on muscle surfaces; buccal cavity; peri-renal; air sac	Brygoo, 1963a
F. philistinae	Subcutaneous tissues and superficial muscle fascia	Schacher and Khalil, 1967

was found in captive snakes by Hull and Camin (1959) and they suggested that occlusion of the portal vein may have led to the death of one snake.

Diagnosis

Diagnosis of filariasis is usually made by detecting microfilariae on fresh or stained blood smears. A drop of blood in saline covered by a cover slip and examined at 10X will usually show moving microfilariae if present. Smears fixed with methanol and stained by the Giemsa method should be examined at 10X, with special attention given to ends and edges of the smear. Identification is difficult from microfilariae alone except for M. oschei, which is readily distinguished by the broad sheath within which the larva lies. Filarial adults found at autopsy should be fixed in warm alcohol-formalin-acetic acid or 70% ethanol and later placed in lactophenol for clearing, after which they can be studied in temporary mounts. Species diagnosis is based upon adult morphology and requires expert assistance usually, as adult filariae can be difficult to identify. It is best to refer specimens stored in 70% ethanol and accompanied by thin blood smears when possible to a helminthologist for identification.

Immunity

There have been no studies on possible immunity by reptilian hosts towards filarial parasites.

M. oschei apparently has low specificity for definitive hosts, as infections were found in seven host species of three families (Telford, 1965b). Frank (1964a) reported successful, though pathogenic, infections of Old World Python spp. with M. oschei. M. seetae is known only from colubrid snakes (Hull and Camin, 1959; Khanna, 1933; Telford, 1965b), parasitizing Pituophis and Elaphe spp. in the southwestern United States and Mexico and T. biscutatus in Mexico. M. colimensis was found in both B. constrictor and T. biscutatus. Other New World and Australian Macdonaldius spp. are known from single hosts only. Brygoo (1963) found F. furcata in five Chamaeleo spp., but the other filariae (Befilaria, Solafilaria, Madathamugadia, F. brevicauda) were recorded from single host species only. F. candezei is known to parasitize the agamid genera Agama and Uromastix, as well as Chamaeleo, in Africa and the Middle East (Brygoo, 1963). F. schikhobalovi has been recorded from both Elaphe and Lacerta spp. in Russia (Yamaguti, 1961). All other described reptilian filariids seem to known from single host species only.

Treatment

There seems to be no published accounts of chemotherapy applied to reptilian filariasis. Possibly the mammalian antifilarial drug diethylcarbamazine would be effective, but dosages would have to be determined.

Telford (1965a) exposed a B. constrictor with a M. oschei infection, in which microfilaremia ranged from 656 to 1,273 microfilaria (mf)/ml to an ambient temperature of 37 C for 144 hours. Afterward, smears made from both cardiac and caudal blood were negative for microfilariae and remained negative with smears taken 2 to 5 days apart for over one month. Over two years later the snake still showed no microfilaremia (G.H. Ball, personal communication). A second boa with far higher microfilaremia, 10,958 to 29,058 mf/ml was exposed to an ambient temperature of 35 C for 96 hours, but no reduction in parasitemia resulted. It was then placed at 37 C for 288 hours until it died. Microfilaremia decreased from 17,250 to 7,210 mf/ml within the first 24 hours and dropped to 90 to 1,200 mf/ml from 48 to 288 hours. At autopsy several hundred adult M. oschei recovered from the post vena cava were dead, non-motile, discolored and decomposing. All microfilariae observed from 144 to 288 hours were distorted or decomposing, but were not completely cleared from the circulating blood. Death of the host may have resulted from an inability to remove decomposing adults and microfilariae before toxic substances resulting from decomposition were fatal to the snake. Extremely heavy filarial infections should perhaps not be treated to avoid a fatal conclusion, inasmuch as reptiles infected naturally by filarial worms seem to survive as well in captivity as those uninfected. Treatment over an extended period might prevent death from decomposition products.

Control

Control can be established by frequent inspection of captive reptiles for ectoparasites, removal of these when found and maintenance of specimens in clean cages screened properly against flying arthropods. Control in nature is not practical.

REFERENCES

Acholonu, A.D., 1974, Haemogregarina pseudemydis n. sp. (Apicomplexa: Haemogregarinidae) and Pirhemocyt chelonarum n. sp. in turtles from Louisiana, J. Protozool., 21:659-664.

Adler, S., and Theodor, O., 1935, Investigations on Mediterranean Kalaazar. X. A note on Trypanosoma platydactyli and Leishmania tarentolae, Proc. Royal Soc. (Ser. B), 116:543-544.

Andrushko, A.M., and Markov, G.S., 1955a, Incidence of infection with blood parasites in reptiles of various biotopes in the Kara-Kum desert, Doklad Akad. Nauk SSR, 104:674-677.

Andrushko, A.M., and Markov, G.S., 1955b, Parasite fauna of blood of lizards in the Kzyl-Kum desert, including protozoa, Vestnik. Leningrad. Univ., Ser. Biol. Geogr. Geol., 9:31-46.

Andrushko, A.M., and Markov, G.S., 1956, Blood parasites of reptiles of the Kara-Kum desert, Vestnik Leningrad. Univ. Ser. Biol., 15:57-65.

Aragao, H. de B., and Neiva, A., 1909, A contribution to the study of parasites of lizards. Two new species of Plasmodium, Pl. diploglossi and Pl. tropiduri n. sp., Mem. Inst. Osw. Cruz., 1:44-50

Arantes, J.B., and da Fonseca, F., 1931, Pesquisas sobre trypanosomas, 1. Trypanosoma butantanense sp. n. parasita da serpente Ophis merremi Wagler, 1924, Mem. Inst. Butantan, 6:215-222.

Arcay de Peraza, L., 1971, The "paranuclear corpuscles" in poikilothermic vertebrates: Description of a new species of Pirhemocyton in Iguana iguana of Venezuela, with remarks on the nature of these organisms and their relation to allied parasites, Mem. Inst. Osw. Cruz., 69:57-69.

Arcay de Peraza, L., Nasir, P., and Diaz, M.T., 1971, The "paranuclear corpuscles" in poikilothermal vertebrates. I. Description of a new species of Toddi from Iguana iguana in Venezuela, Acta Biol. Venezuela, 7:191-199.

Ashford, R.W., Bray, M.A., and Foster, W.A., 1973, Observations on Trypanosoma boueti (Protozoa) parasitic in the skink, Mabuya striata (Reptilia), and the sandfly, Sergentomyia bedfordi, in Ethiopia, J. Zool., London, 171:285-292.

Audy, J.R., Nadchatram, M., and Lim, B.L., 1960, Malaysian parasites, XLIX. Host distribution of Malaysian ticks (Ixodoidea), Inst. Med. Res. Fed. Malaya, Study 29:225-246.

Awerinzew, S.V., 1914, Beitrage zur Morphologie und Entwicklungs geschichte der Protozoen von Deutsch-Ost-Afrika, Zhurnal Mikrobiol., 1:1-9.
Ayala, S.C., 1970a, Haemogregarine from sandfly infecting both lizards and snakes, J. Parasitol., 56:387-388.
Ayala, S.C., 1970b, Lizard malaria in California; Description of a strain of Plasmodium mexicanum and biogeography of lizard malaria in western North America, J. Parasitol., 56:417-425.
Ayala, S.C., 1971, Sporogony and experimental transmission of Plasmodium mexicanum, J. Parasitol., 57:598-602.
Ayala, S.C., 1977, Plasmodia of reptiles, in: "Parasitic protozoa", J.P. Kreier, ed., Academic Press, New York.
Ayala, S.C., 1978, Checklist, host index, and annotated bibliography of Plasmodium from reptiles, J. Protozool., 25:87-100.
Ayala, S.C., and Hutchings, R., 1974, Haemogregarines (Protozoa: Sporozoa) as zoogeographical tracers of Galapagos Island lava lizards and marine iguanas, Herpetologica, 30:128-132.
Ayala, S.C., and Mckay, J.G., 1971, Trypanosoma gerrhonoti n. sp. and extrinsic development of lizard trypanosomes in California sandflies, J. Protozool., 18:430-433.
Ayala, S.C., and Spain, J., 1976, A population of Plasmodium colombiense, sp. n. in the iguanid lizard, Anolis auratus, J. Parasitol., 62:177-189.
Ayala, S.C., Moreno, E., and Bolanos, R., 1978, Plasmodium pessoai sp. n. from two Costa Rican snakes, J. Parasitol., 64:330-335.
Bain, O., 1969, Developpement larvaire de Saurositus agamae hamoni n.s. sp., Eufilariinae parasite d'Agame en Haute-Volta, chez Anopheles stephensi, Ann. Parasitol. Hum. Comp., 44:581-594.
Bain, O., 1970, Etude morphologique du developpement larvaire de Foleyella candezei chez Anopheles stephensi et Aedes aegypti, Ann. Parasitol. Hum. Comp., 45:21-30.
Bain, O., and Chabaud, A.G., 1975, Developpement chez des Moustiques de trois filaires de lezards sud-americains du genre Oswaldofilaria, Ann. Parasitol. Hum. Comp., 50:209-221.
Baker, J.R., 1961, Attempts to find the vector of the Plasmodiidae of the lizard, Agama agama agama, in Liberia, Ann. Rep. Res. Activities Liberian Inst., American Found. Trop. Med., 28-40.

Ball, G.H., 1958, A haemogregarine from a water snake, Natrix piscator taken in the vicinity of Bombay India, J. Protozool., 5:274-281.

Ball, G.H., 1967, Some blood sporozoans from East African reptiles, J. Protozool., 14:198-210.

Ball, G.H., and Oda, S.N., 1971, Sexual stages in the lif history of the hemogregarine, Hepatozoon rarefaciens (Sambon and Seligmann, 1907), J. Protozool., 18:697-700.

Ball, G.H., Chao, J., and Telford, S.R., Jr., 1967, The life history of Hepatozoon rarefaciens (Sambon and Seligmann, 1907) from Drymarchon corais (Colubridae), and its experimental transfer to Constrictor constrictor (Boidae), J. Parasitol. 53:897-909.

Ball, G.H., Chao, J., and Telford, S.R., Jr., 1969, Hepatozoon fusifex sp. n., a hemogregarine from Boa constrictor producing marked morphological changes in infected erythrocytes, J. Parasitol. 55:800-813.

Batelli, C., 1947, Su di un piroplasma della Naja nigricollis (Aegyptianella carpani sp. n.), Riv. Parassitol., 8:205-212.

Belova, E.M., 1966, Culturing of leptomonads from geckoes, Gymnodactylus caspius Eich., Med. Parazit., Moscow, 34:349-351.

Belova, E.M., 1971, Reptiles and their importance in the epidemiology of leishmaniasis, Bull. World Healt Org., 44:553-560.

Belova, E.M., and Bogdanov, O.P., 1968, Leptomonad infections of snakes in Turkmen SSR, Med. Parazit., Moscow, 37:304-306.

Beyer, T.V., and Selivanova, G.V., 1969, Cytophotochemical studies of the nuclear DNA content in haemogregarines from diploid and triploid hosts, the Armenian rock-lizards, Tsitologiya, 11:739-743.

Beyer, T.V., and Sidorenko, N.V., 1972, Cytochemical studies on the haemogregarines of Armenian reptiles. II. Shifts in haemoglobin and total protein contents in the haemogregarine-infected erythrocytes of rock-lizards, Parasitolojia, 6:385-390.

Beyer, T.V., and Sidorenko, N.V., 1973, Cytochemical studies on the haemogregarines of Armenian rock-lizards. III. Dehydrogenase activity in haemogregarines from the peripheral blood of lizards and in infected erythrocytes, Tsitologiya, 15:598-606.

Bird, R.G., and Garnham, P.C.C., 1967, Aegyptianella pullorum Carpano, 1928. Fine structure and taxonomy, J. Protozool, 14:suppl. 42.

Blanc, G., and Ascione, L., 1958, Sur un parasite endoglobulaire du lezard Eremias guttulatus olivieri Augoin den la region de Marrakech (Maroc), Bull. Soc. Pathol. Exot., 51:508-511.

Bonorris, J.S., and Ball, G.H., 1955, Schellackia occidentalis n. sp., a blood-inhabiting coccidian found in lizards in southern California, J. Protozool., 2:31-34.

Booden, T., Chao, J., and Ball, G.H., 1970, Transfer of Hepatozoon sp. from Boa constrictor to a lizard, Anolis carolinensis, by mosquito vectors, J. Parasitol., 56:832-833.

Bray, R.S., 1959, On the parasitic protozoa of Liberia. II. The malaria parasites of agamid lizards, J. Protozool., 6:13-18.

Bray, R.S., 1964, A check-list of the parasitic protozoa of West Africa with some notes on their classification, Bull. Inst. Fr. Afr. Noire (ser. A), 26:238-315.

Brumpt, E., 1914, Le xenodiagnostic. Application au diagnostic de quelques infections parasitaires et en particular a la Trypanosomiase de Chagas, Bull. Soc. Pathol. Exot., 7:706-710.

Brumpt, E., and Lavier, G., 1935, Sur un piroplasmide nouveau parasite de tortue, Tunetella emydis n. g., n. sp., Ann. Parasitol. Hum. Comp., 13: 544-550.

Brygoo, E.R., 1960, Evolution de Foleyella furcata (Von Linstow, 1899) chez Culex fatigans Wiedemann, 1828, Arch. Inst. Pasteur Madagascar, 28:129-138.

Brygoo, E.R., 1963a, Hematozoaires de Reptiles malgaches. I. Trypanosoma therezieni n. sp. parasite des chameleons de Madagascar. Infestation naturelle et experimentale, Arch. Inst. Pasteur Madagascar, 31:133-141.

Brygoo, E.R., 1963b, Contribution a la connaissance de la Parasitologie des chameleons malgaches. Part I., Ann. Parasitol. Hum. Comp., 38:149-334.

Brygoo, E.R., 1963c, Contribution a la connaissance de la Parasitologie des chameleons malgaches. Part II., Ann. Parastiol. Hum. Comp., 38:525-739.

Brygoo, E.R., 1965a, Description de Trypanosoma brazili E. Brumpt, 1914, Arch. Inst. Pasteur Madagascar, 34:41-46.

Brygoo, E.R., 1965b, Hematozoaires de Reptiles Malgaches. IV. Les microfilaires de Befilaria urschi Chabaud, Anderson et Brygoo, 1959 et de Madathamugadia hopluri C., A. et B., 1959, Arch. Inst. Pasteur Madagascar, 34:55-62.

Brygoo, E.R., 1966, Hematozoaires de Reptiles Malgaches. VI. Trypanosoma petteri n. sp. parasite de Phelsuma. Liste des Trypanosomes de Reptiles, Arch. Inst. Pasteur Madagascar, 35:171-184.

Carini, A., 1930, Presence de corpuscules de nature parasitaire probable (Bertariella leptodactyli) dans les hematies du Leptodactylus pentadactylus, Compt. Rend. Soc. Biol. Paris, 103:1312-1313.

Carini, A., 1937, Sur une nouvelle Tunetella d'une tortue du Bresil, Ann. Parasitol. Hum. Comp., 15:537-538.

Carpano, M., 1939, Sui piroplasmidi dei cheloni e su una nuova specie rinvenuta nelle tartarughe Nuttalli guglielmi, Riv. Parassitol., 3:267-276.

Cerruti, C.G., 1931, Su di una Grahamella parassita di Talassochelys caretta (Grahamella talassochelys u. sp.), Arch. Ital. Sci. Med. Colon, 12:321-325.

Chabaud, A.G., and Anderson, R.C., 1959, Nouvel essais de classification des Filaires (Superfamille des Filaroidea) II, Ann. Parasitol. Hum. Comp., 34:64-87.

Chao, J., and Ball, G.H., 1969, Transfer of Hepatozoon rarefaciens (Sambon and Seligmann, 1907) from the indigo snake to a gopher snake by a mosquito vector, J. Parasitol., 55:681-682.

Chatton, E., and Blanc, G., 1914, Sur un Hematozoaire nouveau, Pirhemocyton tarentolae, du Gecko Tarentola mauritanica, et sur les alteracions globulaires quil determine, Compt. Rend. Soc. Biol., 77:496-498.

Chatton, E., and Blanc, G., 1918, Culture du trypanosome de gecko chez la punaise des lits, Bull. Soc. Pathol. Exot., 11:387-391.

Christensen, H.A., and Telford, S.R., Jr., 1972, Trypanosoma thecadactyli sp. n. from forest geckoes in Panama, and its development in the sandfly, Lutzomyia trinidadensis (Newstead) Diptera, Psychodidae, J. Protozool., 19:403-406.

Correa de Meyrelles, C., 1938, Parasites of the genus Bertarellia in the blood of the tortoises of India and Brazil, Proc. Indian Acad. Sci., 7: 49-53.

Da Rocha e Silva, E.O., 1975, Ciclo evolutivo do Hepatozoon triatomae (Sporozoa, Haemogregarinidae) Parasita de triatomineos, Rev. Saude Publ. Sao Paulo, 9:383-391.

De Biasi, P., Pessoa, S.B., and Belluomini, H.E., 1971, Nota sobre a transmissao congenita de hemogregarinas em duas especies de serpentes pe gonhentas viviparas, Atas Soc. Biol., Rio de Janeiro, 15:27-28.

De Biasi, P., Pessoa, S.B., Puorto, G., and Fernandes, W., 1975, Nota sobre formas evolutivas de Trypanosoma de serpentes em meio de cultura, Mem. Inst. Butantan, 39:85-101.

De Giusti, D.L., 1965, Haemoproteus metchinikovi of chelonians, its tissue phases, peripheral parasitemia, host specificity and geographical distribution, Prog. Protozool., 176, Excerpt. Med. Found., Int. Ser. 91.

De Giusti, D.L., 1970, Additional studies on the life cycle of Haemoproteus metchnikovi (Simondia metchnikovi) from the turtle Chrysemys picta marginata, J. Parasitol., 54 (4, Sect. 2, pt. 1):70-71.

De Giusti, D.L., and Dobrzechowshi, D., 1974, The biology of the chelonian haemoproteid, Haemoproteus metchnikovi, in turtle hosts and in the intermediate host, Chrysops callidus, Proc. 3rd Int. Congr. Parasitol., 1:80-81.

De Giusti, D.L., Sterling, C.R., and Dobrzechowski, D., 1973, Transmission of the chelonian haemoproteid, Haemoproteus metchnikovi by a tabanid fly, Chrysops callidus, Nature, 242:50-51.

De Mello, F., 1934, Contribution a l'etude du Cycle Evolutif des Haemocystidium, Arquivos Esc. Med.-Cirurgica Nova Goa, Ser. A, 9:1785-1799.

De Mello, F., and Correa de Meyrelles, C., 1937, On the nature and identification of some roundish bodies found either free or as endoglobular parasites in the blood of Calotes versicolor Daud. subspecies major Blyth, Proc. Indian Acad. Sci. B, 6:98-108.

De Sousa, M.A., and Freire, E.G., 1975, Consideracoes sobre a natureza, desenvolvimento e transmissao de Cytamoeba bacterifera Labbe, 1894 de Leptodactylus ocellatus, Mem. Inst. Osw. Cruz., 73:109-119.

De Sousa, M.A., De Biasi, P., and Pessoa, S.B., 1973, Protistas "incertae sedis" de ofidios do Brasil: Toddia Franca, 1912, Pirhemocyton Chatton and Blanc, 1914 - Estudo comparativo, Mem. Inst. Osw. Cruz., 71:443-468.

Desser, J.S., McIver, S.B., and Ryckman, A., 1973, Culex territans as a potential vector of Trypanosoma rotatorium. I. Development of the flagellate in the mosquito, J. Parasitol., 59:353-358.

Dobell, C.C., 1910, Contributions to the life history of Haemocystidium simondi Castellani et Willey, Festschrift 60 Geburst., R. Hertwigs, 2:124-132.

Du Toit, P.J., 1937, A new piroplasm (Sauroplasma thomasi n. g., n. sp.) of a lizard (Zonurus giganteus, Smith), Onderstepoort J. Vet. Sci. Anim. Industry, 9:289-299.

Dutton, J., Todd, J.T., and Tobey, E.N., 1907, Concerning certain parasitic protozoa observed in Africa, Ann. Trop. Med. Parasitol., 1:287-348.

Edeson, J.F.B., and Himo, J., 1973, Leishmania sp. in the blood of a lizard (Agama stellio) from Lebanon, Trans. Royal Soc. Trop. Med. Hyg., 67:27.

Ewers, W.H., 1968, Blood parasites of some New Guinea reptiles and amphibia, J. Parasitol., 54:172-174.

Fantham, H.B., Porter, A., and Richardson, L.R., 1942, Some haematozoa observed in vertebrates in eastern Canada, Parasitology, 34:199-226.

Franca, C., 1911, Notes sur les hematozoaires de la Guinee Portugaise, Arq. R. Inst. Bact., Camara Pestana, 3:229-238.

Frank, W., 1964a, Biologie von Macdonaldius oschei Chabaud et Frank 1961 (Filarioidea, Onchocercidae) und seine pathogenen wirkungen auf Verschiedene wirte (Reptilia, Ophidia), unter berucksichtigun der biologie des ubertragers, Ornithodoros talaj (Ixodoidea, Argasidae), Z. Parasitol., 24:249-275.

Frank, W., 1964b, Die Entwicklung von Macdonaldius oschei Chabaud et Frank 1961 (Filarioidea, Onchocercidae) in der Lederzecke Ornithodoros talaje Guerin-Meneville (Ixodoidea, Argasidas), Z. Parasitol., 24:319-350.

Frank, W., 1964c, Die Ubertragung der Filarien-Infektionstadien von Macdonaldius oschei Chabaud et Frank 1961 (Filaroidea, Onchocercidae) durch Ornithodoros talaje (Ixodoidea, Argasidae) auf den Endwirt zugleich ein Beitrag zur Biologie des Ubertragers, Z. Parastitol., 24:415-441.

Frank, W., 1974, Sauroplasma and other so-called parasites of reptile blood corpuscles, Proc. 3rd Int. Congr. Parasitol., 3:1666.

Furman, D.P., 1966, Hepatozoon balfouri (Laveran, 1905): Sporogonic cycle, pathogenesis and transmission by mites to jerboa hosts, J. Parasitol., 52:373-382.

Gardener, P.J., 1977, Taxonomy of the genus Leishmania: A review of nomenclature and classification, Trop. Dis. Bull., 74:1069-1088.

Garnham, P.C.C., 1965, Plasmodium wenyoni sp. nov., a malaria parasite of a Brazilian snake, Trans. Royal Soc. Trop. Med. Hyg., 59:277-279.

Garnham, P.C.C., 1966, "Malaria parasites and other Haemoaporidia," Blackwell Sci. Publ., Oxford.

Garnham, P.C.C., 1971, The genus Leishmania, Bull. World Health Org., 44:477-489.

Goodwin, M.H., 1951, Observations on the natural occurrence of Plasmodium floridense, a saurian malaria parasite, in Sceloporus undulatus undulatus, J. Nat. Mal. Soc., 10:57-67.

Goodwin, M.H., and Stapleton, T.K., 1952, The course of natural and induced infections of Plasmodium floridense Thompson and Huff, in Sceloporus undulatus undulatus (Latreille), Amer. J. Trop. Med. Hyg., 1:773-783.

Gorgas Memorial Laboratory, 1964, Blood parasites of reptiles from Almirante, 35th Ann. Rept. (1963), United States Government Printing Office, Washington.

Greiner, E.C., and Daggett, P.M., 1973, A saurian Plasmodium in a Wyoming population of Sceloporus undulatus, J. Herpetol., 7:303-304.

Grewal, M.S., 1955, On a new trypanosome from the blood of an African gecko, Hemidactylus brookii angulatus Gray, 1845, Res. Bull. Punjab Univ. Sci., 106:269-281.

Hannum, C.A., 1943, Nematode parasites of Arizona vertebrates, Univ. Washington Publ. Theses Ser., 7:229-231.

Herban, N., 1971, Blood parasites of Lygosoma laterale Say, 1823 from Louisiana, Amer. Midland Natur., 85:279-284.

Hoare, C.A., 1929, Studies on Trypanosoma grayi. 2. Experimental transmission to the crocodile, Trans. Royal Soc. Trop. Med. Hyg., 23:39-56.

Hoare, C.A., 1930, On a new Dactylosoma occurring in fish of Victoria Nyanza, Ann. Trop. Med. Parasitol., 24:241-248.

Hoare, C.A., 1931a, The peritrophic membrane of Glossina and its bearing upon the life-cycle of Trypanosoma grayi, Trans. Royal Soc. Trop. Med. Hyg., 25:57-64.

Hoare, C.A., 1931b, Studies on Trypanosoma grayi. 3. Life cycle in the tsetse fly and in the crocodile, Parasitology, 28:449-484.

Hoare, C.A., 1932, On protozoal blood parasites collected in Uganda, with an account of the life cycle of the crocodile haemogregarine, Parasitology, 24:210-224.

Hoare, C.A., 1972, "The trypanosomes of mammals. A zoological monograph," Blackwell Sci. Publ., Oxford.

Huff, C.G., and Marchbank, D.F., 1953, Saurian malaria in Panama, Naval Med. Res. Inst. Rept. II:509-516.

Hull, R.W., and Camin, J.H., 1959, Macdonaldius seetae Khanna, 1933 in captive snakes, Trans. Amer. Microscop. Soc., 73:323-329.

Hull, R.W., and Camin, J.H., 1960, Haemogregarines in snakes: The incidence and identity of the erythrocytic stages, J. Parasitol., 46:515-523.

Jakowska, S., and Nigrelli, R.F., 1956, Babesioma, gen. nov., and other babesioids in erythrocytes of cold-blooded vertebrates, Ann. New York Acad. Sci., 64:112-127.

Johnston, M.R.L., 1975, Distribution of Pirhemocyton Chatton and Blanc and other, possibly related, infections of poikilotherms, J. Protozool., 22:529-535.

Jordan, H.B., 1964, Lizard malaria in Georgia, J. Protozool., 11:562-566.

Jordan, H.B., 1975, The effect of host constitution on the development of Plasmodium floridense, J. Protozool., 22:241-244.

Jordan, H.B., and Friend, M., 1971, The occurrence of Schellackia and Plasmodium in two Georgia lizards, J. Protozool., 18:485-487.

Khanna, R.K., 1933, A new filarial worm from a North American snake, J. Helminth., 11:105-108.

Krasilnikov, E.N., 1965, On undescribed blood parasites from the Caucasus, "Gerpetologija', Acad. Nauk Uzbeksoj SSR, Tashkent.

Lainson, R., and Shaw, J.J., 1969a, A new haemosporidian of lizards, Saurocytozoon tupinambi gen. nov., sp. nov., in Tupinambis nigropunctatus (Teiidae) Parasitology, 59:159-162.

Lainson, R., and Shaw, J.J., 1969b, New host records for Plasmodium diploglossi, P. tropiduri Aragao and Neiva, 1909, and P. cnemidophori Carini, 1941, Parasitology, 59:163-170.

Lainson, R., Landau, I., and Shaw, J.J., 1971, On a new family of nonpigmented parasites in the blood of reptiles: Garniidae fam. nov., (Coccidiida: Haemosporidiidea). Some species of the new genus Garnia, Int. J. Parasitol., 1:241-250.

Lainson, R., Landau, I., and Shaw, J.J., 1974a, Further parasites of the family Garniidae (Coccidiida: Haemosporidiidea) in Brazilian lizards. Fallisia effusa gen. nov., sp. nov., and Fallisia modesta gen. nov. sp. nov., Parasitology, 68:117-125.

Lainson, R., Landau, I., and Shaw, J.J., 1974b, Observations on non-pigmented haemosporidia of Brazilian lizards, including a new species of Saurocytozoon in Mabuya mabouya (Scincidae), Parasitology, 69:215-233.

Lainson, R., Shaw, J.J., and Landau, I., 1975, Some blood parasites of the Brazilian lizards Plica umbra and Uranoscodon superciliosa (Iguanidae), Parasitology, 70:119-141.

Lainson, R., Shaw, J.J., and Ward, R.D., 1976, Schellackia landaue sp. nov. (Eimeriorina: Lankesterellidae) in the Brazilian lizard Polychrus marmoratus (Iguanidae): Experimental transmission by Culex pipiens fatigans, Parasitology, 72:225-243.

Landau, I., 1973, Diversite des mecanismes assurant la parennite de l'infection chez sporozoaires coccidiomorphes, Mem. Museum Natur. Hist. Naturelle, Ser. A Zool., 77:1-62.

Landau, I., Lainson, R., Boulard, Y., and Shaw, J.J., 1974, Transmission au laboratoire et description de l'Hemogregarine Lainsonia legeri n. sp. (Lankesterellidae) parasite de lezards bresiliens, Ann. Parasitol. Hum. Comp., 49:253-263.

Landau, I., Michel, J.C., Chabaud, A.G., and Brygoo, E.R., 1972, Cycle biologique d'Hepatozoon domerguei; discussion sur les caracteres fondamentaux d'un cycle de Coccidie, Z. Parasitenk., 38:250-270.

Laird, M., 1950, Haemogregarina tuatarae sp. n., from the New Zealand Rhyncocephalian Sphenodon punctatus (Gray), Proc. Zool. Soc. London, 120:529-533.

Leger, M., 1918, Infection sanguine par Leptomonas chez un saurien, Compt. Rend. Soc. Biol. Paris, 81:772-774.

Lehman, D.L., 1961, Cytamoeba bacterifera Labbe, 1894. I. Morphology and host incidence of the parasite in California, J. Protozool., 8:29-33.

Lewis, J.F., and Wagner, E.D., 1964, Hepatozoon sauromali sp. n., a haemogregarine from the chuckwalla (Sauromalus spp.) with notes on the life history, J. Parasitol., 50:11-14.

Mackerras, M.J., 1953, Lizard filaria: Transmission by mosquitoes of Oswaldofilaria chlamydosauri (Breinl) (Nematoda: Filarioidea), Parasitology, 43:1-3.

Mackerras, M.J., 1961, The haematozoa of Australian reptiles, Australian J. Zool., 9:61-122.

Mackerras, M.J., 1962a, The life history of a Hepatozoon (Sporozoa: Adeleidea) of varanid lizards in Australia, Australian J. Zool., 10:35-44.

Mackerras, M.J., 1962b, Filarial parasites (Nematoda: Filarioidea) of Australian animals, Australian J. Zool., 10:400-457.

Manwell, R.D., 1964, The genus Dactylosoma, J. Protozool., 11:526-530.

Markov, G.S., and Bogdanov, O.P., 1961, Parasites of desert lizards in Central Asia, Uchen. Zapiski Stalingradsk. Gosudarstv. Pedagog. Inst. im. A.S. Serafimovich Kafedry Zool. Fiziol. i Morfol., 13:101-123.

Markov, G.S., Ataev, C., and Bogdanov, O.P., 1968, Information about parasites of the skink Eumeces taeniolatus Blyth, Gerpetologija Srednej Azii, Akad. Nauk Uzbek. SSR, Tashkent.

Markov, G.S., Ivanov, V.P., Krjutchkov, B.P., Lukjanova, Z.F., Nikulin, V.P., and Tchernobaj, V.F., 1964, Protozoa and Acarina parasitizing reptiles of the Caspian Sea region, Uchen Zapuki Volgograd. Gosudarstv. Pedagog. Inst. im. A.S. Serafimovich Kafedry Zool. Fiziol. i Morfol., 16:106-110.

Marquardt, W.C., 1966, Haemogregarines and Haemoproteus in some reptiles in southern Illinois, J. Parasitol., 52:823-824.

Marquardt, W.C., and Yaeger, R.G., 1967, The structure and taxonomic status of Toddia from the cottonmouth snake, Agkistrodon piscivorous leucostoma, J. Protozool., 14:726-731.

Mathis, C., and Leger, M., 1911, Recherches de parasitologie et de pathologie humaines et animales au Tonkin, Paris.

Michel, J.C., 1973, Hepatozoon mauritanicum (Et. et Ed. Sergent, 1904) n. comb., parasite de Testudo graeca: Redescription de la sporogonie chez Hyalomma aegyptium et de la schizogonic tissulaire d'apres le material d'E. Brumpt, Ann. Parasitol. Hum. Comp., 48:11-21.

Miller, W.W., 1908, Hepatozoon perniciosum (n. g., n. sp.) a haemogregarine pathogenic for white rats; with a description of the sexual cycle in the intermediate host, a mite Laelaps echidninus, Bull. United States Hyg. Lab., 46:1-48.

Minchin, E.A., 1907, On a haemogregarine from the blood of a Himalayan lizard (Agama tuberculata), Proc. Zool. Soc. London, 78:1098-1104.

Miyata, A., 1974, The detection of haemogregarines in blood of some Japanese snakes, Trop. Med., 16:71-84.

Miyata, A., 1976, Anuran haemoprotozoa found in the vicinity of Nagasaki city. 2. Dactylosoma ranarum (Kruse, 1890), Trop. Med., 18:135-141.

Miyata, A., and Miyagi, I., 1977, Toddia detected from Rana (Babina) holsti Boulenger, 1892 in Okinawa Island, Trop. Med., 19:123-128.

Miyata, A., Miyagi, I., and Tsukamoto, M., 1978, Haemoprotozoa detected from cold-blooded animals in Ryukyu Islands, Trop. Med., 20:97-112.

Mohiuddin, A., Pal, R.A., and Warsi, A.A., 1967, Haemogregarina echisi n. sp. from the saw-scaled viper Echis carinatus of the Sind region of West Pakistan, J. Protozool., 14:255-259.

Molyneux, D.H., 1977, The attachment of Trypanosoma grayi in the hind-gut of Glossina, Protozoology, 3: 83-86.

Moreno, E., and Bolanos, R., 1977, Haemogregarinas en serpientes de Costa Rica, Rev. Biol. Trop., 25:47-57.

Nadim, A., Seyed Rashti, M.A., and Mesghali, A., 1968, Epidemiology of cutaneous leishmaniasis in Turkmen Sahara, Iran, J. Trop. Med. Hyg., 71: 238-239.

Oda, S.N., Chao, J., and Ball, G.H., 1971, Additional instances of transfer of reptile hemogregarines to foreign hosts, J. Parasitol., 57:1377-1378.

Pandit, C.G., Pandit, .S.R., and Iyer, P.V.S., 1929, A new filaria in Calotes versicolor - Conispiculum guindiensis n. g. n. sp., Indian J. Med. Res., 16:954-958.

Pandit, C.G., Pandit, S.R., and Iyer, P.V.S., 1930, The development of the filaria Conispiculum guindiensis (1929) in C. fatigans with a note on the transmission of the infection, Indian J. Med. Res., 17:421-429.

Peirce, M.A., and Castleman, A.R.W., 1974, An intraerythrocytic parasite of the Moroccan tortoise, J. Wildlife Dis., 10:139-142.

Pelaez, D., Perez-Reyes, R., and Barrera, A., 1948, Estudios sobre hematozoarios. I. Plasmodium mexicanum Thompson and Huff, 1944 en sus huespedes naturales, Anal. Esc. Nac. Cienc. Biol., 5:197-215.

Pereira, N.M., Costa, S.C.G., and Sousa, M.A., 1973, Toddia sp., "corpusculo paranuclear" no sangue de Leptodactylus e Bufo de Brazil - Deseavolvimento e Citoquimica, Mem. Inst. Osw. Cruz., 71:19-31.

Pessoa, S.B., 1967, Sobre um hemoparasita do genero "Toddia" (incerta sedis) encontrado em uma serpente do Brasil "Tomodon dorsatus" (Dumeril et Bibron), Rev. Brasil, Biol., 27:391-394.

Pessoa, S.B., 1968, Sobre uma hemogregarina de Amphisbaena alba, Gaz. Med. Bahia, 68:75-78.

Pessoa, S.B., and Cavalheiro, J., 1969a, Notas sobre hemogregarinas de serpentes Brasileiras. VIII. Sobre a evolucao da "Haemogregarina miliaris" na sansuessuga "Haementeria lutzi"., Rev. Brasil Biol., 29:451-458.

Pessoa, S.B., and Cavalheiro, J., 1969b, Notas sobre hemo gregarinas de serpentes Brasileiras. IX. Sobre a hemogregarina da Helicops carinacauda (Wied), Rev. Goiana Med., 15:161-168.

Pessoa, S.B., and Cavalheiro, J., 1970, Sobre uma nova especie de Haemoproteus, parasita de uma lagartixa, Enyolius catenatus (Wied, 1821) de Sao Paulo (Brasil), Rev. Brasil Biol., 30:403-404.

Pessoa, S.B., and de Biasi, P., 1973a, Consideracoes taxonomicas sobre cistos esquizonicos e sobre gametocitos de Hepatozoon (Sporozoa, Haemogregarinidae) parasitas de serpentes Brasileiras, Mem. Inst. Butantan, 37:291-298.

Pessoa, S.B., and de Biasi, P., 1973b, Nota taxonomica sobre cistos esprorogonicos de algumas especies de Hepatozoon (Sporozoa, Haemogregarinidae) parasites de serpentes Brasileiras, Mem. Inst. Butantan, 37:299-307.

Pessoa, S.B., and Fleury, G.C., 1968, Plasmodium tomodoni sp. n. parasita da serpente Tomodon dorsatus D. and B., Rev. Brasil Biol., 28:525-530.

Pessoa, S.B., and Fleury, G.C., 1969, Duas novas especies de tripanosomas parasitas de serpentes do Brasi Rev. Brasil Biol., 29:81-86.

Pessoa, S.B., and Pimenta de Campos, E., 1966, Sobre um hemoparasita do genero "Pirhaemocyton" (Organis de afinidades incertas) encontrado em serpentes Brasileiras, Rev. Brasil Biol., 26:412-423.

Pessoa, S.B., de Biasi, P., and Puorto, G., 1974a, Nota sobre a frequencia de hemoparasitas em serpente do Brasil, Mem. Inst. Butantan, 38:69-118.

Pessoa, S.B., de Biasi, P., and Puorto, G., 1974b, Transferencia do Hepatozoon tupinambis parasita do lagarto Tupinambis teguixin, para a serpente cascavel (Crotalus durissus terrificus) por intermedio de mosquito Culex fatigans, Mem. Ins Osw. Cruz., 72:295-299.

Pessoa, S.B., Sacchetta, L., and Cavalheiro, H., 1970, Notas sobre hemogregarinas de serpentes Brasileiras. X. Hemogregarinas de Hydrodynastes giga (Dumeril et Bibron) e su evolucao, Rev. Latin Amer. Microbiol., 12:197-200.

Pessoa, S.B., Sacchetta, L., and Cavalheiro, H., 1971, Notas sobre hemogregarinas de serpentes Brasileiras. XV. Sobre uma nova especie do genero Haemogregarina (S.S.) parasita Thamnodynastes pallidus nattereri (Thomberg) e sua evolucao em mosquitoes, Rev. Latin Amer. Microbiol., 13:29-32.

Pienaar, U. de V., 1962, "Haematology of some South African reptiles," Witwatersrand Univ. Press, Johannesberg.

Pringle, G., 1960, Two new malaria parasites from East African vertebrates, Trans. Royal Soc. Trop. Med. Hyg., 54:411-414.

Prod'hon, J., 1970, Saurositus peyrierasi n. sp. Filaire parasite d'Uroplatus fimbriatus a Madagascar, Ann. Parasitol. Hum. Comp., 45:449-454.

Prod'hon, J., and Bain, O., 1972, Development larvaire chez Anopheles stephensi d'Oswaldofilaria bacillaris, Filaire de Caiman sud-americain, et redescription des adultes, Ann. Parasitol. Hum. Comp., 47:745-758.

Reichenow, E., 1910, Haemogregarina stepanowi. Die Entwidklungsgeschichte einer Hamogregarine, Arch. Protistenk., 20:251-350.

Reichenow, E., 1920, Der Entwicklungsgang der Hamococcidien Karyolysus und Schellackia nov. gen., Sitzungsb. Natur. Fr. Berlin, 10:440-442.

Reichenow, E., 1921, Die Hamoccidien der Eidechsen. Vorbermer-Kungun und I. Teil. Die Entwicklungsgeschicte von Karyolysus, Arch. Protistenk, 42: 179-291.

Riding, D., 1930, Haemoproteus of Tarentola annularis, Trans. Royal Soc. Trop. Med. Hyg., 23:635-636.

Robertson, M., 1909, Studies on Ceylon haematozoa. No. 1. The life cycle of Trypanosoma vittatae, Quart. J. Microscop. Sci., 53:665-695.

Robertson, M., 1910, Studies on Ceylon haematozoa. No. 2. Notes on the life cycle of Haemogregarina nicoriae Cast. and Willey, Quart. J. Microscop. Sci., 55:741-762.

Robin, L.A., 1936, Cycle evolutif d'um Hepatozoon de Gecko verticillatus, Ann. Inst. Pasteur Paris, 56:376-394.

Roudabush, R.L., and Coatney, G.R., 1937, On some blood protozoa of reptiles and amphibians, Trans. Amer. Microscop. Soc., 56:291-297.

Rousselot, R., 1953, Notes de parasitologie tropicale. I. Parasites du sang des Animaux, Vigot, Paris.

Saf'janova, V.M., 1966, Serological comparison of leptomonad strains isolated from sandflies with Leishmania tropica and leptomonads of reptiles, Med. Parazit. Moscow, 35:686-695.

Schacher, J.F., and Crans, W.J., 1973, Foleyella flexicauda sp. n. (Nematoda: Filaroidea) from Rana catesbeiana in New Jersey, with a review of the genus and erection of two new subgenera, J. Parasitol., 59:685-691.

Schacher, J.F., and Khalil, G.M., 1967, Foleyella philistinae sp. n. (Nematoda: Filaroidea) from the lizard, Agama stellio, in Lebanon with notes on Foleyella agamae (Rodhain, 1906), J. Parasitol., 53:763-767.

Schacher, J.F., and Khalil, G.M., 1968, Development of Foleyella philistinae Schacher and Khalil, 1967 (Nematoda: Filaroidea) in Culex pipiens molestus with notes on pathology in the arthropod, J. Parasitol., 54:869-878.

Schwetz, J., 1931a, Sur quelques hematozoaires des lezards de Stanleyville et du Lac Albert, Ann. Parasitol Hum. Comp., 9:193-201.

Schwetz, J., 1931b, Les hematozoaires des serpents de Stanleyville, Ann. Parasitol. Hum. Comp., 9: 303-310.

Schwetz, J., 1934, Sur les hematozoires de lezards de Stanleyville, (Deuxieme note), Ann. Parasitol. Hum. Comp., 12:283-285.

Scorza, J.V., 1970, Lizard malaria, Ph.D. dissertation, Univ. London.

Scorza, J.V., 1971, Anaemia in lizard malaria infections, Parassitol., 13:391-405.

Scorza, J.V., and Dagert, C., 1956, Consideraciones sobre les llamados corpusculos paranucleares. Revisio del genero Toddia Franca, 1911 con adicion de tres nueves especies, Bol. Venezuela Lab. Clin., 1:199-210.

Sergent, E., Sergent, E., Lamaire, G., and Senevet, G., 1914, Insect e transmetteur et reservoir de virus du clou de Biskra. Hypothese et experiences preliminaires, Bull. Soc. Pathol. Exot., 7:577-579.

Sergent, E., Sergent, E., Lemaire, G., and Senevet, G., 1915, Hypothese sur le phlebotome "transmetteor" et la tarente reservoir du virus du bouton d'orient, Ann. Inst. Pasteur, Paris, 29:309-322.

Shortt, H.E., 1922, Review of the position of the genus Haemocystidium (Castellani and Willey, 1904), with a description of two new species, Indian J. Med. Res., 9:814-826.

Shortt, H.E., 1962, Exo-erythrocytic schizont of Haemoproteus, parasite of the gecko Hemidactylus sp. in the liver, Trans. Royal Soc. Trop. Med. Hyg., 56:3.

Shortt, H.E., and Swaminath, C.S., 1931, Life history and morphology of Trypanosoma phlebotomi Mackie, 1914, Indian J. Med. Res., 19:541-564.

Stehbens, W.E., and Johnston, M.R.L., 1966, The viral nature of Pirhemocyton tarentolae, J. Ultrastructure Res., 15:543-554.

Sterling, C.R., and de Giusti, D.L., 1972, Ultrastructural aspects of schizogny, mature schizonts and merozoites of Haemoproteus metchnikovi, J. Parasitol., 58:641-652.

Sterling, C.R., and de Giusti, D.L., 1974, Fine structure of differentiating oocysts and mature sporozoites of Haemoproteus metchnikovi in its intermediate host Chrysops callidus, J. Protozool., 21:276-283.

Sulahian, A., and Schacher, J.F., 1968, Brygoofilaria agamae gen. et, sp. n. (Nematoda: Filarioidea) from the lizard Agama stellio in Lebannon, J. Parasitol., 54:831-833.

Svahn, K., 1974, Incidence of blood parasites of the genus Karyolysus (Coccidia) in Scandinavian lizards, Oikos, 25:43-53.

Svahn, K., 1975, Blood parasites of the genus Karyolysus (Coccidia, Adeleidae) in Scandinavian lizards. Description and life cycle, Norwegian J. Zool., 23:277-295.

Telford, S.R., Jr., 1965a, Some observations on the effects of varying ambient temperatures in vivo on filarial worms of snakes, Japan J. Exp. Med., 35:291-300.

Telford, S.R., Jr., 1965b, A study of filariasis in Mexican snakes, Japan J. Exp. Med., 35:565-586.

Telford, S.R., Jr., 1967, Parasitology of the seasnake Laticauda semifasciata in the vicinity of Amami Island, Japan, Japan J. Exp. Med., 37:245-256.

Telford, S.R., Jr., 1969, A new saurian malarial parasite Plasmodium balli from Panama, J. Protozool., 16:431-437.

Telford, S.R., Jr., 1970a, Plasmodium chiricahuae sp. nov. from Arizona lizards, J. Protozool., 17:400-405.

Telford, S.R., Jr., 1970b, A comparative study of endoparasitism among some southern California lizard populations, Amer. Midland Natur., 83:516-554.

Telford, S.R., Jr., 1970c, Saurian malarial parasites in eastern Panama, J. Protozool., 17:566-574.

Telford, S.R., Jr., 1972, The course of infection of Japanese saurian malaria (Plasmodium sasai Telford and Ball) in natural and experimental hosts, Japan J. Exp. Med., 42:1-21.

Telford, S.R., Jr., 1973, Saurian malarial parasites from Guyana: Their effect upon the validity of the family Garniidae and the genus Garnia, with descriptions of two new species, Int. J. Parasitol., 3:829-842.

Telford, S.R., Jr., 1974a, The malarial parasites of Anolis species (Sauria: Iguanidae) in Panama, Int. J. Parasitol., 4:91-102.

Telford, S.R., Jr., 1974b, Zoogeographic patterns of New World saurian malaria in relation to the vector problem, Proc. 3rd Int. Congr. Parasitol., 1: 83-84.

Telford, S.R., Jr., 1975, Saurian malaria in the Caribbean Plasmodium azurophilum sp. nov., a malaria parasite with schizogony and gametogony in both red and white cells, Int. J. Parasitol., 5:383-394.

Telford, S.R., Jr., 1977, The distribution, incidence and general ecology of saurian malaria in Middle America, Int. J. Parasitol., 7:299-314.

Telford, S.R., Jr., 1978a, Intralymphocytic schizonts associated with an initial infection of Saurocytozoon tupinambi in Tupinambis teguixin, Int. J. Parasitol., 8:133-138.

Telford, S.R., Jr., 1978b, Saurian malaria in Texas, J. Parasitol., 64:553-554.

Telford, S.R., Jr., 1978c, A haemoparasite survey of Florida lizards, J. Parasitol., 64:1126-1127.

Telford, S.R., Jr., 1978d, The saurian malarias of Venezuela: Haemosporidian parasites of gekkonid lizards, Int. J. Parasitol., 8:341-353.

Telford, S.R., Jr., 1979a, A taxonomic reconsideration of some Plasmodium species from iguanid lizards, Ann. Parasitol. Hum. Comp., 54:129-144.

Telford, S.R., Jr., 1979b, Evolutionary implications of Leishmania amastigotes in circulating blood cells of lizards, Parasitology, 79:317-324.

Telford, S.R., Jr., 1979c, Two new trypanosomes from Neotropical gekkonid lizards, J. Parasitol., 65: 898-901.

Telford, S.R., Jr., 1980, The saurian malarias of Venezuela: Plasmodium species from iguanid and teiid hosts, Int. J. Parasitol., 10:365-374.

Telford, S.R., Jr., and Ball, G.H., 1969, Plasmodium sasai n. sp. from the Japanese lizard Takydromus tachydromoides, J. Protozool., 16:312-317.

Thompson, P.E., 1944, Changes associated with acquired immunity during initial infections in saurian malaria, J. Infect. Dis., 74:138-150.

Thompson, P.E., 1946a, Effects of quinine on saurian malarial parasites, J. Infect. Dis., 78:160-166.

Thompson, P.E., 1946b, The effects of atabrine on the saurian malarial parasite, Plasmodium floridense, J. Infect. Dis., 79:282-288.

Thompson, P.E., and Huff, C.G., 1944a, A saurian malarial parasite, Plasmodium mexicanum, n. sp., with both elongatum and gallinaceum-types of exoerythrocytic stages, J. Infect. Dis., 74:48-67.

Thompson, P.E., and Huff, C.G., 1944b, Saurian malarial parasites of the United States and Mexico, J. Infect. Dis., 81:68-79.

Thompson, P.E., and Winder, V., 1947, Analysis of saurian malarial infections as influenced by temperature, J. Infect. Dis., 81:84-95.

Uilenberg, G., and Blanc, Ch.P., 1966, Note sur un Hematozoaire d'un Reptile malgache, Uroplatus fimbriatus (Gekkonidae): Sauroplasma sp. (Protozoa incertae sedis), Ann. Parasitol. Hum. Comp., 41:209-212.

Wang, C.C., and Hopkins, S.H., 1965, Haemogregarina and Haemoproteus (Protozoa: Sporozoa) in blood of Texas freshwater turtles, J. Parasitol., 51: 682-683.

Wenyon, C.M., 1926, "Protozoology," Vols I and II, Bailliere, Tindall and Cox, London.

Woo, P.T.K, 1969, The life cycle of Trypanosoma chrysemydis, Canadian J. Zool., 47:1139-1151.

Wood, S.F., 1935, Variations in the cytology of the blood of geckos (Tarentola mauritanica) infected with Haemogregarina platydactyli, Trypanosoma platydactyli and Pirhemocyton tarentolae, Univ. California Publ. Zool., 41:9-22.

Wood, S.F., and Wood, F.D., 1936, Occurrence of haematozoa in some California cold-blooded vertebrates, J. Parasitol., 22:518-520.

Yamaguti, S., 1961, "Systema Helminthum, Vol. 3. The nematodes of vertebrates," Interscience Publ. Inc., New York.

Yap, L.F., Fredericks, H.J., and Omar, I., 1967, A new host for Plasmodium minasense Carini and Rudolph, 1912, Med. J. Malaya, 21:369.

Zuckerman, A., and Lainson, R., 1977, Leishmania, in: "Parasitic protozoa," Vol. 1, J.P. Kreier, ed., Academic Press, New York.

Zwart, P., 1964, Intraepithelial protozoan, Klossiella boae n. sp., in the kidneys of a boa constrictor, J. Protozool., 11:261-263.

NEOPLASIA IN REPTILES

Samuel V. Machotka, II

Hazleton Laboratories America, Inc.

Vienna, Virginia

INTRODUCTION

Neoplasia, though still not thoroughly understood, has been of medical importance since the beginning of recorded history and, undoubtedly, before that. Cancer in man presently ranks as the second largest killer, lagging only behind cardiovascular disease. As a consequence of its obvious impact on human life, millions of dollars and countless research hours have been dedicated to determining causes, treatments and preventions for this dread disease. This interest has spilled over into the comparative study of neoplastic disease in the higher vertebrates. Until the last 50 years, however, cold-blooded vertebrates were neglected in such investigative studies even though more than a century and a half ago the question of brute creatures being subject to diseases resembling cancer in man was posed (Baillie et al., 1806). The fear and disgust for reptiles was documented with Adam and Eve and has been perpetuated to this day, probably contributing to the paucity of studies in reptilian diseases. In addition, there had been a general misconception that reptiles were not susceptible to most forms of neoplasia as it occurs in man. Contrary to that belief are the now numerous reports of neoplasia in reptiles that cover the spectrum of those occuring in man and other warm-blooded vertebrates. As the Book of Ecclesiastes states, "There is no new thing under the sun".

To dispel some of the disquieting thoughts conjured up by a statement attributed to Mark Twain that "There is something fascinating about science. One gets such a wholesale return of conjecture out of such a trifling investment of fact.", a thorough approach to the discussion of neoplasia in reptiles has been prepared.

In order to accomplish this task the subject matter is presented in the following categories. First, a brief historical overview of the applicable literature is described so the reader may appreciate the strides that have been made and see where contributions are needed. Second, review terminology and definitions used by the pathologist and outline methods for classifying neoplastic lesions. Third, present published studies relative to the etiology, transmission and experimental iduction of reptilian neoplasia. Fourth, assemble a current review, by taxonomic/systemic distribution, of the available literature and cases submitted to the Registery for Tumors in Lower Animals (RTLA), Smithsonian Institution, Washington, D.C., and the Registry of Veterinary Pathology, Armed Forces Institute of Pathology (AFIP), Washington, D.C. Fifth, point out diagnostic methods and potential approaches to treatment.

HISTORICAL BACKGROUND

When reviewing the progress of fish pathology in this century, the well-known specialist in fish diseases, Dr. Snieszko stated "anyone expecting to find there is a wealth of publications on fish pathology more than 100 years old will be disappointed" (Mawdesley-Thomas, 1975). If this statement were applied to reptilian pathology and in particular reptilian neoplasia, one would have to think in terms of 25 to 50 years. The earliest published report occurred late in the 19th century (Bland-Sutton, 1885). Since that time, individual cases surfaced in the literature until a voluminous report was prepared on "Tumors of Fishes, Amphibians, and Reptiles" (Schlumberger and Lucke, 1948) in which the authors listed and reviewed eight neoplasms in turtles, two in crocodiles, six in lizards and ten in snakes. The same authors, one year later, published a paper in which they proposed to "first, summarize existing knowledge concerning the occurrence, the varieties, and the behavior of tumors in fishes, amphibians, and reptiles; second, to give a brief account of tumors which have proved favorable material for studies upon neoplasia; and third, to discuss the lines of investigation which have been persued" (Lucke and Schlumberger, 1949). In that paper, previously reported reptilian neoplasms were tabulated and attempts at transplantation of a squamous cell carcinoma from a lizard and melanomas from two pythons were described. One of these authors, sometime later, reported on tumors characteristic for certain animal species (Schlumberger, 1957) in which a short paragraph dealt primarily with papillomas of the green sea turtle, Chelonia mydas. In "The prinicipal diseases of lower vertebrates", a section on tumors was presented in the chapter dealing with non-parasitic and environmental diseases (Reichenbach-Klinke and Elkan, 1965). Shortly thereafter, a paper on "Diseases of captive reptiles" listed neoplasms which occurred in 10 of 1,249 reptiles from the Philadelphia Zoological Garden (Cowan, 1968). More recently, chapters in two books presented overviews of published and unpublished cases (Billups and Harshbarger, 1976; Harshbarger, 1978a). And finally, a complete review of selected cases along with other pertinent material on neoplasia in reptiles has been prepared (Jacobson, 1981).

Reports dealing solely with Serpentes include a review of reported cases and a description of two previously unreported cases (Wadsworth, 1954a), and a subsequent paper by the same author listing previous cases and describing six new cases (Wadsworth, 1956). Ten years later a review of diseases and infections of snakes failed to present any previously unreported cases (Page, 1966). Lastly, a report of a probable mesothelioma in a rattlesnake, Crotalus horridus, and a tabulation of earlier cases was presented (Machotka and Whitney, 1980).

A few reports indicated the numbers of animals that were examined and of those the number with neoplastic lesions. Peyron (1939) disected 4,000 snakes, none of which had a tumor. Bergman (1941) reported 1 of 2,200 free-ranging snakes with a growth, while Ippen (1972) necropsied 1,500 reptiles and found 3 turtles, 2 lizards and 2 snakes with neoplasms. Finally, an extensive tabulation of 28 of 1,233 reptiles with neoplasms was prepared (Effron et al., 1977).

Papers discussing neoplasia in specific organs or organ systems are available. One of the earliest reports was that of Ratcliffe (1943) in which the author described numerous snakes representing at least ten species with pancreatic lesions characterized by abortive hyperplastic regeneration of acinar tissue following unexplained necrosis. In advanced cases he felt these lesions to be adenocarcinomas. Subsequent papers by Schlumberger and Lucke (1948) and by Cowan (1968) related that these lesions were reevaluated as idiopathic, atypical regenerative hyperplasia. Another paper considered the oral neoplasms with a section denoting attempts to transplant portions of squamous cell carcinoma from a tegu, Tupinambi sp., and melanomas from a reticulated python, Python reticulatus (Schlumberger, 1953).

Some fifteen years later in a review of neoplasms of blood cell origin in poikilothermic animals, Dawe (1969) reported the lack of leukemias, leukoses or reticular neoplasms of any sort in reptiles. Shortly thereafter, at a workshop on comparative pathology of hemopoietic and lymphoreticular neoplasms, cases of lymphoid leukemia in C. horridus and reticulum cell sarcoma in a hognose snake, Heterodon platyrhinos, were presented (Dawe and Berard, 1971). It could finally be stated that proliferative disorders morphologically comparable to leukemias and lymphomas in man had been identified in animals of every vertebrate class.

Researchers with interest in the causative aspects of neoplasia have explored reptilian neoplasia as it relates to a possible viral etiology. The discovery that the Schmidt-Ruppin strain of Rous sarcoma virus produced sarcomas in turtles and serpents (Svet-Moldavsky et al., 1967) stimulated the attempts and success in finding "C" type virus particles in spleen-derived cell cultures from a Russell's viper, Vipera russelli, with a myxofibroma (Ziegel and Clark, 1969).

To facilitate the comparative study of tumorigenesis and related disorders in invertebrate and poikilothermic vertebrate animals, The Registry of Tumors in Lower Animals, Smithsonian Institution, Washington, D.C., was established in 1965. The registry provides a collection point for submissions from cases of neoplasia in lower animals. The purpose and functions of the Registry were presented at a symposium on neoplasms and related disorders of invertebrate and lower vertebrate animals (Harshbarger, 1969). It is from this Registry that all materials presented in Figs. 21.1 to 21.18 were derived.

TERMINOLOGY AND CLASSIFICATION

The study of things caused must be appropriately defined and classified. Pathology (as derived from two Greek words, pathos--suffering, disease, and logos--discourse, treatise, expressing in a general way "the study of") may be broadly defined as the study of disease which represents the response by the host to a noxious agent, whether it be physical, chemical, biological or unknown. Comparative pathology then is the pathology of diseases of animals, especially in relation to human pathology, and comparative oncology being, specifically, the study of neoplasia in a comparative way. Neoplasia or, more properly "neoplasm", as defined by the Shorter Oxford Dictionary in 1864, was "a new formation of tissue in some part of the body; a tumor". Since then, numerous authorities have attempted to delineate what a tumor is and have failed. Willis (1967), however, formed the following definition to which most pathologists will subscribe: A tumor is an abnormal mass of tissue, the growth of which exceeds and is uncoordinated with that of the normal tissues, and persists in the same excessive manner after cessation of the stimuli which evoked the change.

Tumor classification and nomenclature is largely based on the fact that in most tumors the neoplastic cells are derived from a single kind of tissue. On the other hand, a few tumors consist of two or more kinds of neoplastic tissue and are named accordingly. This may be called the histogenic method of classification and according to Willis (1967) include the following groups: Group 1 or the tumors of epithelial tissues; Group 2 or tumors of non-hemopoietic mesenchymal tissues; Group 3 or tumors of hemopoietic tissues; Group 4 or tumors of neural tissues; and, Group 5 or special classes of tumors, e.g., melanomas and embryonic tumors of viscera. In lower vertebrates, Group 5 also should contain several tumors of pigmented cells or chromatophores having no domestic animal or human counterpart. Chromatophores are named after the color of the pigment which they contain so black/brown pigment-bearing cells are melanophores, yellow/orange pigment-bearing cells are xanthophores, and orange/red pigment-bearing cells are erythrophores (Alexander and Fahrenbach, 1969). Since all of these cells arise from the neural crest (Bagnara and Hadley, 1973), neoplasms of these cells have been included in this text under the heading of Nervous System/Pigment Cells.

Two difficulties arise in classifying neoplasm histogenically since there is: 1) a lack of exactness in the histological classification and naming of normal tissues as is demonstrated in naming tumors arising from coelomic lining cells i.e., carcinoma, endothelioma, mesothelioma and serosal epithelioma; and, 2) uncertainty regarding the tissues of origin of some kinds of tumors, examples being ovarian tumors and teratomas. Furthermore, it is necessary to have another method of grouping neoplasms which will have more practical value.

This method is designated "behvioristic" classification and refers to the "innocence" or malignancy of a tumor. It may generally be said that innocent or benign tumors cause no harm to their host except by virtue of their position or some accidental complication whereas malignant tumors or "cancer" inevitably prove fatal. Between these two extremes in clinical manifestations are gradations which may only be detectable microscopically. Microscopic criteria used in determining the biologic behavior of neoplasms, though by no means iron-clad, include: 1) the degree of anaplasia or morphologic deviation as neoplastic cells cease to resemble their parent tissue; 2) the rate and mode of growth as by expansion in most benign tumors or by invasion, implantation or metastasis (distant spread via vascular system) in malignant tumors; 3) the mitotic index or frequency of mitoses and more importantly the presence of abnormal appearing mitotic figures in malignancies.

Gross features of benign masses include polypoid or pedunculated appearance, distinct fibrous capsule, etc., while malignant masses may appear sessile or cause ulceration and hemorrhage. Gross determination of innocence or malignance is, however, subject to various pitfalls and should be confirmed or refuted by microscopic examination of the neoplasm.

A classification scheme based on the histogenic and behavioristic characteristics of particular neoplasms has resulted in the ensuing terminology. Most benign tumors are classified by naming the cell from which they arose and adding the suffix "-oma" as in adenoma from glandular tissue, fibroma from fibrous tissue, chondroma from cartilagenous tissue, etc. Most malignant epithelially-derived neoplasms are named by adding the suffix "-carcinoma" as in adenocarcinoma, or simply naming the cell from which it arose followed by carcinoma as in squamous cell carcinoma. Malignant neoplasms derived from mesenchymal tissue or its derivatives are called sarcomas and are named accordingly. Combinations of these classifications do occur and are termed mixed or compound.

ETIOLOGY

Much work has been done and many papers published concerning the cause of neoplasia in man and animals. More than twenty-five years ago, Stolk (1953) stated that "with regard to the aetiology one can divide the malignant tumours in three groups: (1) tumours dependent on genetic and stimulation factors; (2) tumours dependent on genetic factors but not, or only slightly, dependent on stimulation factors; (3) tumours dependent on stimulation factors but not, or only slightly dependent on genetic factors". Genetic factors will be discussed to include genetic, phylogenetic and immunologic factors. The stimulation factors will include pollutants, pesticides and other chemicals in the environment, oncogenic viruses and parasites.

Genetic factors

Whether one of the recognized carcinogens actually produces a tumor depends on the relative susceptability not only of the individual, but of the organ or tissue in question (Smith et al., 1972). To that statement, two neoplasms which are known to have a genetic basis (Hill and Lin, 1977) are basal cell nevus and xeroderma pigmentosum of man. The latter is a hereditarily recessive disease that is due to sensitivity to light; a dermatitis progressing to terminal cancer occurs.

In poikilothermic vertebrates, the undeniable evidence for a primary genetic influence on the development of neoplasia is presented in the form of melanomas in fish, Xiphophorus sp. (Sobel et al., 1975). In addition, it has been reported that male sex hormones appear to augment the development of melanomas in these fish (Siciliano et al., 1971). There has not been documented, however, a neoplasm in reptiles strongly influenced by genetic factors.

It has been concluded by some immunologists that there is a basic relationship between the evolution of the host immune system and the occurrence or progression of neoplasia (Good and Finstad, 1969). Precisely what this relationship is has not been determined though it has been suggested as a partial explanation for the low incidence of neoplasia in more primitive vertebrates with a less sophisticated immune system. This concept seems paradoxical in that development of neoplasia in higher vertebrates is often related to a compromised or incompetent immune system. In concert with this concept are statistical studies which have shown lymphocytes in tumors are an indication of longer patient survival (Smith et al., 1972).

Environmental factors

Discussion of environmental factors may seem inappropriate in that there has been a dearth of neoplasms reported in free-ranging reptiles suggesting that the "wild" or natural environment has little influence on the development of neoplasia in reptiles. Alternative explanations for this observation have been put forth. It serves no purpose to discuss these explanations for they are, so far, purely speculative. That various polluted environments containing carcinogens, whether in the wild or in captivity, do exist cannot be challenged. Nor can the fact that other poikilothermic vertebrates, namely fish and amphibians from highly polluted waters, have been found with cutaneous and oral neoplasms (Lucke and Schlumberger, 1941; Rose and Harshbarger, 1977; Russell and Kotin, 1957).

As previously discussed, sun light has a promoting influence on the development of cancer in people with the heredirary disease xeroderm pigmentosum. A study using the lizard, Lacerta agilis, described the development of hyperkeratosis and carcinoma planocellulare (squamous cell carcinoma) in these animals after they were deprived of sun light for several months (Stolk, 1953). The author attempted to explain this curious twist by hypothesizing man, who is not normally exposed to intensive radiation, may be affected by carcinoma planocellulare, according to the current opinion, in consequence of an excess of light while the same affect occurs in the light-dominated lizard, on the other hand, by too small an amount. Though the author hoped to return to this problem later on additional papers addressing this condition were not found The same author did, however, publish a paper in which he produced cutaneous papillomas on adult female L. agilis by applying a single dose of dimethyl benzanthrocene in acetone to the skin (Stolk, 1963).

Oncogenic viruses

Great detail could be gone into concerning the history and classification of oncogenic viruses. Suffice it to say that the relatively recent interest in viral oncology has resulted in numerous publications relative to this topic. A reasonable overview of the material can be found in pathology texts (Cheville, 1976; Smith et al., 1972). Briefly, without attempting to define much of the subject material, the status of viral oncology as it relates to neoplasia in reptiles will be presented below.

The tumor-producing capabilities of viruses were established early in this century with the discovery that fowl leukosis and fowl sarcoma were caused by RNA viruses (Ellermann and Bang, 1908; Rous, 1910). Further evidence of virally induced neoplasia has progressed slowly but continually. Most of these discoveries were of neoplasia induced by RNA oncornaviruses. These cause cancer in three classes of vertebrates; mammals, birds and reptiles. The pathogenicity and oncogenicity of the Rous or chicken sarcoma virus (Schmidt-Ruppin) for Testudo horsfieldi and Eryx tataricus was first reported by Svet-Moldavsky et al. (1967). Shortly thereafter, this virus was shown to have oncogenic properties in lizards (Veskova et al., 1970) and extended to include additional reptilian species (Trubcheninova et al., 1977).

Previous to these later reports, cultured spleen cells from a V. russelli with a naturally occurring edematous myxofibroma were found to contain a "C" type RNA virus (Zeigel and Clark, 1969) whose biophysical, biological and immunological properties were subsequently studied (Gilden, 1970). The original authors further studied the light and electron microscopic features of the viper spleen derived cell line, concluding that these cells did represent metastatic cells from the primary myxofibroma (Zeigel and Clark, 1971). DNA polymerase (reverse transcriptase), an enzyme thought to be necessary for RNA viruses to induce neoplasia, were found to be a feature of the reptilian type "C" RNA virus (Hatanaka et al., 1970; Twardzik et al., 1974). A "C" type RNA virus also has been demonstrated in cells of an embryonal rhabdomyosarcoma from a corn snake, Elaphe guttata (Lunger et al., 1974).

Among DNA viruses, only herpesviruses have been associated with naturally-occurring neoplasms. More than forty years ago it was found that the renal adenocarcinoma of frogs are virally induced (Lucke, 1938a). Other herpes viruses known to cause or be associated with cancer include Marek's virus disease of chickens, Herpes sairmiri of marmosets and monkeys, and Epstein-Barr herpesvirus of man. Reports of DNA oncogenic viruses associated with neoplasms in reptiles have not yet surfaced.

Parasites

Metazoan parasites have been documented as causes of neoplasia in man (Shistomsoma hematobium, a blood fluke causing carcinoma of the urinary bladder) (Brand, 1975), in rats (Crysticercus fasciolaris causing sarcomatous proliferation in the liver) (Bullock and Curtis, 1920; Dunning, 1946; Dunning and Curtis, 1939), and the dog (Spirocerca lupi causing esophageal fibrosarcomas and osteosarcomas with metastasis to the lung and other viscera) (Seibold et al., 1955). It has not been determined how much of their effect is due to physical or chemical influence. There have been no confirmed cases of parasite induced neoplasia in reptiles though the presence of leeches, Ozobranchus branchiatus (Nigrelli, 1942; Nigrelli and Smith, 1943), and blood flukes, Distom constricum, and their ova have been associated with the fibropapillomas of the sea turtle C. mydras (Smith et al. 1941). A papillomatous change in the gallbladder associated with trematodes in these turtles (Smith et al., 1941) and papillary bile duct carcinoma in a snake, Homalopsis buccata, associated with a trematode (Bergman, 1941) have been reported.

SPONTANEOUSLY OCCURRING NEOPLASIA

The ensuing paragraphs are descriptive lists of selected spontaneously occurring neoplasms in reptiles briefly separated by taxonomic distribution, e.g., turtles (Chelonia), crocodilians (Crocodilia), lizards (Squamata; Lacertilia), snakes (Squamata; Serpentes) and described by systemic distribution, e.g., cardiovascular, digestive, endocrine, hemic and lymphatic, integumentary, musculo-skeletal, nervous/pigment cell, reproductive, respiratory, urinary, so that those having a more traditional pathology background may quickly scan the text for previously documented cases by system. For those more traditional biologists and zoologists the neoplasms have been segregated by the taxonomic classification of the reptile in which they occurred (Tables 21.1-21.4).

The lack of primary central nervous system and rarity of peripheral nervous system neoplasms, the paucity of reproductive system cancer and the abundance of cutaneous lesions especially in turtles and lizards should be pointe out. No doubt these observations reflect previously incomplete necropsy techniques which, with improved gross followed by microscopic evaluation of all tissues, will be altered.

Turtles

Cardiovascular system. The ruptured heart of a Sternotherus niger, "was converted into a soft whitish growth full of very large multinucleated cells" (Plimmer, 1913). A diagnosis of rhabdomyoma was subsequently put forth due to the presence of multinucleate cells and the lack of a similar mass elsewhere (Schlumberger and Lucke, 1948).

Digestive system. A male African soft-shelled tortoise, Malacochersus tornieri, with adenomatous proliferation of the intrahepatic bile ducts (Effron et al., 1977) and papillomas in the gallbladder associated with trematodes, Rhytidoides similis, in C. mydras have been reported (Smith et al., 1941).

A "glandular cancer in the stomach of a tortoise" was reported by Plimmer (1912). A gross description later published, identified the animal as Geochelone elaphantopus in which "there was a large mass, 8 X 5 inches, of new growth springing from the mucosa of the stomach which was very red and swollen" (Scott and Beattie, 1927). The growth was white in color and gelatinous in texture. Microscopic findings were not recorded. A more recent report listed this mass as an adenocarcinoma (Schlumberger and Lucke, 1948). Another gastric carcinoma was described in a black sidenecked turtle, Pelusios subniger, with renal metastasis (Cowan, 1968).

Endocrine system. Parathyroid adenoma was diagnosed in an immature, male South African red-footed tortoise, G. carbonaria, which was presented for examination because

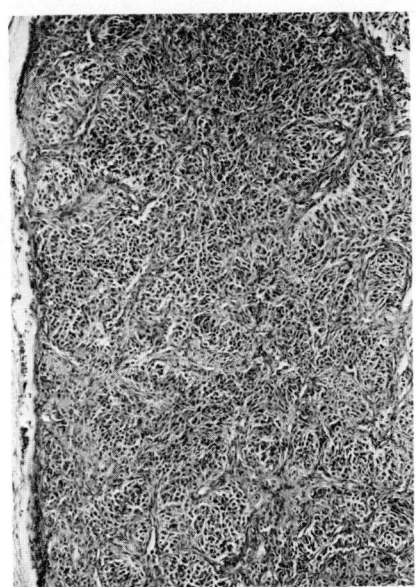

Fig. 21.1. Red-footed tortoise, Geochelone carbonaria, parathyroid adenoma (RLTA 970), contains relatively uniform cells with small, round nuclei and scanty cytoplasm separated into small packets by fibrovascular stroma. H&E X100

Table 21.1. Neoplasms in Turtles (Chelonia).

Taxonomic classification	Neoplasm	Reference
Cheloniidae		
Chelonia mydas	Papillomas, fibromas, fibropapillomas	Lucke, 1938b; Nigrelli, 1942; Nigrelli and Smith, 1943; Smith and Coates, 1938, 1939; Smith et al., 1941; RTLA 12, 121, 651, 1767, 1774, 1856, 1883 and 2097
Chelydridae		
Sternotherus niger	Possible rhabdomyoma	Plimmer, 1913
S. odoratus	Papilloma	Schlumberger and Lucke, 1948
Testudunidae		
Chrysemys picta	Thyroid carcinoma	Ippen, 1972; RTLA 718
C. scripta elegans	Myelogenous leukemia	Frye and Carney, 1972
C. emmys sp.	Verrucal papillomatosis	RTLA 1388
Emys orbicularis	Squamous cell carcinoma	Billups and Harshbarger, 1976; AFIP Registry
	Fibroadenoma, lung	Bresler, 1963
Geochelone carbonaria	Parathyroid adenoma	Frye and Carney, 1975; RTLA 970
G. elephantopus	Carcinoma of stomach	Plimmer, 1912
G. emys	Hematopoietic cell neoplasm	RTLA 1879 and 1880
Malacochersus tornieri	Adenomatous proliferation of bile ducts	Effron et al., 1977
Melanochelys trijuga	Thyroid carcinoma, squamous cell carcinoma (foot)	Cowan, 1968

Terrapene carolina	Renal adenocarcinoma	Ippen, 1972; RTLA 716
Testudo hermanii	Lymphoblastic lymphosarcoma	Ippen, 1972; RTLA 717
T. horsfieldi	Fibroadenoma of lung	Zsvetaeva (cited in Finkelstein, 1944)
Trionychidae		
Trionyx ferox	Lyphoreticular neoplasm	RTLA 654
Chelydae		
Phrynops geoffroanus	Thyroid adenoma	Pick and Poll, 1903
Pelomedusidae		
Pelomedusa subrufa	Myelongenous leukemia	RTLA 1206
Pleusios subniger	Gastric carcinoma	Cowan, 1968

Table 21.2. Neoplasms in Crocodilians (Crocodilia).

Taxonomic classification	Neoplasm	Reference
Alligatoridae		
Alligator mississip- piensis	Seminoma, wart-like growth	Wadsworth and Hill, 1956
Crocodylidae		
Crocodylus acutus	Lipoma or fat storage disease	RTLA 1241
C. porosus	Round cell sarcoma	Scott and Beattie, 1927
	Bony tumors	Kalin, 1937
Crocodylus sp.	Warts	Hansemann (cited in Schlumberger and Lucke, 1948)

Table 21.3. Neoplasms in Lizards (Squamata; Lacertilia).

Taxonomic classification	Neoplasm	Reference
Agamidae		
Hydrosaurus amboinensis	Lymphoblastic lymphoma	Zwart and Harshbarger, 1972; RTLA 291
	Plasma cell tumor	Schmidt, 1977
Uromastix acanthinurus	Lymphosarcoma	Effron et al., 1977
Chamaelenotidae		
Chamaeleo dilepis	Hepatoma	RTLA 462
Cordylidae		
Cordylus polyzonus	Thyroid adenoma	RTLA 633
Helodermatidae		
Heloderma suspectum	Squamous cell carcinoma	Schlumberger (cited in Reichenbach-Klinke and Elkan, 1965)
	Melanoma	Cooper, 1968
Iguanidae		
Anolis carolinensis	Reticulum cell sarcoma	Frye and Dutra, 1974
Basiliscus plumifrons	Fibrosarcoma	RTLA 2069
Cyclura cornuta	Chondro-osteo-fibroma	Rodhain, 1949
C. ricordi	Biliary adenoma	Effron et al., 1977
Iguana iguana	Hepatoma	Stolk, 1964
	Adenocarcinoma arising in a teratoma	RTLA 460
	Lymphoma	RTLA 1385
	Myxoma	RTLA 2073
Lacertidae		
Lacerta agilis	Papilloma	Koch, 1904
	Carcinoma planocellulare	Stolk, 1953

(contd.)

Table 21.3. Neoplasms in Lizards (Squamata; Lactertilia). (Continued)

Taxonomic classification	Neoplasm	Reference
L. muralis	Papilloma	Heller (cited in Schlumberger and Lucke, 1948); Raynaud and Adrian, 1976
L. sicula	Lymphoma, malignant	Lawson, 1962
	Fibrosarcoma/mesenchymosarcoma	Elkan and Cooper, 1976; RTLA 1069
L. viridis	Papilloma	Plehm, 1911; RTLA 482, 1821, and 1917
	Papillomatosis	RTLA 1389 and 1524
	Multiple osteomas	Stolk, 1958
Scincidae		
Eumeces fasciatus	Hepatocarcinoma	Ippen, 1972
Teiidae		
Calopistes maculatus	Renal neoplasm	Hill, 1952
Tupinambis nigropunctatus	Squamous cell carcinoma	Schlumberger and Lucke, 1948
T. rufescens	Parotid carcinoma	Bland-Sutton, 1885
T. teguixin	Hepatoma	Ippen, 1972; RTLA 720
	Squamous cell carcinoma	Schwarz, 1923
Varanidae		
Varanus bengalensis	Lymphoblastic leukemia	RTLA 1499
V. dracoena	Enchondroma	Bland-Sutton, 1885
V. komodoensis	Islet cell tumor, colonic pancreas; carcinoma; metastatic, adenocarcinoma, spleen; pheochromo-	RTLA 1166

	cytoma; multiple follicular adenoma, thyroid; cystic interstitial cell tumor, testis	
V. niloticus	Plasma cell tumor	RTLA 635
V. salvator	Lymphosarcoma	Ippen, 1972; Zwart and Harshbarger, 1972; RTLA 461, 719
Varanus sp.	Osteosarcoma	Frye, 1973

Table 21.4. Neoplasms in Snakes (Squamata; Serpentes).

Taxonomic classification	Neoplasm	Reference
Acrochordiae		
Acrochordus javanicus	Ovarian fibroma	RTLA 532
Boidae		
Constrictor constrictor	Lymphatic leukemia	Frye and Carney, 1973
	Fibrosarcoma	Frye and Dutra, 1973; RTLA 588
	Epidermal papilloma	RTLA 498
	Renal adenocarcinoma	RTLA 1242
	Mesenteric adenocarcinoma; myocardial rhabdomyosarcoma	Elkan and Cooper, 1976
	Anitschkow myocyte tumor	RTLA 1115
	Lipoma	RTLA 1823
	Melanoma, malignant, epitheliod type, amelanotic	RTLA 2070
	Adenomatous polyp, gastric mucosa	Wadsworth, 1956
Eunectes murinus	Lymphosarcoma	Frank and Schepky, 1969
	Granulosa cell tumor	Effron et al., 1977
	Adenoameloblastoma	Kast, 1967; RTLA 441
	Lymphoid leukosis	Finnie, 1972
	Fibroma	Idowu et al., 1975
Python molurus	Intraoral carcinoma	Wilhelm and Emswiller, 1977; AFIP Registry
	Lymphoma, malignant	RTLA 1600

P. m. molurus	Adenocarcinoma, meta- static, liver	AFIP Registry
P. reticulatus	Melanoma, malignant	Schlumberger and Lucke, 1948; AFIP Registry
	Melanoma, non-malignant	Schlumberger and Lucke, 1948; AFIP Registry
	Cloacal transitional cell carcinoma	AFIP Registry
P. sebae	Lymphoma, malignant	RTLA 1960
	Ovarian adenocarcinoma	Bland-Sutton, 1885
	Cystic adenoma, stomach	Vaillant and Pettit, 1902
	Fibroma	Effron et al., 1977
Colubridae		
Arizona elegans occidentalis	Pheochromocytoma	Effron et al., 1977
Dispholidus typus	Biliary adenoma; hepatic hemangioma	Effron et al., 1977
Elaphe guttata	Cloacal carcinoma	Smith and Betz, 1965
	Chondrosarcoma	RTLA 465
	Embryonal rhabdomyo- sarcoma	Lunger et al., 1974
E. obsoleta obsoleta	Intestinal hemagnio- adenocarcinoma	Wadsworth, 1956
	Undifferentiated sarcoma	AFIP Registry
E. o. quadrivittata	Transitional cell carci- noma, oral	RTLA 1937
	Melanoma, malignant	Elkan, 1974; RTLA 507
E. o. rossalleni	Fibroma	Wadsworth, 1956
E. o. spiloides	Cloacal sarcoma	Wadsworth, 1954b
Heterodon nasicus	Lymphosarcoma	Cowan, 1968
H. platyrhinos	Reticulum cell carcinoma	Snyder (cited in Dawe and Berard, 1971); RTLA 664
Homalopsis buccata	Papillary bile duct, carcinoma	Bergman, 1941 (contd.)

Table 21.4. Neoplasms in Snakes (Squamata; Serpentes). (Continued)

Taxonomic classification	Neoplasm	Reference
Lampropelitis getulus	Lymphosarcoma	RTLA 2235
	Adenocarcinoma	Ratcliffe, 1953
L. g. californiae	Undifferentiated sarcoma	RTLA 478
	Squamoid adenocarcinoma, tracheal	Hill, 1977; RTLA 1835
	Lymphosarcoma	Jacobson et al., 1980; RTLA 1770
Masticophis flagellum testaceus	Adenocarcinoma, abdominal	Ball (cited in Wadsworth, 1954a)
Natrix natrix	Renal adenocarcinoma	Patay, 1933
N. stolata	Hemangioendothelioma	Ippen, 1972; RTLA 722
Pituophis melanoleucus	Melanoma, malignant, rhabdomyoma	Ball, 1946; AFIP Registry
	Abdominal sarcoma	Cowan, 1968
	Serosal sarcoma	Ratcliffe, 1953
	Iridophoroma, malignant	RTLA 2131
	Xanthoma	RTLA 1955
	Fibroblastic sarcoma	RTLA 1400; AFIP Registry
	Colonic adenocarcinoma	Jessup (cited in Jacobson, 1980)
P. m. catenifer	Renal cortical adenoma	Effron et al., 1977
	Colonic adenocarcinoma	Cowan, 1968
	Pigmented spindle-cell tumors	RTLA 810
P. m. sayi	Intestinal polyopses/papillomatoses	RTLA 1174
	Subcutaneous sarcoma	AFIP Registry

Species	Tumor	Reference
Pseudoboa cloelia	Pancreatic adenocarcinoma	Ratcliffe, 1935
Ramphiophis rostratus	Hepatoma, benign	Cowan, 1968
Spilotes pullatus	Spinal osteosarcoma	Hill, 1954
	Pancreatic adenocarcinoma	Effron et al., 1977; RTLA 1387
Thamnophis elegans	Chromatophoroma, malignant	Frye et al., 1975; RTLA 1016
T. sirtalis	Granulosa cell tumor	Onderka and Zwart, 1978
	Fibropapilloma	RTLA 95A
	Sertoli cell tumor	RTLA 95B
	Squamous cell carcinoma, cloaca	Froom, 1974
	Cholangioma	RTLA 634
Elapidae		
Naja melanoleuca	Poison gland carcinoma	Hill, 1951
	Osteochondrosarcoma	Wadsworth, 1954a
N. naja	Lymphosarcoma	Cowan, 1968
	Leiomyosarcoma, rectum and liver	RTLA 560
	Carcinoma (pancreas?)	AFIP Registry
	Bile duct adenoma	Cowan, 1968
N. nigricollis	Lymphosarcoma	Effron et al., 1977
N. nivea	Bronchiogenic carcinoma	Effron et al., 1977
Pseudechis porphyriacus	Skin papillomas; adenomatous proliferation of intrahepatic bile duct	Effron et al., 1977
Pseudechis sp.	Fibrosarcoma	Wadsworth, 1956
Viperidae		
Acanthophis antarctieus	Leukemic lymphosarcoma	Effron et al., 1977
	Reticulum cell sarcoma	Griner (cited in Harshbarger and Dawe, 1973) (contd.)

Table 21.4. Neoplasms in Snakes (Squamata; Serpentes). (Continued)

Taxonomic classification	Neoplasm	Reference
Agkistrodon halys brevicaudus	Biliary adenocarcinoma	Effron et al., 1977
A. piscivorous	Spinal neurofibrosarcoma	Wadsworth, 1960
	Intraoral squamous cell carcinoma	
	Sarcoma of the stomach	Cowan, 1968
	Fibroma molle, ovary	Ippen, 1972; RTLA 721
	Plasma cell tumor	RTLA 1176
	Hemangioendothelioma	RTLA 2208
Atheris albolabui	Granulosa-theca cell tumor	Effron et al., 1977
Bitis arietans	Metastatic adeno-carcinoma, liver	AFIP Registry
	Leukemic lymphosarcoma; renal cortical adenoma	Effron et al., 1977
B. gabonica gabonica	Transitional cell tumor, testis	Wadsworth and Hill, 1956
	Biliary adenocarcinoma	Effron et al., 1977
B. nasicornis	Lymphosarcoma	Cowan, 1968; Effron et al., 1977; RTLA 379; AFIP Registry
	Leukemic lymphosarcoma	Effron et al., 1977
	Granulocytic leukemia	Snyder (cited in Dawe and Berard, 1971); RTLA 508
B. atrox	Adenocarcinoma, intra-pancreatic ducts	Effron et al., 1977
Crotalus atrox	Fibrosarcoma	Wadsworth, 1954a

C. horridus	Adenoma of the intestine	Wadsworth, 1956
	Fibroma	Orr et al., 1972
	Fibrosarcoma	RTLA 486
	Lymphoid leukemia	Effron et al., 1977; Griner, 1975; RTLA 378; AFIP Registry
	Mesothelioma/angiosarcoma	Machotka and Whitney, 1980; RTLA 1819
	Adenosarcoma, intestine	Wadsworth, 1956
	Pancreatic adenocarcinoma	AFIP Registry
	Pancreatic duct adenocarcinoma	Effron et al., 1977
C. mitchelli pyrrhus	Undifferentiated sarcoma	RTLA 984
C. ruber	Cloacal hemangioma	Wadsworth, 1956
C. viridis helleii	Fibrosarcoma	Ball (cited in Wadsworth, 1954a)
C. v. viridis		
Sistrurus catenatus catenatus	Ovarian hemangioma	Effron et al., 1977
Vipera berus	Melanoma	Stolk, 1957
	Adenocarcinoma	AFIP Registry
V. palestinae	Myxofibroma	Zeigel and Clark, 1969
V. russelli	Fibrosarcoma	Effron et al., 1977

of lethargy, anorexia and progressive softening and deformation of the carapace and plastron (Frye and Carney, 1975) The tumor mass was delicately encapsulated, measured 0.3 cm in diameter and consisted of cuboidal to columnar or fusiform cells with small round nuclei separated into small packets by a fibrovascular stroma (Fig. 21.1).

A thyroid gland adenoma reported in a fresh water turtle, Phrynops geoffroanus, appeared as an oval, encapsulated mass containing moderate amounts of connective tissue stroma dividing the parenchyma into elongated lobules, comprised of tubuloacinar structures lined by columnar epithelium resting on layers of small polyhedral cells with large nuclei (Pick and Poll, 1903).

Thyroid gland carcinoma has been reported in a Ceylon terrapin, Melanochelys trijuga, without further discussion (Cowan, 1968). Thyroid gland carcinoma also has been

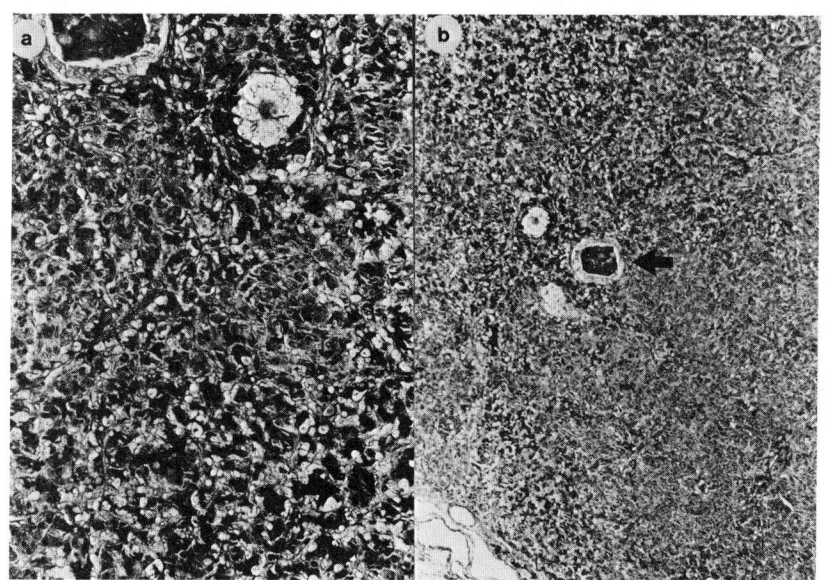

a   b

Fig. 21.2a,b. Ornamental tortoise, Chrysemys picta, thyroid carcinoma (RTLA 718).
   a. Thyroid gland architecture has been obliterated by neoplastic cells. One follicle remains (arrow). H&E X65
   b. Small culusters of dark cells (straight arrow) are separated by larger, vacuolated cells (curved arrow). H&E X160

described in a male Chrysemys picta (Ippen, 1972) which, though later reviewed and considered a parathyroid adenoma (Harshbarger, 1974), has subsequently been reevaluated as a thyroid carcinoma (Harshbarger, 1980b). The thyroid gland architecture was obliterated by invasive cells with vaculated cytoplasm and smaller clusters of dark cells leaving only scattered follicles (Fig. 21.2).

Hemic and lymphatic systems. Systemic lymphoblastic lymphosarcoma has been reported in a male Greek land tortoise, T. hermanii, involving the liver, heart, kidneys, spleen, pancreas and intestinal serosa (Ippen, 1972). Grey-white nodules in the liver and kidney contained large lymphoid cells with vesiculated nuclei (Fig. 21.3). Lymphoreticular neoplasia (granulocytic neoplasm versus a reticulum cell sarcoma) was listed in a Florida soft-shelled turtle, Trionyx ferox (Harshbarger, 1974).

Myelogenous leukemia has been reported in an immature, female Mobile terrapin, C. elegans, which was moribund due to epistaxis of 12 to 14 hours duration (Frye and Carney, 1972). Blood films contained large basophilic and eosinophilic myeloblasts with frequent mitoses. A helmeted turtle, Pelomedusa subrufa, also has been reported with myelogenous leukemia (Harshbarger, 1976). In addition, a hematopoietic cell neoplasm in a Burmese tortoise, G. emys, has been documented (Harshbarger, 1980a).

Integumentary system. C. mydas with papillomas, fibromas and fibropapillomas have long and frequently been documented (Harshbarger, 1974, 1977, 1979, 1980a; Lucke, 1938b; Smith and Coates, 1939). These masses, though occasionally smooth elevations composed of interlacing bands of connective tissue and considered fibromas, are more frequently large cauliflower-like nodules involving the skin around flippers, head, neck and tail (Figs. 21.4, 21.5). Microscopically, these masses are papillary in appearance and comprised of a well-organized layer of keratinizing squamous epithelium overlying a fibrous connective tissue core. Trematode ova, D. constrictum, although noted in more than half of approximately 240 such growths from six turtles, were not considered a primary cause by Smith and Coates (1939). Interestingly, reports of leeches, O. branchiatus, attached to similar fibropapillomas have been published (Nigrelli, 1942; Nigrelli and Smith, 1943). In the areas of leech attachment the tumor's vascularity was increased. Hirudin secreted by the leeches may have improved the tumor's circulation having a direct stimulating effect on its growth. A possible viral etiology with the leeches as

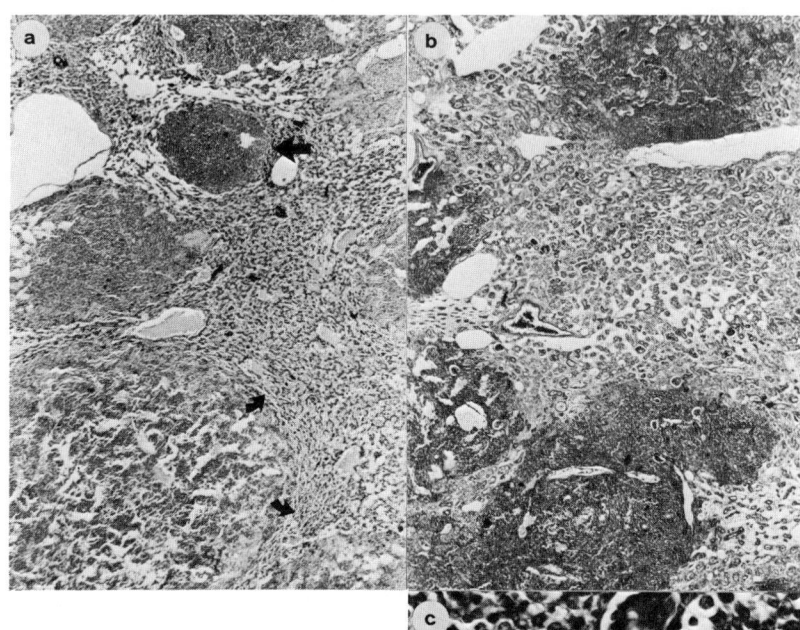

Fig. 21.3a,b,c.
Greek land tortoise, Testudo hermanii, lymphoblastic lymphosarcoma (RTLA 717).
a. Multiple nodules (straight arrow) of neoplastic lymphoblasts have compressed the remaining hepatic parenchyma (curved arrows). H&E X400.
b. Kidney containing nodules of lymphoblasts that have infiltrated between tubules and glomeruli. H&E X25.
c. Higher magnification of kidney nodule (arrow) adjacent to intact glomerulus and tubules. H&E X400.

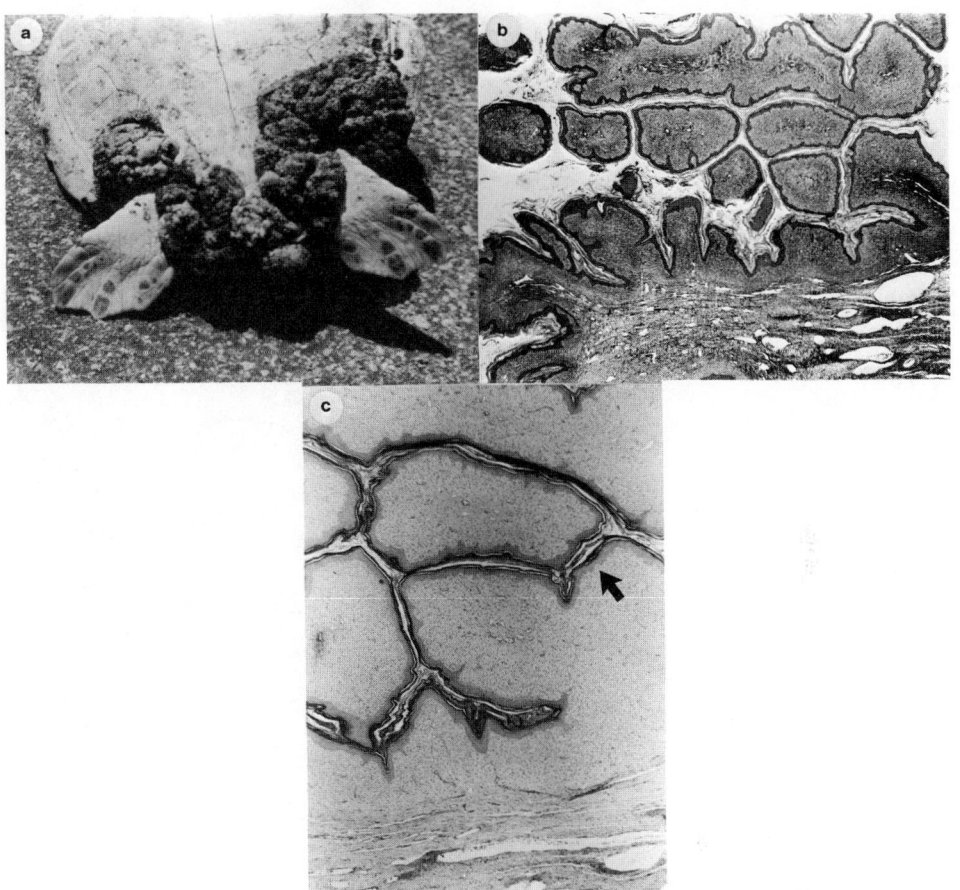

Fig. 21.4a,b,c. Green turtle, Chelonia mydas, fibropapilloma (RTLA 12).
a. Multiple cauliflowed-like nodules associated with rear flippers and tail.
b. Papillary nature of masses is demonstrated. H&E X20.
c. Well-organized layer of keratinizing squamous epithelium (arrow) overlies fibrous connective tissue core. H&E X40.

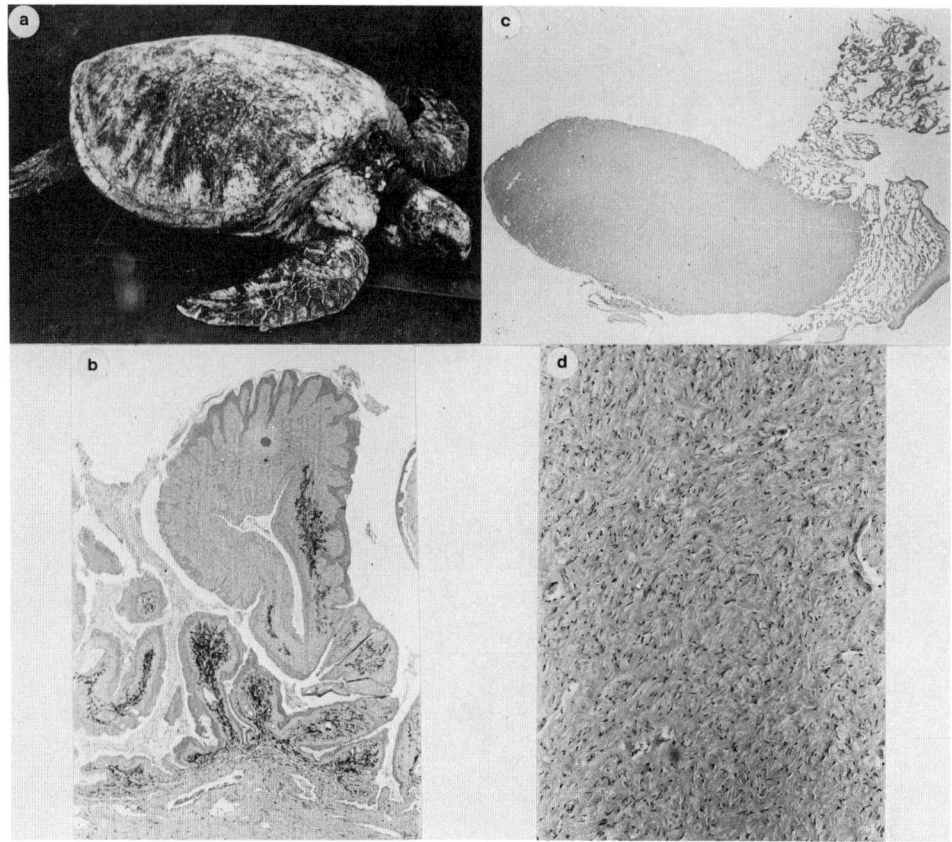

Fig. 21.5a,b,c,d. Green turtle, Chelonia mydas, fibropapillomas (RTLA 1774) and fibromas (RTLA 1856).
  a. One large and multiple smaller nodules near right shoulder and ventrolateral aspect of head.
  b. Fibropapilloma of the skin. H&E X20
  c. Fibroma of the lung. H&E X6
  d. Lung fibroma containing even distribution of fibrocytes separated by abundant fibrous connective tissue. H&E X130

vectors was suggested since the indigenous human population had similar growths.

Cutaneous papillomas on the tail and flippers have been reported in musk turtles, S. odoratus. These lesions with a loose, well vascularized connective tissue core covered by keratinizing squamous epithelium sending long epithelial pegs into the underlying connective tissue resembled the common warts of man (Schlumberger and Lucke, 1948). Verrucal papillomatosis has been listed in a Clemmys sp. (Harshbarger, 1977).

Squamous cell carcinoma on the foot of a G. tritugu has been reported (Cowan, 1968) as has an oral squamous cell carcinoma in an European pond turtle, Emys orbicularis, with metastasis to the liver (Billups and Harshbarger, 1976).

Respiratory system. Three pulmonary neoplasms have been recorded in turtles, two of which were diagnosed as fibroadenomas, the other as a fibroma. The first fibroadenoma occurred in a T. horsfieldi (Finkelstein, 1944) and the second in an E. orbicularis and thought to have arisen from the bronchial epithelium and connective tissue (Bresler, 1963). Fibromas of the lung in C. mydas have been documented (Harshbarger, 1979) and appear as solitary, firm masses containing an even distribution of fibrocytes separated by abundant fibrous connective tissue (Fig. 21.5).

Urinary system. A large female box turtle, Terrapene carolina, contained small grey-white foci scattered throughout the kidneys and liver (Ippen, 1972). The carcinomatous cells were considered of renal epithelial origin and were, therefore, diagnosed as renal adenocarcinoma, metastatic to the liver.

Crocodilians

Digestive system. An American crocodile, Crocodylus acutus, with an intrhepatic lipoma or fat storage disease has been recorded (Harshbarger, 1975).

Hemic and lymphatic systems. A young porose crocodile, C. porosus, was found recumbant and had been ataxic. At necropsy, small and large masses were seen to involve numerous organs (Scott and Beattie, 1927). A small growth located on the ventral surface of the cerebellum had invaded the neural tissue. The right auricle of the heart was occluded by a mass that penetrated the auricular wall and ventricular septum. These masses were primarily comprised of small round cells and a few larger, often multinucleated cells with occasional mitotic figures. Similar cells were noted in the portal spaces and had infiltrated the obliterated hepatic parenchyma. The authors reasoned that the round cell sarcoma was a primary hepatic neoplasm metastatic to the heart and cerebellum. Following evaluation of photomicrographs, others theorized that the tumor may have arisn from blood forming tissues in the liver and was comparable to lymphosarcoma in man (Schlumberger and Lucke, 1948).

Integumentary system. A large Crocodylus sp. with warts similar to cutaneous papillomas in lizards has been described (Schlumberger and Lucke, 1948). An American alligator, Alligator mississippiensis, had a wart-like growth located on the dorsum nasi beyond the right naris (Wadsworth and Hill, 1956).

Musculoskeletal system. Bony tumors and malformation in a C. porosus without further description have been documented (Kalin, 1937).

Reproductive system. The very old and large alligator previously mentioned as having wart-like growths also contained huge tumor masses occupying the dorsal wall of the body cavity which obscured the adrenal glands and testes (Wadsworth and Hill, 1956). The masses contained well-defined groups of large polyhedral cells resembling spermatocytes. The tumor was diagnosed as a seminoma.

Lizards

Digestive system. An early report identified a "spongy" carcinoma in the parotid area of a black-spotted tegu, T. nigropunctatus (Bland-Sutton, 1885).

A Komodo dragon, Varanus komodoensis, with a colonic carcinoma and a metastatic adenocarcinoma in the spleen with numerous other neoplasms to be noted later has been reported (Harshbarger, 1976).

Hepatomas have been described in the common lizard, Iguana iguana (Stolk, 1964), the golden tegu, T. rufescens (Ippen, 1972) and the two-flapped chameleon, Chaemaeleo dilepis (Harshbarger, 1974). In the iguana there were multiple hepatic nodules comprised of disorganized hepatocytes with areas of alveolar to adenomatoid formation and multinucleated giant cells. These features are consistent with a diagnosis of hepatocellular carcinoma. The tegu contained a large mass in the right lobe of the liver and was histologically compatible with a diagnosis of liver cell adenoma as was the hepatoma in the chameleon. A hepatocarcinoma in a male five-lined skink, Eumeces fasciatus, which extended to the serous membrane of the body cavity also has been described (Ippen, 1972). A

Ricord's iguana, Cyclura ricordi, from the Zoological Society of San Diego was listed as having a biliary adenoma (Effron et al., 1977).

Endocrine system. Thyroid gland adenomas have been reported in an African sungazer lizard, Cordylus polyzonus (Harshbarger, 1974) and a Komodo dragon (Harshbarger, 1976). The same Komodo dragon contained a pancreatic islet cell tumor and an adrenal gland pheochromocytoma.

Hemic and lymphatic systems. Lymphoma in an I. iguana has been listed (Harshbarger, 1974).

Malignant lymphomas, lymphosarcomas and leukemia have been reported in lizards. A male ruin lizard, L. sicula, after one month of captivity developed a neck bulge which rapidly increased in size after which another growth formed in the tail (Lawson, 1962). Following the lizard's death, necropsy revealed major organ involvement with similar masses composed of neoplastic lymphoid cells. Thyroid carcinoma in a female water monitor, V. salvator, with masses on the lower jaw and neck which penetrated the trachea (Ippen, 1972) was later reevaluated and diagnosed as a lymphosarcoma with smaller, histiologically similar masses in the heart, pancreas and kidney (Harshbarger, 1974). The kidney and thyroid contained interstitial infiltrates of neoplastic lymphocytes (Fig. 21.6). A probable lymphosarcoma has been detailed in a male V. salvator, but concomitant parasitic infestations and disseminated septic necrosis have made this diagnosis less than definative (Zwart and Harshbarger, 1972). A lymphosarcoma in a spiny-tailed agamid, Uromastix acanthinurus, was listed (Effron et al., 1977). Lymphoblastic lymphoma in a female water dragon, Hydrosaurus amboinensis, with hepatosplenomegally and swollen, pale kidneys (Zwart and Harshbarger, 1972) and lymphoblastic leukemia in a Bengal monitor, V. bengalensis (Harshbarger, 1977) have been described.

Plasma cell tumors have been listed (Harshbarger, 1974) in a Nile monitor, V. niloticus, and described in a sub-adult female H. amboinensis (Schmidt, 1977). The water lizard, found dead after 1.5 years in captivity, had 1 to 2 mm diameter grey-white nodules in the lungs and liver, and a 2 x 2.5 cm grey-white ulcerated mass in the wall of the stomach. The lung, liver and gastric lesions contained numerous round to oval cells with eccentric nuclei, distinct cytoplasmic borders, few mitotic figures and minimal stroma. Electron microscopic examination revealed that these cells had typical features

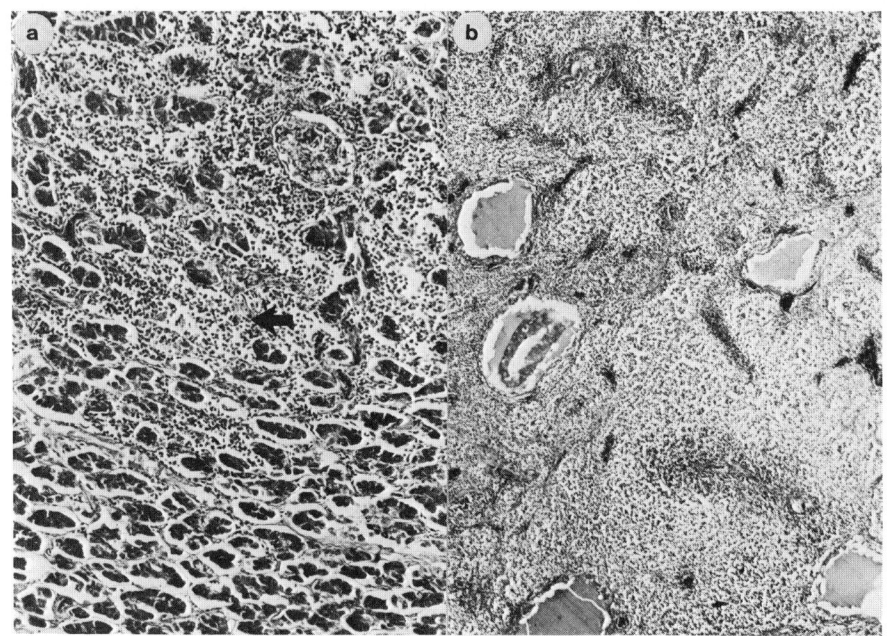

Fig. 21.6a,b. Varanus salvator, lymphocytic lymphoma (RTLA 719).
  a. Kidney containing interstitial infiltrates of neoplastic lymphocytes (arrow) H&E 70
  b. Thyroid gland containing few follicles separated by infiltrates of neoplastic lymphocytes. H&E X70

of plasma cells including extensive rough endoplasmic reticulum and prominent clumped central and peripheral nuclear chromatin.

Reticulum cell sarcoma has been described in a mature female Anolis carolinensis which had a 2 x 7 mm flesh-colored soft mass in the left mandibular-labial fold (Frye and Dutra, 1974). The fairly well demarked, though not encapsulated mass, consisted of cells with moderate amounts of finely vacuolated cytoplasm without distinct cell borders, large vesicular nuclei and mitotic figures; delicately and irregularly separated by argylophilic strands.

Integumentary system. Epidermal papillomas in lizards, as fibropapillomas in turtles, have long and frequently been reported and often referred to as "pox".

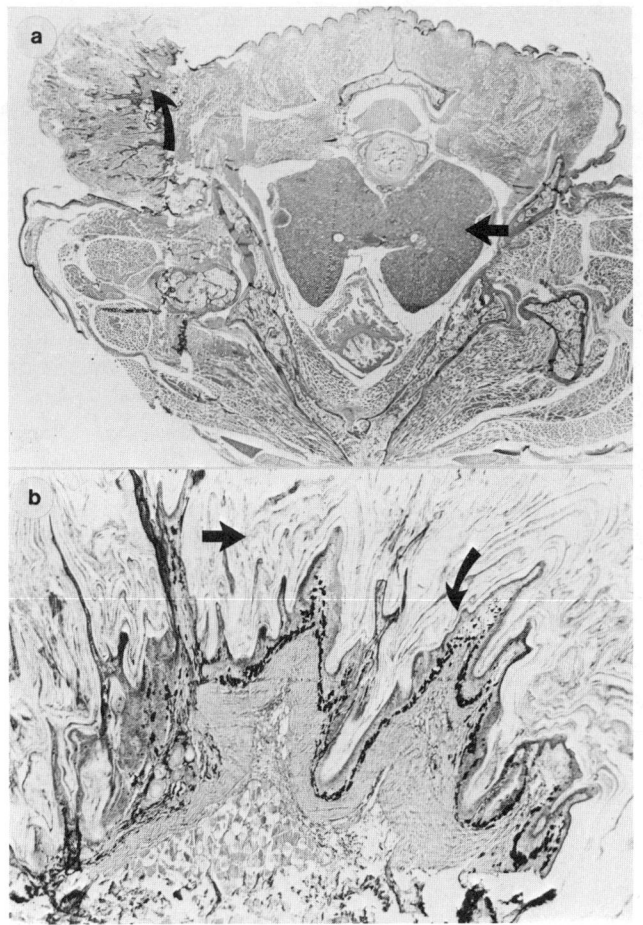

Fig. 21.7a,b. Green lizard, Lacerta viridis, epidermal papilloma (RTLA 1821).
a. Whole body cross-section at level of kidney (straight arrow) with keratogenous mass (curved arrow) protruding from skin. H&E X6
b. Abundant keratin (straight arrow) produced by delicate finger-like projections of squamous epithelium (curved arrow) on a fibrous base. H&E X40

The first report documented numerous papillomas of the head and thorax of a sand lizard, L. agilis (Koch, 1904). Similar lesions were observed in an emerald lizard, L. Viridis and were limited to the skin surface and usually consisted of abundant keratin produced by finger-like projections of squamous epithelium on a fibrous base (Fig. 21.7). In their more advanced forms, these lesions have been descriptively called "tree bark tumors" which consist of a mixed fibroepithelial papilloma involving the epidermis and corium (Klein, 1952). Papillomas described as keratinized inguinal masses resembling keratinizing condylomata acumenata of man, have been reported in several wall lizards, L. muralis (Schlumberger and Lucke, 1948). More recently, a detailed record of papillomas in wall lizards has been prepared (Raynaud and Adrian, 1976). Masses in females were most commonly near the tail base whereas lesions in males were usually more anterior. This distribution of lesions was thought to be related to the reproductive and aggressive behavior of the males. Papillomatosis in emerald lizards also has been listed (Harshbarger, 1977).

Squamous cell carcinomas have been described in the gila monster, Heloderma suspectum, T. nigropunctatus, T. teguixin and L. agilis by varaous authors (Schlumberger, 1958; Schlumberger and Lucke, 1948; Schwarz, 1923; Stolk, 1953). The cutaneous mass in the gila monster was described as an epithelioma on the foot. However, squamous epithelium had invaded the fibromuscular tissue and underlying bone suggesting a malignant neoplasm. There were two oral masses in the T. nigropunctatus which were smooth, pink and firm. The animal died two years and eight months later from an accidental injury. There was local infiltration by the tumor, but no metastases. The neoplasm was composed of squamous epithelium and delicate connective tissue trabeculae, prominent intercellular bridges and frequent cell aggregates containing epithelial "pearls" characteristic of squamous cell carcinomas. Mitotic figures were numerous as were giant, pleomorphic nuclei. The right forefoot of the T. teguixin had a spherical, 3 cm mass which had nearly destroyed the metacarpal and proximal two phalanges of the fifth and fourth toes and had microscopic features of squamous cell carcinoma. Carcinoma planocellulare (squamous cell carcinoma) was described in seven L. agilis as small nodules in the skin (Stolk, 1953).

Soft-tissue tumors reported in lizards consist of fibrosarcoma/mesenchymosarcoma and a myxoma. A L. sicula had a large solid swelling of the left foreleg (Elkan and Cooper, 1976). The mass surrounded the leg and extended into the mediastinum, dorsal aorta, lungs and stomach. The original diagnosis of mesenchymosarcoma has been termed a fibrosarcoma (Harshbarger, 1975). A fibrosarcoma in a Basiliscus plumifrons and an I. iguana with a myxoma have been listed (Harshbarger, 1980a).

Musculoskelatal system. Multiple enchondromas in an Indian monitor, V. dracoena, were located in the distal metaphysis of the right humerus, in the left humerus, metacarpal bones, the hyoid bone and two cervical vertebrae (Bland-Sutton, 1885). The neoplasms consisted of hyaline cartilage. Since this animal was described as having rickets, the condromatous condition may have been a nutritionally-related disorder.

An osteochondrosarcoma from the neck of a monitor has been briefly cited (Frye, 1973) as has a chondro-osteofibroma in a rhinocerous iguana, C. cornuta (Rodhain, 1949). Numerous small tumors in the tail of a female L. viridis which were shown to originate in the vertebral column (Stolk, 1958), contained osteoblasts, fibroblasts, bundles of collagen and small fragments of bone allowing a diagnosis of osteomata or, in more current terminology, osteosarcomas.

An interesting subspecialty of pathology, termed paleopathology, consists of evaluating the remains of ancient life forms. A product of this interest is the report of an osteoma on the third dorsal vertebrae of a large mosasaur, an extinct aquatic reptile which lived during the latter part of the Cretaceous age (Moodie cited in Stolk, 1958). Tumor-like lesions were observed in the caudal vertebrae of three dinosaurs, Diplodocus Sp., which in general are not considered as true neoplasms. These masses were originally interpreted as excess calus formation following a fracture, osteomyelitis and hemangioma (Hatcher, 1901; Holland, 1906; Moodie cited by Stolk, 1958). A more recent report concludes that they were hemagiomas (Stolk, 1958), whereas in an earlier review Schlumberger and Lucke (1948) felt the original descriptions strongly suggested that the lesions were benign overgrowths following fracture, rather than neoplasms.

Nervous system/pigment cells. After 18 years in captivity, a H. suspectum developed a small tail mass which enlarged over a five year period (Cooper, 1968). Surgical removal of the mass, which contained multiple nodules of brown pigmented cells and therefore considered a melanoma, was successful.

Reproductive system. A mucin producing adenocarcinoma in an ovarian teratoma was listed for an I. iguana (Harshbarger, 1974). The mass was a huge dark polycystic structure involving the left ovary (Fig. 21.8). Epithelially-lined, mucin-containing cysts, bone, fibrous

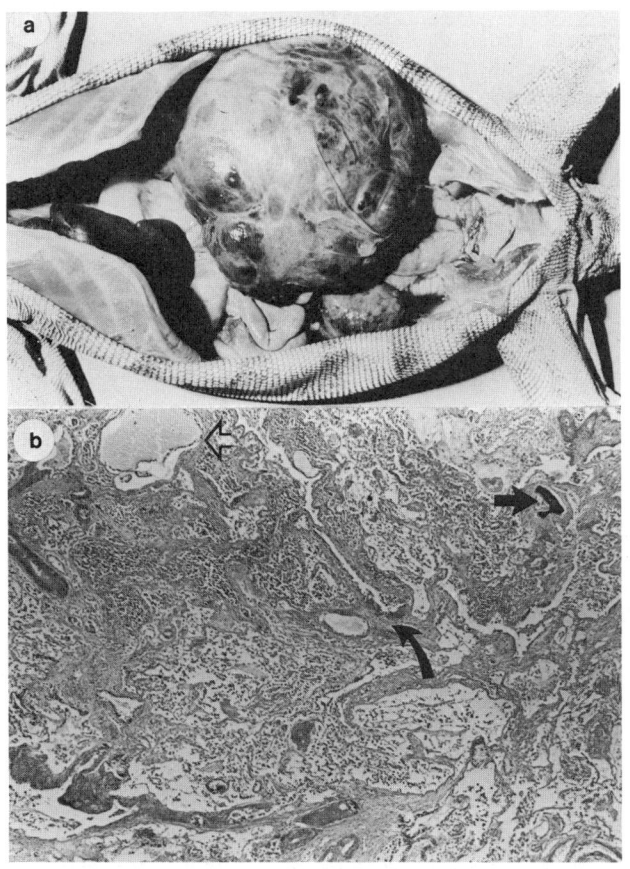

Fig. 21.8a,b. Common iguana, Iguana iguana, teratoma (adenocarcinoma) ovary (RTLA 460).
a. Large polycystic abcominal mass involvin left ovary.
b. Mass consisted of epithelially-lined mucin containing cysts (open arrow), bone (closed arrow), fibrous connective tissue (curved arrow) and extensive necrotic debris. H&E X40

connective tissue and extensive necrotic debris were components of the tumor. A V. komodoensis, previously described with numerous other neoplasms, also contained a cystic interstitial cell tumor of one testicle (Harshbarger, 1976).

Urinary system. A renal neoplasm in a brown-spotted lizard, Calopistes maculatus, was noted as having involved the posterior portion of both kidneys, but its histological make-up was not described (Hill, 1952).

Snakes

Cardiovascular system. A myocardial tumor situated in the external layer of the heart was described in a female Constrictor constrictor which, after initially feeding normally, eventually refused to eat, showed signs of lack of tonus, imbalance, inability to climb, became moribund, convulsive and died (Elkan and Cooper, 1976). The well-vascularized mass displaced the adjacent myocardium without infiltrating. The neoplasm was considered a rhabdomyosarcoma due to the presence of numerous abnormal mitotic figures and cross-striated fibers demonstrated with phosphotungstic acid hematoxylin stain (PTAH). An Anitchkow monocyte tumor in another snake of the same species has been listed (Harshbarger, 1976).

Hemangioma and hemangioendotheliomas have been documented in various serpents. Hepatic and ovarian hemangiomas have been listed in a male boomslang, Dispholidus typus, and a female massasauga, Sistrurus catenatus, respectively (Effron et al., 1977). Hemangioendothelioma in a water moccasin, Agkistrodon piscivorus, was listed (Harshbarger, 1980a) as was a metastasizing hemangioendothelioma in a Natrix natrix (Ippen, 1972). The tumor was considered of hepatic or splenic origin with pulmonary, cardiac and renal metasteses. An immature Southern Pacific rattlesnake, C. viridis helleri, had an elongated pericloacal, hemangiomatous growth containing cystic areas which was diagnosed as a cystic hemangioma (Wadsworth, 1956).

Digestive system. Transitional cell carcinomas have Been listed in a yellow rat snake, E. obsoleta quadrivittata (Harshbarger, 1979), and described in a female gaboon viper, Bitis gabonica, which had a bloody exudate from the glottis and a coagulum in the buccal cavity (Wadsworth and Hill, 1956). There was a necrotic encrustation of the right mandibular ramus and a pigeon egg-sized swelling in the left ramus. Histologic examination revealed numerous blood vessels separated by spindle-shaped and round cells. The only reported case of a poison gland carcinoma was noted in a black-and-white cobra, Naja melanoleuca, with metastases to the cervical lymph nodes (Hill, 1952). A tumor originating from the buccal mucous membrane in an Indian python, Python molurus, had a pronounced tendency to gland-like formation and was designated an adenoameloblastoma due to its histological resemblence to the odontogenic tumors of ectoderma origin known to occur in man (Kast, 1967). Another intraoral carcinoma has been described in a 9 kg, 2.7 m long female P. molurus with erosion of the dorsal palate, maxillary, suborbital and nasal tissues and 1 to 1.5 cm white nodules metastatic to the liver (Wilhelm and Emswiller, 1977).

Gastric neoplasms reported include a cystic adenoma appearing as a 28 cm mucosal mass in an African rock python, P. sebae (Valliant and Pettit, 1902), a benign adenomatous polyp in an anaconda, Eunectes murinus, which presented as a pea-shaped polypoid nodule attached to the mucosa (Wadsworth, 1956), and a gastric sarcoma listed in an A. piscivorus (Cowan, 1968).

Intestinal and cloacal neoplasms are not uncommon in serpents. Benign intestinal polyposes/papillomastosis in a bullsnake, Pituophis melanoleucus sayi, has been listed (Harshbarger, 1976) as has an intestinal adenoma in a C. horridus (Wadsworth, 1956). Adenocarcinomas of the intestine/colon occurred in a C. horridus atricaudatus and a black rat snake, E. obsoleta (Wadsworth, 1956). Colonic adenocarcinomas were identified in P. m. catenifer (Cowan, 1968; Jessup cited in Jacobson, 1980). A rectal mass in a N. naja with metasteses to the liver was diagnosed as a leiomyosarcoma (Harshbarger, 1974). The hepatic nodules compressed surrounding liver cords and contained "cigar" shaped nuclei arranged in whorls (Fig. 21.19). Transitional cell carcinoma was listed as occurring in the cloaca of a 15 year old female reticulated python, P. reticulatus (Billups and Harshbarger, 1976). Squamous cell carcinoma in an eastern garter snake, Thamnophis sirtalis sirtalis, was described as infiltrating the cloaca (Froom, 1974). A cloacal carcinoma (Smith and Betz, 1965) and a cloacal sarcoma (Wadsworth, 1954b) have been reported in a corn snake, E. g. gutta, and a western hognose snake, H. nasicus, respectively.

A single case of hepatocellular neoplasia (benign hepatoma) has been reported in a massurana, Pseudoboa cloelia, which was exhibited for approximately 11.5 years (Cowan, 1968). Biliary neoplasms have frequently been documented. They include a bile duct adenoma in a male black-necked cobra, N. nigricollis (Cowan, 1968), a female red-bellied black snake, Pseudechis porphyriacus, with adenomatous proliferation of intrahepatic bile ducts, a male D. typus with a biliary adenoma (Effron et al., 1977) and cholangioma in a T. sirtalis (Harshbarger, 1974). Examination of 2,200 free-ranging snakes revealed a single

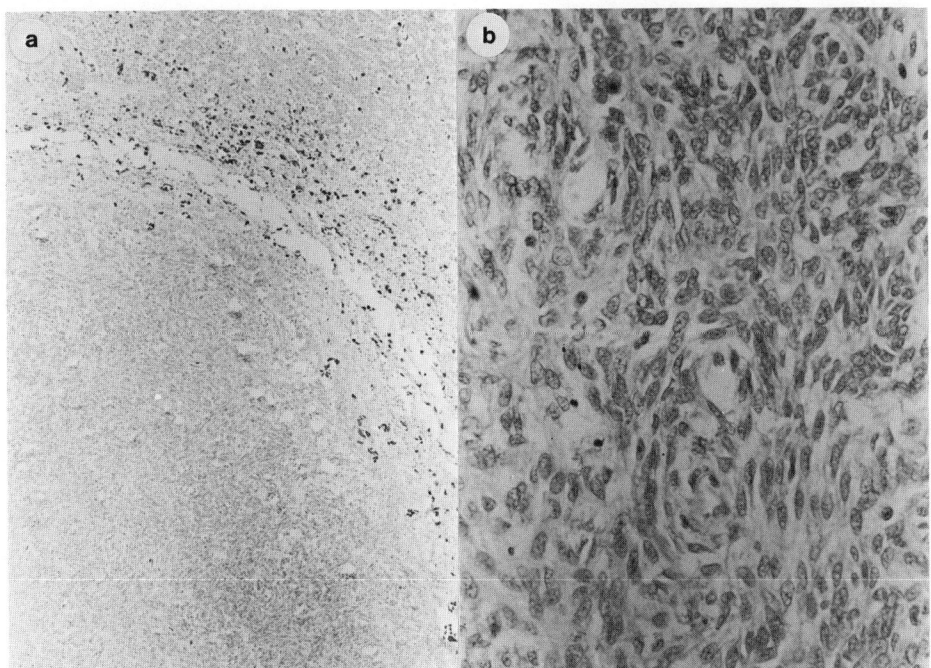

Fig. 21.9a,b. Cobra, Naja naja, leiomyosarcoma (RTLA 560).
a. Liver parenchyma (upper right) is compressed by metastatic, nodular mass of cells arranged in whorls. H&E X70
b. Closely spaced cells with "cigar" shaped nuclei. H&E X400

neoplasm in the East Indian water snake, H. buccata (Bergman, 1941). Though the growth was only a small mass protruding into the bile duct and associated with a trematode, it was considered a bile duct papillary carcinoma. A scirrhous biliary adenocarcinoma in a female B. gabonica has been noted (Effron et al., 1977) as has an adenocarcinoma of possible bile duct origin in a 10 year old female Palestine viper, V. palestinae (Billups and Harshbarger, 1976). Cystic mucinous adenocarcinoma metastatic to the liver and adenocarcinoma metastatic to the liver, intestine and kidney with primary site not determined have been recorded in a seven year old male P. m. molurus and a three year old female puff adder, B. arietans (Billups and Harshbarger, 1976). Lastly, an undifferentiated abdominal sarcoma with osseous metaplasia involving the liver has been listed in an E. o. obsoleta (Machotka and Whitney, 1980).

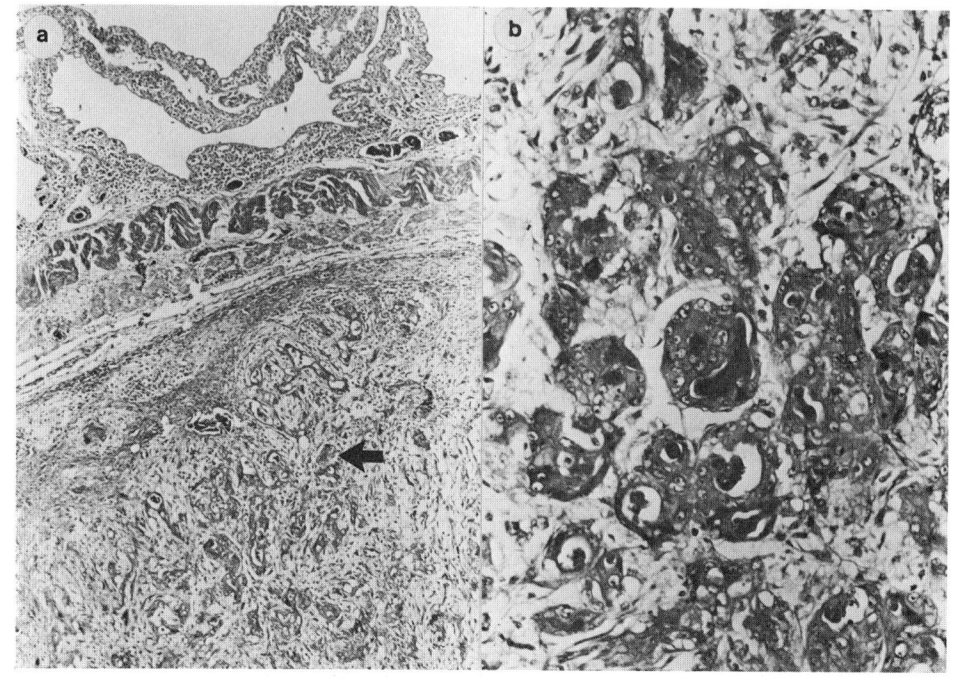

Fig. 21.10a,b. Spilotes pullatus, pancreatic adenocarcinoma (RTLA 1387).
 a. Neoplastic epithelium in small clusters (arrow) separated by loose fibrous connective tissue. H&E X50
 b. Anaplasia, disorderly arrangement with some acinar/ductular formation and invasiveness are demonstrated. H&E X16

All pancreatic neoplasms described in serpents have been carcinomas or adenocarcinomas of the acinar or ductular epithelium. Pancreatic adenocarcinomas have been listed in C. horridus (Billups and Harshbarger, 1976), Spilotes pullatus, C. mitchelli pyrrhus and Bothrops atrox with marked connective tissue development (Effron et al., 1977) and a P. melanoleucus which at necropsy was found to have a greatly enlarged pancreas (Ratcliffe, 1935). Histologically prepared sections of the latter case demonstrated irregular groups of large poorly-formed acini or tubules composed of one or more layers of pleomorphic cells with large basophilic nuclei and occasional mitoses replacing the normal pancreatic parenchyma. A similar lesion is presented in Fig. 21.10 from a S. pullatus. A later publication detailed the occurrence of pancreatic adenocarcinomas or atypical regeneration in various stages of development in 45 snakes from several families, most frequently Crotalidae and Colubridae (Ratcliffe, 1943). Subsequently, the author re-evaluated his findings and considered these lesion instead to be regenerative (Schlumberger and Lucke, 1948).

Miscellaneous abdominal/mesenteric growths from various snakes have appeared in the literature. A small adenocarcinomatous mass was noted in mesenteric adhesions from a C. constrictor which had a myocardial rhabdomyosarcoma (Elkan and Cooper, 1976). A coachwhip snake, Masticophis flagellum testaceus, also has been listed with an abdominal adenocarcinoma of undetermined origin (Ball cited in Wadsworth, 1954a). An angiosarcoma was listed in a 15 year old male, dark phase C. horridus which had been in captivity for 14 years (Harshbarger, 1978b). A

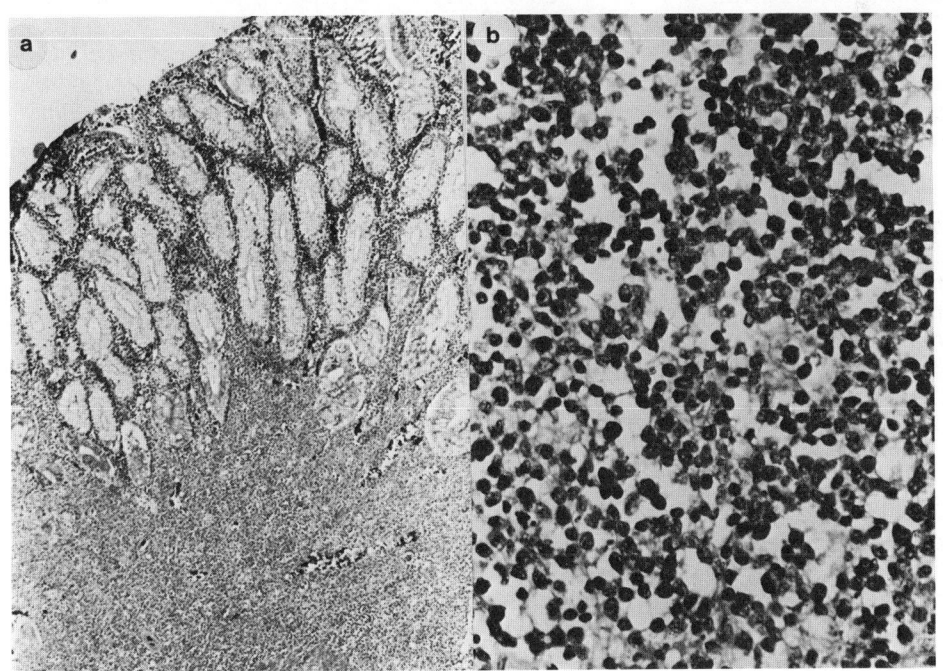

Fig. 21.11a,b. Rhinocerus viper, Bitis nasicornis, lymphosarcoma (RTLA 379).
a. Intestinal epithelium overlies sheets of neoplastic cells. H&E X70
b. Morphologically uniform cells with small round nuclei and scanty cytoplasm. H&E X400

detailed gross and microscopic description of this neoplasm was presented (Machotka and Whitney, 1980) which the authors felt was consistent with a diagnosis of mesothelioma. Another sarcoma of the serous surfaces in a male P. melanoleucus was listed and may represent a mesothelioma (Ratcliffe, 1953).

Endocrine system. Adrenal gland pheochromocytoma in a male California glossy snake, Arizona elegans occidentalis, is the lone endocrine tumor reported in snakes (Effron et al., 1977).

Hemic and Lymphatic Systems. Lymphoid neoplasia in serpents has been variously described as lymphosarcoma, malignant lymphoma, leukemic lymphocarcoma, lymphatic leukemia, lymphoid leukemia and lymphoid leukosis. Lymphosarcomas have been noted by Cowan (1968) in the liver, lung and kidneys of a H. platyrhinos, heart and liver of N. naja, and in the spleen, gut wall, liver, kidney and adrenal glands of B. nasicornis. Lymphosarcoma has been listed in a female N. nigricollis and a female B. nasicornis (Effron et al., 1977). Typical microscropic appearance of these cancers is presnted in a B. nasicornis with an intestinal mass containing sheets of neoplastic lymphocytes (Fig. 21.11). A well described lymphosarcoma with lymphoblasts predominating occurred in the liver of an E. murinus which had secondary deposits in the thyroid, spleen, pancreas and kidney (Frank and Schepky, 1969). A P. molurus from the San Diego Zoo contained a large, dark multinodular intermandibular growth comprised primarily of cells with round nuclei and a moderate quantitiy of cytoplasm which were considered typical of malignant lymphoma (Fig. 21.12) (Harshbarger, 1978b). Another python, P. reticulatus, was listed with a malignant lymphoma (Harshbarger, 1979). A California king snake, Lampropeltis getulus californiae, has been listed (Harshbarger, 1979) and later described (Jacobson et al., 1980). Major organs were infiltrated with lymphoblastic cells often containing Cowdry Type A intranuclear inclusions. Electron microscopy demonstrated intracytoplasmic virus-like particles in the neoplastic cells.

Leukemic lymphosarcomas were noted in three female snakes, a death adder, Acanthophis antarcticus, a B. arietans and a B. nasicornis from the Zoological Society of San Diego (Effron et al., 1977). Lymphoid/lymphoblastic leukemia was characterized in a 1 kg, 2.98 m P. molurus after a 10 mm, flat, pink lesion was observed adjacent to the larynx and pharynegeal cavity (Finnie, 1972). Additional lesions were present in the esophageal and

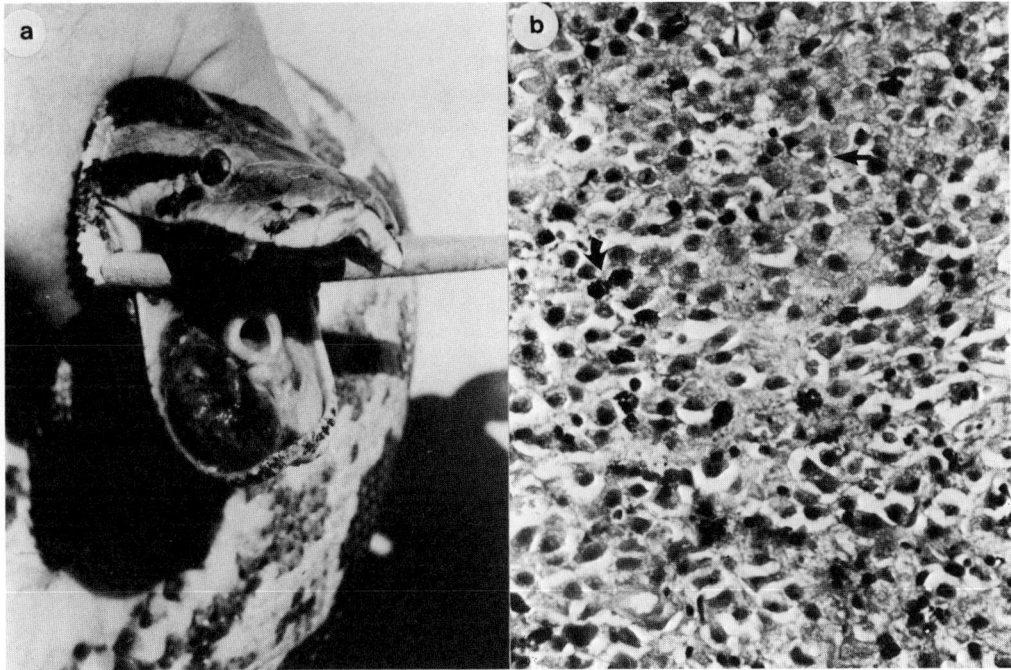

Fig. 21.12a,b. Indian rock python, Python molurus, malignant lymphoma (RTLA 1600).
  a. Large, dark, multinodular mass between the mandibles.
  b. Mass primarily contains cells with round nuclei and moderate cytoplasm (straight arrow); granulated inflammatory cells (curved arrow) scattered throughout the mass; and large vacuoles which are probable post-mortem or fixation artifacts. H&E X400

tracheal mucosa. All major organs contained lymphoblastic cell infiltrates. Blood films demonstrated numerous lymphocytic-type cells, many of which were lymphoblasts. Acute lymphatic leukemia in an immature male C. constrictor was diagnosed following examination of blood films revealing all stages of mitosis in lymphocytes (Frye and Carney, 1973). The immature lymphocytes tended to adhere to each other in a raft-like fashion. Lymphoid leukemia (lymphocytic lymphosarcoma) in a male C. horridus has been presented (Billups and Harshbarger, 1976; Effron et al., 1977; Griner, 1975; Harshbarger, 1974) with involvement of the liver (Fig. 21.13), lung, intestine, kidney, spleen, pancreas and heart. Hepatic involvement also occurred in a case of granulocytic leukemia from a B. nasicornis

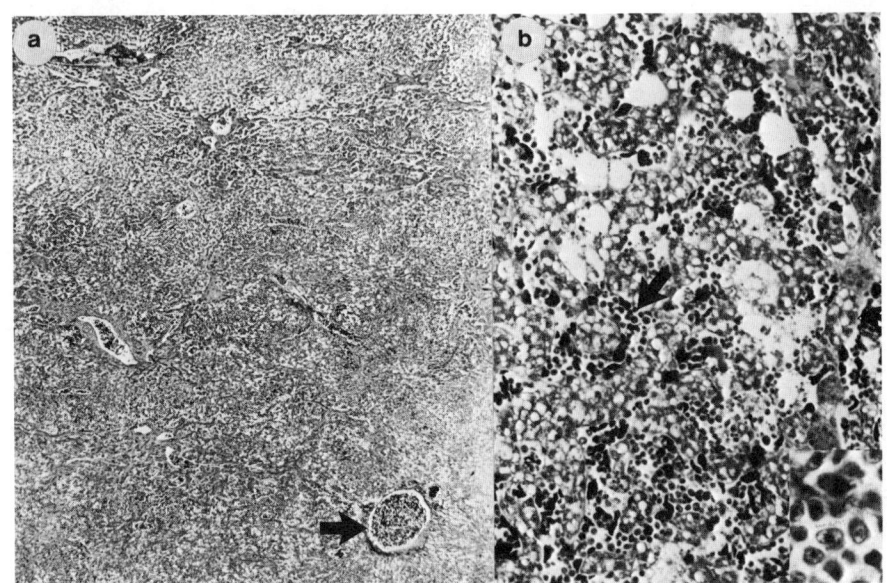

Fig. 21.13a,b. Timber rattlesnake, Crotalus h. horridus, lymphoblastic leukemia (RTLA 378).
a. Lymphoblastic cells located in liver sinusoids and larger vessels (arrow). H&E X20
b. Sinusoidal leukemic cells (straight arrow) separate cords of vacuolated hepatocytes (curved arrow). H&E X160 Insert: Leukemic cells contain moderately large, generally round nuclei; apparent lack of cytoplasm is a fixation stain artifact. H&E X400

(Fig. 21.14) (Synder cited in Dawe and Berard, 1971). A single case of plasma cell tumor (leukemic) in Serpentes has been listed from an A. piscivorus (Harshbarger, 1976).

Two cases of reticulum cell sarcoma have been documented. One occurred in a H. platyrhinos (Synder cited in Dawe and Berard, 1971) and the other in an A. antarcticus (Griner cited in Harshbarger and Dawe, 1973).

Integumentary system. Numerous cutaneous and soft tissue neoplasms with benign and malignant features have been characterized in snakes. The cutaneous lesions have generally been benign with occasional exceptions and include papillomas of the skin (Effron et al., 1977),

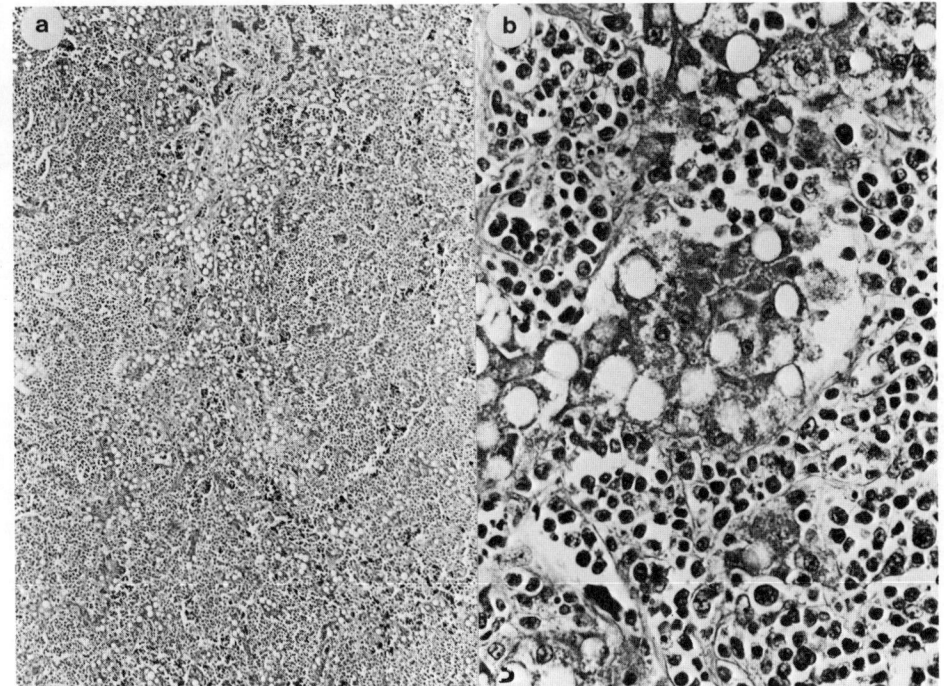

Fig. 21.14a,b. Rhinocerous viper, Bitis nasicornis, granulocytic leukemia (RTLA 508).
a. Extensive infiltrate of neoplastic cells has obliterated normal liver architecture. H&E X70
b. Leukemic cells shown surrounding hepatocytes or biliary epithelium contain varied sized/shaped nuclei. H&E X400

epidermal papillomas and fibropapillomas (Harshbarger, 1974) and an intraoral squamous cell carcinoma (Wadsworth, 1960) in P. porphyriacus, C. constrictor, T. sirtalis and A. piscivorus, respectively.

Fibromas in various locations have been described in pythons (Effron et al., 1977; Idowu et al., 1975), a C. horridus (Orr et al., 1972) and an E. o. spiloides (Wadsworth, 1956). The C. horridus is of particular interest since it represents the first report of in vitro cultivation of fibroma cells from a primary lesion. Another interesting lesion in a V. russelli has been diagnosed as an edematous myofibroma from the precardiac region (Ziegel and Clark, 1969) with intravascular clusters of neoplastic cells in other organs. Splenic cell cultures from this snake contained a budding "C" type virus and

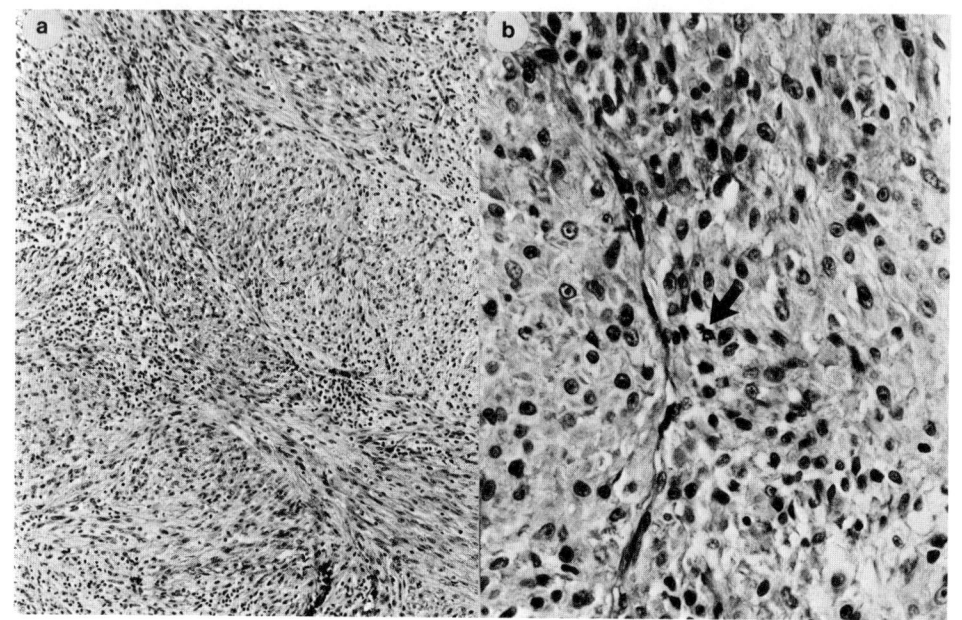

Fig. 21.15a,b. Timber rattlesnake, Crotalus h. horridus, fibrosarcoma (RTLA 486).
  a. Round, oval to stellate-appearing nuclei arranged in streams separate nodules of similar cells. H&E X100
  b. Nuclei frequently contain prominent nucleoli and bizzare mitoses (arrow). Moderately abundant ground substance is evident. H&E X400

documents the first evidence for the existence of this type of virus from a poikilothermic animal. Because the oncogenic potential of RNA-containing viruses of the C-type has been reported for other vertebrate species (Beard, 1964; Rich and Moloney, 1966), various biological and biophysical properties of the reptilian virus were studied and found to conform with those of avian and murine C-type viruses (Gilden, 1970).

Fibrosarcomas have been noted in V. russelli (Effron Et al., 1977), C. constrictor (Frye and Dutra, 1973), C. horridus (Harshbarger, 1974) (Fig. 21.15), C. atrox and C. v. viridis (Wadsworth, 1954a). Pseudechis sp. was Mentioned as having a subcutaneous fibrosarcoma (Wadsworth 1956). A lipoma and a xanthoma (not considered a neoplasm in other species) have been listed for C. constrictor and

P. melanoleucus, respectively (Harshbarger, 1978, 1979). Three undifferentiated sarcomas have been noted in L. getulus californiae and C. ruber (Harshbarger, 1974, 1975) and in P. melanoleucus sayi (Machotka and Whitney, 1980).

Musculoskeletal system. Muscle tumors in snakes have proven to be rare. A leiomyosarcoma from the rectum metastatic to the liver of a cobra and a myocardial rhabdomyosarcoma in a Boa constrictor have been discussed above. There remains only two other reported muscle neoplasms. One, a rhabdomyosarcoma in the left anterior portion of the palate in a P. melanoleucus, appeared as a 1.5 cm spherical, non-pigmented, broadly based sessile mass (Ball, 1946). Lunger et al. (1974) described an embryonal rhabdomyosarcoma in an E. guttata, captive for 13 years. Electron microscopic examination revealed viral particles

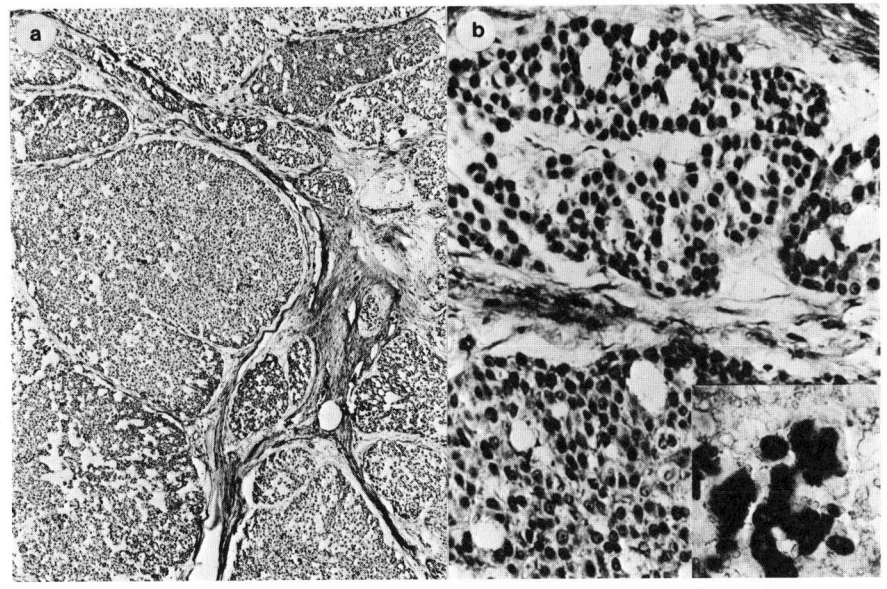

Fig. 21.16a,b. Corn snake, Elaphe g. guttata, chondrosarcoma (RTLA 465).
    a. Multiple nodules of neoplastic chondrocytes. H&E X40
    b. Nodules comprised of cells with small round nuclei and scanty cytoplasm. H&E X250 Insert: Associated with these cells are abundant calcium salts. Alizarin red S X200

in various stages of maturation morphologically resembling avian and mammalian C-type RNA viruses.

Skeletal lesions (Fig. 21.16) reported in snakes include an E. guttata with a chondrosarcoma (Harshbarger, 1974), a rufous-beaked snake, Ramphiophis rostratus, with Spinal osteosarcoma (Hill, 1954) and a N. melanoleuca with spinal osteochondrosarcoma (Wadsworth, 1954a).

Nervous system/pigment cells. Not a single report of central nervous system neoplasia has been reported in serpents, and only one peripheral nervous system tumor was reported, that a neurofibrosarcoma involving the spine in A. halys brevicaudus (Effron et al., 1977).

Pigment cell tumors are included here since these cells originate from the neural crest early in the embryo development. Non-malignant melanomas were reported in a P. reticulatus which had been on display at the Philadelphia Zoological Gardens for 20 years (Schlumberger and Lucke, 1948). This animal had a swelling in the right side of the upper jaw that measured 6 x 3x 2 cm, was firm, pale and fibrous appearing. There were two smaller black masses, one 2.4 m from the tip of the tail and the other 1.2 m from the head. Histologically, the tumors were composed of non-invading, spindle-shaped cells grouped in interlacing bundles with abundant melanin evident in the smaller growths.

Malignant melanomas were described in paired male and female P. melanoleucus after they had been in captivity and on display at the San Diego Zoological Gardens for 3 years (Ball, 1946). The female had a dark, rapidly growing mass on the tail which was amputated. Two years later a swelling developed anterior to the cloaca reaching a size of 11 x 6 x 5 cm within six months. Two metastatic nodules were noted in the liver at necropsy. The neoplastic cells were spindle-shaped, contained fine pigmented cytoplasmic granules and tended to be arranged in interlacing bundles with occasional palisading. The male developed a melantotic mass in the upper labial fold after six years in captivity. There were histological similarities to the aforementioned mass, but without metastases. This animal also had a palatine rhabdomyosarcoma previously described. A widespread malignant melanoma in a male Everglades rat snake, E. obsoleta rossaleni, was thoroughly described (Elkan, 1974). Extensive involvement of all major organs including the epidermis, longitudianl muscles along the body, oral cavity including the pulp of the maxillary teeth, the vertebral bone marrow, lung, heart,

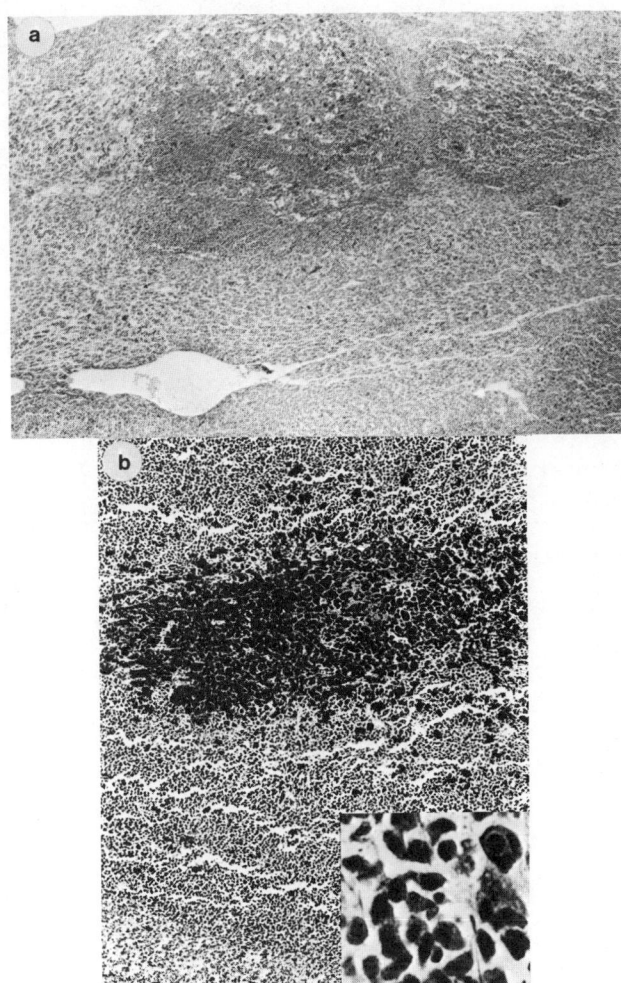

Fig. 21.17a,b. Everglades rat snake, Elaphe obsoleta rossaleni, malignant melanoma (RTLA 507).
a. Two dark, cellular masses in the liver. H&E X30
b. These masses contain cells with abundant black, cytoplasmic pigment that frequently obscures the nucleus. H&E X70 Insert: Other cells contain less cytoplasmic pigment that is distinguishable as finely stippled black specks. H&E X400

kidneys and liver as is demonstrated in Fig. 21.17. Malignant melanomas have been listed in a boa (Harshbarger 1980a) and thoroughly characterized in a 50 to 60 year old, 5.4 m female P. reticulatus (Schlumberger and Lucke, 1948). Other pigmented tumors have been described as malignant chromatophoroma in a terrestrial garter snake, T. elegans terrestris (Frye et al., 1975), malignant iridophoroma in P. melanoleucus and pigmented spindle-cell tumor in a Pacific gopher snake, P. m. catenifer (Harshbarger, 1974, 1980a).

Reproductive system. All but one gonadal neoplasm have been recorded in the ovary. Granulosa-theca cell and granulosa cell tumors of the ovary were listed in Atheris albolabui and E. murinus, respectively (Effron et al., 1977). A granulosa cell tumor in a six year old female garter snake with renal metasteses has been extensively characterized (Onderka and Zwart, 1978). The earliest record of an ovarian neoplasm was diagnosed as an adenocarcinoma in a P. sebae which had been on display at the London Zoological Gardens for 15 years (Bland-Sutton, 1885). Although there were enormous numbers of yellowish-white nodules in the liver, lung and kidneys, the author concluded that "the ovaries may have been the starting place of the mischief" since they contained several orange-sized nodules and the relation of the blood stream to the organs. Ovarian fibromas have been diagnosed in an elephant trunk snake, Acrochordus javanicus (Harshbarger, 1974) and an A. piscivorus (Ippen, 1972). A hemangioma in an ovary of a C. horridus was presented under the cardiovascular system.

The only documented case of testicular neoplasia was noted in a T. sirtalis and was diagnosed as a sertoli cell tumor (Harshbarger, 1974).

Respiratory system. The only bona fide pulmonary growth has been diagnosed in a male cape cobra, N. nivea, as a bronchogenic adenocarcinoma (Effron et al., 1977). Another mass occurred as a 2.5 x 1.5 x 1.0 cm, ulcerated, firm enlargement of the right maxilla in a newly captured L. getulus and was considered to be a squamous cell carcinoma (Hill, 1977). Further evaluation revealed that this mass contained a mucin-producing adenomatous component and was listed as a squamous (versus mucoepidermoid) carcinoma of probable salivary gland origin (Harshbarger, 1978b). Subsequently, this author examined sections of the mass and while attempting to find a suitable field for photomicrography found a few of the glandular structures to be lined by a ciliated squamoid epithelium. The

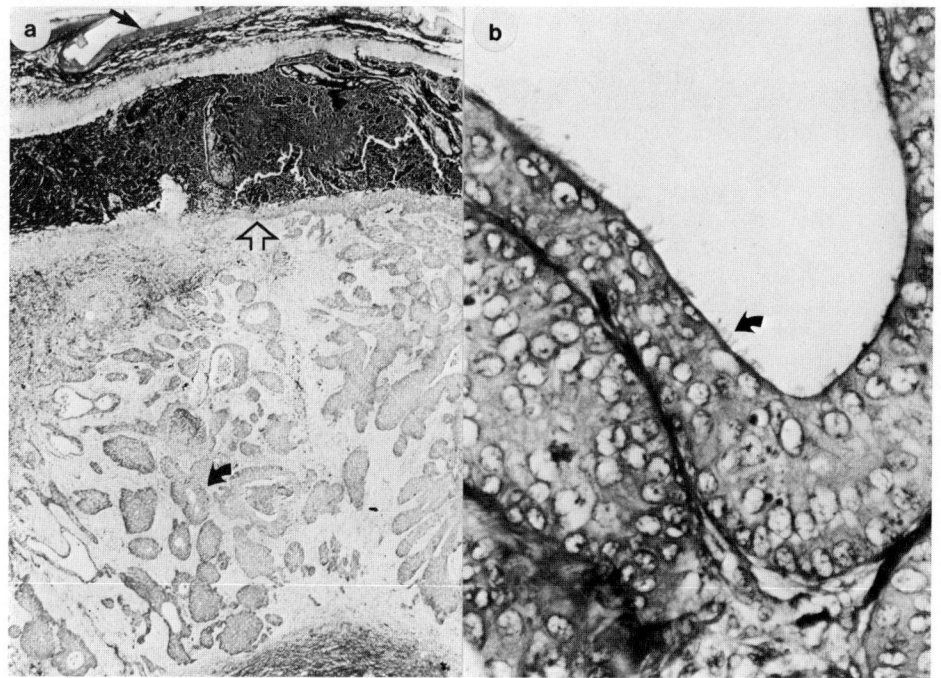

Fig. 21.18a,b. Lampropeltis getulus, squamoid adenocarcinoma, probable tracheal origin (RTLA 1835).
a. Superficial epithelium (closed arrow) covering pool of keratogenous and cellular debris surrounded by epithelium (open arrow). Cords and small islands of epithelium, sometimes with lumina (curved arrow), are separated by fibrous connective tissue. H&E X30
b. Small dermal tubule composed of multilayered ciliated epithelium (arrow). H&E X1020

features of this mass, now considered a squamoid adenocarcinoma of probable tracheal origin (Fig. 21.18).

Urinary system. Renal cortical adenomas have been listed in an albino P. m. annectens and a B. arietans From the Zoological Society of San Diego (Effron et al., 1977). Renal adenocarcinoma has been recorded in a C. constrictor (Harshbarger, 1976) and a N. natrix characterized by atypical epithelial cells in an acinar arrangement into which papillary projections protruded (Patay, 1933).

DIAGNOSIS AND TREATMENT

Rational treatment of a condition, be it neoplastic or non-neoplastic, requires a timely, definitive diagnosi Though the pathologist is frequently considered a diagnos tition, e.g. the diagnostic pathologist, when it comes to neoplasia, it should be remembered that he primarily confirms the diagnosis, with a few embellishments. The clinician more often deals with a living patient whereas the pathologist frequently examines the tissues of dead animals. So basically, there is an artifical separation of the diagnostic process to clinical and pathological with much of the diagnostic burden falling on the shoulder of the clinician.

Clinical evaluation must begin with the taking of an exhaustive historical record. History of the patient includes: its environment (captive or free-ranging); age or physical dimensions if age is not known; sex; species; feeding habits; duration of illness or presence of tumor if visible with a description of its gross features and growth characteristics; and, finally the signs of illness exhibited by the patient. Clinical procedures useful in detecting neoplasia include a thorough physical examination, obtaining blood which on blood film preparation may reveal hematopoietic neoplasia (Frye and Carney, 1972, 1973), biopsy sampling and radiography to detect the presence or extent of the neoplastic process.

Unfortunately, the animal may be dead or presented in a moribund state so that it dies shortly thereafter and the clinician must become a prosector. The fact that the animal may have died from some known traumatic injury should not deter the performance of a complete necropsy, including the central nervous system. Knowledge of reptilian anatomy may be obtained by reading various texts (Ashley, 1955; Chiasson, 1962; Harris, 1963; Oldham, 1970; Weickert, 1951). For information on necropsy techniques the reader is referred to Dolensek (1971), Jacobson (1978) and Chapter 29 of this text. Necropsy technique, though important, should not overshadow keen observation and description of necropsy findings for these facts may well be necessary in determining a definitive diagnosis. Lastly, in order for the pathologist to satisfactorily evaluate the tissues submitted, they must be properly collected and preserved in a sufficient quantity of fixative such as 10% neutral buffered formalin.

The diagnostic process now continues with the histopathological evaluation of tissues submitted. The pathologist routinely has access to light microscopy and special stains which will, in most cases, prove sufficient for diagnostic interpretation. In more troublesome cases the diagnosis is not so easily determined and may require utilization of transmission and scanning electron microscopes.

Further sophistications of the diagnostic process including viral isolation, immunologic detection of specific tumor antigens and initiation of tissue cultures may be warranted in specific instances.

Treatment of neoplasms in reptiles can, as in other animals, include sugery, irradiation and chemotherapy. The decision to attempt treatment and which mode of therapy to utilize will depend on patient factors, type, location and extent of neoplasia. As is the case for other animal patients, the cost of the procedure utilized will be a determining factor. Surgical treatment is the most likely to be employed and has been reported (Idowu, 1975; Schwarz, 1923).

REFERENCES

Alexander, N.J., and Fahrenbach, W., 1969, The dermal chromatophores of Anolis carolinensis (Reptilia, Iguanidae), Amer. J. Anat., 126:41-56.
Ashley, L.M., 1955, "Laboratory anatomy of the turtle," Wm.C. Brown Co., Dubuque.
Bagnara, J.T., and Hadley, M., 1973, "Chromatophores and color change," Prentice-Hall Inc., Englewood Cliffs.
Baillie, Sims, Willan, Sharpe, Home, Pearson, Abernethy, and Denman, 1806, Institution for investigating the nature of cancer, Edinburgh Med. J., 2: 382-389 (reprinted in Int. J. Cancer, 2:281-285, 1967).
Ball, H.A., 1946, Melanosarcoma and rhabdomyoma in two pine snakes (Pituophis melanoleucus), Cancer Res., 6:134-138.
Beard, J.W., 1964, "International conference on avian tumor viruses," Nat. Cancer Inst. Monogr., 17, United States DHEW, Washington.
Bergman, R.A.M., 1941, Tumoren biji Slangen, Geneesk. Tijdschr. Ned. Indie, 81:557-577.
Billups, L.H., and Harshbarger, J., 1976, Reptiles, in: "Handbook of laboratory animal science," E.C. Melby and N.H. Altman, eds., CRC Press, Cleveland.

Bland-Sutton, J., 1885, Tumors in animals, J. Anat. Physiol., 19:415-475.

Brand, K.G., 1975, Foreign body induced sarcomas, in: "Cancer," F.F. Becker, ed., Plenum Publ. Corp., New York.

Bresler, V.M., 1963, Opukhol-legkogo u cherepakhi Emys orbicularis, Vop. Onkol., 9:87-91.

Bullock, F.D., and Curtis, M., 1920, Experimental production of sarcoma of the liver of the rat, Proc. New York Pathol. Soc. N.S., 20:149-175.

Cheville, N.F., 1976, "Cell pathology," Iowa State Univ. Press, Ames.

Chiasson, R.B., 1962, "Laboratory anatomy of the alligator," Wm.C. Brown Co., Dubuque.

Cooper, R.H., 1968, Melanoma in Heloderma suspectum, Cope, Proc. Indiana Acad. Sci., 78:466-467.

Cowan, D.F., 1968, Diseases of captive reptiles, J. Amer. Vet. Med. Ass., 153:848-859.

Dawe, C.J., 1969, Neoplasms of blood cell origin in poikilothermic animals: A review, in: "Comparative morphology of hematopoietic neoplasms," C. Lingeman and F. Garner, eds., Nat. Cancer Inst. Monogr., 32, United States DHEW, Washington.

Dawe, C.J., and Berard, C., 1971, Workshop on comparative pathology of hematopoietic and lymphoreticular neoplasms, J. Nat. Cancer Inst., 47:1365-1390.

Dolensek, E.P., 1971, Necropsy techniques in reptiles, J. Amer. Vet. Med. Ass., 159:1616-1617.

Dunning, W.F., 1946, Multiple peritoneal sarcoma in rats from intraperitoneal injection of washed ground Taenia larvae, Cancer Res., 6:668-670.

Dunning, W.F., and Curtis, M., 1939, Malignancy induced by Cysticercus fasciolaris: Its independence of age of the host when infested, Amer. J. Cancer, 37:312-328.

Effron, M., Griner, L., and Berirschke, K., 1977, Nature and rate of neoplasia in captive wild mammals, birds and reptiles at necropsy, J. Nat. Cancer Inst., 59:185-198.

Elkan, E., 1974, Malignant melanoma in a snake, J. Comp. Pathol., 84:51-57.

Elkan, E., and Cooper, J., 1976, Tumors and pseudotumors in some reptiles, J. Comp. Pathol., 86:337-348.

Ellerman, E., and Bang, O., 1908, Experimentelle leukamie bei huhnern, Zentralbl. Bakteriol., 46:595-609.

Finkelstein, E.A., 1944, Opukholevii Rost Besspozvonochnykh i Nizshikh Pozvonochnykh, USP Sovrem. Biol., 17:320-348.

Finnie, E.P., 1972, Lymphoid leukosis in an Indian python (Python molurus), J. Pathol., 107:295-297.

Frank, W., and Schepky, A., 1969, Metastasierendes lymphosarkom bei einer riesenschlange, Eunectes murinus (Linnaeus, 1758), Pathol. Vet., 6:437-443.

Froom, B., 1974, A pet melanistic garter snake dies of cancer, Canadian Amphibian Reptile Conserv. Soc., 12:1-6.

Frye, F.L., 1973, "Husbandry, medicine and surgery in captive reptiles," V.M. Publ. Inc., Bonner Springs.

Frye, F.L., 1981, "Biomedical and surgical aspects of captive reptile husbandry," V.M. Publ. Inc., Bonner Springs.

Frye, F.L., and Carney, J., 1972, Myelopproliferative disease in a turtle, J. Amer. Vet. Med. Ass., 161:595-599.

Frye, F.L., and Carney, J., 1973, Acute lymphatic leukemia in a boa constrictor, Vet. Med. Small Animal Clin., 68:653-654.

Frye, F.L., and Carney, J., 1975, Parathyroid adenoma in a tortoise, Vet. Med. Small Animal Clin., 70: 582-584.

Frye, F.L., and Dutra, F., 1973, Fibrosarcoma in a boa constrictor, Vet. Med. Small Animal Clin., 69: 245-246.

Frye, F.L., and Dutra, F., 1974, Reticulum cell sarcoma in an American anole, Vet. Med. Small Animal Clin., 69:897-899.

Frye, F.L., Carney, J., Harshbarger, J., and Zeigel, R., 1975, Malignant chromatophoroma in a western terrestrial garter snake, J. Amer. Vet. Med. Ass., 167:557-558.

Gilden, R.V., 1970, Reptilian C-type virus: Biophysical, biological and immunological properties, Virology, 41:187-190.

Good, R.A., and Finstad, J., 1969, Essential relationship between the lymphatic system, immunity and malignancy, in: "Neoplasms and related disorders of invertebrates and lower vertebrate animals," C.J. Dawe and J.C. Harshbarger, eds., Nat. Inst. Cancer Monogr., 31, United States DHEW, Washington.

Griner, L.A., 1975, Hematopoietic neoplasia in animals of the San Diego Zoological Gardens, XII Internationalen Symposiums uber die Erkrankungen der Zootiere, Akademie der Wissenschaften der DDR, Berlin.

Harris, V.A., 1963, "Anatomy of the rainbow lizard," Hutchinson Trop. Monogr., Hutchinson Co., London.

Harshbarger, J.C., 1969, The registry of tumors in lower animals, in: "Neoplasms and related disorders of invertebrates and lower vertebrate animals," C.J. Dawe and J.C. Harshbarger, eds., Nat. Cancer Inst. Monogr., 31, United States DHEW, Washington.

Harshbarger, J.C., 1974, "Activities report registry of tumors in lower animals, 1965-1973," Smithsonian Inst., Washington.

Harshbarger, J.C., 1975, "Activities report registry of tumors in lower animals, 1974 supplement," Smithsonian Inst., Washington.

Harshbarger, J.C., 1976, "Activities report registry of tumors in lower animals, 1975 supplement," Smithsonian Inst., Washington.

Harshbarger, J.C., 1977, "Activities report registry of tumors in lower animals, 1976 supplement," Smithsonian Inst., Washington.

Harshbarger, J.C., 1978a, Neoplasms in reptiles, in: "Pathology of laboratory animals," K. Berirschke F. Garner, T. Jones, and C. Kozma, eds., Springer-Verlag, Inc., New York.

Harshbarger, J.C., 1978b, "Activities report registry of tumors in lower animals, 1977 supplement," Smithsonian Inst., Washington.

Harshbarger, J.C., 1979, "Activities report registry of tumors in lower animals, 1978 supplement," Smithsonian Inst., Washington.

Harshbarger, J.C., 1980a, "Activities report registry of tumors in lower animals, 1979 supplement," Smithsonian Inst., Washington.

Harshbarger, J.C., 1980b, Personal communication, National Museum of Natural History, Smithsonian Inst., Washington.

Harshbarger, J.C., and Dawe, C., 1973, Hematopoietic neoplasms in invertebrate and poikilothermic vertebrate animals, in: "Unifying concepts of leukemia. Bibliography of haematology No. 39," R.M. Dutcher, ed., S. Karger, Basel.

Hatanaka, M., Huebner, R., and Gilden, R., 1970, DNA polymerase activity associated with RNA tumor viruses, Proc. Nat. Acad. Sci., 67:143-147.

Hatcher, J.B., 1901, Diplodocus, Marsh, its osteology taxonomy, and probable habits with a restoration of the skeleton, Marsh Mem. Carnegie Museum, Pittsburg, 1:36.

Hill, H.Z., and Lin, H., 1977, Carcinogenesis and tumor growth, in: "Clinical pathology," J. Horton and G. Hill, eds., W.B. Saunders Co., Philadelphia.

Hill, J.R., 1977, Oral squamous cell carcinoma in a California king snake, J. Amer. Vet. Med. Ass., 171:981-982.

Hill, W.C.O., 1952, Report of the society's prosector for the year 1951, Proc. Zool. Soc. London, 122: 515-532.

Hill, W.C.O., 1954, Report of the society's prosector for the year 1953, Proc. Zool. Soc. London, 125: 533-539.

Holland, W.J., 1906, The osteology of Diplodocus, Marsh Mem. Carnegie Museum, Pittsburg, 2:225.

Idowu, A.L., Goldong, R., Ikede, B., Hill, D., Cunningham, J., and Akerele, S., 1975, Oral fibroma in a captive python, J. Wildlife Dis., 11:201-204.

Ippen, R., 1972, Ein beitrag zu den spontantumoren bei Reptilien, XIV Internationalen Symposiums uber die Erkrankungen die Zootiere, Akademie der Wissenschafter der DDR, Berlin.

Jacobson, E.R., 1978, Reptile necropsy protocol, J. Zoo Animal Med., 9:7-13.

Jacobson, E.R., 1981, Neoplastic diseases of the Reptilia, in: "Diseases of the Reptilia," J.E. Cooper and O.F. Jackson, eds., Academic Press, New York.

Jacobson, E.R., Seely, J., and Novilla, M.N., 1980, Lymphosarcoma associated with virus-like intra-nuclear inclusions in a California king snake (Colubridae: Lampropeltis), J. Nat. Cancer Inst., 65:577-579.

Kalin, J.A., 1937, Uber Skeltanomalien bei Crocodiliden, Z. Morph. Okol. Tiere, 32:327-337.

Kast, A., 1967, Malignes adenoameloblastoma des gaumens bei einer tiger-python, Frankfort Z. Pathol., 7:135-140.

Klein, B.M., 1952, Die Borkengeschwulst der Eidechsen, Mikrokosmos, 42:49-52.

Koch, J., 1904, Demostration einiger geschwulste bei tieren, Verh. Dtsch. Ges. Pathol., 7:136-147.

Lawson, R., 1962, A malignant neoplasm with metastases in the lizard, Lacerta sicula cetti Cara., British J. Herpetol., 3:22-24.

Lucke, B., 1938a, Carcinoma in the leopard frog. Its probable causation by a virus, J. Exp. Med., 68:457-468.

Lucke, B., 1938b, "Studies on tumors in cold-blooded vertebrates," Ann. Tortugas Lab., Carnegie Inst., Washington.

Lucke, B., and Schlumberger, H., 1941, Transplantable epithelioma of the lip and mouth of catfish. I. Pathology. Transplantation to anterior chamber of eye and into cornea, J. Exp. Med., 74:397-408.

Lucke, B., and Schlumberger, H., 1949, Neoplasia in cold-blooded vertebrates, Physiol. Rev., 29:91-126.

Lunger, P.D., Hardy, W., Jr., and Clark, H., 1974, C-type particles in a reptilian tumor, J. Nat. Cancer Inst., 52:1231-1235.

Machotka, S.V., and Whitney, G., 1980, Neoplasms in snakes Report of a probable mesothelioma in a rattlesnake and a thorough tabulation of earlier cases in: "The comparative pathology of zoo animals," R.J. Montali and G. Migaki, eds., Smithsonian Inst. Press, Washington.

Mawdesley-Thomas, L.E., 1975, Neoplasia in fish, in: "The pathology of fishes," W.E. Ribelin and G. Migaki, eds., Univ. Wisconsin Press, Madison.

Nigrelli, R.F., 1942, Leeches (Ozobranchus branchiatus) on fibro-epithelial tumors of marine turtles (Chelonia mydas), Anat. Rec., 84:539-540.

Nigrelli, R.F., and Smith, G., 1943, The occurrence of leeches, Ozobranchus branchiatus (Menzies), on fibroepithelial tumors of marine turtles (Chelonia mydas), Zoologica (New York), 28:107-108.

Oldham, J.C., Smith, H., and Miller, S., 1970, "A laoboratory perspectus of snake anatomy," Stipes Publ. Co., Champaign.

Onderka, D.K., and Zart, P., 1978, Granulosa cell tumor in a garter snake (Thamnophis sirtalis), J. Wildlife Dis., 14:218-220.

Orr, H.C., Harris, L., Jr., Bader, A., Kirschstein, R., and Probst, P., 1972, Cultivation of cells from a fibroma in a rattlesnake, Crotalus horridus, J. Nat. Cancer Inst., 48:259-264.

Page, L.A., 1966, Diseases and infections of snakes: A review, Bull. Wildlife Dis. Ass., 2:121-126.

Patay, R., 1933, Sur un cas d'epithelioma du rein chez Tropidontus natrix L. (Ophidien: Colubridae), C.R. Seances Soc. Biol., 144:865-867.

Peyron, A., 1939, Sur la frequence des tumeurs dans les divers ordres do vertebres a sang froid les especes, C.R. Acad. Sci., 209:261-263.

Pick, L., and Poll, H., 1903, Uber einige bemerkenswerthe tumorbildugen aus der thierpathologie, insebesonders uber gutartige und krebsige nuebildungen bei kaltblutern, Berl. Klin. Wochenschr., 40: 518-521.

Plimmer, H.G., 1912, Report on the deaths which occurred in the zoological gardens during 1911, Proc. Zool. Soc. London, 1:235-240.

Plimmer, H.G., 1913, Report on the deaths which occurred in the zoological garden during 1912 together with the blood parasites found during the year, Proc. Zool. Soc. London, 2:141-149.

Ratcliffe, H.L., 1935, Carcinoma of the pancreas in Say's pine snake, Pituophis sayi, Amer. J. Cancer, 24:78-79.

Ratcliffe, H.L., 1943, Neoplastic diseases of the pancreas of snakes (Serpentes), Amer. J. Pathol., 19:359-369.

Ratcliffe, H.L., 1953, "Deaths and diseases in the animal collection: Neoplasms," Rep. Penrose Res. Lab., Philadelphia.

Raynaud, A., and Adrian, M., 1976, Lesions cutanees a structure papilomateuse associees a des virus chez le lezard vert (Lacerta viridis Laur.), C.R. Acad. Sci. Paris, 283D:845-847.

Reichenbach-Klinke, H., and Elkan, E., 1965 "The principal diseases of the lower vertebrates," Academic Press, New York.

Rich, M.A., and Moloney, J., 1966, "Conference on murine leukemia," Nat. Cancer Inst. Monogr. 22, United States DHEW, Washington.

Rodhain, J., 1949, Tumeurs chondro-osteo-fibreuses multiples chez le lezard Cyclura cornuta, Rev. Belge. Pathol., 19:317-320.

Rose, F.L., and Harshbarger, J.C., 1977, Neoplastic and possibly related skin lesions in neotenic tiger salamanders from a sewage lagoon, Science, 196:315-317.

Rous, P., 1910, A transmissable avian neoplasm (sarcoma of the common fowl), J. Exp. Med., 12:697-705.

Russell, F.E., and Kotin, P., 1957, Squamous papilloma in the white croaker, J. Nat. Cancer Inst., 18:857-861.

Schlumberger, H.G., 1953, Comparative pathology of oral neoplasms, Oral Surg. Oral Med. Oral Pathol., 6:1078-1094.

Schlumberger, H.G., 1957, Tumors characteristic for certain animal species: A review, Cancer Res., 17:823-832.

Schlumberger, H.G., 1958, Krankeiten der Fische, Amphibien und Reptilien, in: "Pathologie de Laboratoriumstiere," Vol. 2., P. Cohrs, R. Jaffe, and H. Messen, eds., Springer, Berlin.

Schlumberger, H.G., and Lucke, B., 1948, Tumors of fishes, amphibians and reptiles, Cancer Res., 8:657-753.

Schmidt, R.E., 1977, Plasma cell tumor in an East Indian water lizard (Hydrosaurus amboinensis), J. Wildlife Dis., 13:47-48.

Schwarz, E., 1923, Ueber swei geschwuelste bei kalt-bluetern, Z. Krebsforsch., 20:353-357.
Scott, H.H., and Beattie, J., 1927, Neoplasm in a porose crocodile, J. Pathol. Bacteriol., 30:61-66.
Seibold, H.R., Bailey, W., Hoerlein, B., Jordan, E., and Schwabe, C., 1955, Observations on the possible relation of malignant esophageal tumors and Spirocerca lupi lesions in dogs. Amer. J. Vet. Res., 16:5-14.
Siciliano, M.J., Perlmutter, A., and Clark, E., 1971, Effect of sex on the development of melanoma in hybrid fish of the genus Xiphophorus, Cancer Res., 31:725-729.
Smith, G.M., and Betz, T., 1965, A case of fatal cloacal tumor in a snake, Brit. J. Herpetol., 3:199-201.
Smith, G.M., and Coates, C., 1938, Fibro-epithelial growth of the skin in large marine turtles, Chelonia mydas (Linnaeus), Zoologica (New York), 23:93-98
Smith, G.M., and Coates, C., 1939, The occurrence of trematode ova, Hapalotrema constrictum (Leared), in fibroepithelial tumors of the marine turtle, Chelonia mydas (Linnaeus), Zoologica (New York), 24:379-382.
Smith, G.M., Coates, C., and Nigrelli, R., 1941, A papillomatous disease of the gallbladder associated with infection by flukes, occurring in the marine turtle, Chelonia mydas (Linnaeus), Zoologica (New York), 26:13-16.
Smith, H.A., Jones, T., and Hunt, R., 1972, "Veterinary pathology," Lea and Febiger, Philadelphia.
Sobel, H.J., Marquet, E., Kallman, K., and Corley, G., 1975, Melanomas in platy/swordtail hybrids, in: "The pathology of fishes," W.E. Ribelin and G. Migaki, eds., Univ. Wisconsin Press, Madison.
Stolk, A., 1953, Hyperkeratosis and carcinoma planocellulare in the lizard, Lacerta agilis L., Proc K. Ned. Akad. Wer. Ser. C Biol. Med. Sci., 56:157-163.
Stolk, A., 1957, Tumors in reptiles. I. Melanoma of the skin of the viper, Viper berus, Proc. Med. Akad. Amsterdam, 60C:557-566.
Stolk, A., 1958, Tumors of reptiles, 4 multiple osteomas in the lizard, Lacerta viridis, Beaufortia, 7:1-9.
Stolk, A., 1963, Mast cell reaction during chemical skin carcinogenesis of the lizard, Lacerta agilis, Experientia, 19:20-21.

Stolk, A., 1964, Succinic dehydrogenase activity in the nucleolus of the normal and tumorous liver cells of the common iguana (Iguana iguana), Acta Morphol. Nee-Scand., 5:302-315.

Svet-Moldavsky, G.J., Trubchenivova, L., and Ravkina, L., 1967, Pathogenicity of the chicken sarcoma virus (Schmidt-Ruppin) for amphibians and reptiles, Nature, 214:300-302.

Trubcheninova, L.P., Knutoryansky, A., Svet-Moldvasky, G., Kuznetsova, L., Sokolov, P., and Belianchykova, N., 1977, Body temperature and tumor virus infection. I. Tumorignicity of Rous-sarcoma virus for reptiles, Neoplasms, 24:13-19.

Twardzik, D.R., Papas, T., and Portugal, F., 1974, DNA polymerase in virions of a reptilian type C virus, J. Virol., 13:166-170.

Vaillant, L., and Pettit, A., 1902, Lesions stomacles observees chez un Python de seba, Bull. Bus. Hist. Natur., 8:593-595.

Veskova, T.K., Trubcheninova, L., and Dook, L., 1970, Tumors in reptiles inoculated with chicken Rous sarcoma material, Folia Biologica (Praka), 16:353-355.

Wadsworth, J.R., 1954a, Neoplasms of snakes, Univ. Pennsylvania Bull. Vet. Ext. Quart., 133:65-74.

Wadsworth, J.R., 1954b, Some neoplasms of captive wild animals, J. Amer. Vet. Med. Ass., 125:121-123.

Wadsworth, J.R., 1956, Serpentine tumors, Vet. Med., 51:326-328.

Wadsworth, J.R., 1960, Tumors and tumor-like lesions in snakes, J. Amer. Vet. Med. Ass., 137:419-420.

Wadsworth, J.R., and Hill, W.C.O., 1956, Selected tumors from the London Zoo menagerie, Univ. Pennsylvania Vet. Ext. Quart., 141:70-73.

Weickert, C.K., 1951, "Anatomy of the chordates," McGraw-Hill Co., Inc., New York.

Wilhelm, R.S., and Emswiler, B., 1977, Intraoral carcinoma in a Burmese python, Vet. Med. Small Animal Clin., 72:272-273.

Willis, R.A., 1967, "Pathology of tumors," 4th ed., Appleton-Century-Crofts, New York.

Zeigel, R.F., and Clark, H., 1969, Electron microscopic observations on a "C"-type virus in cell cultures derived from a tumor-bearing viper, J. Nat. Cancer Inst., 43:1097-1102.

Zeigel, R.F., and Clark, H., 1971, Histologic and electron microscopic observations on a tumor-bearing viper: Establishment of a "C"-type virus producing cell line, J. Nat. Cancer Inst., 46:309-313.

Zwart, P., and Harshbarger, J., 1972, Hematopoietic neoplasms in lizards: Report of a typical case in *Hydrosaurus amboiensis* and of a probable case in *Varanus salvator*, Int. J. Cancer, 9:548-553.

LUCKE TUMOR OF FROGS

Robert G. McKinnell

Department of Genetics and Cell Biology

University of Minnesota

INTRODUCTION

The Lucke renal adenocarcinoma of the Northern leopard frog, Rana pipiens, has been studied more than any other neoplasm that afflicts amphibians. Abundant scientific literature relates, in part, to the biology of the species and is, in part, due to the biology of the tumor.

In former years, R. pipiens was plentiful and with this abundance was associated abundant tumors. The leopard frog has been described as "the most common frog in North America east of the Sierra Nevada Mountains" (Dickerson, 1906); "it is abundant throughout Minnesota" (Breckenridge, 1944); it "occurs in abundance in the vicinity of streams, ponds or lakes" (Smith, 1961); and "it is the commonest amphibian in its range, it is the most used amphibian in biological teaching and experiment, it is the amphibian most used for human food" (Wheeler and Wheeler, 1966). In the early 1970s, it was estimated that 20 million amphibians were used for educational purposes alone (Nace et al., 1974) and it is clear that the overwhelming majority of these animals were leopard frogs. Associated with the heavy use of R. pipiens for instructional use was a reliable system of collectors and retail dealers. Many of the collectors and dealers were knowledgeable concerning the source of tumor-bearing frogs and who needed them. Further, the dealers were sympathetic with the use of frog tumors for cancer research. Because of the abundance of frogs and because of knowledgable and cooperative dealers, it was not at all difficult to obtain Lucke tumors a decade or so ago.

There are a number of reasons why scientists might become interested in the biology of the Lucke renal adenocarcinoma. However, the principal reason for interest thus far relates to the Lucke tumor herpesvirus (LTHV). The Lucke tumor was the first neoplasm to be associated in a causal way with a herpesvirus. As will be shown below, the frog renal adenocarcinoma was a tumor rich with herpesvirus that could be induced to replicate by a change of environmental temperature. Harvest of oncogenic viruses was simple and frog embryos proved to be vulnerable to virus infection which induced tumors at metamorphosis. Characterization of the interrelationships of virus with tumor cells, virus replication and tumor induction by LTHV became the principal occupation of Lucke frog tumor biologists during the period from Tweedell's (1967) discovery that virus-containing tumor homogenates are oncogenic to the present time.

However, while the relationships of LTHV to the tumor were being investigated, as profitable an area of research as it was, other exceedingly important aspects of frog tumor biology were not being exploited. It will be the purpose of this chapter to review what is known about the tumor and its virus and to point out potentially profitable areas of research that have been inadequately studied.

The tumor was described first by Smallwood (1905) who noticed an unusual frog in a teaching laboratory at Syracuse University, Syracuse, New York. The frog had a bilateral renal tumor which Smallwood believed to be of adrenal origin. Murray (1908) illustrated the histology of Smallwood's tumor and concluded that "the cells do not present the slightest trace of the characteristic granules of the adrenal tissue." Lucke (1934a) also illustrated Smallwood's tumor and concurred with Murray that the tumor was renal. Downs (1932), like Smallwood, also preceded Lucke with a report of a frog neoplasm. A tumor was discovered in a R. pipiens intended for student use at the University of Alberta, Edmonton. Downs thought it to be of gut epithelial origin. Lucke obtained a slide from Downs and illustrated in his 1934 paper a portion of the growth with tumor epithelium adjacent to normal kidney tubules. Lucke judged the Downs tumor to be of renal origin. It is clear that Lucke was not the first to report and illustrate the frog tumor which bears his name, but he was certainly the first to describe it properly (Lucke, 1934a).

Lucke reported that some nuclei of the frog tumors displayed peripheralization of chromatin and contained acidophilic intranuclear inclusion bodies. Because of the inclusion bodies, Lucke called attention to the fact that there was a "filterable virus" associated with the neoplasm. The herpesvirus of the Lucke tumor was not revealed with electron microscopy until 1956, some 22 years after Lucke's 1934 paper, when proper fixation, embedding and thin section technique became generally available (Fawcett, 1956). Thus, Lucke was not only first with the correct histopathology of the tumor, but he also correctly surmised in the 1934 paper that a virus was associated with the neoplasm.

Geographic distribution of spontaneous tumors

The leopard frog complex is a group of closely related species that range across North America, east of the Rocky Mountains from Hudson Bay in the north to Costa Rica in the south (Conant, 1975; Wright and Wright, 1949). Despite the superficial similarity of these widely distributed frog species, it seems likely that spontaneous renal tumors are confined to limited populations of Northern leopard frogs ranging from Minnesota to northern Vermont.

Probably because most of the scientists who have worked with the Lucke tumor were primarily concerned with the virus, little attention has been paid to geographic pathology, i.e., distribution of tumor-susceptible populations of frogs. Lucke stated on several occasions that tumor-bearing frogs were common in Vermont, northern New England and adjacent parts of Canada (Lucke, 1934a, 1952; Lucke and Schlumberger, 1942). Unfortunately, Lucke did not provide collecting data from northern New England and Canada, nor did he provide collecting sites to substantiate his assertion that tumor-bearing frogs could be obtained from the Mississippi Valley, North Dakota and Indiana (Lucke, 1952). By the 1960s, however, frog tumor biologists began to venture forth from the laboratory to rivers, swamps and other damp areas. R. pipiens were collected in April 1961 at four sites north of Alburg, Vermont. Renal tumors were detected in frogs collected at three of the four sites (Auclair, 1961). Renal tumors have been found in abundance in midwestern R. pipiens obtained from commercial sources (McKinnell, 1965) or in frogs collected by this author from a number of localities in Minnesota (McKinnell, 1969; McKinnell and Ellis, 1972a, 1972b; McKinnell and Zambernard, 1968; McKinnell et al., 1972; Zambernard and McKinnell, 1969). Tumor-bearing frogs have been collected at Milford,

Michigan (Nace and Richards, 1969). Spontaneous tumors were not found in leopard frogs from northwest Montana, North Dakota and Louisiana (McKinnell and Duplantier, 1970; Mateyko, 1957).

Geographic origin of tumor-susceptible frogs

R. pipiens from the midwestern part of the United States were shown to be susceptible to renal tumors under certain experimental conditions (Rose, 1952; Rose and Rose, 1952, Tweedell, 1955, 1965). However, little direct information was known about tumor susceptibility of frogs from known collecting sites until frogs were collected by K.A. Rafferty, Jr., and R.G. McKinnell from eastern South Dakota to Quebec Province, Canada. R. pipiens from South Dakota, Minnesota, two sites in Wisconsin, New York, Vermont and Quebec Province became afflicted with renal tumors when held in the laboratory under tumor promoting conditions for eight months. Tumors failed to appear in frogs collected in Michigan (Rafferty, 1967). R. pipiens from North Dakota and R. utricularia from Louisiana were induced to develop renal adenocarcinoma under experimental conditions (McKinnell and Duplantier, 1970).

Perhaps not related to susceptibility in nature, but nevertheless of interest with regard to the species specificity of LTHV, is the report that R. palustris, R. clamitans and hybrids of R. pipiens with R. paulstris develop renal tumors when injected with LTHV-containing homogenates of tumor cells (Mulcare, 1969).

Seasonal distribution

It is difficult to interpet the significance of tumor prevalence almost a half century after the fact, especially when the data are reported by an investigator who, as many biologists are wont to do, used commercially obtained animals. Nevertheless, Lucke (1934a) stated that there was no seasonal fluctuation in prevalence of tumors. In contrast to Lucke, seasonal variation in tumor prevalence among Minnesota frogs was reported by McKinnell (1967). McKinnell (1965) reported that 79 of 884 R. pipiens from the north central United States were afflicted with renal adenocarcinoma. With this high tumor prevalence (8.9%), ecological factors could be correlated with tumor distribution. Of 1,081 frogs collected during the summer of 1965, no tumors were detected. This was puzzling because evidence was available that many of the frogs in dealers facilities were afflicted with tumors. The dealer's frogs that were examined in November 1963 were freshly caught. Perhaps a seasonal fluctuation in prevalence could have been the reason why tumors were not found among summer collections. Subsequent collections of early spring frogs at the time of emergence from hibernation, and collections made just prior to hibernation, were tumor positive (Table 22.1) (McKinnell, 1967, 1969; McKinnell and McKinnell, 1968).

There is at present no adequate explanation to account for the annual fluctuation of tumor prevalence. It is reasonable to postulate that the warm temperature encountered by a tumor-bearing frog during the early spring permits the tumor to grow rapidly resulting in that frog being at a selective disadvantage after the breeding season. Surely a frog with a rapidly growing tumor cannot evade a predator with the same efficiency as a frog unaffected by tumor burden. Tumors appearing de novo during the summer would be quite small at first, difficult to detect at autopsy and would not seriously affect the survivability of the host. Growth would be rapid during late summer and early autumn because of warm weather. Thus, frogs collected at the onset of hibernation would be expected and were shown to have tumors.

Knowledge of seasonal variation of tumor prevalence permitted studies related to herpesvirus replication (McKinnell and Ellis, 1972a, 1972b; McKinnell and Zambernard, 1968; McKinnell et al., 1972; Zambernard and McKinnell, 1969).

Declining tumor abundance

Geographic pathology and seasonal fluctuations in abundance have been considered above. A third change is being observed at the present time. That change is a drop in prevalence over the past several years (Fig. 22.1). Tumor prevalence was 8.5% in 1963 (McKinnell, 1965), between 1966 and 1968 it fell to 6.3%, it became 2.9% in 1970-1971, and prevalence then dropped to 0.0% in 1977 and remained there through 1979 (McKinnell et al., 1979, 1980). As in the case with seasonal fluctuation in prevalence, the cause of the annual decrease in prevalence is at present unknown. Rafferty (1964) considered the possibility of crowding as being a factor in tumor agent transmission as did DiBerardino and King (1965a) and de Thé (1978). Rafferty pointed out correctly that traditional tumor sources have been areas of exceptionally dense frog populations. What was true in 1964 has changed in the past decade and a half. Minnesota,

Table 22.1. Seasonal Variation in Tumor Prevalence Among Minnesota Leopard Frogs.[a]

	Spring				Summer				Fall		
Year	No. Frogs	No. Tumors	%	Year	No. Frogs	No. Tumors	%	Year	No. Frogs	No. Tumors	%
1966	212	6	2.8	1965	1,081	0	0.0	1967	150	9	6.0
1967	279	12	4.3	1966	473	1	0.2	1968	534	21	3.9
1968	88	11	12.5	1967	550	2	0.4				
Total	579	29	5.0		2,104	3	0.1		684	30	4.4

[a] The results of 3,367 autopsies of frogs collected in Minnesota are summarized. Prevalence of tumors among spring and fall frogs (5% and 4.4% respectively) exceeds tumor prevalence in summer frogs (0.1%). This difference is statistically significant. The apparent increase in tumor prevalence during the spring was interpreted as reflecting enhanced capability of finding tumor-positive geographic locations (McKinnell, 1969).

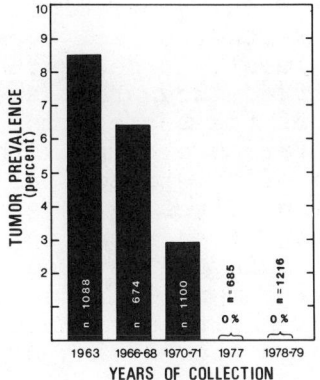

Fig. 22.1. Reduced prevalence of renal adenocarcinoma in leopard frogs, Rana pipiens, collected in Minnesota.

an area with over 15,000 lakes and therefore a rich environment suitable for frogs, no longer is host to hoards of R. pipiens.

The diminution of frog abundance has led to prohibition of commercial harvesting of R. pipiens measuring 15.24 cm or more (body plus leg length) in Minnesota since 1975. The Department of Natural Resources prohibited frog harvests because population assessments showed an annual decline dating since about 1971. For example, an average of 7.5 mature frogs were sighted per 1,000 yards walked by Department of Natural Resources personnel in 12 Minnesota counties in 1975. The Department judged from these data that frog populations were reduced that year. The summer of 1976 census revealed that the numbers of frogs were reduced by another 50% in the 12 counties surveyed in 1975. The census of the summer of 1977 showed additional and continued decline statewide except for isolated populations.

Our field notes from many years of collecting agree with the data of the Department of Natural Resources. McKinnell and McKinnell (1968) obtained 72 mature R. pipiens in approximately four hours in Kandiyohi County on July 2, 1965. This contrasts with a futile two hour collecting effort at the same site on June 5, 1977, when no frogs were seen. Thus, there has been an unparalleled diminution of frogs over the past several years and the decrease in frog density may be causally related to the diminution of tumor prevalence (McKinnell et al., 1979, 1980, 1982).

Whether or not populations of frogs recover to their former numbers and whether or not Lucke tumor prevalence regains its former level, it seems that population dynamics and tumor frequency are inadequately understood and studied facets of the Lucke tumor. Surely, cancer in animals and man is far more complex than simply the presence or absence of an etiological agent. The victim, whether animal or man, lives in an environment which may modify the capability of an agent in exerting its oncogenic effect. Stated in the reverse, host susceptibility may vary as the environment is altered. There may be a lesson to be learned with environmental studies of a spontaneous tumor of a free-living population of frogs.

ETIOLOGY

The etiological agent of the renal adenocarcinoma of R. pipiens is the Lucke tumor herpesvirus. While scientific proof of the etiology of the tumor was not available until much later, Lucke (1934a) recognized that a virus was associated with the frog tumor. Lucke illustrated acidophilic nuclear inclusions in tumor cells and stated "as yet no intranuclear inclusion bodies have been produced by agents other than viruses and such bodies are at present widely regarded as indicative of the action of a filterable virus" (Lucke, 1934a). He later wrote "the outstanding characteristic of the frog tumor is the frequent presence of acidophilic intranuclear inclusion bodies which in their general appearance are like those found in herpes and certain other diseases known to be due to viruses" (Lucke and Schlumberger, 1942). Similar statements appeared elsewhere (Lucke, 1938, 1952). Although Lucke lacked the methodology to establish a causal relationship of the virus to the tumor, he clearly was aware of the virus and its possible significance.

There is seasonal variation of the acidophilic intranuclear inclusion bodies; they are more common during winter and spring and less common during summer and autumn (Lucke, 1934a, 1952). There are seasonal fluctuations of temperature and one could propose that the variation in commonness of nuclear inclusions described by Lucke was related to temperature. All frog tumors maintained in the laboratory at cold temperatures (5 C) for two or more months had nuclear inclusions; no nuclear inclusions were detected in renal tumors maintained at 20 to 25 C (Roberts, 1963).

The expected significance of the inclusion bodies

was revealed with transmission electron microscopy of the renal tumor. "Virus-like" particles of inclusion-containing tumor cells, that were strikingly similar to particles of cells known to be infected with herpes simplex, were described (Fawcett, 1956). Later, the particles were identified as herpesviruses because of their 95 to 110 nm diameter (Fawcett, 1956), DNA core (Zambernard and Vatter, 1966a), and capsid symmetry calculated to contain 162 capsomeres with facets forming a polygon of icosahedral symmetry (Lunger, 1964).

It was stated above that some tumors had acidophilic intranuclear inclusion bodies and the inclusion bodies were related to both season and temperature. Is the LTHV similarly seasonal and temperature dependent? The answer to that question is yes. Frog tumors collected in late summer and early autumn were devoid of LTHV detectable with transmission electron microscopy (Zambernard and McKinnell, 1969) but LTHV were common in frogs during hibernation (Fig. 22.2) (McKinnell and Ellis, 1972b; McKinnell and Zambernard, 1968). The relationship of virus to season and temperatue is reviewed elsewhere (McKinnell, 1973, 1981a; McKinnell and Ellis, 1972a).

The virus may be present in many tumors but is it the etiological agent? Oocytes and prefeeding embryos of R. pipiens were exposed to tumor homogenates containing herpesviruses. Many of the experimental animals developed typical renal tumors at metamorphosis. Control tadpoles injected with homogenates devoid of LTHV did not develop renal tumors (Tweedell, 1967, 1969, 1978; Tweedell and Wong, 1974). One might argue that intact tumor cells are transplanted with LTHV homogenate and that the tumors observed in the experimental animals were therefore transplanted tumors and not induced by the LTHV. A virus-containing homogenate from a diploid tumor was injected into triploid embryos. Only triploid tumors ensued (Fig. 22.3). The diploid chromosome number of R. pipiens is 26 (DiBerardino, 1962). The experimental tumors had 39 chromosomes, the triploid number (Fig. 22.4), thus proving that the tumors were induced, not transplanted (McKinnell and Tweedell, 1970). LTHV, partially purified by zonal centrifugation, retained its oncogenecity (Mizell et al., 1969).

Koch's postulates were fulfilled with regard to the LTHV and the Lucke renal adenocarcinoma because of three procedures: visualization of viruses with the electron microscope, detection of viral transcripts in "virus-free" tumors and the virus injection procedure of Tweedell.

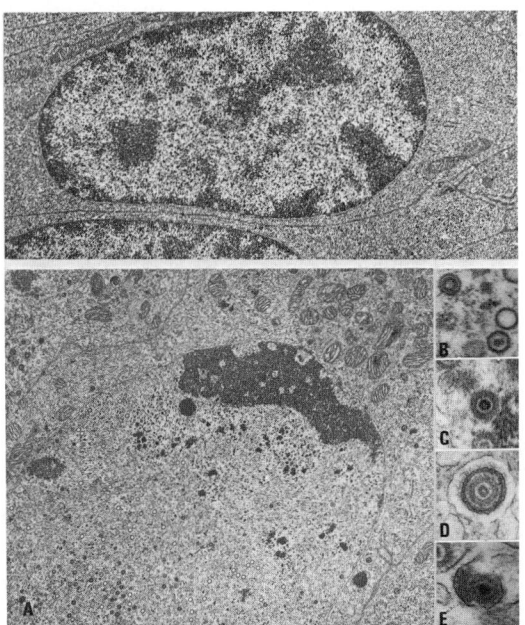

Fig. 22.2. Top. "Virus-free" renal tumor obtained from a prehibernating frog.
Bottom. (A) Spontaneous renal tumor containing intranuclear herpesviruses. Ontogenetic stages of herpesvirus replication shown on right. (B) Three types of nuclear virus: empty capsid, capsid with double-walled core. (C) Cytoplasmic virus with dense core. (D) Cytoplasmic virus with envelope. (E) Extracellular enveloped virus. (from McKinnell et al., 1972)

The first of Koch's postulates related to the presence of the agent in all cases of the disease. Virus particles, as stated above, are present in all renal tumors a few days after the onset of hibernation (McKinnell et al., 1972), during hibernation and persist for more than a month after the frog leaves hibernation (McKinnell and Ellis, 1972a, 1972b; McKinnell and Zambernard, 1968). Thus, all renal tumors in the cold have the LTHV. However, as stated above, frogs collected during warm periods of the year are devoid of LTHV (Zambernard and McKinnell, 1969). Do "virus-free" renal tumors have LTHV in a latent state? The detection of LTHV-specific transcripts of viral DNA (Collard et al., 1973) and the demonstration of virus-associated membrane

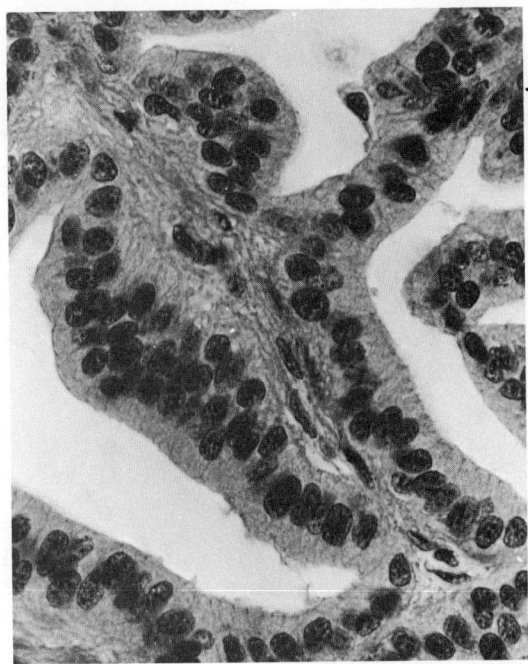

Fig. 22.3. Renal adenocarcinoma of a triploid frog induced by injection of Lucke tumor herpesvirus. While cell size is greater, the tumor does not appear to differ in other aspects from its diploid counterpart. Note well differentiated columnar epithelium. (from McKinnell and Tweedell, 1970)

antigens (Naegle and Granoff, 1977) in "virus-free" tumors, provides an affirmative answer to that question. Thus, LTHV is present in all tumors as detected either directly by electron microscopy or indirectly by virus-specific gene products.

The agent can be propagated in a cell culture and recovered from that culture (Tweedell, 1978). The agent appears to be relatively abundant, i.e., it was estimated that there is an average of 5×10^{11} virions per gram of cold Lucke tumor (Toplin et al., 1969) from tumors of animals exposed to low temperature in nature or to cold laboratory conditions (McKinnell and Cunningham, 1982; Morek, 1972; Stackpole, 1969). Harvest of viruses from cells comprises a modified second postulate of Koch. Homogenates of the cold tumor contain LTHV which will induce tumors in susceptible tadpoles (McKinnell and

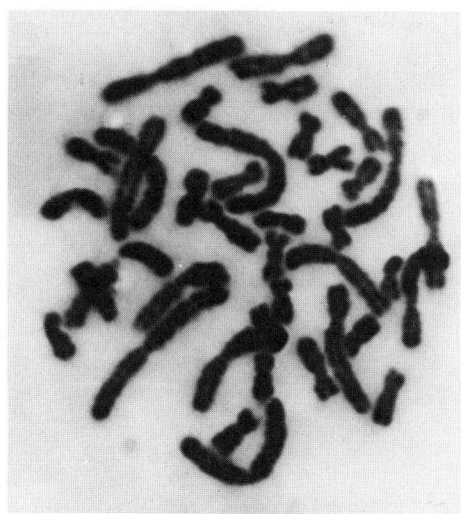

Fig. 22.4. Metaphase plate of induced triploid (3n=39) renal adenocarcinoma. (photo courtesy of Dr. M.A. DiBerardino, from McKinnell and Tweedell, 1970)

and Tweedwell, 1970; Tweedwell, 1967, 1969) which upon chilling yield the agent LTHV. Recovery of the agent in the experimentally produced tumors fulfills the last of Koch's postulates (Naegele et al., 1974). A final word concerning etiology: it goes without saying that other factors such as age at the time of exposure, crowding, temperature, etc., interact with the etiological agent and the susceptible host to result in the formation of a tumor (de The, 1978).

TRANSMISSION

The LTHV is probably transmitted from tumor-bearing adults to gametes or immature offspring while the adults occupy breeding ponds during the spring. Leopard frogs leave overwintering lakes ansd streams in Minnesota during early spring when they migrate to nearby temporary ponds where, after a variable period of time, amplexus occurs, and release of gametes occurs with fertilization. It is postulated that infection with LTHV occurs in the period of time that adults occupy breeding ponds for the following reasons. Infection cannot occur if mature viruses are not present. Mature viruses are not present during warm months (Zambernard and McKinnell, 1969). Maturation of LTHV occurs after tumor-bearing frogs enter hibernation

(McKinnell et al., 1972), but release of mature LTHV from the tumor is dependent upon an increase of environmental temperature (Zambernard and Vatter, 1966b). No increase in temperature will be encountered by frogs until they leave hibernation the following spring because water temperatures under an ice sheet are very constant. As breeding ponds become warm, mature LTHV are released from tumors (McKinnell and Ellis, 1972b). Viruses can be detected in the urine of frogs (Granoff and Darlington, 1969). In short, LTHV are mature and being released while adults are present in breeding ponds. Since oocytes and young embryos are susceptible to LTHV infection resulting in tumor formation (Tweedell, 1967, 1969), it would seem that virus replication and release are precisely timed to coincide with the production of susceptible stages of the host.

PATHOLOGY

The normal mesonephric kidney of R. pipiens is a brick red, dorso-ventrally flattened, elongate organ which parallels the antero-posterior body axis. A strip of bright yellow adrenal cells that parallels the major body axis occurs on the ventral aspect of the mesonephros.

Lucke tumors of the mesonephros may be recognized grossly because they are cream colored nodules, lumps or bulges in the matrix or on the surface of the organ. Tumor masses may occur singly or in multiples and may be either unilateral or bilateral. Spontaneous tumors occur in both sexes with little regard to size of the host other than that requisite for maturity (McKinnell, 1965); induced tumors differ in that they occur in the pronephric or mesonephric kidney of juvenile frogs (Tweedell, 1969).

The tumor has the microscopic appearance of enlarged tubules or irregularly shaped acini composed of tall epithelial cells. The epithelium rests on connective tissue stroma that is extensive in some tumors and minimal in others. The tumor cells often appear as a well differentiated simple epithelium or as an epithelium comprised of several layers of columnar cells. Neoplasms probably arise as a transformation of cells of the proximal tubules (Rafferty, 1964). A notable feature of many tumors is the presence of acidophilic intranuclear inclusion bodies. The tumor is not encapsulated. Variations in histopathology are described at length elsewhere (Duryee, 1956; Duryee et al., 1960; Granoff, 1973; Lucke, 1934a; Rafferty, 1972).

James Ewing (1916) wrote in the first issue of the American Journal of Cancer that metastases are the "most convincing evidence of lawless growth." Lucke (1952) stated "the cardinal sign of malignancy is metastasis." Before describing metastasis of the Lucke tumor, it is appropriate to point out the scarcity of spontaneous metastasis in the small rodents which are used extensively in cancer research (Foulds, 1969; Gorelik et al., 1980; Kim, 1979; Spreafico and Garattini, 1978; Wallace, 1961). The rarity of mouse tumor metastasis is emphasized to point out the difficulty of conducting research on the most malignant aspect of cancer with mammals. However, metastasis occurs spontaneously in the Lucke renal adenocarcinoma (Lucke, 1934b; Lucke and Schlumberger, 1949; McKinnell and Cunningham, 1982; Schlumberger and Lucke, 1948, 1949).

Organ sites of decreasing frequency of metastasis are: liver, lung, mesentery, parietal peritoneum, pancreas, urinary bladder, spleen, ovary and nerve (Lucke and Schlumberger, 1949). Clearly, the most useful aspect of spontaneous metastasis in the Lucke tumor is the fact that frogs are ectothermic vertebrates. Accordingly, tumor-bearing animals can be held at various temperatures and their bodies will shortly assume the environmental temperature. Low temperature (7 to 18 C) discourages metastasis and warm temperature (28 C) enhances metastasis (Lucke and Schlumberger, 1949). Up to 75% of well fed tumor-bearing frogs have multiple metastatic growths when maintained in the laboratory for about 50 days at 28 C. An exceptionally important and previously unexploited aspect of the Lucke tumor is the study of cellular and biochemical changes that occur at permissive temperatures.

It is doubtful if many human tumors are caused by viruses. However, most human cancer fatalities are attributable to metastasis. The study of Lucke tumor metastasis may prove in the future to be more significant than the study of its virus.

The diploid chromosome number of R. pipiens is 26 (DiBerardino, 1962). It would be appropriate to ascertain whether or not the chromosome constitution of the renal adenocarcinoma is similar to or differs from the normal diploid cells. Early studies of cultured renal adenocarcinoma cells reported a diploid chromosome number (Duryee and Doherty, 1954; Freed and Cole, 1961; Lucke, 1939). Tumor cells grow not only in the culture dish but also as grafts in the anterior eye chamber (Fig. 22.5) (Lucke and Schlumberger, 1939; Schlumberger and

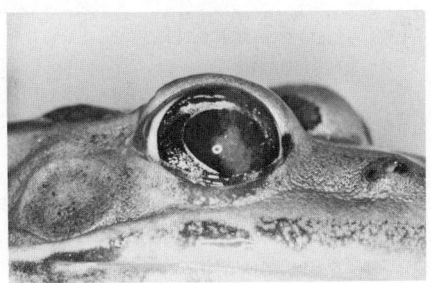

Fig. 22.5. Renal adenocarcinoma growing in the anterior eye chamber of a normal adult Rana pipiens (from McKinnell, 1978).

Lucke, 1949). Chromosomes from cells of normal embryos were compared with chromosomes from cells of a primary renal tumor and fragments of that tumor grown in the anterior eye chamber. Eighty-five to 90% of the tumor cells were diploid (387 metaphase plates from 1 primary and 11 anterior eye chamber grafts were studied). Karyotypic analysis of the diploid tumor cells showed non-specific structural abnormalities in 14% of the tumor cells compared with only 2% in the chromosomes of normal cells (DiBerardino et al., 1963). Later the chromosomes of nine primary renal tumors which were not cultured or grafted, revealed that the tumors are predominantly diploid although karyotypic study revealed aberrations in a number of metaphases varying in individual tumors from 0 to 75% (DiBerardino and Hoffner, 1969). The significance of tumor cell chromosome constitution to problems of experimental developmental biology are discussed elsewhere (DiBerardino, 1979; DiBerardino and King, 1965b).

While intact tumors and grafts of tumors tend to retain a near euploid chromosome number, in vitro cultured cell lines of the renal adenocarcinoma may become heteroploid (Przybelski and Tweedell, 1978; Rafferty, 1969). One aneuploid "tumor" cell line (Kucera and Simonson, 1974) is neither from the Lucke tumor nor is it derived from the frog R. pipiens (Freed et al., 1978).

IMMUNITY

It has been known for a number of years that adult mammals are frequently less susceptible to virus infection leading to tumorigenesis than neonatal mammals (Law and

Ting, 1965; McCoy et al., 1972). Related to the observation in mammals is the oncogenic effectiveness of LTHV in inducing tumors in embryos of R. pipiens (McKinnell and Tweedell, 1970; Mizell et al., 1969; Tweedell, 1967, 1969, 1978; Tweedell and Wong, 1974). It has been shown that prefeeding embryos at the onset of feeding and a larval stage just beginning to develop hind limbs are equally tumor-prone when injected with LTHV; however, a more advanced premetamorphosis larval stage did not develop tumors when exposed to LTHV (Mizell et al., 1978).

Does the presence of a thymus have an effect on susceptibility of a tadpole to LTHV injection? No is the answer to that question. Larvae thymectomized at Taylor-Kollros (1946) stages I, II and III were no different in their susceptibility to LTHV than normal immunocompetent animals (Rollins-Smith and Cohen, 1979, 1982).

A Lucke tumor virus associated membrane antigen has been demonstrated (Naegele and Granoff, 1977) and an immunofluorescent antiserum has been prepared against LTHV (Tweedell and Mizell, 1979).

While fragments of the Lucke tumor can be cultured in the anterior eye chamber (DiBerardino et al., 1963; Lucke and Schlumberger, 1939, 1940; Schlumberger and Lucke, 1949), only 22% of first-set alloimplants and 5% of second-set alloimplants survive more than 40 days in this so-called immunologically privileged site. However, more than 70% of tumor implants survived for more than 40 days when hosts were treated with corticosterone or aldosterone. The tumor fragments also enjoyed enhanced growth in the steroid treated animals (Rollins-Smith and McKinnell, 1980). More general comments concerning the immune response of lower vertebrates to tumors are found elsewhere (Balls and Ruben, 1976).

TEMPERATURE AND THE LUCKE TUMOR

Special properties of the Lucke renal adenocarcinoma associated with temperature need to be emphasized. Acidophilic nuclear inclusions are common in tumors of cold frogs and rare in tumors of warm frogs. Herpesviruses, as detected by electron microscopy, are similarly common in tumors of cold frogs but absent in tumors of warm frogs. Tumor fragments transplanted to the anterior eye chamber grow more rapidly at elevated temperatures than at reduced temperatures (Lucke and Schlumberger, 1940) as do tumor cells in vitro (Lucke et al., 1953). Finally, metastasis, the most malignant aspect of cancer, is enhanced by an increase in temperature. Manipulation of temperature therefore can become a powerful aid in experimental analysis of a number of critical biological phenomena of this spontaneous tumor in a natural population of a vertebrate.

NUCLEAR TRANSPLANTATION (CLONING) OF THE LUCKE TUMOR

The frog cloning procedure involves the insertion of a nucleus into a previously activated and enucleated mature eggs (Briggs and King, 1952; Fischberg et al., 1958). The procedure is useful as a bioassay for characterizing the developmental capabilities of nuclei obtained from a variety of sources. Normal undamaged nuclei from early embryos will substitute for a zygote nucleus and program viable gametes and normal progeny (Gurdon, 1962; McKinnell, 1962). Transplanted nuclei of the Lucke tumor, while not competent to program for normal development as many transplanted young embryonic nuclei do, nevertheless program for substantial early development. Swimming tadpoles ensue from tumor nuclear transplantation which shows that genetic information for many tissues and organs is present in tumor cells, and further, the genetic information is capable of being reactivated by interaction with enucleated egg cytoplasm (DiBerardino and King, 1965b; King and DiBerardino, 1965; King and McKinnell, 1960; McKinnell et al., 1969, 1976). These experiments and their significance to the understanding of neoplasia in terms of the differentiated state are reviewed elsewhere (McKinnell, 1978, 1979, 1981b).

REFERENCES

Auclair, W., 1961, Monolayer culture of Rana pipiens kidney and ecological factors, in: "Frog kidney adenocarcinoma conference," W.R. Duryee and L. Warner, eds., National Institutes of Health, Bethesda.

Balls, M., and Ruben, L.N., 1976, Phylogeny of neoplasia and immune reactions to tumors, in: "Comparative immunology," J.J. Marchalonis, ed., John Wiley, New York.

Breckenridge, W.J., 1944, "Reptiles and amphibians of Minnesota," Univ. Minnesota Press, Minneapolis.

Briggs, R., and King, T.J., 1952, Transplantation of living nuclei from blastula cells into enucleated frogs' eggs, Proc. Nat. Acad. Sci., 38:455-463.

Collard, W., Thornton, H., Mizell, M., and Green, M., 1973, Virus-free adenocarcinoma of the frog (summer phase tumor) transcribes Lucke tumor herpesvirus-specific RNA, Science, 181:448-449.

Conant, R , 1975, "A field guide to reptiles and amphibians," 2nd ed., Houghton Mifflin, Boston.

de The, G., 1978, Co-carcinogenic events in herpesvirus oncogenesis: A review, Int. Agency Res. Cancer Sci. Publ., 24:933-945.

DiBerardino, M.A., 1962, The karyotype of Rana pipiens and investigation of its stability during embryonic differentiation, Dev. Biol., 5:101-126.

DiBerardino, M.A., 1979, Nuclear and chromosomal behavior in amphibian nuclear transplants, Int. Rev. Cytol., Suppl., 9:129-160.

DiBerardino, M.A., and Hoffner, N., 1969, Chromosome studies of primary renal carcinoma from Vermont Rana pipiens, in: "Biology of amphibian tumors," M. Mizell, ed., Springer-Verlag, New York.

DiBerardino, M.A., and King, T.J., 1965a, Renal adenocarcinoma promoted by crowded conditions in laboratory frogs, Cancer Res., 25:1910-1912.

DiBerardino, M.A., and King, T.J., 1965b, Transplantation of nuclei from the frog renal adenocarcinoma. II. Chromosomal and histologic analysis of tumor nuclear-transplant embryos, Dev. Biol., 11:217-242.

DiBerardino, M.A., King, T.J., and McKinnell, R.G., 1963, Chromosome studies of a frog renal adenocarcinoma line carried by serial intraocular transplantation, J. Nat. Cancer Inst., 31:769-789.

Dickerson, M.C., 1906, "The frog book," Doubleday, Page and Co., New York.

Downs, A.W., 1932, An epithelial tumor of the intestine of a frog, Nature, 130:778.

Duryee, W.R., 1956, Precancer cells in amphibian adenocarcinoma, Ann. New York Acad. Sci., 63:1280-1302.

Duryee, W.R., and Doherty, J.K., 1954, Nuclear and cytoplasmic organoids in the living cell, Ann. New York Acad. Sci., 58:1210-1231.

Duryee, W.R., Long, M.E., Taylor, H.C., McKelway, W.P., and Ehrmann, R.L., 1960, Human and amphibian neoplasms compared, Science, 131:276-280.

Ewing, J., 1916, Pathological aspects of some problems of experimental cancer research, Amer. J. Cancer, 1:71-86.

Fawcett, D.W., 1956, Electron microscope observations on intracellular virus-like particles associated with the cells of the Lucke renal adenocarcinoma, J. Cell Sci., 2:725-741.

Fischberg, M., Gurdon, J.B., and Elsdale, T.R., 1958, Nuclear transplantation in Xenopus laevis, Nature, 181:424.

Foulds, L., 1969, "Neoplastic development," Academic Press, London.

Freed, J.J., and Cole, S.J., 1961, Chromosome studies on haploid and diploid cell cultures from Rana pipiens, Amer. Soc. Cell Biol., 1:62.

Freed, J.J., Toji, L.H., and Green, A.E., 1978, On the "Lucke tumor" origin of cell line LT-1, J. Nat. Cancer Inst., 60:493-495.

Gorelik, E., Fogel, M., Segal, S., and Feldman, M., 1980, The control of tumor metastasis, in: "Differentiation and neoplasia," R.G. McKinnell, M. DiBerardino, M. Blumenfeld, and R. Bergad, eds., Springer-Verlag, Heidelberg.

Granoff, A., 1973, The Lucke renal adenocarcinoma of the frog, in: "The herpesviruses," A. Kaplan, ed., Academic Press, New York.

Granoff, A., and Darlington, R.W., 1969, Viruses and renal carcinoma of Rana pipiens. VIII. Electron microscopic evidence for the presence of herpes virus in the urine of a Lucke tumor-bearing frog, J. Virol., 38:197-200.

Gurdon, J.B., 1962, Adult frogs derived from the nuclei of single somatic cells, Dev. Biol., 4:256-273.

Kim, A., 1979, Factors influencing metastasis of breast cancer, in: "Breast cancer," Vol. 3, W.L. McGuire, ed., Plenum Publ. Corp., New York.

King, T.J., and DiBerardino, M.A., 1965, Transplantation of nuclei from the frog renal adenocarcinoma. I. Development of tumor nuclear-transplant embryos, Ann. New York Acad. Sci., 126:115-126.

King, T.J., and McKinnell, R.G., 1960, An attempt to determine the developmental potentialities of the cancer cell nucleus by means of transplantation, in: "Cell physiology of neoplasia," Univ. Texas Press, Austin.

Kucera, L.S., and Simonson, J., 1974, Isolation and characterization of a cell line from the cocultivation of Lucke renal tumor cells and nontransformed feeder cells, J. Nat. Cancer Inst., 53:415.

Law, L.W., and Ting, R.C., 1965, Immunologic competence and induction of neoplasms by polyoma virus, Proc. Soc. Exp. Biol. Med., 119:823-830.

Lucke, B., 1934a, A neoplastic disease of the frog, Rana pipiens, Amer. J. Cancer, 20:352-379.

Lucke, B., 1934b, A neoplastic disease of the kidney of the frog, Rana pipiens. II. On the occurrence of metastasis, Amer. J. Cancer, 22:326-334.

Lucke, B., 1938, Carcinoma of the leopard frog: Its probable causation by a virus, J. Exp. Med., 68:457-468.

Lucke, B., 1939, Characteristics of frog carcinoma in tissue culture, J. Exp. Med., 70:260-276.

Lucke, B., 1952, Kidney carcinoma of the leopard frog: A virus tumor, Ann. New York Acad. Sci., 54:1093-1109.

Lucke, B., and Schlumberger, H., 1939, The manner of growth of frog carcinoma, studied by direct microscopic examination of living intraocular transplants, J. Exp. Med., 70:257-269.

Lucke, B., and Schlumberger, H., 1940, The effect of temperature on the growth of frog carcinoma. I. Direct microscopic observations on living intraocular transplants, J. Exp. Med., 72:321-330.

Lucke, B., and Schlumberger, H., 1942, Common neoplasms in fish, amphibians and reptiles, J. Tech. Methods and Bull. Int. Ass. Med. Museums, 22:2-17.

Lucke, B., and Schlumberger, H., 1949, Induction of metastasis of frog carcinoma by increase of environmental temperature, J. Exp. Med., 89:269-278.

Lucke, B., Berwick, L., and Nowell, P., 1953, The effect of temperature on the growth of virus-induced frog carcinoma. II. The temperature coefficient of growth in vitro, J. Exp. Med., 97:505-509.

Lunger, P.O., 1964, The isolation and morphology of the Lucke frog kidney tumor virus, J. Virol., 24:138-145.

Mateyko, G.M. 1957, Studies on renal neoplasms in Western frogs, Anat. Rec., 128:587.

McCoy, J.L., Fefer, A., Ting, R.C., and Glynn, J.P., 1972, The development of specific cellular and humoral immunity in mice infected with Rauscher leukemia virus as neonates or adults, Cancer Res., 32:1671-1678.

McKinnell, R.G., 1962, Intraspecific nuclear transplantation in frogs, J. Hered., 53:199-207.

McKinnell, R.G., 1965, Incidence and histology of renal tumors of leopard frogs from the north central states, Ann. New York Acad. Sci., 126:85-98.

McKinnell, R.G., 1967, Evidence for seasonal variation in incidence of renal adenocarcinoma in *Rana pipiens*, Proc. Minnesota Acad. Sci., 34:173-175.

McKinnell, R.G., 1969, Lucke renal adenocarcinoma: Epidemiological aspects, in: "Biology of amphibian tumors," M. Mizell, ed., Springer-Verlag, New York.

McKinnell, R.G., 1973, The Lucke frog kidney tumor and its herpesvirus, Amer. Zool., 13:97-114.

McKinnell, R.G., 1978, "Cloning: Nuclear transplantation in amphibia," Univ. Minnesota Press, Minneapolis.

McKinnell, R.G., 1979, The pluripotential genome of the frog renal tumor cell as revealed by nuclear transplantation, Int. Rev. Cytol., Suppl., 9:179-188.

McKinnell, R.G., 1981a, The Lucke renal adenocarcinoma: Environmental influences on the biology of the tumor with an appendix concerning chemical mutagenesis, in: "Phyletic approaches to cancer," C.J. Dawe, J.C. Harshbarger, S. Kondo, T. Sugimura, and S. Takayama, eds., Japan Sci. Soc. Press, Tokyo.

McKinnell, R.G., 1981b, Amphibian nuclear transplantation: State of the art, in: "New technologies in animal breeding," B.G. Brackett, G.E. Seidel, and S.M. Seidel, eds., Academic Press, New York.

McKinnell, R.G., and Cunningham, W.P., 1982, Herpesviruses in metastatic Lucke renal adenocarcinoma, Differentiation, 22:41-46.

McKinnell, R.G., and Duplantier, D.P., 1970, Are there renal adenocarcinoma-free populations of leopard frogs?, Cancer Res., 30:2730-2735.

McKinnell, R.G., and Ellis, V.L., 1972a, Epidemiology of the frog renal tumour and the significance of tumour nuclear transplantation studies to a viral aetiology of the tumour--A review, Int. Agency Res. Cancer Sci. Publ., 2:187-197.

McKinnell, R.G., and Ellis, V.L., 1972b, Herpesviruses in tumors of postspawning *Rana pipiens*, Cancer Res., 32:1154-1159.

McKinnell, R.G., and McKinnell, B.K., 1968, Seasonal fluctuation of frog renal adenocarcinoma prevalence in natural populations, Cancer Res., 28:440-444.

McKinnell, R.G., and Tweedell, K.S., 1970, Induction of renal tumors in triploid leopard frogs, J. Nat. Cancer Inst., 44:1161-1166.

McKinnell, R.G., and Zambernard, J., 1968, Virus particles in renal tumors obtained from spring Rana pipiens of known geographic origin, Cancer Res., 28:684-688.

McKinnell, R.G., Deggins, B.A., and Labat, D.D., 1969, Transplantation of pluripotential nuclei from triploid frog tumors, Science, 165:394-396.

McKinnell, R.G., Gorham, E., and Binger, D.G., 1982, Variation in the incidence of renal adenocarcinoma among Rana pipiens held under tumor-promoting conditions, Amer. Midland Natur., 108:111-116.

McKinnell, R.G., Gorham, E., and Martin, F.B., 1980, Continued diminished prevalence of the Lucke renal adenocarcinoma in Minnesota leopard frogs, Amer. Midland Natur., 104:402-404.

McKinnell, R.G., Steven, L.M., and Labat, D.D., 1976, Frog renal tumors are composed of stroma, vascular elements and epithelial cells. What type nucleus programs for tadpoles with the cloning procedure?, in: "Progress in differentiation research," N. Müller-Berat, ed., North Holland, Amsterdam.

McKinnell, R.G., Ellis, V.L., Dapkus, D.C., and Steven, L.M., Jr., 1972, Early replication of herpesviruses in naturally occurring frog tumors, Cancer Res., 32:1729-1732.

McKinnell, R.G., Gorham, E., Martin, F.B., and Schaad, J.W., 1979, Reduced prevalence of the Lucke renal adenocarcinoma in populations of Rana pipiens in Minnesota, J. Nat. Cancer Inst., 63:821-824.

Mizell, M., McCue, R., and Charbonnet, L., 1978, "Neonatal" tumour induction: The emerging immune surveillance mechanism and amphibian embryo tumorigenesis, Int. Agency Res. Cancer Sci. Publ., 24:835-844.

Mizell, M., Toplin, I., and Issacs, J.J., 1969, Tumor induction in developing frog kidneys by a zonal centrifuge purified fraction of the frog herpes-type virus, Science, 165:1134-1137.

Morek, D.M., 1972, An organ culture study of frog renal tumor and its effects on normal frog kidney in vitro, Ph.D. Dissertation, Univ. Notre Dame, Norte Dame.

Mulcare, D.J., 1969, Non-specific transmission of the Lucke tumor, in: "Biology of amphibian tumors," M. Mizell, ed., Springer-Verlag, New York.

Murray, J.A., 1908, The zoological distribution of cancer, Imperial Cancer Res. Fund Sci. Rep., 3:41-60.

Nace, G.W., and Richards, C.M., 1969, Development of biologically defined strains of amphibians, in: "Biology of amphibian tumors," M. Mizell, ed., Springer-Verlag, New York.

Nace, G.W., Culley, D.D., Emmons, M.B., Gibbs, E.L., Hutchinson, V.H., and McKinnell, R.G., 1974, "Amphibians. Guidelines for the breeding, care and management of laboratory animals," Nat. Acad. Sci., Washington.

Naegele, R.F., and Granoff, A., 1977, Viruses and renal adenocarcinoma of Rana pipiens. XV. The presence of virus-associated membrane antigen(s) on Lucke tumor cells, Int. J. Cancer, 19:414-418.

Naegele, R.F., Granoff, A., and Darlington, R.W., 1974, The presence of the Lucke herpesvirus genome in induced tadpole tumors and its oncogenicity: Koch-Helne postulates fulfilled, Proc. Nat. Acad. Sci., 71:830-834.

Przybelski, R.J., and Tweedell, K.S., 1978, Karyotype analysis of a pronephric tumor cell line, Exp. Cell Biol., 46:289-297.

Rafferty, K.A., Jr., 1964, Kidney tumors of the leopard frog: A review, Cancer Res., 24:169-185.

Rafferty, K.A., Jr., 1967, The biology of spontaneous renal carcinoma of the frog, in: "Renal neoplasia," J.S. King, ed., Little, Brown and Co., Boston.

Rafferty, K.A., Jr., 1969, Mass culture of amphibian cells: Methods and observations concerning stability of cell type, in: "Biology of amphibian tumors," M. Mizell, ed., Springer-Verlag, New York.

Rafferty, K.A., Jr., 1972, Pathology of amphibian renal carcinoma--A review, Int. Agency Res. Cancer Sci. Publ., 2:159-170.

Roberts, M.E., 1963, Studies on the transmissibility and cytology of the renal adenocarcinoma of Rana pipiens, Cancer Res., 23:1709-1714.

Rollins-Smith, L.A., and Cohen, N., 1979, Effect of early thymectomy on development of Lucke tumors in virus-injected tadpoles, Amer. Zool., 19:858.

Rollins-Smith, L.A., and Cohen, N., 1982, Effect of thymectomy on development of Lucke renal adenocarcinomas in virus-infected leopard frog tadpoles, J. Nat. Cancer Inst., 68:133-138.

Rollins-Smith, L.A., and McKinnell, R.G., 1980, The influence of glucocorticoids on survival and growth of allografted tumors in the anterior eye chamber of leopard frogs, Develop. Comp. Immunol., 4:283-294.

Rose, S.M., 1952, Interaction of tumor agents and normal cellular components in amphibia, Ann. New York Acad. Sci., 54:1110-1119.

Rose, S.M., and Rose, F.C., 1952, Tumor agent transformations in amphibia, Cancer Res., 12:1-12.

Schlumberger, H.G., and Lucke, B., 1948, Tumors of fishes, amphibians and reptiles, Cancer Res., 8:657-754.

Schlumberger, H.G., and Lucke, B., 1949, Serial intraocular transplantation of frog carcinoma for fourteen generations, Cancer Res., 9:52-60.

Smallwood, W.M., 1905, Adrenal tumors in the kidney of the frog, Anat. Anz., 26:652-658.

Smith, P.W., 1961, "The amphibians and reptiles of Illinois," Illinois Natur. Hist. Sur. Bull., 28:Article 1.

Spreafico, F., and Garattini, S., 1978, Chemotherapy of experimental metastasis, in: "Secondary spread of cancer," R.W. Baldwin, ed., Academic Press, London.

Stackpole, C.W., 1969, Herpes-type virus of the frog renal adenocarcinoma. I. Virus development in tumor transplants maintained at low temperature, J. Virol., 4:75-93.

Taylor, A.C., and Kollros, J.J., 1946, Stages in the normal development of Rana pipiens larvae, Anat. Rec., 94:7-23.

Toplin, I., Brandt, P., and Sottong, P., 1969, Density gradient centrifugation studies on the herpes-type virus of the Lucke tumor, in: "Biology of amphibian tumors," M. Mizell, ed., Springer-Verlag, New York.

Tweedell, K.S., 1955, Adaptation of an amphibian renal carcinoma in kindred races, Cancer Res., 15:410-418.

Tweedell, K.S., 1965, Renal tumors in a western population of Rana pipiens, Amer. Midland Natur., 73:285-292.

Tweedell, K.S., 1967, Induced oncogenesis in developing frog kidney cells, Cancer Res., 27:2042-2052.

Tweedell, K.S., 1969, Simulated transmission of renal tumors in oocytes and embryos of Rana pipiens, in: "Biology of amphibian tumors," M. Mizell, ed., Springer-Verlag, New York.

Tweedell, K.S., 1978, Pronephric tumour cell lines from herpesvirus-transformed cells, Int. Agency Res. Cancer Sci. Publ., 24:609-616.

Tweedell, K.S., and Mizell, M., 1979, Detection of Lucke herpesvirus antigens in infected frog pronephric cells, Arch. Virol., 59:239-249.

Tweedell, K.S., and Wong, W.Y., 1974, Frog kidney tumors induced by herpesvirus cultured in pronephric cells, J. Nat. Cancer Inst., 52:621-624.
Wallace, A.C., 1961, Metastasis as an aspect of cell behavior, Canadian Cancer Conf., 4:139-165.
Wheeler, G.C., and Wheeler, J., 1966, "The amphibians and reptiles of North Dakota," Univ. North Dakota Press, Grand Forks.
Wright, A.H., and Wright, A.A., 1949, "Handbook of frogs and toads of the United States and Canada," Cornell Univ. Press, Ithaca.
Zambernard, J., and McKinnell, R.G., 1969, "Virus-free" renal tumors obtained from prehibernating leopard frogs of known geographic origin, Cancer Res., 29:653-657.
Zambernard, J., and Vatter, A.E., 1966a, The fine structural cytochemistry of virus particles found in renal tumors of leopard frogs. I. An enzymatic study of the viral nucleoid, J. Virol., 28: 318-324.
Zambernard, J., and Vatter, A.E., 1966b, The effect of temperature change upon inclusion-containing renal tumors of leopard frogs, Cancer Res., 26:2148-2153.

PHYSICAL INFLUENCES

John E. Cooper

Comparative Pathology

Royal College of Surgeons of England

INTRODUCTION

The term "physical influences" covers traumatic and chemical injuries, electrocution, exposure to excessive heat or cold, changes in humidity, drowning and irradiation. Although the amphibians and reptiles are discussed together, and, indeed, have much in common, it must be borne in mind that they are in separate Classes and differ in many respects. Space does not permit discussion of their respective defence mechanisms but they are an important consideration when reviewing physical influences. Much of the emphasis of the chapter is on captive animals since there is a paucity of information on diseases of free-ranging amphibians and reptiles.

TRAUMA

Etiology

Trauma is a common cause of injury in amphibians and reptiles both in the wild and in captivity. In the case of the reptiles such incidents may not be accidental. Ever since the Biblical serpent was "cursed above all cattle, and above every beast of the field" deliberate slaughter of snakes and other reptiles has been characteristic of many races of mankind. Although the killing of venomous snakes is, on occasion, justifiable, many of those which suffer this fate are non-poisonous and some have an important role to play in the control of pests.

Free-living amphibians and reptiles are subject to injury or death due to motor vehicles. Newly metamorphosed frogs and toads, for example, may be killed in thousands as they attempt to cross a busy highway. Predation may represent an important factor in the control of populations, as has been reported for free-ranging garter snakes, *Thamnophis* sp. (Aleksiuk, 1977). The significance of injuries in free-living populations is far from clear, but surveys, for example in crocodilians, suggest that they may be of some importance (Webb and Messel, 1977).

Traumatic injuries also are surprisingly common in captivity and are usually associated with poor management. A common example in the past was the practice of tethering pet tortoises by a string attached to the shell. The string could twist around a leg and, if not removed, cause tissue damage and gangrene. Poorly designed cages are commonly responsible for cuts or abrasions while in larger enclosures an animal may damage itself as a result of a fall from a wall or roof. Snakes and lizards can damage their rostrum by rubbing it on the front of the cage and frogs by jumping against cage walls. A surprisingly large number of injuries are associated with poor handling techniques and these are usually due to unobservant or inexperienced personnel. Examples here range from grabstick damage (Fig. 23.1)(Cooper, 1973) to the trapping of a tail when the lid of a vivarium is closed or damage to a newt or salamander when stones in the enclosure are moved. Skin damage in amphibians can easily follow rough handling and many authors emphasise the need to exercise care when dealing with these animals (Universities Federation for Animal Welfare, 1976). Bite wounds are another common cause of injury in captivity and may result in the loss of a tail tip or digit; infection can quickly supervene. Traumatic injuries can be internal; a physical blow may cause internal hemorrhage or rupture of an organ. An animal may ingest stones or sharp objects when feeding and these can damage, or even perforate, the alimentary tract.

Diagnosis

The clinical features of traumatic injury vary enormously. Minor injuries may be manifested only as mild abrasions or areas of bruising. More severe lesions may be very obvious, for example, when a digit is crushed or broken, and there may be evidence of locomotory disturbance. Hemorrhage and fluid loss are a feature of many traumatic injuries and extensive internal damage may be accompanied by abdominal swelling and pale mucous

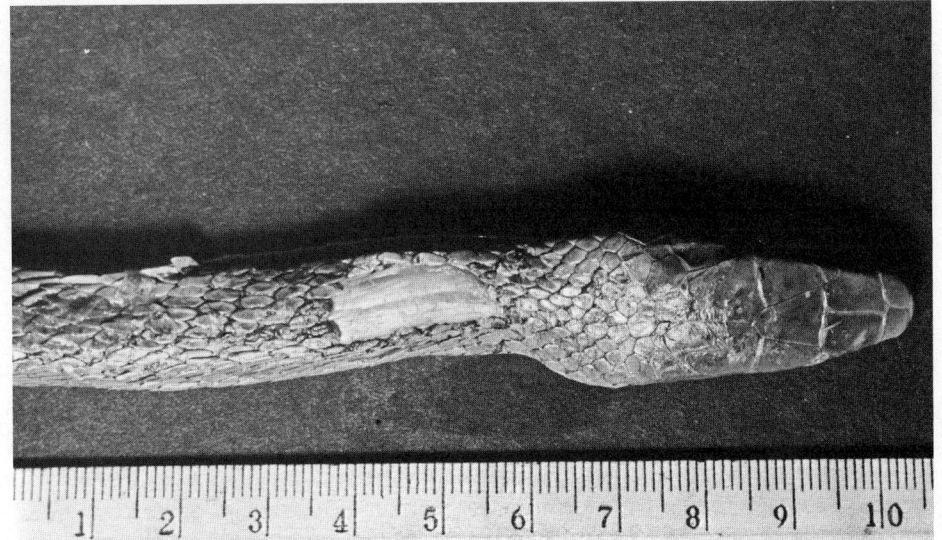

Fig. 23.1. Jameson's mamba, Dendroaspis jamesoni, showing damage to the neck following handling with a metal grabstick.

membranes. Wounds in amphibians can very rapidly become infected and it may be the infection that is first noticed rather than the injury. Fungi, such as Saprolegnia spp., are early invaders and can be one cause of so-called "newt-pest" (Vogel, 1964); more chronic lesions may be associated with Mycobacterium spp. (Temple and Fowler, 1978).

Diagnosis is based upon history and clinical examination. Palpation is important and radiography is helpful both in confirming skeletal damage and detecting internal lesions. In the case of post-mortem material, radiography is valuable and it is also advisable to skin the animal in order to search for such lesions as subcutaneous bruising.

Treatment

Treatment depends upon the severity of the injury. Mild skin wounds should be cleaned and bathed with saline and/or a dilute cetrimide solution. Attempts must be made to prevent recurrence, for example, by the provision of cover in which animals can hide and thus avoid rostral damage. In the case of more severe injuries, debridement and/or suturing may be necessary and these should usually be carried out under general anesthesia. Sutures are best left for at least four weeks before removal and in the case of the reptiles special care should be taken to use strong silk or nylon for the skin.

Fractures are commonly encountered in reptiles and amphibians and many will heal spontaneously; however, deformity and distortion may result. Limb fractures should be immobilised using modifications of techniques employed in mammals and birds, for example, external splints or internal pinning, plating or wiring. The "shells" of chelonians can be repaired using dental repair material (Wallach, 1969) or epoxyresin (Frye, 1973; Jackson, 1978; Zeman et al., 1967). Limbs can be amputated and most tetrapod species manage surprisingly well with only three legs. A common form of injury in free-ranging frogs and toads is a crushed foot or leg and the limb must be removed promptly if infection is not to supervene. In amphibians there is a tendency for regeneration to occur; for example, new fingers or toes may grow following an injury and on occasion supernumerary digits may be the result. Such regeneration is not usually a feature in reptiles although some lizards will readily shed their tails which then regrow.

Internal injuries may necessitate laparotomy and surgery though the prognosis is not good. Details of anesthetic and surgical techniques will not be given in this chapter; instead, reference should be made to such works as those by Cooper (1979), Cooper and Jackson (1981), Frye (1973), Nace et al. (1974) and Wallach (1969).

Fluid therapy has an important role to play in amphibians and reptiles and the author's approach is to give dextrose-saline (5% dextrose in 0.85% saline) subcutaneously, at up to 4% of bodyweight, to all cases where hemorrhage, contusion or fluid loss is suspected. Such treatment is of value in the management of other physical diseases, such as burns and frostbite.

ELECTROCUTION

Etiology

Electrocution is not common in free-ranging amphibians and reptiles but does occasionally occur; for example, if a snake slithers over an electric rail or while climbing comes into contact with powerlines. Such incidents are almost invariably fatal.

In captivity electrocution is more common and is usually associated with defects in the animal's cage or enclosure. The most common cause is a faulty connection or a piece of exposed wire in a heating appliance. Again, death is often the sequel, especially in the case of amphibians and aquatic reptiles where the effect of the current is exacerbated by the presence of water. Occasionally, however, the animal may survive the incident.

Diagnosis

The clinical features of electrocution vary considerably. Occasionally the victim will show signs of incoordination or flaccidity with no evidence of external lesions; such cases usually recover within 4 to 5 days. More often burns are present and these are discussed in more detail later in this chapter.

Diagnosis of electrocution is usually based upon the history. Frequently, the incident results in the light or heat source being extinguished; on examination black carbon deposits may be found on it or nearby objects. Care must be taken when investigating problems involving electricity since the current may still be flowing and thus present a hazard to the herpetologist; the electricity should first be turned off at the source.

Post-mortem examination of electrocution cases may yield useful information. Burns can be seen on the skin and may again be associated with black carbon deposits. Careful examination may reveal petechial hemorrhages under the skin, in the muscles and internal organs.

Treatment

Therapy is rarely necessary in electrocution cases as they are usually fatal. If the incident has occurred within the previous hour attempts at resuscitation are advisable even if the animal appears to be dead; oxygen can be administered and artifical respiration initiated by squeezing the thorax or tilting the body. In cases where there are only localised lesions treatment should be as for burns.

HYPERTHERMIA

Etiology

Exposure to high temperatures can result in death, systemic disturbances or localized burns. Amphibians and reptiles are ectothermic and thus have limited internal control of their body temperature. However, as will be mentioned later, representatives of both groups may show a physiological response to variation in temperature, so called "thermal acclimation" (Feder, 1978; Jacobson and Whitford, 1970).

There are various terms that are used in connection with the temperature relations of amphibians and reptiles. The "normal activity range" relates to the range of temperatures at which a given species is usually active. The "preferred body temperature" (PBT) lies within this range and is the temperature or range of temperatures which the animal will choose in a temperature gradient. It should be noted that the PBT can be influenced by a number of factors including the sex of the animal and the season of the year (Patterson and Davies, 1978), while other studies have indicated that both reptiles and amphibians infected with a pathogenic bacterium prefer a higher temperature (Kluger, 1977; Vaughn et al., 1974). It is postulated that the latter phenomenon may be of relevance to the evolution of fever. The "critical thermal maximum" lies a few degrees above the upper limit of the normal activity range and is the point at which the animal will die (Cowles and Bogert, 1944; Lowe and Vance, 1955). However, this can be influenced by thermal acclimation in certain species, for example Thamnophis proximus (Jacobson and Whitford, 1970).

There is much published information on metabolism and a review of this subject can be found elsewhere (Bennett and Dawson, 1976). It should be noted that studies on animals in the laboratory have yielded information of great practical value to those who keep amphibians and reptiles in captivity. Similar work should be encouraged on uncommon species in zoological collections although the numbers involved are rarely statistically significant (Gans, 1979).

Overheating or heat stress is a common cause of morbidity in both free-ranging and captive amphibians and reptiles. Free-ranging amphibians are particularly susceptible to the heat of the sun and large numbers succumb in the summer on sun-baked roads or dried-up ponds. Reptiles, having a dry protective skin, are less at risk but they too may die, especially during periods of drought or in bushfires. On the Island of Aldabra in the Indian Ocean, giant tortoises, Geochelone gigantea, grazing on the coast seek the shade of bushes when the temperature is high; those that are unable to reach the shade quickly perish (Swingland and Frazier, 1979). In captivity the usual causes of overheating are a faulty vivarium heater or undue exposure to sunlight in an outside reptiliary or glass-fronted cage; failure to provide hiding places is often an important contributory factor. In the case of reptile eggs overheating may be due to an incorrect or faulty setting on an incubator.

Chemical burns can occur following exposure to acid or alkali. This is uncommon in the wild but may be encountered in captivity; for example, if a cage is not well rinsed after disinfection.

Signs and diagnosis

The clinical signs of overheating vary markedly. In severe cases of heat stress the animal is found dead or comatose. Overheated reptile eggs fail to hatch and become desiccated and crumpled; exposure to less critical temperatures can result in low hatchability and possibly developmental abnormalities (Vinegar, 1973). In the case of hatched or metamorphosed animals the first clinical sign of overheating is increased activity; the animal moves rapidly and excitedly around its enclosure but intermittent attempts are usually made to find a sheltered or cooler place (Burke and Pough, 1976). Respiration is often accelerated. Loss of righting reflex is a well recognised feature of overheating in certain amphibians and has prompted study on the role of fatigue in temperature resistance (Burke and Pough, 1976). Finally, the animal appears to collapse and quickly dies. Localised overheating will result in skin burns but it should be noted that some species, in particular certain reptiles, appear to have a high threshold of response to thermal energy and will continue to sit or lie on a heater long after it has caused severe skin damage. There may be a difference between dorsal and central radiant energy receptors in different species. Some reptiles are obviously thigmothermic and respond to substrate heat while others respond more to dorsal heat arriving as radiant energy. Skin burns can cause dehydration and this is usually a marked clinical feature in amphibians.

It is of interest to note that Daugherty et al. (1978) recorded a difference in response of male and female frogs, Rana pretiosa, in their response to thermal stress; frogs exposed to water at 45 to 50 C initially showed rapid escape movements but after five seconds adopted two different sterotyped positions. The humanitarian aspects of the work can be questioned but Daugherty

(1979) believes that frogs treated in this way are insensitive to pain.

Diagnosis of overheating is based upon a combination of history, clinical observation and, where appropriate, post-mortem examination. Post-mortem findings in cases of heat stress are not marked but amphibians show a very dry skin and in both amphibians and reptiles there is dehydration. Care must be taken not to confuse with these cases those animals that have died for another reason and then been left for several hours in a heated cage before necropsy; the latter also appear very desiccated but, in addition, show marked autolysis. At post-mortem examination of animals exposed to a gradual rise in temperature there may be signs indicative of increased activity, such as ulcerative lesions on the rostrum. There may be marks on the wall of the vivarium, suggesting that the animal had been rubbing against it. Burns are usually apparent as areas of burnt, sometimes charred, skin or ulceration. Wound infection is a common sequel in cases which are not treated promptly; Pseudomonas, Aeromonas and other gram-negative bacilli can rapidly produce a dermatitis followed by a generalized septicemia.

Treatment

Treatment of overheating must be carried out promptly. The comatose or apparently dead amphibian or reptile may respond to bathing in cool physiological saline; administration of fluids by subcutaneous injection is advisable and a cool water enema may be benefical. Skin burns must be cleaned using a broad spectrum disinfectant, preferably quaternary ammonium or ampholytic, and there should be debridement or surgical removal of necrotic tissue (Vozenilek, 1978). In the case of reptiles it is often wise to cover and dress the fresh wound in order to prevent the entry of pathogenic bacteria; once healing has commenced in 10 to 14 days such dressings can be removed. Wounds on amphibians are not easy to cover and instead it is preferable, where practicable, to maintain them in a salt solution, 0.6 to 1.0% which is changed daily. In both groups of animals suturing of burn wounds can accelerate healing and reduce the risk of infection but must follow complete excision of necrotic material. Some burns cannot be sutured and the wound must granulate. It should be dressed and kept clean. Prevention of infection depends upon good hygiene. The vivarium should be cleaned daily and particular attention should be paid to water bowls in which Pseudomonas and other organisms will rapidly multiply. If antibiotic treatment is deemed necessary a careful choice must be made; where infection has already occurred, culture and antibiotic sensitivity should be performed. Antibiotics which regularly prove of value in such cases include tetracyclines, topically and by injection, and neomycin, topically on small burns only. Gentamicin is frequently the agent of choice following in vitro tests, but must be admistered cautiously and at specified intervals (Holt, 1981). Vaccination is proving of value in preventing Pseudomonas infection in human burn patients (Jones et al., 1978) and may have a part to play in lower vertebrates (Addison and Jacobson, 1974; Cooper and Leakey, 1976).

Chemical burns can be treated in the same way as those produced by heat, but it is important to remove any residual chemical by washing and irrigating the wound in normal saline.

A surgical adhesive called "Opsite" (Smith and Nephew) has proved useful in the treatment of burns in reptiles in Britain (Cooper, 1981). This protects the wound but permits gaseous exchange.

Mention should be made of the healing of burns. Healing is often by second intention, with the formation of granulation tissue. As a result, the normal scalation in reptiles is often lost and evidence of an earlier burn may be an area of shiny, scaleless and often colorless skin. In amphibians a similar lesion may result but a feature here can be a pigmented scar rather than a colorless one. In both groups the presence of a scar can initially interfere with the sloughing of the skin; layers of skin which accumulate over the lesion should be removed by bathing.

Many of the problems associated with too high or too low temperatures in captive amphibians and reptiles could be avoided if herpetologists provided their charges with a "temperature gradient" so that the animals can select their own PBT. The value of such a design has been emphasised by many authors over the past few years (Nace, 1977; Peaker, 1969).

HYPOTHERMIA

Etiology

Maintaining amphibians and reptiles below their PBT can produce both systemic and local effects. Hypothermia at a temperature above freezing will cause "chilling" while the outcome of exposure to more extreme temperatures may be frostbite or death. There is a "critical thermal minimum" for species and this, like the "critical thermal maximum", can be altered by thermal acclimation (Jacobson and Whitford, 1970).

Low temperatures are another hazard facing free-ranging animals although many of those living in temperate climates are able to tolerate cold by appropriate behavioral changes or hibernation. It is increasingly recognised that hibernation is a specific physiological response. There are, for example, changes in the hematological picture of hibernating tortoises, Testudo spp. (Will, 1978) and it should not be assumed that hibernation and cold-induced torpor are the same. Hibernation will not be discussed in detail. Low temperatures can occur under conditions of captivity when there is a power failure or when a vivarium or incubator is maintained at an inadequate temperature. Refrigeration is sometimes used as a means of immobilising animals in transit, for example recently imported tortoises, but it is a practice to be deprecated. Exposure of amphibians and reptiles to very low or near freezing temperatures occurs in captivity and in the wild but will only be discussed in the context of the former.

Signs and diagnosis

The clinical signs of chilling are a marked reduction in activity. The animal is lethargic, anorexic and responds only slightly or slowly to stimuli. It is likely to be found in the warmest part of its cage and is often pressed tightly against the wall or another area which offers insulation. Upper respiratory signs can be a feature of chilling; in chelonians, for example, there may be a serous discharge from the nares and in crocodilian species the shedding of "tears" from the eyes is sometimes seen (Vogel, 1964). If the low temperatures persist the eyelids may become sealed, the nares blocked and infection supervene. Wallach (1971) suggested that exposure to cold temperatures in an animal that has recently fed can cause fermentation of the stomach/intestinal contents with resultant abdominal distention and discomfort. Eggs of reptiles which become chilled usually fail to hatch and there may be excessive growth of fungi on the surface. In the case of amphibians death is less likely but development is retarded. At near freezing temperatures the affected animal may be torpid and careful examination will be needed to distinguish it from a dead specimen; gently stroking or squeezing of a limb will usually elict a response in amphibians, lizards and chelonians while in snakes squeezing of the tail is a useful indicator. It can be difficult to diagnose frostbite until the affected tissues begin to slough; prior to this it may be possible to detect a change in color, hyperemia or darkening and lack of use of the area. At temperatures below freezing the animal is likely to die but localized frostbite is a common occurrence. Frostbite usually affects appendages such as crests, flaps, digits, limbs and tip of tail. Tissues that are affected by frostbite but which do not become necrotic may lose their pigment and remain as pale areas. This has been used to advantage in that freeze-branding can be used to mark both amphibians and reptiles (Honegger, 1979).

Diagnosis of hypothermia depends largely upon an adequate history. Affected animals are cold to the touch and, in advanced cases, gangrenous changes may be apparent in the extremities. Post-mortem examination often adds little to the diagnosis although hydropericardium, ascites and pulmonary congestion may be a feature of chilling.

Treatment

Treatment of the chilled animal consists of warming it to its correct temperature. If chilling has been prolonged over 24 hours the warming process should be carried out slowly, over 3 to 4 hours. Usually there are no immediate clinical complications to chilling but after a few days respiratory infection may occur. Every effort should be made to encourage the recently chilled animal to feed and at the first sign of secondary respiratory infection antibiotic therapy should commence.

In the case of frostbite surgery may be indicated. It is preferable that appendanges affected by ischemia are amputated rather than sloughed naturally. Although amputation can be carried out on the conscious animal, anesthesia is desirable since the site of the operation is proximal to the junction of normal and ischemic tissue. Hemostasis is important and asepsis is vital if bacterial infections are not to supervene.

Prevention of chilling and frostbite in captive animals is not easy but a special point should be made to check all heating appliances at daily intervals. In the case of outside enclosures adequate cover must be provided, especially in cold weather, to enable the animals to hide and protect themselves.

CHANGES IN HUMIDITY

Etiology

Amphibians, and to a lesser extent reptiles, are susceptible to changes in humidity. In the wild, these animals are able to resist such changes by behavioral means, such as seeking a drier or more humid environment but this is often not possible in captivity. There are physical adaptation; for example, the presence of ground substance which can very effectively bind water in the skin of many species (Elkan, 1976). As a general rule, a relative humidity of 60 to 80% is satisfactory for an amphibian and 40 to 60% for a reptile but there is considerable species variation. In Europe, Bufo spp. are able to tolerate a lower relative humidity than frogs, Rana spp. Some species of amphibian may favor a fluctuation in humidity (Jordan, 1969) and this is a strong argument for providing a varied environment for animals in captivity.

Signs and diagnosis

Clinical signs associated with a low relative humidity are usually restricted to the integument. Amphibians will show a dry and very hard skin in which lesions, such as "cracks" or ulcerations, may appear. In reptiles dysecdysis is more likely. In more severe cases the animal becomes dehydrated and death can occur. High relative humidity is rarely a cause of disease in amphibians although it is the author's opinion that fungal infections may be more prevalent in frogs and toads kept under such conditions. In reptiles excessive humidity may result in "blister disease", a condition characterised by the presence of fluid filled vesicles in the skin. Such lesions may be extensive and involve all parts of the body.

Diagnosis of disease associated with changes in humidity is based upon clinical history and the presence of skin lesions. There are no characteristic post-mortem signs.

Treatment

Prevention of diseases associated with unsatisfactory humidity is not always easy. However, it is useful to create an environment in the vivarium such that the animal can find its own optimum humidity.

PHYSICAL INFLUENCES

DROWNING

Etiology

Drowning occurs from time to time in free-ranging amphibians and reptiles but is, for obvious reasons, more common in the latter. Mass mortalities may result when areas are flooded intentionally, for example, during the construction of a dam or reservoir, or if natural habitats fill with water during periods of heavy rain or following snowfalls (Aleksiuk, 1977; Kraemer and Bell, 1980; Magnusson, 1982). In captivity drowning can occur in poorly constructed enclosures or when an animal is unable to climb out of a waterbowl. Chelonians are inclined to fall into ponds when drinking during hot weather. Nevertheless, as will be emphasized later, both groups of animals are remarkably resistant to hypoxia and will survive incidents that would rapidly prove fatal to a mammal or bird.

Drowning of adult amphibians can sometimes occur when they are anesthetised in water, as with MS222 (Sandoz). Water can be inhaled if the anesthetised animal's nostrils sink below the surface. For this reason anesthesia in a shallow container is advisable.

Diagnosis

The clinical features of drowning are usually a water-logged, often edematous, animal which is flaccid and may appear to be dead. The word "appear" is used intentionally since some supposedly fatal cases will recover. The cause of the edema is uncertain, but is assumed to be diffusion of fluid into the tissues. The results can be bizarre, with swollen, distorted areas of the body, extrusion of the hemipenes and early rectal prolapse. Such severe cases rarely survive.

The diagnosis of drowning is based upon the history rather than specific clinical signs or post-mortem findings. Usually the animal is found submerged in the water. The tissues may be swollen, as described above, and the buccal and nasal cavities may contain water. Inhaled water is seen in the respiratory tract and often the stomach at post-mortem examination.

Determination of whether or not a drowned animal is alive is far from easy and the author has learnt from experience that it is wiser to err on the side of optimism. Recovery is possible even in animals in which there is no palpable heartbeat, although it must be admitted that use has not been made of electrocardiography on such occasions.

Treatment

Treatment of drowning necessitates the immediate removal of the amphibian or reptile from the water and the clearing of the fluid from the respiratory tract. The latter is best accomplished by holding the animal upside-down and gently "milking" out water through the nares and mouth. The nasal and buccal cavities must be kept clear of saliva and mucus and every effort made to maintain an airway. Attempts at artifical respiration, by squeezing the animal's thorax or rocking it up and down, are helpful. However, the best approach appears to be the administration of oxygen. Intubation should be carried out or, failing this, the animal should be exposed for several hours to an atmosphere rich in oxygen in an anesthetic chamber or a plastic container fashioned for the purpose (Cooper, 1979). Amphibians often respond to being placed in shallow water through which oxygen has been bubbled.

It is impossible to state categorically for how long treatment must continue before one assumes that the patien is dead. Experience with two tortoises, T. graeca, which were rescued after several hours in a garden pond, suggest that oxygen and supportive treatment should be continued for at least 36 hours. Even then full clinical recovery may be slow, with the return of reflexes, sensation and activity over a period of several days.

IRRADIATION

Etiology

Exposure to radiation occurs in free-ranging animals and has been the subject of some research (Brisbin et al., 1974; Cosgrove, 1971). In captivity it is unlikely to be significant unless the animal is part of an experiment involving irradiation. However, radiography is now a commonplace diagnostic procedure for amphibians and reptiles and should be considered a potential hazard; repeated X-ray examination must be avoided. Exposure to ultra-violet light is also worthy of mention in view of the widespread use of such lighting in vivaria. There is evidence that a certain amount of ultra-violet light is beneficial to reptiles (King, 1971) and to amphibians

(Temple and Fowler, 1978) but there appear to have been no statistically significant studies on the responses of amphibians and reptiles to artifical ultra-violet lighting. Papers in the International Zoo Yearbook, for example, have reported "success" using such lighting for small groups of animals, the latter showing an improvement in condition, behavior or reproduction (Laszlo, 1969). Other authors have been less enthusiastic but have been unable to demonstrate any dangers with artifical sources of ultra-violet light so long as it is used sensibly (Kauffeld, 1969; Logan, 1969). More work is needed on this subject and it is probably wise to restrict the use of such lighting, especially in amphibians, until reliable data are available.

Signs and diagnosis

The clinical signs of irradiation in amphibians and reptiles are documented in a number of publications and a useful review is that by Cosgrove (1971). Clinical features include lethargy, anorexia, skin burns, enteritis and death. LD_{50} values range from 1000 rads for adult box turtles, *Terrapene carolina*, to 300 to 400 rads for snakes.

Diagnosis is based upon the history and post-mortem findings. The latter are characterised by changes in organ size and histopathology reveals loss of cellularity in the spleen, bone marrow and gonads. There is a marked leukopenia and secondary bacterial infections may be a feature.

Treatment

Treatment is of limited value. The animal must be removed from the source of the irradiation and subjected to palliative treatment, such as cleaning of wounds, administration of fluids and nursing.

REFERENCES

Addison, J.B., and Jacobson, E.R., 1974, An autogenous bacterin for a chronic mouth infection in a reticulated python, J. Zoo Animal Med., 5:10-11.

Aleksiuk, M., 1977, Sources of mortality in concentrated garter snake populations, Can. Field-Naturalist, 91:70-72.

Bennett, A.F., and Dawson, W.R., 1976, Metabolism, *in*: "Biology of the Reptilia," Vol. 5, C. Gans and W.R. Dawson, eds., Academic Press, New York.

Brisbin, I.L., Station, M.A., Pinder, J.E., and Geiger, R.A., 1974, Radiocesium contamination of snakes from contaminated and non-contaminated habitats of AEC Savannah River Plant, Copeia 1974:501-506

Burke, E.M., and Pough, F.H., 1976, The role of fatigue in temperature resistance of salamanders, J. Thermal. Biol., 1:163-167.

Cooper, J.E., 1973, Veterinary aspects of recently captured snakes, British J. Herpetol., 5:368-374.

Cooper, J.E., 1979, Anaesthesia of exotic species, in: "A manual of anaesthesia for small animal practice," C.M. Ash and R.M. Furber, eds., British Small Animal Vet. Ass., London.

Cooper, J.E., 1981, Use of a surgical adhesive drape in reptiles, Vet. Rec., 108:56.

Cooper, J.E., and Jackson, O.F., 1981, "Diseases of the Reptilia," Academic Press, London.

Cooper, J.E., and Leakey, J.H.E., 1976, A septicaemic disease of East African snakes associated with Enterobacteriaceae, Trans. Royal Soc. Trop. Med. Hyg., 70:80-84.

Cosgrove, G.E., 1971, Reptilian radiobiology, J. Amer. Vet. Med. Ass., 159:1678-1684.

Cowles, R.B., and Bogert, C.M., 1944, A preliminary study of the thermal requirements of desert reptiles, Bull. Amer. Mus. Nat. Hist., 83:265-296.

Daugherty, C.H., 1979, Personal communication, Dept. of Biology, Northern Michigan Univ., Marquette.

Daugherty, C.H., Wishard, L.N., and Daugherty, L.B., 1978, Sexual dimorphism in an anuran response to severe thermal stress (Amphibia, Anura), J. Herpetol., 12:431-432.

Elkan, E., 1976, Ground substance: An anuran defence against dessication, in: "Physiology of the Amphibia," B. Lofts, ed., Academic Press, New York.

Feder, M.E., 1978, Environmental variability and thermal acclimation in neotropical and temperate zone salamanders, Physiol. Zool., 51:7-16.

Frye, F.L., 1973, "Husbandry, medicine and surgery in captive reptiles," V.M. Publ. Inc., Bonner Springs.

Gans, C., 1979, On exhibiting reptiles, Int. Zoo Yearbook, 19:1-14.

Holt, P.E., 1981, Drugs and dosages, in: "Diseases of the Reptilia," J.E. Cooper and O.F. Jackson, eds., Academic Press, London.

Honegger, R.E., 1979, Marking amphibians and reptiles for future identification, Int. Zoo Yearbook, 19:14-22.

Jacobson, E.R., and Whitford, W.G., 1970, The effect of acclimation on physiological responses to temperature in the snakes, *Thamnophis proximus* and *Natrix rhombifera*, Comp. Biochem. Physiol., 35:439-449.

Jackson, O.F., 1978, Tortoise shell repair over two years, Vet. Rec., 102:284-285.

Jones, R.J., Roe, E.A., and Gupta, J.L., 1978, Low mortality in burned patients in a *Pseudomonas* vaccine trial, Lancet, ii:401-403.

Jordan, T., 1969, Notes on keeping arboreal and terrestrial amphibians in captivity, Int. Zoo Yearbook, 9: 14-16.

Kauffeld, C., 1969, The effect of altitude, ultra-violet light and humidity on captive reptiles, Int. Zoo Yearbook, 9:8-9.

King, F.W., 1971, Housing, sanitation and nutrition of reptiles, J. Amer. Vet. Med. Ass., 159:1612-1615.

Kluger, M.J., 1977, Fever in the frog *Hyla cinerea*, J. Thermal. Biol., 2:79-81.

Kraemer, J.E., and Bell, R., 1980, Rain-induced mortality of eggs and hatchlings of loggerhead sea turtles (*Caretta caretta*) on the Georgia coast, Herpetologica, 36:72-77.

Laszlo, J., 1969, Observations on two new artifical lights for reptile displays, Int. Zoo Yearbook, 9:12-13.

Logan, T., 1969, Experiments with Gro-lux light and its effect on reptiles, Int. Zoo Yearbook, 9:9-11.

Lowe, C.H., and Vance, V.J., 1955, Acclimation of the critical thermal maximum of the reptile *Urosaurus ornatus*, Science 122:73-74.

Magnusson, W.E., 1982, Mortality of eggs of the crocodile *Crocodylus porosus* in northern Australia, J. Herpetol., 16:121-130.

Nace, G.W., 1977, Breeding amphibians in captivity, Int. Zoo Yearbook, 17:44-50.

Nace, G.W., Culley, D.D., Emmons, M.V., Gibbs, E.L., Hutchinson, V.H., and McKinnell, R.G., 1974, "Amphibians: Guidelines for the breeding, care and management of laboratory animals," Inst. Lab. Animal Resources, Nat. Acad. Sci., Washington.

Patterson, J.W., and Davies, P.M.C., 1978, Preferred body temperature: Seasonal and sexual differences in the lizard *Lacerta vivipara*, J. Thermal. Biol., 3:39-41.

Peaker, M., 1969, Some aspects of the thermal requirements of reptiles in captivity, Int. Zoo Yearbook, 9:1-8.

Swingland, I.R., and Frazier, J.G., 1979, The conflict between feeding and overheating in the Aldabran tortoise, Proc. Cotswold Herpetol. Symp., Oxfordshire, England.

Temple, R., and Fowler, M.E., 1978, Amphibians (Amphibia), in: "Zoo and wild animal medicine," M.E. Fowler, ed., W.B. Saunders, Philadelphia.

Universities Federation for Animal Welfare, 1976, "The UFAW handbook on the care and management of laboratory animals," 6th ed., Churchill, Livingstone.

Vaughn, L.K., Bernheim, H.A., and Kluger, M.J., 1974, Fever in the lizard Dipsosaurus dorsalis, Nature 252:473-474.

Vinegar, A., 1973, The effects of temperature on the growth and development of embryos of the Indian python, Python molurus, Copeia 1973:171-173.

Vogel, Z., 1964, "Reptiles and amphibians: Their care and behaviour," Studio Vista, London.

Vozenilek, P., 1978, Leceni Spaleniny u Python molurus vittatus, Fauna Bohemiae Septentrionalis, 3:57.

Wallach, J.D., 1969, Medical care of reptiles, J. Amer. Vet. Med. Ass., 155:1017-1034.

Wallach, J.D., 1971, Environmental and nutritional disease of captive reptiles, J. Amer. Vet. Med. Ass., 159:1632-1643.

Webb, G.J.W., and Messel, H., 1977, Abnormalities and injuries in the estuarine crocodile, Crocodylus porosus, Australian Wildlife Res., 4:311-319.

Will, R., 1978, The structural transformation of phagocytic cells, an old phylogenetic principle - Part I: The monocyte, Vet. Med. Rev., 2:204-211.

Zeman, W.V., Falco, F.G., and Falco, J.J., 1967, Repair of the carapace of a box turtle using a polyester resin, Lab. Animal Care, 17:424-425.

AGING AND DEGENERATIVE DISEASES

Gerald E. Cosgrove and Marilyn P. Anderson

Pathology Department, Zoological Society of San Diego and School of Medicine, University of California-San Diego

AGING

The duration of life in free-living amphibians and reptiles is not really known, but extrapolations can be made from information from captive animals, where the most extensive records are those from zoos (Anon., 1966; Bowler, 1977; Shaw, 1969). Aging degenerative diseases occur in all classes of vertebrates (Andrew, 1971). This chapter will mention some expected diseases of this type in free-ranging herptiles, but specific information on most is almost completely lacking. The fate of aged herptiles in captivity indicates what could occur in wild populations. Arteriosclerosis and gout could be considered the most prominent diseases of this type, but they are covered in the nutritional chapters of this volume.

Criteria of age

Gibbons (1976) gives a very good summary of some of the aging techniques and their value and pitfalls. These have included the external annuli or shell growth rings of turtles, cortical stratification or growth rings on bone, decrease of collagen in skin and fibrous tissue, tendon ossification, changes in epiphyseal centers of bone and relative body size. In their multivolume work on the biology of reptiles, Gans and Parsons (1969-1979) cite numerous references to aging changes that are encountered in specific organ systems (Enlow, 1969; Zangerl, 1969).

Attempts to correlate the age of individual herptiles found in the wild with the presence or absence of degenerative (or other) diseases or aging morphologic changes are certainly of value and very rare to date. The best are probably those related to ecologically oriented studies of reptile populations irradiated in the wild and then followed by demographic field studies (Turner et al., 1973).

Maximum ages

Extremely wide ranges of maximum age are known to occur in reptiles and amphibians (Anon., 1966; Bowler, 1977). Species of captive tortoises have the greatest known maximum ages of vertebrates, about 150 years (Comfort, 1961), while crocodilians fall far short of that, e.g., Alligator mississippiensis circa 51 years, and lizard maxima are about 28 years, e.g., Heloderma suspectum (Anon., 1966; Bowler, 1977). Extensive records of captive snake survival are available and indicate maxima of about 39 years for Boidae, 29 years for Elapidae 25 years for Colubridae and 30 years for Viperidae (Anon., 1969; Bowler, 1977; Shaw, 1969).

AMYLOIDOSIS

Amyloid is a variable complex of pathological proteins classified into different groups based on the chemical properties of the constituent fibrils. It is deposited extracellularly as a homogeneous eosinophilic material in a wide variety of tissue locations usually associated with blood vessels. It appears with a number of pathological conditions in a wide variety of vertebrates. Chronic diseases such as neoplasms or infections with gradual protracted tissue breakdown, apparently predispose. In vertebrates, marked species and even individual susceptibilities to amyloid deposition occur. In reptiles it seems to be of rare occurrence and in amphibians it is doubtful if confirmed cases have occurred (Gruys, 1979).

Incidence

While apparently unreported from free-ranging herptiles, occasional reports indicate its presence in captive animals. In a zoo necropsy series (Cowan, 1968) it was found in 2 of 886 snakes with no occurrences in 363 reptiles of other orders. More surprising was the report of Trautwein and Pruksaraj (1967) of the occurrence of amyloidosis in 30 of 52 tortoises, Testudo hermanii,

AGING AND DEGENERATIVE DISEASES

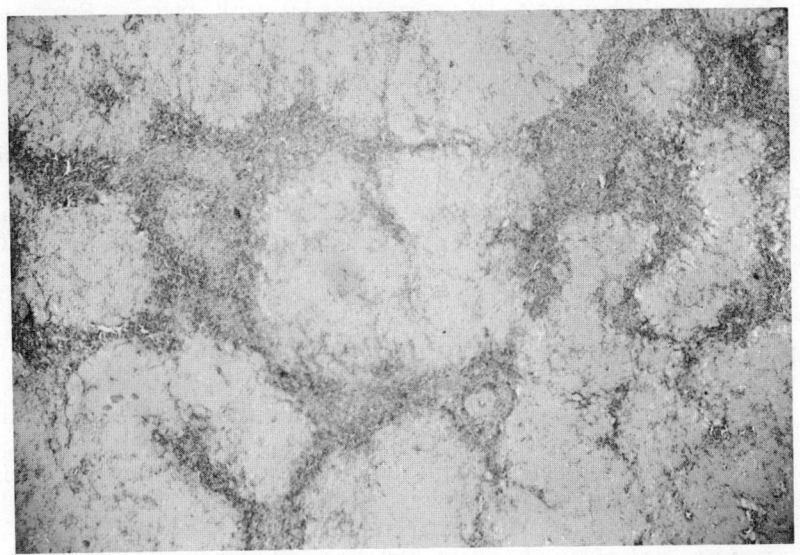

Fig. 24.1.   Severe splenic amyloidosis in an adult male, captive spiny-tailed iguana, Ctenosaura acanthura. Large deposits of amyloid have replaced the splenic white pulp nodules. H&E X45

kept in captivity. The involvement was splenic, with additional deposits around cerebral blood vessels in two cases. In the San Diego Zoo records there are scattered cases of amyloidosis in a variety of reptiles (Griner, 1980). In the authors' personal files cases are very rare, but there is an interesting one with glomerular deposits in a 10 year old American alligator. This rare but widespread occurrence suggests that amyloidosis will be found or has been overlooked in free-ranging herptiles.

Pathology

Amyloid occurs most commonly in the spleen, liver, renal glomeruli and intestinal mucosa, but can occur in many other sites, e.g., pancreas, heart, lymph node, brain, muscle, adrenal gland, etc. The acellular deposits of amyloid stain reddish-pink with routine H&E tissue stains. They occur in association with vascular channels, as irregular ring-like zones around the periphery of the white pulp nodules in the spleen (Fig. 24.1), beneath the lining of the hepatic or adrenal sinusoids, around renal glomerular vessels, around small blood vessels in the submucosa or diffusely in the lamina propria of the gut, and in the myocardium. The relationship to amyloid of other vertebrates is apparently unknown. Further study by modern differential staining techniques and electronmicroscopy are needed.

The chief pathological effects seem to be space occupancy, with compression and gradual elimination of functional elements of the invaded tissues. The presence of amyloid in a tissue does not seem to involve an inflammatory response. The surrounded or infiltrated cells survive for a long time.

GLOMERULOSCLEROSIS

A few surveys of zoo or captive herptiles indicate the presence of glomerulosclerosis, but there seem to be no reports of this condition in free-ranging animals (Cosgrove and Jared, 1974; Cowan, 1968; Zwart, 1964). It is manifested by the deposition or accumulation of hyaline or fibrous tissue in the glomeruli; however, the location of fibrosis in glomeruli is variable, suggesting that this is a complex of diseases of varying etiology possibly related to aging, immunological, degenerative, infective, arteriosclerotic or other factors.

Incidence

In reptiles glomerulosclerosis has been found by Cowan (1968) in the Philadelphia Zoo series, principally in snakes but also in one alligator, and by Zwart (1964) in various morphological forms in over 20% of his zoo reptiles. It occurred in the amphibian Xenopus, in a study of 369 captive specimens with brief to long periods of captivity (Cosgrove and Jared, 1974). In none of these studies is there a published breakdown of the types of glomerulosclerosis by species affected, time in captivity, age or associated diseases etc., all of which may be important in understanding this disease complex.

Pathology

Morphologic manifestations are variable as suggested by the names used by various authors. Zwart (1964) separated four types of "glomerulitis": membranous, acute, chronic intracapillary and chronic extracapillary. Cowan (1968) separated glomerulitis from glomerular sclerosis. Cosgrove and Jared (1974) used the term nephritis with glomerular hyalinization. The relation to glomerular changes in other vertebrates, results of special staining or electronmicroscopy techniques, are not clear yet.

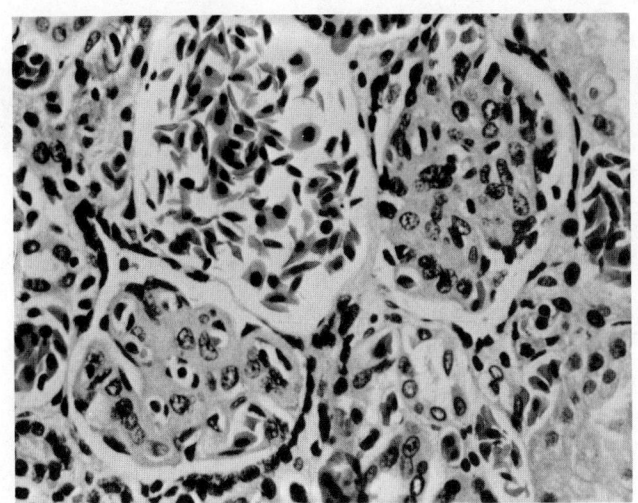

Fig. 24. 2. Two glomeruli from a young adult male Fire salamander, Salamandra salamandra, zoo-kept for over six months. The lower one has excessive homogeneous interstitial tissue. H&E X200

Histologically, the glomerular changes consist of varying degrees of tuft hypercellularity, focal or diffuse thickening of capillary walls and thickening of tubular, arteriolar and glomerular capillary basement membranes. Eventually, glomeruli may become acellular and sclerotic (Fig. 24.2). Atrophic tubular changes may follow the glomerular lesion.

HYPERPLASTIC PANCREATIC REGENERATION

This disease of the pancreas of snakes is very poorly understood. It was reported by Ratcliffe (1935) and with further accumulation of cases he was able to review the Philadelphia Zoo experience and delineate the problem more clearly (Ratcliffe, 1943). Cowan (1968), reviewing 66 years of reptile necropsies at the Philadelphia Zoo, updated the work of Ratcliffe. The published reports deal with this disease largely in captive snakes, where it was present in 33% of snakes dying after prolonged captivity and in 4% of snakes captive 90 days or less. However, Ratcliffe (1943) did obtain the pancreases of presumably wild-caught eastern diamondback rattlesnakes, Crotalus adamanteus, and cottonmouths, Agkistrodon piscivorus, from a Florida canning plant, and the disease

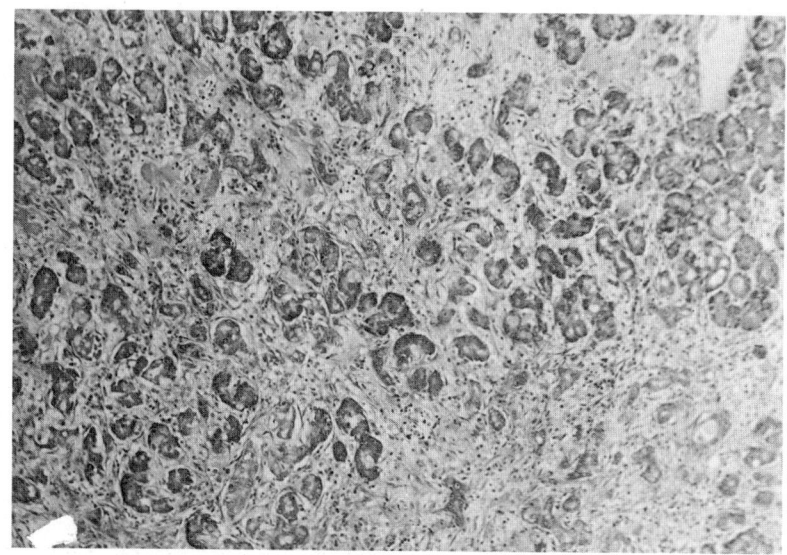

Fig. 24.3. Pancreas of a large adult male black rat snake
Elaphe o. obsoleta, captive about two months.
The pancreatic interstitial tissue has markedl
increased fibrous tissue and infiltrate of
inflammatory cells. Acini are distorted.
H&E X80

was found in 3 of 56 rattlesnakes. Otherwise, it seems
to be unrecorded from free-ranging snakes. The authors
find it sporadically in various species of captive snakes
and from an extensive experience at the San Diego Zoo
(Griner, 1980) it is known to be present in snakes of a
wide range of families and species.

Pathology

Involved pancreases may have a variety of gross
pathological changes involving color, size and consistency
which reflect the range of histological changes found.
The earliest stages consist of necrosis of areas of gland
acini with early stromal edema progressing rapidly to
widespread leukocytic infiltrate. As necrotic epithelial
elements disappear, the stromal component is more prominent
and beginning fibrosis, and a wider variety of inflammatory
cells are the chief features (Fig. 24.3). With further
progression, epithelial regenerative activities result in
atypical, irregular adenomatous areas usually surrounded
by extensive fibrous stroma. This succession of events
with considerable variation in individual snakes, has led

to the use of different terms to designate the condition such as atypical regenerative pancreatitis, atypical regenerative hyperplasia, hyperplastic pancreatic regeneration, post-necrotic fibrosis and hyperplasia, and even adenocarcinoma of the pancreas. The latter is Ratcliffe's term (1935, 1943) but in spite of the atypical hyperplasia apparently no cases have been found where invasion or metastasis occurred. The cause of this disease is not known, but it is apparently largely associated with conditions of captivity. As wider experience with pathology of free-ranging reptiles is gained, the incidence in them may become clear.

REFERENCES

Andrew, W., 1971, "The anatomy of aging in man and animals," Grune and Stratton, New York.
Anon., 1966, A survey of recent longevity records for reptiles and amphibians in zoos, Int. Zoo Yearbook, Vol. VI, Zool. Soc., London.
Bowler, J.K., 1977, "Longevity of reptiles and amphibians in North American collections," Misc. Publ. Herpetol. Circ. 6, Soc. Study Amphibians and Reptiles.
Comfort, A., 1961, The life span of animals, Sci. Amer., 205:108-119.
Cosgrove, G.E., and Jared, D.W., 1974, Diseases and parasites of Xenopus, the clawed toad, in: "Proceedings of the Gulf Coast regional symposium on diseases of aquatic animals," R.L. Amnorski, M.A. Hood, and R.R. Miller, eds., Center for Wetland Res., Louisiana State Univ., Baton Rouge.
Cowan, D.F., 1968, Diseases of captive reptiles, J. Amer. Vet. Med. Ass., 153:848-859.
Enlow, D.H., 1969, The bone of reptiles, in: "Biology of the Reptilia," Vol. I, C. Gans, A.d'A. Bellairs, and T.S. Parsons, eds., Academic Press, New York.
Gans, C., and Parsons, T.S., 1969-1979, "Biology of the Reptilia," Vols. I-X, Academic Press, New York.
Gibbons, J.W., 1976, Aging phenomena in reptiles, in: "Special review of experimental aging research," M.F. Elias, B.E. Eleftheriou, and P.K. Elias, eds., Exper. Aging Res., Inc., Bar Harbor.
Griner, L.A., 1980, Personal communication, Zool. Soc. San Diego, San Diego.
Gruys, E., 1979, A comparative approach to secondary amyloidosis: Mini review, Develop. Comp. Immunol., 3:23-36.

Ratcliffe, H.L., 1935, Carcinoma of the pancreas in Say's pine snake, *Pituophis sayi*, Amer. J. Cancer, 24: 78-79.

Ratcliffe, H.L., 1943, Neoplastic disease of the pancreas of snakes (Serpentes), Amer. J. Pathol., 19: 359-368.

Shaw, C.E., 1969, Longevity of snakes in North American collections as of 1 January 1968, Der Zool. Garten, 37:193-196.

Trautwein, C., and Pruksaraj, D., 1967, Uber amyloidose bei Schildkroten, Dtschr. Teirarztl. Wochenschr. 74:184-186.

Turner, F.B., Licht, P., Thrasher, J.D., Medica, P.A., and Lannom, J.R., Jr., 1973, Radiation-induced sterility in natural populations of lizards (*Crotaphytus wizlizenii* and *Cnemidophorus tigris*), *in*: "Third national radioecology symposium," Vol. 2, USAEC Rept. CONF-710501-p2, Oak Ridge.

Zangerl, R., 1969, The turtle shell, *in*: "Biology of the Reptilia," Vol. I, C.Gans, A.d'A. Bellairs, and T.S. Parsons, eds., Academic Press, New York.

Zwart, P., 1964, Studies on renal pathology in reptiles, Pathol. Vet., 1:542-556.

NUTRITIONAL DISORDERS IN REPTILES

Fredric L. Frye

School of Veterinary Medicine

University of California

INTRODUCTION

Reptiles have been kept in captivity and studied for many years, however, the longevity of these captive animals was, until recently, generally rather short because of a lack of knowledge with respect to their specific nutritional, temperature, humidity, photoperiod and other vital husbandry requirements. Many professional and prescient amateur herpetologists have, through their observations and published reports, contributed to the fund of available information relating to captive reptile husbandry.

It should be obvious that each of the foregoing factors beneath the umbrella term "husbandry" is intimately related to the other. For example, unless the preferred temperature, humidity and photoperiod are furnished, the captive reptile eventually will cease to feed voluntarily whether or not its preferred dietary items are provided.

For purposes of exposition and brevity, this discussion must be limited to induced dietary deficiencies, their etiology, pathologic features and prevention and/or treatment. Fortunately, most of the known macrodeficiency-related conditions are recognized easily and the majority are amenable to control and therapy, if diagnosed before irreversible alterations occur.

WATER DEPRIVATION AND DEHYDRATION

Under most conditions, even the best- or most ill-fed

reptile will succumb to the effects of inadequate water (moisture) intake long before the metabolic effects of starvation are recognized. Many desert dwelling species may not have the opportunity to actually imbibe water per se except during rare rainfall, and must rely upon the moisture content of their preferred dietary items. Most of the insectivorous lizards and many herbivorous chelonians are examples of animals whose access to or preference for fluid water is limited by their arid habitat. Those reptiles which normally dwell in tropical rain forests may not accept water from containers; their water must be supplied as droplets on the foliage. These droplets can be produced most conveniently by mist nozzles or hand-held spray bottles used once or twice daily. Ant or termite eating lizards and snakes may or may not accept water from containers, but usually will lap small quantities of water applied as droplets to their lips by pipette. Vegetarian species whose natural succulent diets are replaced by less moisture laden plant materials will require supplemental water. Most tortoises will learn to drink from shallow containers. The water level, however, must be sufficient to allow tha animal to submerge its nostrils.

The reptilian renal system excretes metabolic (and catabolic) nitrogenous waste products principally in the form of uric acid salts. To be sure, smaller volumes of allantoin, ammonia and urea may be processed, but these are minor. Because of the relative insolubility of urates adequate plasma volume and consequent renal perfusion are essential to maintaining clearance of these materials. Furthermore, most reptiles have evolved mechanisms for the reabsorption and conservation of water from their wastes. Extrarenal salt-secreting glands further aid in water conservation and salt elimination.

The overt signs of water deprivation are related to dehydration: loss of skin and subcutaneous turgor, dryness and wrinkling of the integument beyond the normally dry, non-mucous state. There may be multiple small indentations or other deformities in the spectacle shields covering the corneas of those species lacking movable eyelids. Anorexia and lassitude usually are exhibited. As dehydration progresses, hemoconcentration ensues with concomitant reduction in renal perfusion and increased cardiac load.

As the plasma uric acid concentration increases, microcrystals of the uric acid salts begin to be deposited in a wide variety of tissues. Specific sites which appear to be particularly prone to such deposition are the kidneys, liver, pericardial sac, synoviae and submucosal

NUTRITIONAL DISORDERS IN REPTILES

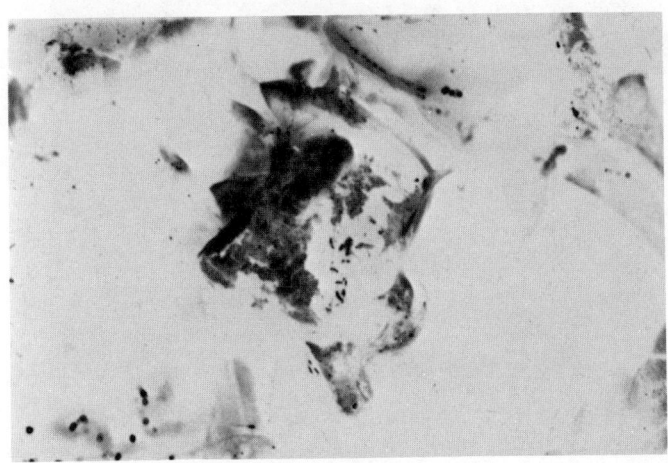

Fig. 25.1. Deposition of urates within the pericardial sac of a desert tortoise, Gopherus agassizi. Note the chalky-white material upon the epicardial surface.

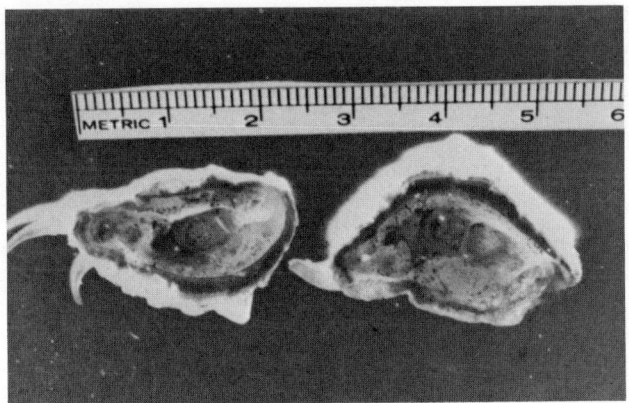

Fig. 25.2. Articular and periarticular gout involving the joints of the G. agassizi in Fig. 25.1. Note the urates in and around the articulations and soft tissues.

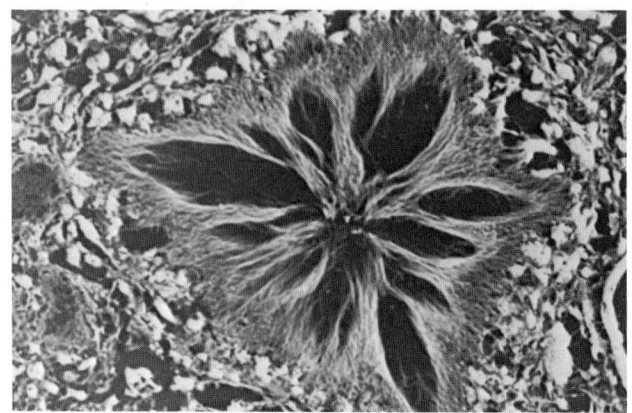

Fig. 25.3. Photomicrograph of a classical gouty tophus in the renal tissue of a snake. Note the granulomatous reaction elicted by the presence of urate microcrystals within soft tissues. The urates are often lost during fixation and processing, leaving a starburst pattern of the surrounding inflammatory tissues. H&E X110

connective tissues (Figs. 25.1 and 25.2). Presence of urate microcrystals provides characteristic granulomatous lesions called tophi which usually possess a starburst appearance (Fig. 25.3). If the individual survives long enough, these tophi may become heavily mineralized with calcium salts.

Obviously, the best means for preventing dehydration is to provide adequate ingested moisture in a form or application appropriate for the particular species and artifical habitat. Reptiles already exhibiting clinical signs of dehydration must be rehydrated. Often this may be accomplished merely by placing small volumes of water on the lips or into the mouth at frequent intervals. Severely dehydrated and weakened animals probably will require intracoelomic or subcutaneous injection of half-strength physiological solutions such as Hartmann's or Ringer's. Intravenous infusion may be employed, if practicable. These debilitated animals must be handled with a minimum of additional stress.

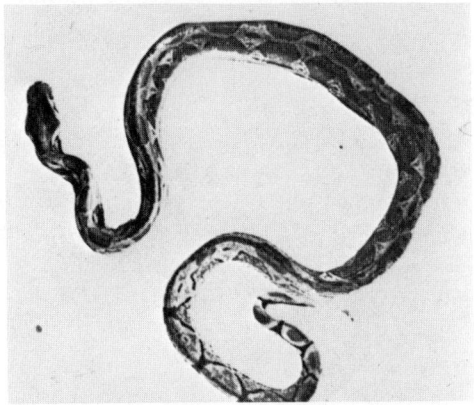

Fig. 25. 4. A severely under-nourished Boa constrictor. Note the shrunken and wrinkled appearance of paravertebral musculature and integument.

STARVATION

Starvation is a rather commonly encountered problem in captive reptiles and generally results from either the lack of sufficient total digestible nutrients available or the failure to consume those food items provided.

The clinical appearance of the affected animal closely resembles starvation in the higher vertebrates. The body weight is subnormal, the musculature appears wasted, some degree of enopthalmos usually is noted, and the skin may be overly wrinkled or folded (Fig. 25.4).

During post-mortem examination, the musculature will be found to be dimished markedly and may present a watery appearance. Those adipose depots remaining may have a gelatinous consistency. The liver mass may be reduced markedly (Figs. 25.5 and 25.6).

One of the histopathological hallmarks of starvation is serous atrophy of body fat, particularly within the coelomic cavity. Omental, perirenal and pericardial fat deposits will be diminished and appear whispy or delicate. The normally plump fat cells will be much reduced in size or collapsed altogether. The interstitial connective tissue will appear greatly increased in comparison to that found in normal fat (Fig. 25.7).

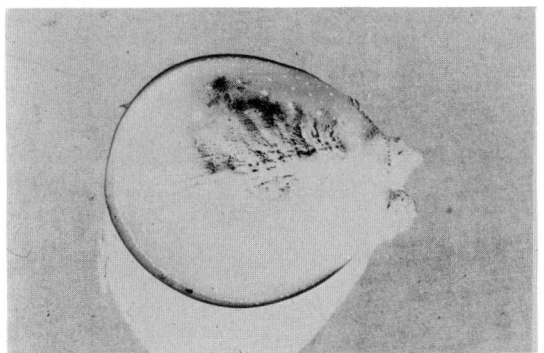

Fig. 25.5. A markedly underfed soft-shelled turtle, Trionyx sp. Note the prominent vertebral column and ribs.

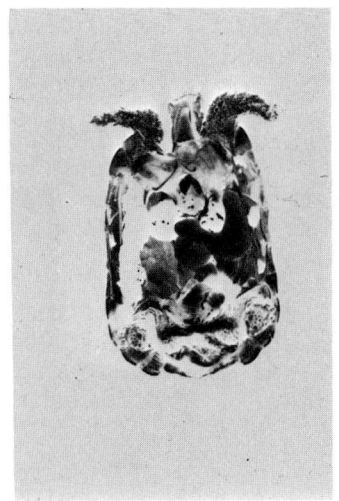

Fig. 25.6. Post-mortem specimen of a Gopherus sp. which had starved to death. Note the markedly diminished hepatic mass, lack of intracoelomic fat and muscle atrophy.

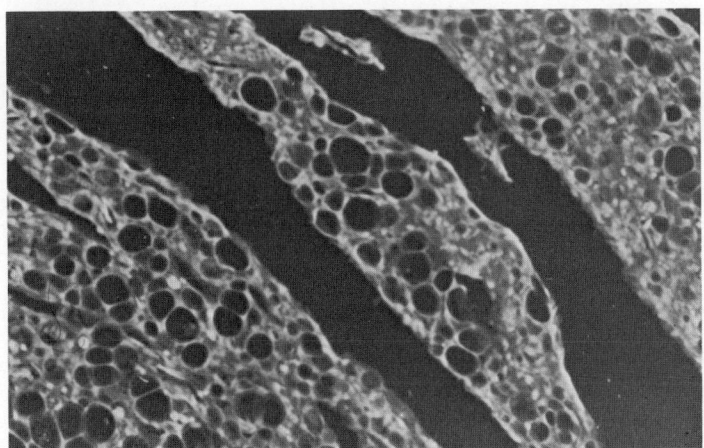

Fig. 25.7. Photomicrograph of coelomic adipose tissue from a cachectic snake. Note the serous atrophy of the tissue resulting in a diminution of intracellular lipid and the relative increase in connective tissue. H&E X80

Treatment for the severly undernourished reptile consists of gently hand- or tube-feeding small volumes of high calorie, highly digestible artifical diet substitutes or small meals of natural diet items, depending upon the circumstances and the availability of food items. For the first few days, the quantity of food must be limited; it is better to administer frequent small meals than solitary large ones. Often, these animals will be dehydrated as well as starved and must be given sufficient water or other appropriate fluid. The immediate environmental temperature should be adequate to assure proper enzymatic digestion of the ingesta. As soon as practicable, natural diet items should be employed in place of artifical substitutes.

A given reptile may exhibit periodic anorexia. For example, most snakes refuse to feed as they prepare to shed their old epidermis. This behavior is normal and the snakes' appetitites return immediately after completion of ecdysis. Other reptiles will, from time to time, refuse even previously favored food items. The etiology of this anorexia may be manifold: improper environmental temperature, humidity, or photoperiod; handling or other physical disturbances; psychological stress or competition by cagemates; infectious disease, protozoan or metazoan parasitism; and, simple overfeeding, all have been identified as causes for appetite loss in reptiles. It is beyond the scope of this chapter to discuss the definitive diagnosis of any or all of these etiologies, but they are addressed elsewhere (Frye, 1981).

VITAMIN-ASSOCIATED CONDITIONS

Several specific syndromes related to hyper- and hypovitaminosis have been identified and described in captive reptiles (Anderson and Capen, 1936; Frye, 1973, 1974, 1981 Frye and Schelling, 1973; Jensen and With, 1939; Pallaske, 1961; Reichenbach-Klinke and Elkan, 1965; Schuchman and Taylor, 1970; Wallach, 1966, 1968, 1971; Wallach and Hoff, 1982).

Vitamin A

Hypovitaminosis A is the most frequently encountered vitamin deficiency in captive reptiles, especially in young aquatic and semi-aquatic turtles. This fact is due to the practice of feeding diets of meat or fish to the exclusion of any green vegetable material.

The clinical signs of hypovitaminosis A are usually, but not always, related to the physiological failure of one or more epithelialized organ systems. The respiratory, ocular, endocrine, gastro-intestinal and genitourinary systems are, in declining order, involved most frequently. Alteration in the normally delicate mucosal surfaces together with diminished cellular and humoral immunity predisposes the vitamin A-deficient animal to infection. Specialized glandular tissues undergo squamous metaplastic and hyperkeratotic changes which diminish or abolish altogether their normal secretory products. The irritants and potential pathogens which abound in the animal's environment soon are given the opportunity to produce their effects. Ciliated columnar epithelial surfaces in the respiratory tract and the lacrimal and nasal glandular tissues are exquisitely sensitive to these alterations (Figs. 25.8, 25.9 and 25.10). The serous and mucus-secreting glands soon become filled with inspissated and keratin debris. The keratinized mouth parts often become overgrown.

Treatment consists of injectible water-miscible vitamin A. Oral supplementation with commercial vitamin A preparations also may be employed. Because overdosage of vitamin A is potentially toxic, careful attention to

NUTRITIONAL DISORDERS IN REPTILES

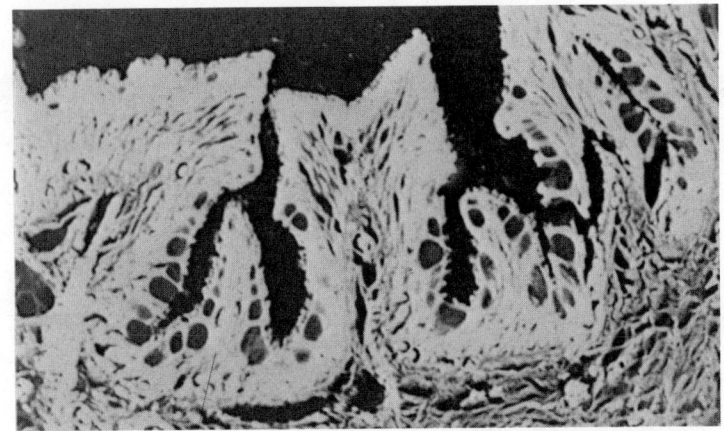

Fig. 25.8. Photomicrograph of the upper respiratory epithelium of a Gopherus sp. exhibiting mild hypovitaminosis-A. Note the partial loss of cilia and mild squamous metaplasia. H&E X80

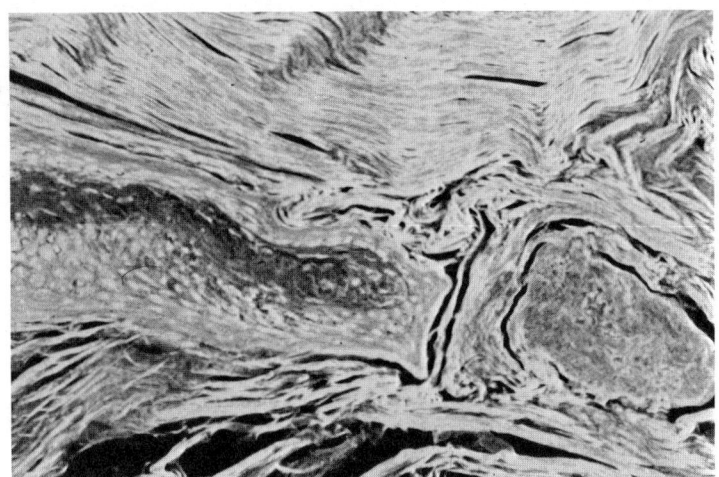

Fig. 25.9. Photomicrograph of the upper respiratory epithelium from a severely vitamin-A-deficient Gopherus sp. Note the advanced squamous metaplasia involving the surface epithelium and associated nasal glands which are filled with heavily keratinized debris. H&E X40

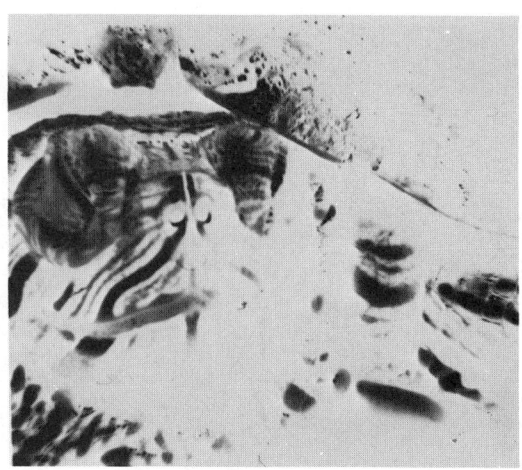

Fig. 25.10. An immature red-eared slider turtle, Chrysemy scripta elegans, exhibiting moderate blepharitis associated with a diet deficient in vitamin A.

dosage is essential. Specific therapeutic dosages of 50 to 50,000 I.U. may be indicated, depending upon body weight and severity of clinical manifestations.

The diet must be improved by the addition of fresh green leafy vegetable matter. Properly prepared alfalfa leaves, pellets or meal usually are accepted well. Aquatic chelonians often readily ingest pond weeds and grasses, watercress, Swiss chard, etc.

Vitamin B

Presently recognized deficiencies of the B-complex vitamins are limited to induced hypovitaminosis B_1 (thiamine) and induced biotin deficiency. Both of these clinical entities are the direct result of narrowly restricted diets. In thiamine deficiency, induction is related to the presence of significant levels of the enzyme thiaminase (found in fresh or thawed frozen fish), ingestion of which soon results in the loss of labile endogenous thiamine.

Clinical signs of thiamine deficiency are central or peripheral neuritis. Early signs of this deficiency are fine muscle tremors and/or fasciculation. Occasionally, the eyes may be withdrawn into their respective orbits.

Replacement therapy utilizing thiamine hydrochloride is often successful.

Induced biotin deficiency arises from the feeding of fresh, uncooked hen's eggs to the exclusion of other sources of animal protein. The anti-biotin substance, avidin, is present in ovalbumin. This condition is observed most commonly in Gila monsters, Heloderma suspectum, Mexican beaded lizards, H. horridum, tegus, Tupinambis spp. and some monitor lizards, Varanus spp. The author also has examined large skinks, especially Tiliqua spp., which had been fed only beaten raw egg and suffered from this condition.

Characteristically, the affected reptile appears well nourished, although one of the earliest signs of clinical biotin deficiency is anorexia. At the same time, generalized muscle asthenia may be observed and usually is interpreted by the owner or keeper as lethary. Upon close examination, the animal is found to be almost incapable of voluntarily moving its limbs.

Under natural conditions, those reptiles subsisting upon a diet rich in avian eggs usually consume fertilized ova which often contain advanced embryos; furthermore, the volume of albumen often is greatly reduced in these incubated eggs. The tissues of the ingested embryo apparently furnish adequate levels of biotin to prevent avidin-induced deficiency. Also, many of these reptiles will voluntarily ingest small birds and mammals, carrion and even fruits in addition to their egg diet.

Prevention and therapy for induced biotin deficiency consists of adding other non-egg sources of animal protein such as immature rodents or chopped meat. Commercially prepared multi-B complex vitamin compounds also may be added to the captive diet.

Deficiencies of niacin, nicotinic acid, riboflavin and other members of the vitamin B-complex group may occur in reptiles, but have yet to be described.

Vitamin C

Ascorbic acid (vitamin C) deficiency occasionally is observed in captive reptiles. It is the opinion of several investigators working in the field of reptile husbandry that the actual incidence is much higher than one would expect. Wallach (1971) suggested that subclinical vitamin C deficiency might be indirectly responsible for the fre-

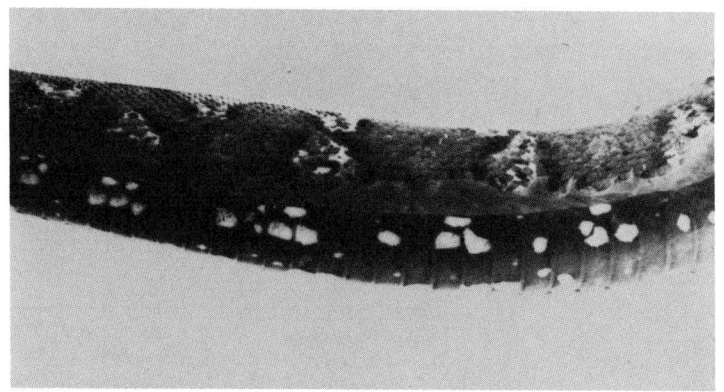

Fig. 25.11. A spontaneous integumentary and subcutaneous rupture in a Boa constrictor due to a deficiency in ascorbic acid. This lesion occurred as the snake was attempting to swallow a small rat. After surgical repair and supplementation with ascorbic acid, the ruptured area healed well and has not been followed by further skin failure.

quent epizootic incidence of infectious ulcerative stomatitis ("mouth rot") in captive snakes. Advanced vitamin C deficiency may result in spontaneous skin rupture (Fig. 25.11). Wallach has emphasized the importance of preformed ascorbic acid and its ascorbate salts within the bowel contents of prey species. It has been demonstrated that some vitamin C is synthesized in the reptilian kidney.

When small rodents are selected as prey for captive reptiles and are separated from their food for several hours, whatever intestinal contents present may have been voided as feces; the available preformed vitamin C is lost. Therefore, vitamin C deficiency in reptiles may be prevented by utilizing recently fed rodents and birds as food prey.

Supplemental vitamin C may be provided either by placing ascorbic acid in tablet form into the oral or body cavities of small rodents, or by injecting sodium ascorbate directly into the reptile itself. Presently, the dosages of ascorbic acid are empirical, but range between 1 to 2 mg to several grams daily, depending upon the body weight of the animal, its physical condition and captive diet.

Vitamin D

Under natural habitat conditions, reptiles obtain adequate levels of vitamin D (usually in the active form, vitamin D_3) from their normally varied diets, and from the formation of 1,25 dihydroxyergocalciferol through the irradiation of cholesterol in the integumentary layers. A cogent discussion of these pathways was published by Fowler (1978).

Currently, most captive reptiles are maintained under artifical lighting which fails to produce radiant light energy of adequate wave length or intensity to induce the irradiation of endogenous cholesterol. Laszlo (1969, 1975, 1976, 1977) has described his work in providing practical and affordable artifical illumination for captive reptiles. Even with totally inadequate artifical lighting, clinical manifestations of hypovitaminosis D may not be apparent if the diet contains sufficient preformed vitamin D_3.

Of equal interest to the comparative medical investigator is the problem of excessive vitamin D, for with an overzealous approach to providing adequate vitamin D comes the pathophysiological difficulties and induced lesions of hypervitaminosis D. In a sincere effort to assure adequate intake, the amateur (and, all too often, the professional) herpetologist will supplement the diet excessively with commercial vitamin D_3, fish liver oil, vitamin D-containing mineral mixes, etc. In addition, natural and/or artificial light may produce endogenous synthesis of vitamin D_3. The result is gross overdosage-induced vitamin D toxicity and pathologic mineralization of soft tissues, particularly those containing smooth muscle (Figs. 25.12, 25.13 and 25.14).

It should be obvious that common sense and prevention are vital to successful captive reptile management. The dosage of vitamin D_3 must be calculated very carefully by taking into consideration effective artificial illumination, the calcium:phosphorus ratio of the diet, and the potential for growth. The actively growing animal will, of course, require higher respective levels of vitamin D_3 than the mature animal which only must maintain its skeleton.

Vitamin E

Hypovitaminosis E is an interesting syndrome in reptiles. First described by Wallach (1968), steatitits is observed most frequently in captive aquatic and semi-

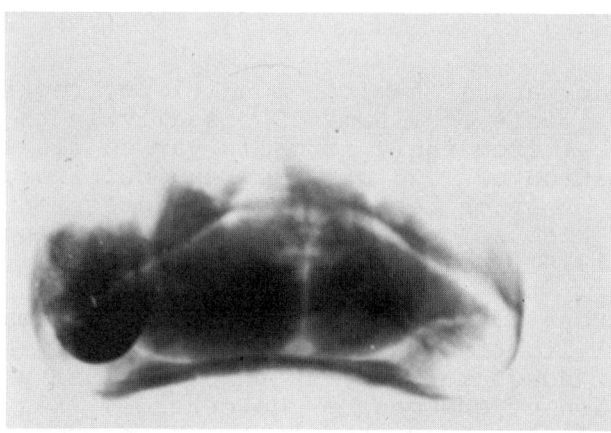

Fig. 25.12. Radiograph of a gopher tortoise, Gopherus polyphemus, affected by severe hypervitaminosis-D resulting from massive overdosages of vitamin D-containing supplements and excessive exposure to ultraviolet light radiation. Note the markedly radiodense pulmonary fields.

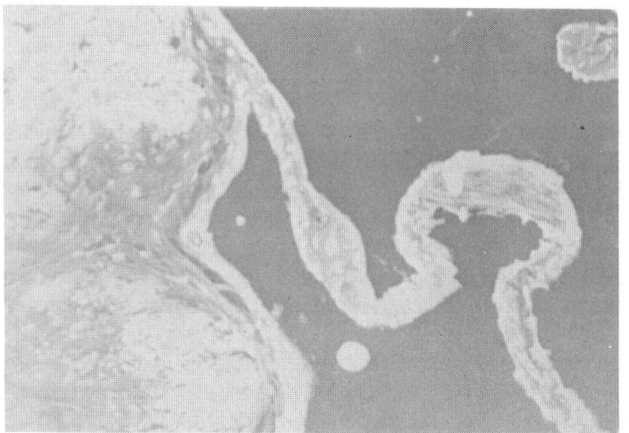

Fig. 25.13. Photomicrograph of pulmonary smooth muscle from Gopherus polyphemus. Note the dark-staining highly mineralized smooth muscle fibers. H&E X40

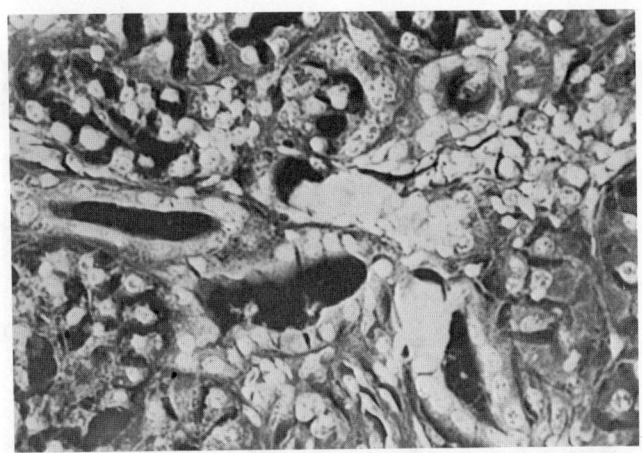

Fig. 25.14. Photomicrograph of the kidney from Gopherus polyphemus. Note the multifocal mineralized renal tubules and interstitial connective tissue. H&E X160

aquatic chelonians and crocodilians, especially those whose diet consists of oil-laden fish such as dark-meat tuna, mackeral, mullet and smelt. The present author has observed severe induced vitamin E deficiency-related steatitis in a Boa constrictor fed an exclusive diet of grossly obese rats which had eaten only sunflower seeds.

The etiology of induced steatitis is related directly to the ingestion of unsaturated or rancid fatty acids over a sufficient time to exhaust endogenous vitamin E. Without the antioxidant activity of vitamin E, these fatty acids undergo peroxidation which, in turn, induces the synthesis of ceroid, a waxy brown pigment. Ceroid is reactive and induces a granulomatous inflammatory response into the areas where this pigment is deposited (Figs. 25.15 to 25.19).

The disease may be prevented by providing a varied and fresh diet which does not contain significant amounts of rancid or unsaturated lipids. Supplemental dosages of vitamin E moieties have not, to date, been determined but since these substances possess only a minimum potential for toxicity, a dose of 50 to 800 I.U. once to three times weekly would be adequate for most reptiles at risk.

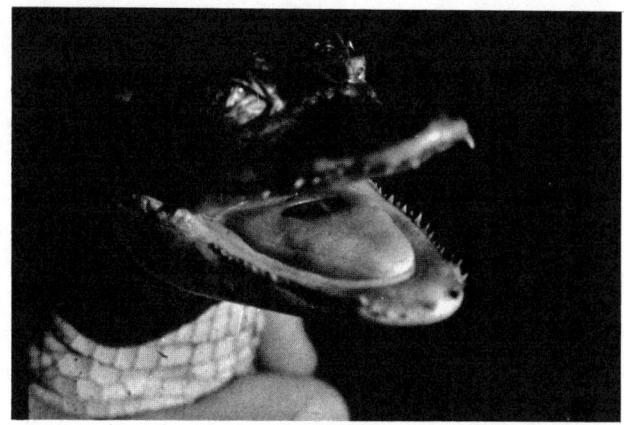

Fig. 25.15. Steatitis in a young caiman, Caiman sp. Ante-mortem appearance of animal. Note the ulcerated lesion on the posterior-dorsal aspect of the tongue.

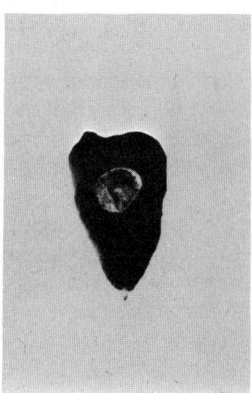

Fig. 25.16. Same caiman as in Fig. 25.15. Post-mortem specimen illustrating the extent of the lingual ulceration which overlies a grossly altered fat pad within the tongue base.

NUTRITIONAL DISORDERS IN REPTILES   649

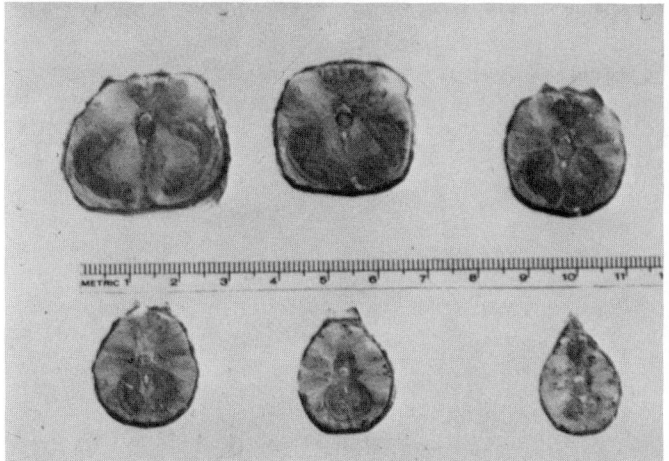

Fig. 25.17. Serial sections of the tail from the caiman in Fig. 25.15. Note the dry waxy texture of the caudal fat bodies.

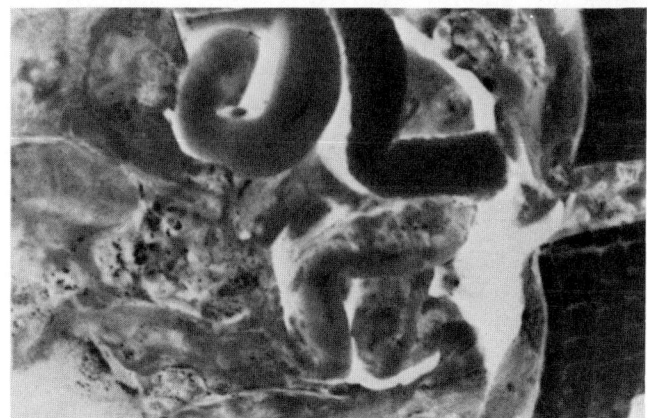

Fig. 25.18. Post-mortem specimen from Caiman sp. which illustrates the multifocal distribution of granulomatous ceroid lesions characteristic of chronic hypovitaminosis E-induced steatitis.

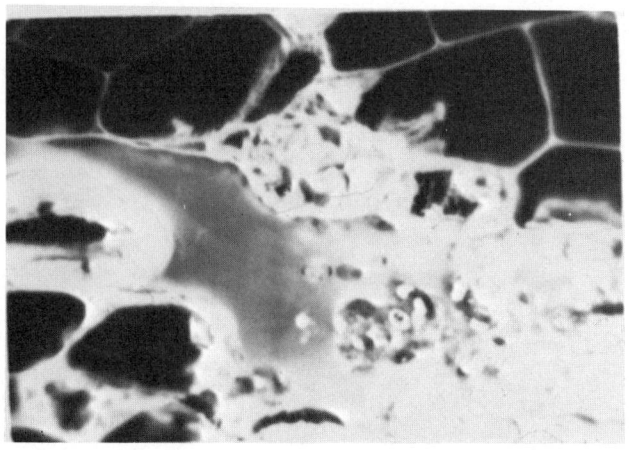

Fig. 25.19. Photomicrograph of steatitic fat from the same caiman illustrated in Fig. 25.18. Note the lakes of dark-staining ceroid pigment and ceroid-laden histiocytic macrophages. Reticulin stain, X220

Lastly, muscle lesions consistent with "white muscle" disease have been observed in some reptiles. The relationship between vitamin E and selenium in the pathogenesis of this myopathy is currently under study.

Vitamin K

Hypovitaminosis K is a rarely observed nutritional problem, usually restricted to captive crocodilians. The few cases seen by the author were confined to American alligators, Alligator mississippiensis.

Clinical manifestations have been limited to spontaneous hemorrhage, most typically from the dental alveoli. Treatment consisted of injections of vitamin K. After the bleeding stopped, oral vitamin K was added to the diet and has proven to be entirely successful. The dosage depends upon the body weight(s) of the animal(s) at risk and the form of synthetic vitamin K employed.

METABOLIC BONE DISEASE

Metabolic bone disease is, perhaps, the most common nutritional deficiency affecting captive reptiles. It is usually the direct result of diets whose overall calcium to phosphorus ratio is seriously skewed toward an overabundance of phosphorus. Much research has been published on this subject (Anderson and Capen, 1976; Collins, 1971, Fowler, 1978; Frye, 1973, 1974, 1981; Ippen, 1965; Reichenbach-Klinke and Elkan, 1965; Wallach, 1968, 1971; Wallach and Hoff, 1982; Zwart and van der Watering, 1969). It is far beyond the scope of this chapter to discuss this important group of bone disorders fully, therefore attention will be focused upon fibrous osteodystrophy, the most frequently encountered of the metabolic bone diseases within the complex.

Variously called secondary nutritional hyperparathyroidism, osteomalacia, renal rickets, osteogenesis imperfecta, cage paralysis, osteodystrophia fibrosa cystica, etc., this author prefers the specific term fibrous osteodystrophy for it most properly denotes the pathological lesions exhibited in affected individuals.

The etiology may involve disorders originating in the parathyroid glands, intestine, kidneys, liver, thyroid gland(s) and bone. Realizing fully that many more factors may enter the equation yielding the final answer. For the purposes of exposition, comments will be confined to that form of fibrous osteodystrophy which results from dietary imbalances in calcium and phosphorus.

Since the ion product(s) of total skeletal calcium and phosphorus in most vertebrate species are in a ratio of approximately 2:1, it would appear reasonable that the available dietary ratio of these elements also should be in a range of 1:1 to 2:1. Simple stoichiometric chemistry predicts that an excess of either calcium or phosphorus will create an imbalance. In clinical practice, one usually finds diets containing gross excesses of phosphorus ion products. Muscle meats and many vegetables contain extremely low quantities of available calcium but are well endowed with excessive phosphorus.

When gross imbalances in the calcium:phosphorus ratio exist, the relatively insoluble salt, calcium phosphate (which is minimally absorbed from the gut), is favored within the intestine. Excess phosphate ion can be absorbed thus resulting in hyperphosphatemia. The parathyroid glands are stimulated to secrete parathormone, thus inducing the leaching of calcium from the hydroxyapatite crystals in mature bone matrix. As resorption continues, the bone is weakened and, concomitantly, is partially replaced by fibrocollagenous connective tissue. Affected bones tend to be larger in diameter with irregular outline and a characteristically spongy consistency (Fig. 25.20). Radiographs demonstrate normal medullary cavities surrounded by massively expanded cortical bone of greatly diminished radiodensity (Fig. 25.21). These bones are deformed easily, and pathological fractures of weight-bearing long bones and vertebrae are common sequelae to this disorder.

Ingestion of excessive dietary calcium ion products (with respect to phosphorus) is possible, but very unusual. When it does occur, the parafollicular cells or "C" cells of the thyroid gland(s) and ultimobranchial bodies are stimulated to secrete a hormone-like substance, calcitonin which acts to inhibit calcium ion resorption from hyroxyapatite, i.e., it is antagonistic to the action of parathormone and, thus, reduces plasma calcium levels.

The plasma calcium concentration usually is elevated in fibrous osteodystrophy until late in the course of the disease, at which time it may be so low that hypocalcemic muscle tremors, tetany or asthenia occur. Death from cardiac failure usually ensues when the plasma calcium reaches such precipitous levels. Even the novice herpetologist usually would have noted the gross abnormal skeletal lesions by this time.

Interestingly, even advanced cases of fibrous osteodystrophy often yield to therapy. Crocodilians and lizards, particularly herbivorous iguanas, respond well to oral and injectable calcium salts such as calcium lactate and calcium gluconate. Oral calcium carbonate is useful also. Vitamin D_3 also should be provided to ensure adequate uptake from the intestinal mucosa. The diet must be corrected to restore the intake of available calcium and phosphorus to an appropriate physiological ratio.

Affected chelonians, because of their bony carapaces and plastrons, are not as fortunate as their saurian and crocodilian cousins. With treatment and the restoration of proper balance of calcium and phosphorus, these animals tend to exhibit rapid growth, but for reasons of geometry, they expand in a dorso-ventral direction more rapidly than in a linear fashion. This growth results in some rather spherical turtles (Figs. 25.22 and 25.23). Some of these turtles grow into ball-like creatures; their legs no longer can propel them on terrestrial surfaces because their feet cannot come into firm contact with the substrate. Even these sadly mishapen chelonians may be salvaged if they are fed corrective diets and provided with mostly aquatic environments in which ramps upon which they may rest are provided.

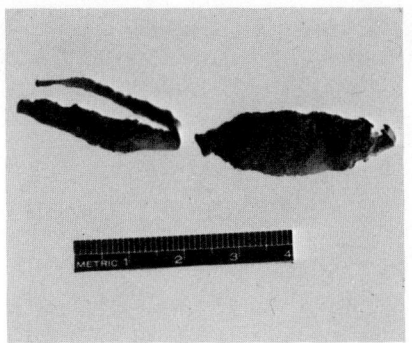

Fig. 25.20. Osteologic preparation of the femur, tibia and fibula from an osteodystrophic iguana. Note the grossly swollen, yet spongy appearance of the bones.

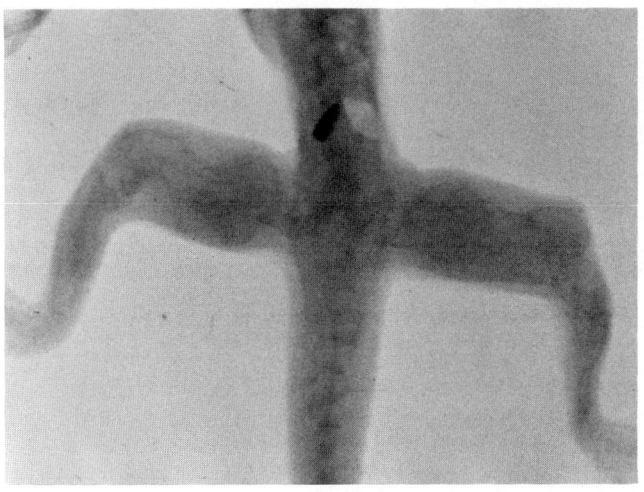

Fig. 25.21. Radiograph of the rear limbs of another iguana exhibiting severe, chronic fibrous osteodystrophy.

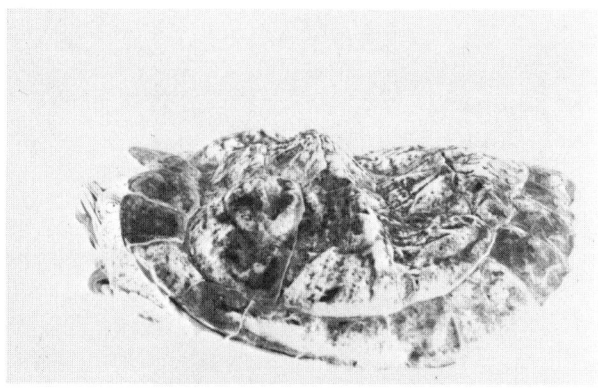

Fig. 25.22. An example of a semi-aquatic turtle which illustrates very severe fibrous osteodystrophy. Note the collapse of the carapace overlying the brachial and pelvic girdles. The musculature in these areas, exerting tension on the softened bone, creates these collapsed lesions. The spinal column of these animals tend to be severely deformed.

TRACE MINERALS

Sodium chloride is required by reptiles and usually is provided by their dietary items. Many reptiles possess salt glands which actively secrete sodium chloride and potassium ions. In order to replace these secreted products, some exogenous source of these ions must be furnished. A means for this supplementation will be offered in the following discussion.

Iodine is another micronutrient required for the maintenance of health and reproductive potential in captive reptiles. To be sure, certain reptile species appear to exhibit particularly high requirements in comparison with other species and these needs may, as previously speculated (Frye and Dutra, 1974), reflect an evolutionary bias. For example, the giant terrestrial tortoieses from the Galapagos and Aldrabra island groups appear to be affected most frequently by hypothyroid goiters. The complete etiology of these thyroid disorders remains speculative because the role of their captive diets also must be considered. The etiology rests upon two points: 1) typi-

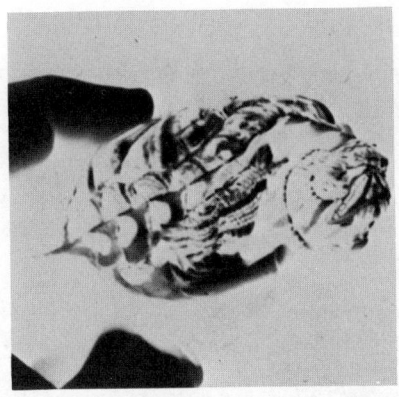

Fig. 25.23. Another turtle of the same species as shown in Fig. 25.22 which has responded to treatment for severe fibrous osteodystrophy. Note the tendency of the animal to grow into a spherical shape. The interface between the carapace and plastron has migrated dorsally from its normal ventro-lateral position. This turtle could barely propel itself on firm substrates because its feet no longer touched the surface.

cally, these animals are fed diets rich in goitrogenous vegetables such as kale, cabbage, broccoli, Brussel's sprouts, bok choy, nappa, etc., and 2) they possess a particularly high metabolic requirement for iodine per se. Both populations of these giant chelonians originated on volcanic island groups, the native flora of which contain known halogen-sequestering plants.

Histologically, the hypoiodine-induced goitrous thyroid consists of irregularly shaped follicles lined by tall columnar epithelial cells possessing basally located nuclei and scanty, often highly vaculated, colloid (Fig. 25.24). This is in marked contrast to the normal (euthyroid) gland which is more regular in size and outline, and is formed from follicles lined by a single layer of cuboidal to almost squamous epithelial cells and contain abundant, homogenous colloid (Fig. 25.25).

Prevention and effective treatment of hypoiodine-induced thyroid goiters entails the inclusion of non-

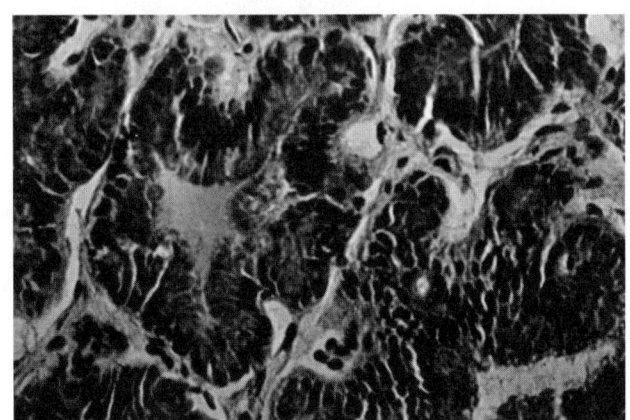

Fig. 25.24. Photomicrograph of a hypoiodine-induced goitrous thyroid gland from a semi-aquatic turtle. Note the irregular follicles lined by tall columnar epithelial cells bearing basally located nuclei and scanty, vacuolated colloid. H&E X220

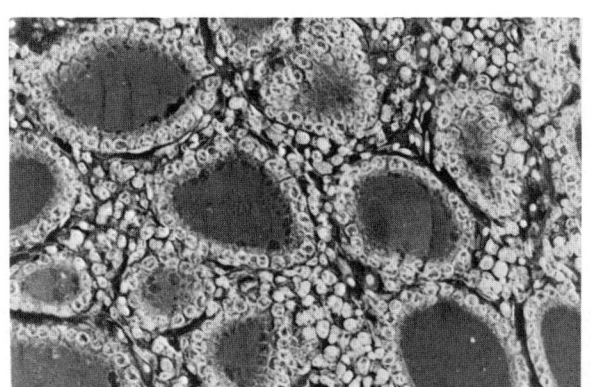

Fig. 25.25. A normal thyroid from another turtle of the same species, age and sex as the one in Fig. 25.24. Note the more regular follicular outline. These follicles are lined by cuboidal glandular epithelium and contain abundant, homogeneous colloid. H&E X220

goitrogenic vegetables and staples in the captive diet plus supplementation of sodium iodide or potassium iodide as a top dressing. Although providing adequate sodium chloride, iodized salt may not contain sufficient iodide ion. Additional iodine may be furnished by sodium iodide, potassium iodide or commerical iodinated casein. Several proprietary animal feed manufacturers produce trace mineralized salt mixes which have proven quite satisfactory for these tortoises.

Other trace minerals such as cobalt, copper, magnesium, manganese, zinc, etc., may or may not be present in sufficient quantities in the diet. Again, trace-mineral mixes furnish them in a palatable and efficiently delivered form.

HYPOGLYCEMIA

Captivity-related hypoglycemia in crocodilians has been described (Coulson and Hernandez, 1953; Wallach, 1971). This disorder usually is related to fasting and/or stress. The clinical signs are widely dilated pupils, fine muscle tremors, generalized weakness and sluggish to totally absent righting reflex.

Recommended treatment consists of oral glucose at a dosage of 3 gm/kg body weight and, of course, the removal of the stressful stimuli (Wallach, 1971).

OBESITY

Obesity is a common problem of long time captive reptiles. Considering the fact that these animals do not have to forage actively for their livelihood, it is not surprising to observe grossly overweight captive reptiles, especially crocodilians and some heavy-bodied sluggish snakes and lizards.

With chronic ingestion of an excessive energy-rich diet, surplus nutrients are stored as lipids in the coelomic fat bodies, subcutis, tail fat depots, perirenal and pericardial fat, and in the parenchymatous visceral organs. It is not unusual for a liver of an obese reptile to be so fat-laden that at necropsy it actually floats in aqueous fluids such as formalin (Figs. 25.26 and 25.27).

The frequency of feeding must be matched closely to the metabolic needs, growth and activity of the particular

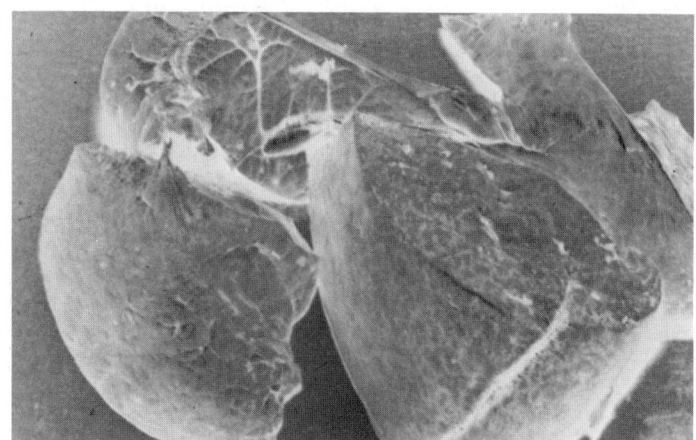

Fig. 25.26. Post-mortem specimen of a massively fatty liver from a Gopherus agassizi. Characteristically, such livers are pale-colored and often are so fat-laden that they actually float in aqueous solutions.

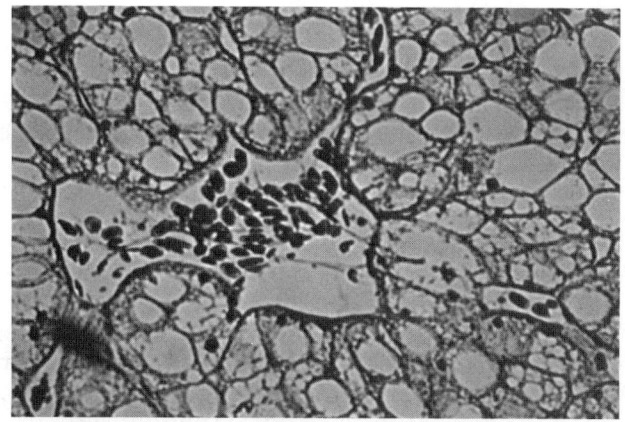

Fig. 25.27. Photomicrograph of a histologic section from the liver illustrated in Fig. 25.26. Note the massive degree of hepatocellular lipid vacuolation and swelling. H&E X160

animal. Whereas almost daily feeding for highly active and foraging snakes, lizards and some turtles is recommended, an interval of 4 to 6 weeks would be more appropriate for some of the very large adult boas, pythons, anacondas and vipers. Since there are no absolute rules governing the proper feeding frequency, common sense and experienced judgement must be relied upon.

REFERENCES

Anderson, M.P., and Capen, C.C., 1976, Fine structural changes of bone cells in experimental osteodystrophy of green iguanas, Virch. Arch. B, 20: 168-184.
Appleby, E.C., and Siller, W.B., 1960, Some cases of gout in reptiles, J. Pathol. Bacteriol., 80:427-430.
Collins, D., 1971, Quantities of calcium carbonate needed to balance calcium-phosphorus ratios of various meats, J. Zoo Animal Med., 2:25.
Derickson, W.K., 1976, Lipid storage and utilization in reptiles, Amer. Zool., 16:711-723.
Dunson, W.A., 1969, Reptilian salt glands, in: "Exocrine glands," S.Y. Botelho, F.P. Brooks and W.H. Shelley, eds., Univ. Pennsylvania Press, Philadelphia.
Fowler, M.E., 1978, Metabolic bone disease, in: "Zoo and wildlife medicine," M.E. Fowler, ed., W.B. Saunders, Philadelphia.
Frye, F.L., 1973, "Husbandry, medicine and surgery in captive reptiles," V.M. Publ., Inc., Bonner Springs.
Frye, F.L., 1974, The role of nutrition in the successful management of captive reptiles, Proc. California Vet. Med. Ass. 86th Meeting Sci. Seminar.
Frye, F.L., 1981, "Biomedical and surgical aspects of captive reptile husbandry," V.M. Publ., Inc., Bonner Springs.
Frye, F.L., 1983, Principles of basic and applied nutrition in the husbandry of captive reptiles, in: "Zoo and wildlife medicine," Vol. 2, M.E. Fowler, ed., W.B. Saunders, Philadelphia.
Frye, F.L., and Dutra, F.R., 1974, Hypothyroidism in turtles and tortoises, Vet. Med. Small Animal Clin., 69:990-993.
Frye, F.L., and Schelling, S.H., 1973, Steatitis in a caiman, Vet. Med. Small Animal Clin., 68:143-145.
Ippen, R., 1965, Considerations of the comparative pathology of bone diseases in reptiles, Zentralbl. Alleg. Pathol., 108:424-434.

Jensen, H.B., and With, T.K., 1939, Vitamin A and carotenoids in the liver of mammals, birds, reptiles and man, with particular regard to the intesity of the ultraviolet absorption and the Carr-Proce reaction of vitamin A, Biochem. J., 33:1771-1786

Laszlo, J., 1969, Observations on two artifical lights for reptile displays, Int. Zoo Yearbook, 9:13.

Laszlo, J., 1975, The effect of light and temperature on reptilian mating and reproduction; recent developments, Proc. Amer. Ass. Zoo Parks Aquar., 1975-1976.

Laszlo, J., 1976, Notes on photobiology, hibernation and reproduction of snakes, Proc. 1st Reptile Symp., Frederick.

Laszlo, J., 1977, Notes on thermal requirements of reptile and amphibians in captivity: The relationship between temperature ranges and life zone concept Proc. Amer. Ass. Zoo Parks Aquar. Regional Conf. 1977.

Pallaske, G., 1961, Hypervitaminosis D in a lizard, Berl. Munch. Tierarztl. Wchnschr., 74:132.

Reichenbach-Klinke, H.H., and Elkan, E., 1965, "The principal diseases of lower vertebrates, Academi Press, New York.

Schmidt-Nielsen, K., 1964, "Desert animals," Oxford Univ. Press, New York.

Schmidt-Nielsen, K., Borut, P., Lee, P., and Crawford, E., 1963, Nasal salt excretion and the possible function of the cloaca in water conservation, Science, 142:1300-1301.

Schuchman, S.M., and Taylor, D.O.N., 1970, Arteriosclerosi in an iguana (Iguana iguana), J. Amer. Vet. Med. Ass., 157:614-616.

Templeton, J.R., 1964, Nasal salt exretion in terrestrial lizards, Comp. Biochem. Physiol., 11:223-229.

Wallach, J.D., 1966, Hypervitaminosis D in green iguanas, J. Amer. Vet. Med. Ass., 149:912-914.

Wallach, J.D., 1968, Steatitis in captive crocodilians, J. Amer. Vet. Med. Ass., 153:845-847.

Wallach, J.D., 1971, Environmental and nutritional diseases of captive reptiles, J. Amer. Vet. Med. Ass., 159:1632-1643.

Wallach, J.D., and Hoessle, C., 1968, Fibrous osteodystrophy in green iguanas, J. Amer. Vet. Med. Ass., 153:863-865.

Wallach, J.D., and Hoff, G.L., 1982, Metabolic and nutritional diseases of reptiles, in: "Noninfectious diseases of wildlife," G.L. Hoff and J.W. Davis, eds., Iowa State Univ. Press, Ames.

IMMUNOLOGIC ASPECTS OF INFECTIOUS DISEASES

George V. Kollias, Jr.

College of Veterinary Medicine

University of Florida

INTRODUCTION

Reptiles and amphibians have been reported to harbor and maintain susceptibility to a wide range of potentially pathogenic agents (Ahne, 1977; Anver et al., 1976; Brock et al., 1976; Cooper et al., 1978; Cosgrove and Jared, 1974; Dondaldson et al., 1975; Glorioso et al., 1974; Kwapinski et al., 1974; Marcus, 1971; McKenzie and Green, 1976; Mizell, 1968; Page, 1966; Reichenbach-Klinke and Elkan, 1965; Scherr and Rippon, 1959; Telford, 1971; Vogel, 1958). Antigenic components from bacterial and viral agents have been shown to stimulate agglutinating and neutralizing antibody production in lower vertebrates, including all orders of reptiles and some amphibians (Good and Papermaster, 1964). Cell-mediated immune responses to such agents in these species have only recently been investigated.

Continued research in the areas of comparative immunology and infectious diseases has not only provided new insights into the immunologic capabilities of reptiles and amphibians in response to mycotic, bacterial, viral, protozoan and metazoan parasites, but has contributed to the understanding of the ontogeny and phylogeny of immune responsiveness (Table 26.1).

Factors such as nutrition, population dynamics and other ecological factors have a profound effect on immune responsiveness. Local immune mechanisms, the mononuclear phagocytic system and polymorphonuclear leukocytes

Table 26.1. The T-cell and B-cell Dichotomy in Vertebrates: Some Characteristics of the Immune System of Poikilotherms and Mammals (from Manning, 1979).

	Fish	Urodeles	Anurans	Reptiles	Mammals
Demonstration of both thymus-dependent and thymus-independent responses to mitogens and to antigens			+		+
Separable populations of hapten and carrier reactive cells	+	+	+		+
Heterogeneity in mitogen responses of lymphocytic populations	+	+	+	+	+
Readily detectable endogenous immunoglobulin on thymocytes	+	+	+	−	−
Presence of low molecular weight class of immunoglobulin	−	−	+	+	+

A blank space indicates that sufficient information is not yet available.

Table 26.2. Summary of the Major Lymphoid Tissues of Poikilothermic Vertebrates (from Manning, 1979).

	Thymus	Bone marrow	Gut-associated lymphoid nodules	Major secondary lymphoid organs
Agnathans	No true thymus	Lacking	Lacking	Scattered foci including kidney in hagfish
Fish	Present	Usually lacking	Lacking	Spleen, kidney, head kidney
Urodeles	Present	Usually lacking	Lacking	Spleen plus peri-hepatic plasmocytes
Anurans	Present	Present	Present	Spleen, primitive lymph nodes, kidney
Reptiles	Present	Present	Present	Spleen, primitive lymph nodes

probably play a significant role in the immune defense system of reptiles and amphibians. Major lymphoid tissues have been identified in many ectothermic vertebrates, the structure and function of which is currently under investigation(Table 26.2).

The purpose of this chapter will be to review some of the basic humoral, cellular and environmental factors involved in the reptilian and amphibian immune response to bacterial, and to a lesser extent, to viral agents. In conclusion, aspects of these factors requiring more complete characterization for further understanding of host-parasite interactions in these species will be considered.

REPTILES

Humoral immune mechanisms

The role of humoral factors in systemic infection is largely related to augmentation of phagocytic function through the processes of chemotaxis and opsonization. However, some mechanisms of antimicrobial activity independent of phagocytosis may be mediated by humoral factors. One such mechanism includes complement-mediated bacteriolysis.

A principal component of the host immune response to viruses includes specific antibody formation. Antibodies are considered to function by preventing adsorption and elution of viruses from host cells. The mechanism by which viruses are neutralized by secretory IgA and humoral antibodies is not well understood in mammals. Description and function of secretory antibody in poikilothermic vertebrates is currently under investigation. Antibodies are not considered to have an important opsonic function for viruses. Host cells infected with surface maturing viruses (rhabdo-, myxo- and paramyxoviruses) or with viruses that direct the placement of viral glycoproteins onto the cell membrane are lysed by complement in the presence of antibody. Such cell fragments are then phagocytosed and further degradated by macrophages.

With these factors in mind, it is first important to consider immune ontogeny as well as immunoglobulin structure and function in the four orders of reptiles.

Ontogeny

Relatively little is known concerning the development

of immunologic capacities in reptiles. Kanakambika and
Muthukkaruppan (1972) studied the immune response of
hatchling garden lizards, Calotes versicolor, by injection
Of 25% sheep red blood cells (SRBC) in saline. Lizards
as young as 24 hours old were capable of mounting an
immune response as indicated by the production of significant numbers of plaque-forming cells in their spleens.
Attempts to induce graft-versus-host reactions by injecting newly hatched lizards intraperitoneally with adult
lizard spleen cells were unsuccessful, indicating immunologic maturation at a young age. It is clear from their
work that antibody-forming capacity, as judged by the
ability to respond to SRBC is already developed at the
time of hatching in C. versicolor. In addition, it was
shown that the rate of reaction to antigen seen in hatchlings is comparable to that of adult lizards.

Maung (1963) demonstrated that eggs acquired from
female tortoises, Testudo ibera, that were injected with
Brucella abortus antigen contained agglutinins to the
homologous antigen. These antibodies can be found in
the yolk at one-sixteenth the concentration of that
in serum, in eggs exceeding 0.6 cm in diameter and are
of the tortoise macroglobin type. Maung concluded that
agglutinins are transmitted from the maternal circulation
to the yolk of the ovarian eggs.

Immunoglobulins

Immunoglobulins are present in the plasma of all
reptiles. The role of specific antibody in immunity to
bacterial and viral infections is well documented
(Campbell, 1976; Fudenberg et al., 1976). Metchinkoff
(1901) appears to have been the first to show an immune
response in a reptile. He found that crocodiles could
produce antibody to both tetanus and cholera toxins.
Later, Grasset and Zontendyk (1935) attempted to confirm
the capacity of crocodiles, tortoises and lizards to
produce antitoxins to tetanus as well as to diphtheria
toxins, but they did not observe a good quantitative
response, even in crocodiles. Downs (1928) succeeded in
inducing anaphylaxis in turtles with mammalian serum
proteins and observed the production of precipitins in
some cases.

In the python, Morelia argus, circulating antibodies
were shown to react with antigens of specific infecting
nematodes (Timourian et al., 1961). Twenty-five percent
of the serum samples from a wide variety of North American

snakes contained agglutinating antibodies against Leptospira (White, 1963). Autoantibodies, present in plasma of the gila monster, Heloderma suspectum, and various snakes are known to neutralize toxins in their respective venoms (see Chapter 27). Ophisaurus apodus was shown to be capable of producing soluble antigen-antibody complexes to bovine gamma-globulin (BGG) and swine serum (Hemmerling 1970). Chelydra serpentina responded with low-titered neutralizing and/or precipitating antibody to amphibian cytoplasmic viruses (Kaminski and Karzon, 1969). Neutralizing antibody to eastern equine encephalitis (EEE) virus has been detected in several species of reptiles in the southern United States. These finding were substantiated by the detection of neutralizing antibody in ten reptile species experimentally inoculated with EEE virus. Repeated inoculations of EEE virus produced results varying from no response to anamnestic-type response within 24 hours of inoculation (Karstad, 1961). Similar findings have been reported in garter snakes, Thamnophis spp., infected with western equine encephalitis (WEE) virus (Gebhardt et al., 1973; Thomas and Eklund, 1962). The role of hibernation in snakes and the persistent arbovirus infections has been reviewed (Karstad, 1963).

To summarize, turtles, tortoises, snakes, lizards and crocodilians are capable of mounting an immune response to a wide variety of antigenic constituents of infectious agents by the production of specific antibodies (Coe, 1972; Coe et al., 1976; Cohen et al., 1971; Ferris, 1961; Gresikova Kohutova and Albect, 1959; Kendall and Minton, 1973; Pavlov et al., 1961). The interaction between two component lymphoid systems for the production of such immunoglobulins still awaits elucidation as well as in vivo and in vitro studies on the effects of these immuno-competent cells on various infectious agents.

Immunoglobulin classes

In the order Rhynchocephalia, the tuatara, Sphenodon punctatum, has been shown to possess an 18S gamma M and 7S immunoglobulins of distinct classes. Both of these antibodies have been shown to be produced in response to Salmonella adelaide flagella. The 7S protein did not show any antibody activity during the immunization period which extended over 8 months. The 18S immunoglobulin appeared to be structurally similar to mammalian IgM. In addition, the observations suggest that the tuatara 7S immunoglobulin might have a similar size to the turtle 7S immunoglobulins (Marchalonis et al., 1969).

The immunoglobulins of the chelonia have been the most extensively studied. Grey (1963) described two immunoglobulin classes in Chrysemys picta. In that same year, Maung (1963) described three serum components that appeared in response to B. abortus antigens when injected Into T. ibera. The fastest moving component (I) corresponded in mobility to mammalian gamma-globulin. The slowest moving component (III) had a velocity intermediate between those of mammalian beta and gamma-globulins. The other component (II) moved with an intermediate velocity, but was not present in all test animals. He stated that the response to immunization was slow with antibody appearing under most favorable conditions at 4 weeks. The production of a secondary response to the same antigen could not be attained. In 1966, Ambrosius (cited in Cooper, 1976) described two immunoglobulin types, corresponding to subclasses of IgG in mammals, in a tortoise. Later in 1972, Benedict and Pollard described three classes of immunoglobulins in Chelonia mydas. When the turtles were immunized with either bovine serum albumin (BSA) or 2,4 dinitrophenylbovine gamma-globulin (DNP-BGG) in complete Freund's adjuvant, a 17S, 7S and a third group of immunoglobulin with a sedimentation coefficient of 5.7 were produced. In contrast to Maung's earlier work, a definite anamnestic response could be elicited with the antigens utilized.

To help substantiate the work of Benedict and Pollard, Leslie and Clem (1972) characterized three immunoglobulin classes in C. scripta. BGG and DNP were used as antigens. The sedimentation coefficients of the three immunoglobulins were 17S, 7.5S and 5.7S, with molecular weights of 850,000, 180,000 and 120,000 respectively. Again in 1972, Coe presented information on the response of C. picta to four purified protein antigens. Specific antibody production was consistently detected and antigen binding was related to four immunoglobulin (Ig) precipitin lines called Ig1, Ig2, Ig3 and Ig4 in turtle serum. Antibody activity was detected first in the Ig1 or Ig2 and then later in the course of immunization in Ig3 and Ig4. Ig1 was about 19S in size, and was the only Ig absent from turtle lymph. Not only did the immunoglobulins described differ in molecular size, they also revealed differences in body fluid distribution and inductive period. The radioimmuno-electrophoretic technique used aided in differentiating Ig from other serum proteins such as "transferrin", which has a slow gamma mobility in the turtle (Coe, 1972). Coe concluded by suggesting the presence of a "surprisingly complex IgG system involving four different serum proteins" in C. picta. If this is true, it may indicate that the reptiles possess greater diversity in immuno-globulin structure than all the vertebrates except the mammals (Cooper, 1976). Most recently a preliminary study indicated the presence of a secretory IgM in C. picta (Portis and Coe, 1975).

The crocodilians may represent an interesting transitional order among the Reptilia from an immunological standpoint. Good et al. (1966) stated that they represent a sequential step in the evolutionary development of the lymphoid system, in which the lymphoepithelial tissue found in the pharyngeal region of alligators appears to be the evolutionary precursor of the tonsils of mammals. Reports on the ability of crocodilians to produce antibody have been fragmentary. As previously mentioned, Metchinkoff in 1901 was probably the first to show that crocodilians are capable of mounting an immune response to both tetanus and cholera toxins (Maung, 1963).

Evans reported the production of antibody to flagellar antigen of S. typhosa by Caiman sclerops (Evans et al., 1965). Lerch et al. (1967) immunized young alligators, Alligator mississippiensis, with keyhole limpet hemocyanin (a molluscan respiratory protein designated KLH). Circulating antibody was first observed 20 days after intracardiac injection and disappeared from circulation by the 45th day. A second series of injections given to four animals produced circulating antibody to KLH in 48 hours. Although primarily qualitative, the conclusion drawn was that alligators possess an immunologic memory and are capable of mounting a secondary response, at least to KLH. The immunoglobulins characterized corresponded to an IgG_1 (gamma 1-globulin) and an IgG_2 (gamma 2-globulin). Baril et al. (1961) had previously reported that the gamma-globulin fractions of alligator serum contained 7S and 19S components. Saluk et al. (1970) stated that the 7S and 19S immunoglobulins of the alligator were antigenically distinct. The light chains of its 7S protein consisted of two antigenically distinct polypeptides, analogous to the kappa and lambda chains of human immunoglobulins.

The superorder Squamata represents the group that has contributed most to the understanding of the reptilian immune response, although structural data on saurian immunoglobulins are rather meager. Evans (1963a,b) reported that Sauromalus obesus and Dipsosaurus dorsalis, produced a good antibody response to S. typhosa H antigen (STH) at 35 C. Through the use of fluorescein-labeled anti-BSA, antibody forming cells were shown within the spleen and liver of D. dorsalis. Studies of antisera from D. dorsalis and S. obesus through the use of paper electrophoresis revealed that antibodies were located in the slowest-migrating component at pH 8.6. Evans stated that although electrophoretic patterns of these species may be quite different from those of mammals, the antibody-containing fraction seemed to be analogous to the gamma-globulin fraction of higher vertebrates. Sedimentation of these immunoglobulins was not carried out utilizing ultracentrifugation, but the immunoelectrophoretic patterns revealed that antibody activity was associated with lines comparable to the 7S or 19S gamma-globulin of mammals (Evans, 1963a,b). In addition to his earlier work, Evans et al. (1965) demonstrated antibodies with similar electrophoretic mobilities to those of D. dorsalis and S. obesus, against flagellar antigen of S. typhosa in Phrynosoma solare and Iguana iguana. Antibodies to KLH and T_2 coliphage also were produced in S. obesus (Evans et al., 1965). Tait(1969) demonstrated the production of antibodies to SRBC, a thymus-dependent antigen, in Egernia cunninghami at 30 C. Antibodies appeared in the plasma within 9 days and reached their highest titer in 3 weeks. O. apodus developed a high molecular weight (16S-alpha$_2$-globulin) and a low molecular weight (LMW) (7S-beta$_1$-globulin) antibody to pig serum and bovine gamma-globulin. A clear anamnestic response was demonstrable with both antigens following secondary immunization. On immunization with small quantities of BGG (0.001 mg and 0.01 mg) antibodies were detectable earlier than with higher doses (100 mg). The antibody response with 100 mg was more prolonged and qualitatively much greater (Hemmerling and Ambrosius, 1971). Both a high and low molecular weight antibody to T_4 bacteriophage have been isolated from the green iguana. The iguana LMW immunoglobulin was larger than human IgG, with sedimentation coefficients of 7.3 to 7.8S. The iguana LMW immunoglobulin appeared to be similar in structure to the turtle 7S LMW immunoglobulins (Kubo et al., 1973). Wright and Schapiro (1973) have shown that D. dorsalis is capable of an adaptive immune response. A single intracoelomic injection of KLH results in the production of passive hemagglutinating and precipitating antibody. An enhanced secondary response to a second injection, given 60 days later, suggests the existence of immunological memory. Antibody synthesized during both primary and secondary responses appears to be a 2-mercaptoethanol-sensitive, LMW beta globulin. It is of interest to note that the antibody synthesized during the primary response in D. dorsalis is a LMW beta globulin.

Until recently little investigation into the immune responsiveness of the order Serpentes has been undertaken. Early evidence for the occurrence of natural or induced antibodies in snakes has been limited to only a few studies. Erythrocyte agglutinins and lysins were reported in snake serum, but their antibody activity was not determined (Bond, 1939; Dujarric De La Riviiere et al., 1974; Timourian et al., 1961). In the early 1960s, Frair demonstrated that rat snakes, Elaphe obsoleta obsoleta, produced high antibody titers to various antigens when maintained near the upper limits of their temperature range (cited in Fenner et al., 1974). In addition, Evans et al. (1965) induced the production of antibodies to flagellar antigen of S. typhosa in Nerodia sipedon and E. o. quadrivittata. An extensive study of the immune response of snakes was carried out by Salanitro and Minton (1973). They immunized E. vulpina, E. obsoleta and Coluber constrictor with BSA or KLH in Freund's adjuvant. Serum antibody, specific for the immunizing antigen, was first detected 4 weeks after immunization. Two weeks after secondary immunization an increase in antibody activity was noted and persisted for 4 months. Evidence for immunologic memory was based on a shorter induction period and higher antibody level following secondary immunization with KLH. Sucrose density gradient centrifugation of whole serum confirmed that snake antibody to BSA was of the 7S type. Sedimentation coefficients of approximately 19S were calculated for the major portion of antibody to KLH. The authors concluded their work by suggesting that a transition in antibody activity from a "heavy, to a light-sedimenting" fraction may be occurring in the anti-KLH serum. This transition presumably is analogous to the IgM-IgG shift in mammals (Kendall and Minton, 1969, 1973). Most recently a third immunoglobulin, secretory IgM, has been defined in the garter snake, T. ordinoides (Portis and Coe, 1975). This species has been determined to have three antigenically distinct serum Ig classes: a 20.5S macroglobulin (called IgM) and two approximately 9S gamma-globulins, Ig-1 and Ig-2. IgM recovered in bile and succus entericus (SE), as compared with IgM from serum, revealed no extra antigenic fragment. Sucrose density gradient analysis revealed distinct differences in molecular size between serum and secretory IgM. The results of the study may indicate that IgM served the function of a secretory immunoglobulin before the evolution of the alpha-heavy chain gene. The biological role of this immunoglobulin remains to be elucidated in reptiles.

Additional work by Coe et al. (1976) with T. ordinoides revealed three immunoglobulin classes. These included IgM (20S), Ig-1 (9S) and Ig-2 (8.5S). When snakes were immunized with egg albumin, human gammaglobulin and KLH in Freund's adjuvant. Early antibody (day 31 after immunization) was frequently IgM, whereas Ig-2 and especially Ig-1 were detectable for the longest duration (992 days). After immunization with antigen in Freund's adjuvant, Ig-1 serum concentration showed the greatest increase, from almost undetectable levels to the most prominent immunoglobulin in immune serum. Preliminary observations with the rabbit anti-snake Ig used in this study indicate that Ig of other snakes are electrophoretically and antigenically similar to those described in garter snakes.

Complement and the reptilian immune response

Antibodies to cell wall antigens of gram-negative bacteria may cause bacteriolysis in the presence of complement. Most studies demonstrating lysis by antibody and complement have employed microorganisms passaged in vitro for some time. Few studies have examined the bacterial susceptibility to lysis in agents isolated from recent reptilian infections or from animal passage. Other functions that complement may play in mediating immune reactions in reptiles include: virolysis; cytolysis; recruitment and enlistment of other humoral and cellular effector systems; inducement of the release of histamine from mast cells; directed migration of leukocytes; and, release of lysosomal constituents from phagocytes (Fudenberg et al., 1976).

Immune hemolytic systems involving complement have been studied in turtles, snakes and lizards (Dessauer, 1974). Flexner and Noguchi (1901) first demonstrated the presence of hemolytic complement activity in snake serum. Studies by Bond and Sherwood (1939) showed that snake sera from 13 different species had natural hemolysin and complement activity for human and sheep erythrocytes. Recently, Day et al. (1970a) demonstrated hemolytic complement activity in cobra and turtle sera using rabbit hemolysin. The lytic activity seemed to be analogous to the complement system of higher vertebrates because it was heat labile, temperature dependent, potentiated by antibody and inhibited by EDTA. The complement activity could be depleted by immune complexes, endotoxin, lipopolysaccharides (LPS) and cobra venom factor (CVF). The CVF induced passive lysis of unsensitized erythrocytes was not supported by cobra or turtle sera (Day et al., 1970b).

If the passive lysis assay was performed in two steps, with frog sera supplying the terminal complement components, then the reptilian sera were active in CVF induced passive lysis of unsensitized erythrocytes. These studies suggest that reptilian serum contains complement components analogous to the classical complement system and an alternate complement pathway that can interact with cobra venom factor and lipopolysaccharides (Ballow, 1977).

There are only a few reports of in vitro studies involving the reptilian complement system and its interaction with infectious agents. Schwab and Reeves (1966) have demonstrated complement-mediated bacteriolysis with serum from Tiliqua rugosa, in a hemolytic complement assay. Lizard serum was shown to be capable of lysing Escherichia coli (BV), E. coli (Lilly), S. typhimurium (M206 and C5), S. gallinarum (9240) and S. paratyphi (BIS and BIR). Both hemolytic and bacteriocidal activity showed temperature dependence. Heating serum at 45 C for 30 minutes showed 70% inactivation while heating at 40 C for 30 minutes caused a 30% inactivation. The reactions revealed that killing of these gram-negative bacteria was mediated by the antibody-complement system and that lysozyme was not found to participate. A second study has shown that normal serum from C. picta and C. serpentina possessed bacteriocidal activity towards Leptospira (Charon et al., 1975). Leptospires from both the parasitic and biflexa complexes were killed by these sera at high dilutions. Antibody was shown to participate with complement in the killing activity. Further support that C. picta serum contained leptospiral antibodies was found by the detection of serotype-specific agglutinins.

Additional factors mediating humoral immune responses

It is clear from the foregoing discussion that reptiles respond to an initial exposure of antigen by the production of antibodies. These antigens may be simple proteins, protein-hapten conjugates or complex antigenic configurations, such as those found in bacterial cell walls and viral capsids or envelopes. The maximal titers obtained are comparable to those obtained in mammals, although the rate of synthesis is dependent on temperature, season, species and age under study.

Temperature has been shown to be an important factor in regulating the immune responsiveness of ectothermic vertebrates (Avtalion et al., 1976). Early researchers recognized that in ectotherms temperature was a significant factor in controlling the elicitation of antibody responses to bacteria (Allen and McDaniel, 1937; Bisset, 1948). Evans (1963a,b) noted that D. dorsalis was capable of producing antibody to the H-antigen of S. typhosa relatively rapidly, provided the ambient temperature was kept at 35 C. Antibody responses at 40 C were moderately good, but at 25 C they were poor to undetectable. If lizards were immunized at 25 C and then acclimatized to 35 C, antibody production would be equivalent to that of lizards immunized initially at 35 C. Low ambient temperature has been shown to be a factor in the survival of certain infectious agents in ectothermic vertebrates as well as affecting their immune response to these agents (Karstad, 1963). Later work by Evans et al. (1965) utilizing STH antigen and the chuckwalla, S. obesus, revealed similar antibody responses to varying temperatures as those seen with D. dorsalis. E. cunninghami injected with SRBCs and maintained at 30 C produced specific antibody in 9 days that reached peak titer in 3 weeks. In the group held at 25 C antibodies appeared more slowly and attained a lower maximal titer. Antibodies were not detected in the group maintained at 20 C during the first 30 days, but were present in low titers by the 54th day (Tait, 1969).

There is mounting ultrastructural evidence that plasma cells of ectothermic vertebrates store large quantities of immunoglobulin, and a secondary antigenic challenge may trigger the mechanism for antibody release resulting in rapid increase of antibody at high titers. Not only may temperature affect the release of such stored antibody, but also it may influence the maturation of antibody producing cells in early stages of development and differentiation (Borysenko, 1976).

It is generally known that reptiles kept at suboptimal temperatures often adapt poorly to new captive environments or are more susceptible to infectious diseases of varying types than are reptiles kept at optimal temperatures. From the above discussion it is clear that alterations in temperature may have a profound effect on reptilian immune responsiveness. Metabolic pathways affected by temperature (digestive enzymes, intermediary metabolism, etc.) are additionally affected. These factors also contribute to an enhanced susceptibility to infectious disease.

It has been demonstrated that reptiles respond to antigens more rapidly and effectively in spring and summer than in fall and winter (Dessauer, 1974). E. cunninghami was not responsive to SRBCs during winter months (Tait,

1969). The tortoise, T. ibera, maintained between 18 and 30 C, responded much more slowly to the B. abortus antigen when challenged in the winter than in the summer (Maung, 1963), which suggests additional factors independent of temperature are important in immune responsiveness.

The mechanisms acting to alter immune responsiveness at varying seasons recently have been studied in several species. The kinetics and magnitude of humoral immune responses correlate with lymphoid tissue structure which in turn is affected by seasonal variations (Hussein et al., 1978a,b, 1979a,b).

Cell-mediated aspects

Compared with the humoral aspects of immunity to infectious agents in reptiles, very little information is available concerning cell-mediated immune (CMI) responses. Most studies involving CMI have been concerned with transplantation immunity (Borysenko, 1970).

First-set skin allograft rejections on adult snapping turtles, several species of lizards, caimans and garter snakes were shown to be temperature-dependent (Borysenko, 1969a,b, 1970; Cooper, 1968, 1969; Manickavel and Muthukkaruppan, 1969; Maslin, 1967).

Acquired resistance to a broad range of intracellular parasites has its origin in a CMI response involving both macrophages and lymphocytes. During the induction of immunity, macrophages probably facilitate the engagement of antigen-sensitive T-lymphocytes, although the mechanism by which this is accomplished is unclear in mammals as well as in reptiles. Antigen-activated T-cells, the specific mediators of cellular resistance to infection, are generated in regionally stimulated lymphoid tissue and then released into the general circulation. Interactions between mononuclear phagocytes and sensitized lymphocytes occur during expression of cellular resistance to infection. In mammals, sensitized lymphocytes produce soluble factors (lymphokines) which help amplify the immune response in many ways (Drutz, 1976). Such factors have not been characterized as products of reptilian lymphocytes, but probably are present.

If the ability to reject allografts is an index of CMI, then other mechanisms may be operable in young snapping turtles to prevent infection with organisms that CMI is primarily responsible for eliminating. Borysenko (1969a) has shown that the snapping turtle matures immunologically in its capacity to reject skin grafts several months after hatching. It takes newly hatched turtles over 90 days to reject skin allografts and xenografts. By 4 to 6 months of age, snapping turtles reject skin allografts and xenografts at about the same rate as do adult turtles. Although it is well documented that thymus-derived lymphocytes exist in reptiles, little information is available concerning their distribution in peripheral lymphoid organs. Pitchappan and Muthukkaruppan (1977) have described the distribution of thymus-derived lymphocytes in the spleen of C. versicolor. Their study revealed the existence of red and white pulp in the spleen. The red pulp consisted of collagenous, fibrous septae containing lymphocytes, erythrocytes and sinuses. The white pulp is enclosed by fibrous septae, containing lymphocytes, reticular cells and arterioles. The region around the arteriole in the white pulp was depleted of lymphocytes either one month after adult thymectomy or after antithymocyte serum treatment. Therefore, this peri-arteriolar region may be designated as a thymus-dependent area, as described previously in higher vertebrates (Pitchappan and Muthukkaruppan, 1977). From a morphologic standpoint, similar distributions of cells have been noted in the tuatara (Marchalonis et al., 1969), in turtles and snakes (Borysenko and Cooper, 1972), in the snapping turtle (Borysenko, 1976) and in T. rugosa (Wetherall and Turner, 1972). Further studies are needed to determine if functional T-lymphocytes populate these regions. It is of interest to note in the above study by Pitchappan and Muthukkaruppan that in the lizard one month after adult thymectomy, the plaque-forming cell response to SRBCs was enhanced. This event provides evidence for another subpopulation of thymus-derived cells, which are involved in modulating the level of antibody response (Pillai and Muthukkaruppan, 1977). This work substantiates recent studies in mammals, wherein the importance of a subpopulation of T-cells in regulating the level of antibody response for both thymus-dependent and thymus-independent antigens has been demonstrated.

Migration inhibition of sensitized spleen cells has been shown to be an in vitro manifestation of CMI to SRBCs in C. versicolor (Jayarman and Muthukkaruppan, 1978). Development of assays such as this for other species of reptiles will aid in the understanding of their immune responses to a wide variety of pathogenic agents that are acted upon by cell-mediated phenomena.

Little work has been conducted to evaluate the in vitro responses of reptilian macrophages and lymphocytes and their interactions with various infectious agents (e.g., lymphocyte transformation by pre-sensitized T-lymphocytes, macrophage cytotoxicity assays, etc.). Several investigators have evaluated a rosette-forming cell assay and a migration inhibition technique for use as T-cell identification and function tests (Jayarman and Muthukkaruppan, 1978; Pillai and Muthukkaruppan, 1977).

AMPHIBIANS

Phagocytosis

Studies in the late 19th century by Metchnikoff (1893) and others utilized amphibians and other ectotherms to investigate the ability of phagocytes to engulf, process and ultimately destroy bacterial agents. Organisms such as Bacillus anthracis were studied in amphibian systems shortly after World War II (Bisset, 1947). Until recently, investigation into this area of amphibian immunity had been largely neglected. A recent study revealed the ability of phagocytic cells from the dorsal lymph sac of Rana pipiens to engulf Staphylococcus epidermidis. This process results in a rapid increase in the numbers of circulating macrophages (Everly and Hansen, 1965). Carbon clearance studies have revealed no significant differences between frogs and chickens in phagocytic capability relative to ectothermic and endothermic temperature regulation (Kent, 1966). Unlike other immunologic functions (e.g., complement activation, antibody synthesis) in amphibians, phagocytosis appears not to be a temperature dependent system (Avtalion et al., 1976).

Humoral factors

The complement system in anurans and urodeles is important in the immune response to infectious agents through the mediation of cell lysis, chemotaxis and phagocytosis. This system in amphibians is analogous to that of mammalian systems, including the presence of an alternate pathway (Day et al., 1970b; Legler et al., 1969). As mentioned above, complement activation is temperature dependent in ectotherms. Serum from R. pipiens exposed to low ambient temperatures exhibited a diminution in the ability to produce red cell cytolysis. Assay for complement components revealed quantitative differences at varying temperatures (Green and Cohen, 1977).

Temperature dependence

Humoral and cell-mediated anuran immune responses are temperature dependent. There are, however, inconsistencies in the literature concerning this phenomena (Avtalion et al., 1973). The opinion of two authors, Wright and Cooper (1980), states that this is due to lack of consideration by others of each species' ecological habitat, e.g., hibernators versus non-hibernators, and generalizations grouping all ectothermic vertebrates together. Recent investigation has shown that in non-hibernating anurans there is no temperature sensitive phase in their immune responses (Wright and Cooper, 1980). Hibernating anurans, by contrast, do appear to have thermal sensitive phases in their immune responses expressed only during the hibernation period. This phenomena appears to be related only to the physiology of hibernation and not to immunity per se.

Immunoglobulins and antibody production

Experimental studies involving immunoglobulin characterization and antibody production to various antigens has been limited in urodeles as compared to anurans (Ambrosius et al., 1970; Ching and Wedgewood, 1967; Houdayer and Fougerean, 1972; Tournefier and Charlemagne, 1975). Studies of the mudpuppy, Necturus maculosus, revealed a serum immunoglobulin with a molecular weight of 900,000 (Marchalonis and Cohen, 1973). After disulfide bond reduction and analysis, the molecule resolves into polypeptide chains resembling light chains and mu-type heavy chains of molecular weight 22,000 and 70,000. This immunoglobulin appears to be antigenically related to the IgM-like immunoglobulins of the toads, Bufo marinus and Xenopus laevis. Unlike the anurans, Necturus does not possess detectable amounts of LMW immunoglobulins. Generally, the urodeles exhibit a slow, prolonged response to bacteria and bacteriophages. The antibody produced is invariably IgM, regardless of the antigen utilized. In contrast to the anurans, there have been no structurally distinct antibodies identified in urodeles (Turner, 1979).

Early studies with anurans revealed that they were capable of eliciting antibody responses to a wide variety of bacterial agents, including salmonellae and pseudomonads. Early studies have demonstrated that frogs could be protected against developing "red-leg" by immunizing experimentally with heat-killed Aeromonas hydrophila (Kulp and Borden, 1942). Anurans elicit a variety of antibody responses depending upon the type of antigen employed. Agglutinating antibodies against bacteria may persist in the serum for months and are exclusively high molecular weight (19S) IgM. Responses to viruses and foreign serum proteins are more specific and involve 19S IgM followed by a distinct 7S, non-mu-immunoglobulin of uncertain designation (Atwell and Marchalonis, 1976; Rosenquist and Hoffman, 1972). The 7S immunoglobulin was later designated IgY (Marchalonis and Germain, 1980).

The 19S and 7S immunoglobulins of Xenopus represent two distinct immunoglobulin classes that are characteristic of anuran amphibians. The proteins are antigenically related, as their light chains are identical in molecular weight of 23,000. The heavy chains differ, though, in that the 19S heavy chains resemble the mu-chain of IgM immunoglobulins of other vertebrates with a molecular weight of 71,300. However, the heavy chain of the light 7S immunoglobulin is comparable to the gamma-chain of IgG in molecular weight of 52,700 and electrophoretic behavior (Cooper, 1976).

Studies have implicated antigens eliciting both IgM and IgG responses are capable of evoking a secondary response, whereas antigens evoking IgM only will not. For example, antibodies to bacteriophage f2 occur in the serum of B. marinus 14 days after primary immunization and reach peak levels at 6 weeks. Although both IgM and IgG antibodies were present, most of the antibody activity persisted in the IgM fraction until 8 weeks after immunization. Following a second injection of antigen 4 weeks after primary immunization, total serum-antibody activity markedly increased, and IgG antibody occurred as early as 4 weeks after the second antigen injection (Lin et al., 1971). In contrast, Marchalonis (1971) did not detect evidence of immunologic memory in antibody production when B. marinus was challenged with S. adelaide. BGG has been shown to induce immunoglobulin production in B. marinus homologous to mammalian IgM (19S) and IgG (7S). The conversion from 19S to 7S antibody activity occurred approximately one month after primary immunization (Lykakis, 1969). R. catesbeiana immunoglobulins have been shown to have the same chain structures as those of mammals. The molecular weights of light chains of both immunoglobulins was 20,000. Heavy chains of the IgG class have molecular weights of 72,100 and those of the IgG class 53,600. The carbohydrate content of the IgG immunoglobulin is 2.1% and that of the IgM protein is 10.8%. The amino acid compositions of both classes are similar to those of mammals (Marchalonis and Edelman, 1966). Studies with viral and protozal antigens in

have only been successful in evoking strong antibody
responses when adjuvants were employed. Explanations for
such low antigenicity as compared to bacterial antigens
have not been presented (Turner, 1979).

Few studies have attempted to isolate secretory antibody structurally comparable to mammalian IgA. There is
no strong evidence indicating that such an immunoglobulin
exists in urodeles or anurans. Jurd (1977) has reported
that antibodies in the bile and gut secretions of Xenopus
resembled circulating antibody in their structure, but
could find no immunoglobulin in the mucus of the skin.

Immediate-type hypersensitivity reactions, possibly
related to mammalian IgE-like immunoglobulin, have been
reported in R. pipiens. Repeated injections of killed
S. typhi were given subcutaneously at 3 to 4 day intervals
and later challenged with a soluble form of the antigen.
Several frogs exhibited immediate but usually non-fatal
flaccid paralysis (Cohen et al., 1971). Although the
physical signs were similar to those of histamine induced
reactions, the investigators were unable to implicate any
particular cell type or organ in this study.

Cell-mediated responses

The majority of studies involving cell-mediated
responses in amphibians have centered around tissue grafting techniques, immunologic tolerance induction and
immunologic ontogeny (Horton, 1980). The immunologic
phenomena associated with graft rejection and tolerance
induction, including specificity, memory and the rejection
process, are similar to those seen in other vertebrates.
These processes in anuran amphibians are to a great extent
temperature dependent (Wright and Cooper, 1980).

There have been few experimental studies involving
amphibian CMI responses to bacterial agents. The majority
of studies have related to mycobacterial agents, which are
commonly present in aquatic environments. The amphibian
host response to mycobacterial agents differs from that
seen in other higher vertebrates. These infections often
appear secondary to other bacterial infections or neoplastic diseases and appear to be of low pathogenicity
(Clothier and Balls, 1973). Experimental host response
appears to be related to the number of organisms present
(Turner, 1979). These studies correlate with other investigators who demonstrated a macrophage inhibition factor
in B. bufo following sensitization with BCG vaccine. The
studies suggest that a lymphokine (e.g., macrophage

activating factor) plays a role in the amphibian defense against mycobacterial infection (Droessler and Ambrosius, 1972).

Cell-mediated responses of anurans to viral associated neoplasms have been examined to a limited extent. Lymphosarcomas of X. laevis and axolotls, Ambystoma mexicanum, have been studied (Balls and Ruben, 1976).

Immunologic ontogeny and metamorphosis

Metamorphosis in anuran amphibians represents a period of increased susceptibility to infectious agents due to the lack of specific acquired immunity and immaturity of cells and organs of the lymphoreticular system. Larval humoral and CMI responses are similar to those of adult anurans, although there is a time sequence in which there appears to be immune suppression (DuPasquier and Weiss, 1973). An example of this occurs with Xenopus larvae. Hatching occurs about 2 days after fertilization, but the ability to reject skin allografts only occurs when the thymus if fully developed 10 days later (Horton, 1969) Additional studies have shown that response to SRBCs in the spleen of larval Xenopus only occurs if antigen is given at day 18 or beyond, when complete lymphocytic differentiation has occurred in this organ (Kidder et al., 1973).

It becomes apparent that other cellular and possibly humoral factors play a role in protecting larval forms against a wide variety of pathogenic agents in the aquatic environment. Further studies are necessary to determine which mechanisms are functional at this point in development.

SUMMARY

Studies conducted by a number of investigators have revealed that reptiles and anuran amphibians are capable of mounting an immune response to varied antigenic components, including complex antigens associated with infectious agents.

Immunoglobulins have been identified in the yolks of eggs from pre-immunized chelonians. The biological role and temporal relationships involving the catabolism of these immunoglobulins in the neonatal reptile are largely unknown. Hatchling C. versicolor are capable of mounting a thymus-dependent immune response to SRBCs as early as 24 hours of age. C. serpentina may require several months post-hatching to reject skin allografts (another thymus-dependent immune reaction) and produce antibody-producing, plaque-forming cells in the spleen. Probable differences occur not only in the maturation of immune responsiveness between aquatic and terrestrial reptiles and amphibians, but also between orders. Other mechanisms must be operative in order to provide adequate protection of immature reptiles and amphibians from infectious disease.

Although immunoglobulins have been characterized for the Rhyncocephalia, Crocodilia, Squamata, Chelonia and for anuran amphibians, little is yet known about their biological functions. Studies of immunoglobulin subclasses may help to elucidate some of these functions, such as predilection for transmission to the yolk, interaction with the complement system and distribution in the various body compartments. The rate of antibody response depends upon the species being examined as well as a number of other factors. Turtles in general have been reported to respond more slowly to antigens than other reptiles. Maximum responses in lizards were reached in 3 to 4 weeks, whereas turtles require 10 to 20 weeks when challenged with similar antigens. Rates of clearance of heterologous proteins in turtles and snakes show marked differences. Immunoglobulin catabolism has rarely been investigated. Recent serological evidence has adequately demonstrated that several species of lizards, the tortoise, the alligator and one species of anuran, produce good secondary responses that are quantitatively higher and/or qualitatively different from the primary response. Success in demonstrating immunologic memory is closely dependent on the type of antigen utilized, dose, immunization schedule, route and environmental conditions. The fact that some species are capable of storing preformed immunoglobulin and then releasing it upon antigenic stimulation or proper environmental conditions suggests that immunological memory may be redefined for reptilian and other species of ectothermic vertebrates.

The effects of temperature and season of the year play a definite role in the immune responsiveness of reptiles and amphibians. Temperature effects on the humoral immune response have been extensively investigated but the case is not so for cell-mediated responses and other immunologic amplification systems, such as complement. The mechanisms involving seasonal variation in immune responsiveness warrant further investigation.

A complement system, including the classical pathway and components of an alternate pathway, has been defined in some reptilian and anuran amphibian species. The kinetics, which include the effects of temperature, biological role and auxilliary functions of this system are open to investigation.

Studies in transplantation and tolerance induction have provided insights into some aspects of the CMI response of reptiles and amphibians. Thymus-derived lymphocytes have been characterized in C. versicolor and anuran amphibians, but little is known about their distribution, maturation, sub-populations and movement through central and peripheral lymphoid organs and aggregates. To aid in understanding the interactions between the CMI response and infectious agents, further in vivo and in vitro studies need to be conducted. Again, much variation will probably be shown depending on the environmental conditions chosen and the species examined. There are still many factors associated with immune responsiveness during metamorphosis of amphibians and early development of reptilian species that require elucidation.

REFERENCES

Ahne, W., 1977, Review of viruses of poikilothermic vertebrates, Tier Praxis, 5:529-540.

Allen, F.W., and McDaniel, E.C., 1937, A study of the relation of temperature to antibody formation in cold-blooded animals, J. Immunol., 32:143-152.

Ambrosius, H., Hemmerling, J., Richter, R., and Schimke, R., 1970, Immunoglobulins and the dynamics of antibody formation in poikilothermic vertebrates (pisces, urodela, reptilia), in: "Developmental aspects of antibody formation and structure," J. Sterzl and I. Riha, eds., Academic Press, New York.

Anver, M.R., Parks, J.S., and Rush, H.G., 1976, Dermatophilosis in the marble lizard (Calotes mystaceus), Lab. Animal Sci., 26:817-823.

Atwell, J.L., and Marchalonis, J.J., 1976, Immunoglobulin class of lower vertebrates distinct from IgM immunoglobulin, in: "Comparative immunology," J.J. Marchalonis, ed., Blackwell, Oxford.

Avtalion, R.R., Weiss, E., and Moalem, T., 1976, Regulatory effects of temperature upon immunity in ectothermic vertebrates, in: "Comparative immunology," J.J. Marchalonis, ed., Blackwell, Oxford.

Avtalion, R.R., Wojdani, A., Malik, Z., Shahrabani, R., and Duczyminer, M., 1973, Influence of environmental temperature on the immune response in fish, Current Topics Microbiol. Immunol., 61:1-36.

Ballow, M., 1977, Phylogenetics and ontogenetics of the complement systems, in: "Comprehensive immunology, Vol. II, Biological amplification systems in immunology," Plenum Publ. Corp., New York.

Balls, R., and Ruben, L.N., 1976, Phylogeny of neoplasia and immune reactions to tumors, in: "Comparative immunology," J.J. Marchalonis, ed., Blackwell, Oxford.

Baril, E., Palmer, J., and Bartel, H.H., 1961, Electrophoretic analysis of young alligator serum, Science, 133:278-279.

Benedict, A.A., and Pollard, L.W., 1972, Three classes of immunoglobulins found in the sea turtles, Chelonia mydas, Folia Microbiol., 17:75-78.

Bisset, K.A., 1947, Bacterial infection and immunity in lower vertebrates and invertebrates, J. Hyg., 45:128-134.

Bisset, K.A., 1948, The effect of temperature upon antibody production in cold-blooded vertebrates, J. Pathol. Bacteriol., 60:87-92.

Bond, R.G., 1939, Serological studies of the Reptilia. I. Hemagglutinins and hemagglutinogens of snake blood, J. Immunol., 36:1-9.

Bond, R.G., and Sherwood, N.P., 1939, Serological studies of the Reptilia. II. The hemolytic property of snake serum, J. Immunol., 36:11-16.

Borysenko, M., 1969a, Skin allograft and xenograft rejection in the snapping turtle, Chelydra serpentina, J. Exp. Zool., 170:341-358.

Borysenko, M., 1969b, The maturation of the capacity to reject skin allografts and xenografts in the snapping turtle, Chelydra serpentina, J. Exp. J. Exp. Zool., 170:359-364.

Borysenko, M., 1970, Transplantation immunity in Reptilia, Transplant Proc., 2:299-306.

Borysenko, M., 1976, Changes in spleen history in response to antigenic stimulation in the snapping turtle, Chelydra serpentina, J. Morphol., 149:223-241.

Borysenko, M., and Cooper, E.L., 1972, Lymphoid tissue in the snapping turtle, Chelydra serpentina, J. Morphol., 138:487.

Brock, J.A., Nakamura, R.M., and Miyahara, A.Y., 1976, Tuberculosis in pacific green turtles, Chelonia mydas, Trans. Amer. Fish Soc., 105:564-566.

Campbell, P.A., 1976, Immunocompetent cells in resistance to bacterial infections, Bacteriol. Rev., 40: 284-313.

Charon, N.W., Johnson, R.C., and Muschel, L.H., 1975, Antileptospiral activity in lower-vertebrate sera, Infect. Immun., 12:1386-1391.

Ching, Y.C., and Wedgwood, R.J., 1967, Immunologic response in the axolotl, Siredon mexicanum, J. Immunol., 99:191-200.

Clothier, R.H., and Balls, M., 1973, Mycobacteria and lymphoreticular tumors in Xenopus laevis, the South African clawed toad. I. Isolation, characterization and pathogenicity for Xenopus, Oncology, 28:445-457.

Coe, J.E., 1972, Immune response in the turtle, Chrysemys picta, Immunology, 23:45-52.

Coe, J.E. Leong, D., Portis, J.L., and Thomas, L.A., 1976, Immune response in the garter snake, Immunology, 31:417-424.

Cohen, N., 1971, Reptiles as models for the study of immunity and its phylogenesis, J. Amer, Vet. Med. Ass., 159:1662-1671.

Cohen, S.G., Sapp, T.M., and Shaskas, J.R., 1971, Phylogeny of hypersensitivity. I. Anaphylactic responsiveness of the frog, Rana pipiens, J. Allergy, 47:121-130.

Cooper, E.L., 1968, Chronic allograft rejection in the iguana, Ctenosaura pectinata, Proc. Soc. Exp. Biol. Med., 128:150-154.

Cooper, E.L., 1969, Skin transplant rejection in apodan amphibians and lacertilian reptiles, Amer. Zool., 9:333-337.

Cooper, E.L., 1976, The immunoglobulins in: "Comparative immunology," J.J. Marchalonis, ed., Blackwell, Oxford.

Cooper, J.E., Needham, J.R., and Griffin, J., 1978, A bacterial disease of Darwin's frog (Rhinoderma darwini), Lab. Animal, 12:91-93.

Cosgrove, G. E., and Jared, D.W., 1974, Diseases and parasites of Xenopus, the clawed toad, in: "Proceedings of the Gulf Coast regional symposium on diseases of aquatic animals," R.L. Amborski, M.A. Hood, and R.R. Miller, eds., Louisiana State Univ. Press, Baton Rouge.

Day, N.K.B., Gewurz, H., Johannsen, R., Finstad, J., and Good, R.A., 1970a, Complement and complement-like activity in lower vertebrates and invertebrates, J. Exp. Med., 132:941-950.

Day, N.K.B., Good, R.A., Finstad, J., Johannsen, R., and Pickering, R.J., 1970b, Interactions between endotoxic lipopolysaccharides and the complement system in the sera of lower vertebrates, Proc. Soc. Exp. Biol. Med., 133:1397-1401.

Dessauer, H., 1974, Plasma proteins of Reptilia, in: "Chemical zoology section II-Reptilia," M. Florkin and B.T. Scheer, eds., Academic Press, New York.

Donaldson, M., Heyman, D., Dempster, R., and Garcia, L., 1975, Epizootics of fatal amebiasis among exhibited snakes: Epidemiologic, pathologic and chemotherapeutic considerations, Amer. J. Vet. Res., 36:807-817.

Downs, C.M., 1928, Anaphylaxis. Vii. Active anaphylaxis in turtles, J. Immunol., 15:77-81.

Droessler, K., and Ambrosius, H., 1972, Specific cell-mediated immunity in batrachians: I. Delayed hypersensitivity to B.C.G. in the toad (Bufo bufo), ACTA Biol. Med. Germ., 29:441-445.

Drutz, D., 1976, Immunity and infection, in: "Basic and clinical immunology," H.H. Fudenberg, D.P. Stites, J.L. Caldwell, and V. Wells, eds., Lange Medical Publ., Los Altos.

Dujarric De la Riviiere, R., Eyquem, A., and Fine, J., 1974, Les hemagglutinines et hemagglutinogens du sange de Vipera aspis, Experimentia, 10:159-165.

DuPasquier, L., and Weiss, N., 1973, The thymus during the ontogeny of the toad, Xenopus laevis: Growth, membrane-bound immunoglobulins and mixed lymphocyte reaction, European J. Immunol., 3:773-777.

Evans, E.E., 1963a, Antibody response in amphibia and reptiles, Proc. Soc. Exp. Biol., 22:1132-1137.

Evans, E.E., 1963b, Comparative immunology antibody response in Dipsosaurus dorsalis at different temperatures, Proc. Soc. Exp. Biol. Med., 112:531-533.

Evans, E.E., Kent, S.P., Attkeberger, M., Seibert, C., Bryant, R.E., and Booth, B., 1965, Antibody synthesis in poikilothermic vertebrates, Ann. New York Acad. Sci., 126:629-646.

Everly, M.E., and Hanson, R.J., 1965, Bacterial (staphylococci) phagocytosis in the dorsal lymph sac of Rana pipiens, Proc. Indiana Acad. Sci., 75:56-60.

Fenner, F., McAuslan, B.R., Mims, C.A., Sambrook, J., and White, D.O., 1974, "The biology of animal viruses," 2nd ed., Academic Press, New York.

Ferris, D.H., 1961, Research into the nidality of Leptospira ballum in campestral hosts, including the hog-nosed snake, Heterodon platyrhincos, Cornell Vet., 51:405-419.

Flexner, S., and Noguchi, H., 1901, Snake venom in relation to hemolysis, bacteriolysis and toxicity, J. Exp. Med., 6:277-301.

Fudenberg, H.H., Stites, D.P., Caldwell, J.L., and Wells, V., 1976, The complement systems, in: "Basic and clinical immunology," H.H. Fundenberg, D.P. Stites, J.L. Caldwell and V. Wells, eds., Lange Medical Publ., Los Altos.

Gebhardt, L.P., St. Jeor, S.C., Stanton, G.J., and Stringfellow, D.A., 1973, Ecology of western encephalitis virus, Proc. Soc. Exp. Biol. Med., 142:731-733.

Glorioso, J.C., Amborski, R.L., Amborski, G.F., and Culley, D.D., 1974, Microbiological studies on septicemic bullfrogs (Rana catesbeiana), Amer. J. Vet. Res., 35:447-450.

Good, R.A., and Papermaster, B.W., 1964, Ontogeny and phylogeny of adaptive immunity, Adv. Immunol., 4:1-115.

Good, R.A., Finstad, J., Pollara, B., and Gabrielason, A.E., 1966, "Phylogeny of immunity," Univ. Florida Press, Gainsville.

Grasset, E., Zoutendyk, A., and Schoafsma, A., 1935, Sur la production d-agglutinines antibacteriennes chez les reptiles, Compt. Rend. Soc. Biol., 119:67-70.

Green, N., and Cohen, N., 1977, Effect of temperature on serum complement levels in the leopard frog, Rana pipiens, Develop. Comp. Immunol., 1:59-64.

Gresikova Kohutova, M., and Albect, P., 1959, Experimental pathogenicity of the tick-borne encephalitis virus for the green lizard, Lacerta viridis, J. Hyg. Epidemiol. Microbiol. Immunol., 3:258-263.

Grey, H.M., 1963, Phylogeny of the immune responses. Studies on some physical, chemical and serologic characteristics of antibody produced in the turtle, J. Immunol., 91:819-825.

Hemmerling, J., 1970, Soluble antigen-antibody complexes: Studies on Ophisaurus apodus (Reptilia, Lacertilia, Anguidae), Allerg. Immunol., 17:154-160.

Hemmerling, J., and Ambrosius, H., 1971, Contributing to the immunobiology of poikilothermic vertebrates. VII. Immunoglobulins and antibody formation by scheltopusik, Ophisaurus apodus (Reptilia, Lacertilia, Anguidae), ACTA Biol. Med. Germ., 27:783-793.

Horton, J.D., 1969, Ontogeny of the immune response to skin allografts in relation to lymphoid organ development in the amphibian, Xenopus laevis Daudin, J. Exp. Zool., 170:449-466.

Horton, J. D., 1980, "Development and differentiation of vertebrate lymphocytes," Elseiver/North-Holland Biomedical Press, New York.

Houdayer, M., and Fougereau, M., 1972, Phylogenie des immunogloulines: La reaction immunitaire de l'axolotl, Ambystoma mexicanum, cinetique de la response immunitaire et caracterisation des anticorps, Ann. L'Inst. Pasteur, 123:3-28.

Hussein, M.F., Badir, N., El Ridi, R., and Akef, M., 1978a, Differential effect of seasonal variation on lymphoid tissue of the lizard, Chalcides ocellatus, Develop. Comp. Immunol., 2:297-310.

Hussein, M.F., Badir, N., El Ridi, R., and Akef, M., 1978b, Effect of seasonal variation on lymphoid tissues of the lizards, Mabuya quinquetaeniata Light and Uromastyx aegyptia Forsk, Develop. Comp. Immunol., 2:469-478.

Hussein, M.F., Badir, N., El Ridi, R., and Akef, M., 1979a, Lymphoid tissues of the snake, Spalerosophis diadema, in the different seasons, Develop. Comp. Immunol., 3:77-88.

Hussein, M.F., Badir, N., El Ridi, R., and El Deeb, S., 1979b, Effect of seasonal variation on immune system of the lizard, Scincus scincus, J. Exp. Zool., 209:91-96.

Jayarman, S., and Muthukkaruppan, V.R., 1978, Detection of cell-mediated immunity of sheep erythrocytes by the capillary migration inhibition technique in the lizard, Calotes versicolor, Immunology, 34:231-240.

Jurd, R.D., 1977, Secretory immunoglobulins and gut-associated lymphoid tissue in Xenopus laevis, in: "Developmental immunobiology," J.B. Solomon and J.R. Horton, eds., Elseiver/North-Holland Biomedical Press, New York.

Kaminski, S., and Karzon, D.T., 1969, Comparative immune response to amphibian cytoplasmic viruses assayed by the complement fixation and gel immunodiffusion tests, J. Immunol., 103:260-267.

Kanakambika, P., and Muthukkaruppan, V., 1972, Immunological competence in the newly hatched lizard, Calotes versicolor, Proc. Soc. Exp. Biol. Med., 140:21-23.

Karstad, L., 1961, Reptiles as possible reservoir hosts for eastern encephalitis virus, Trans. North Amer. Wildlife Natur. Res. Conf., 26:186-202.

Karstad, L., 1963, Influence of low body temperatures on establishment of prolonged infections in animal reservoirs, Sci. Proc. 100th Ann. Meeting Amer. Vet. Med. Ass., New York.

Kendall, S., and Minton, S.A., 1969, Serum profiles of certain reptile sera and preliminary observations on antibody formation in snakes, Proc. Indiana Acad. Sci., 78:113-114.

Kendall, S., and Minton, S.A., 1973, Immune responses of snakes, Copeia, 1973:504-515.

Kent, R., 1966, Uptake of carbon particles by the RES of the fowl, the frog, and the chick embryo, J. Reticuloendotheilal Soc., 3:271-293.

Kidder, G.M., Ruben, L.N., and Stevens, J., 1973, Cytodynamics and ontogeny of the immune response of Xenopus laevis against sheep erythrocytes, J. Embryol. Exp. Morphol., 29:73-85.

Kubo, R.T., Zimmerman, B., and Grey, H.M., 1973, Phylogeny of immunoglobulins, in: "The antigens," Vol.1, M. Sela, ed., Academic Press, New York.

Kulp, W.L., and Borden, D.G., 1942, Further studies on Proteus hydrophilus, the etiological agent in "red-leg" disease of frogs, J. Bacteriol., 44: 673-685.

Kwapinski, J.B.G., Kwapinski, E.H., and McClurg, N.M., 1974, The growth of Mycobacterium leprae in snakes, Canadian J. Microbiol., 20:420-422.

Legler, D.W., Evans, E.E., Weinheimer, P.F., Acton, R.T., and Attleberger, M.H., 1969, Immunoglobulin and complement systems of amphibian serum, in: "Biology of amphibian tumors," M. Mizell, ed., Springer-Verlag, New York.

Lerch, E.G., Huggins, S.E., and Bartel, A.H., 1967, Comparative immunology. Active immunization of young alligators with hemocyanin, Proc. Soc. Exp. Biol. Med., 124:448-451.

Leslie, G.A., and Clem, L.W., 1972, Phylogeny of immunoglobulin structure and function. VI. 17S, 7S5 anti-DNP of the turtle, Pseudemys scripta, J. Immunol., 108:1656-1664

Lin, H.H., Caywood, B.E., and Rowlands, R.T., Jr., 1971, Primary and secondary immune responses of the marine toad (Bufo marinus) to bacteriophage f2, Immunology, 20:373-380.

Lykakis, J.J., 1969, The production of two molecular classes of antibody in the toad, Xenopus laevis, homologous with mammalian IgM (19S) and IgG (7S) immunoglobulins, Immunology, 16:91-98.

Manickavel, V., and Muthukkaruppan, V.R., 1969, Allograft rejection in the lizard, Calotes versicolor, Transplantation, 8:307-310.

Marchalonis, J.J., 1971, Immunoglobulins and antibody production in amphibians, Amer. Zool., 11:171-181.
Marchalonis, J.J., and Cohen, N., 1973, Isolation and partial characterization of immunoglobulin from a urodele amphibian (Necturus maculosus), Immunology, 24:395-407.
Marchalonis, J.J., and Edelman, G.M., 1966, Phylogenetic origins of antibody structure. II. Immunoglobulins of the primary response of the bullfrog, Rana catesbeiana, J. Exp. Med., 124:901-913.
Marchalonis, J.J., and Germain, R.N., 1980, Antibody memory, and tolerance in the marine toad (Bufo marinus), in: "Phylogeny of immunological memory," M.J. Manning, ed., Elsevier/North Holland Biomedical Press, New York.
Marchalonis, J.J., Ealey, E.H.M., and Diener, E., 1969, Immune response of the tuatara, Sphenodon punctatum, Australian J. Exp. Biol. Med. Sci., 47:367-380.
Marcus, L.C., 1971, Infectious diseases of reptiles, J. Amer. Vet. Med. Ass., 159:1626-1631.
Maslin, T.P., 1967, Skin grafting in the bisexual teiid lizard, Cemidophorus sexlineatus and in the unisexual C. tesselatus, J. Exp. Zool., 166:137-150.
Maung, R.T., 1963, Immunity in the tortoise, Testudo iberia, J. Pathol. Bacteriol., 85:51-66.
McKenzie, R.A., and Green, P.E., 1976, Mycotic dermatitis in captive carpet snakes, J. Wildlife Dis., 12:405-408.
Metchnikoff, E., 1893, "Lectures on the comparative pathology of inflammation," Dover, New York. (1968 republication of 1893 edition)
Mizell, M., 1968, "Recent results in cancer research: Biology of amphibian tumors," Springer-Verlag, New York.
Page, L.A., 1966, Diseases and infections of snakes: A review, Bull. Wildlife Dis. Ass., 2:111-126.
Pavlov, P., Dimov, D., Tchilev, D., and Janvev, J., 1961, Tularemia antibodies in tortoises in Bulgaria, Ann. Inst. Pasteur, 100:261-263.
Pillai, P., and Muthukkaruppan, V., 1977, The kinetics of rosette-forming cell responses against sheep erythrocytes in the lizard, J. Exp. Zool., 199:97-104.
Portis J., and Coe, J.E., 1975, IgM, the secretory immunoglobulin of reptiles and amphibians, Nature, 258:547-548.

Rosenquist, G.L., and Hoffman, R.Z., 1972, The production of anti-DNP antibody in the bullfrog, Rana catesbeiana, J. Immunol., 108:1499-1505.

Reichenbach-Klinke, H., and Elkan, E., 1965, "The principal diseases of lower vertebrates," Academic Press, New York.

Salintino, S.K., and Minton, S.A., Jr., 1973, Immunological response of snakes, Copeia, 1973:504-515.

Saluk, P.H., Krauss, J., and Clem, L.W., 1970, The presence of two antigenically distinct light chains in alligator immunoglobulins, Proc. Soc. Exp. Biol. Med., 133:365-369.

Scherr, G.H., and Rippon, P.R., 1959, Experimental histoplasmosis in cold-blooded animals, Mycopathol. Mycol. Appl., 11:241-249.

Schwab, G.E., and Reeves, P.R., 1966, Comparison of the bacteriocidal activity of different vertebrate sera, J. Bacteriol., 91:106-112.

Tait, N.N., 1969, Immune response of the lizard, Egernia cunninghami, Physiol. Zool., 42:29-35.

Telford, S.R., 1971, Parasitic diseases of reptiles, J. Amer. Vet. Med. Ass., 159:1644-1652.

Thomas, L.A., and Eklund, C.M., 1962, Overwintering of western equine encephalomyelitis virus in garter snakes experimentally infected by Culex tarsalis Proc. Soc. Exp. Biol. Mcd., 109:421-424.

Timourian, H., Dobson, C.J., and Sprent, J.F.A., 1961 Precipitating antibodies in the carpet snake against parasitic nematodes, Nature, 192:996-997.

Tournefier, A., and Charlemangne, J., 1975, Antibodies against Salmonella and SRBC in urodele amphibians: Synthesis and characterization, in: "Immunologic phylogeny," W.H. Hildemann and A.A. Benedict, eds., Plenum Publ. Corp., New York.

Turner, R.J., 1979, Antimicrobial responses in amphibia, J. Royal Soc. Med., 72:697-701.

Vogel, H., 1958, Mycobacteria for cold-blooded animals, Amer. Rev. Tuberc. Pulmonary Dis., 77:823-838.

Wetherall, J.D., and Turner, K.J., 1972, Immune response in the lizard, Australian J. Exp. Biol. Med. Sci., 50:79-95.

White, F.H., 1963, Leptospiral agglutinins in snake serums, Amer. J. Vet. Res., 24:179-182.

Wright, R., and Cooper, E.L., 1980, Temperature and immunological memory in anuran amphibians, in: "Phylogeny of immunological memory," M.J. Manning, ed., Elsevier/North Holland Biomedical Press, New York.

Wright, R., and Schapiro, H., 1973, Primary and secondary
    immune responses of the desert iguana, *Diposo-
    saurus* *dorsalis*, Herpetologica, 29:275-280.

RESISTANCE OF REPTILES TO VENOMS

Van B. Philpot, Jr. and Rune L. Stjernholm

Philpot Memorial Laboratory, Houston, MS, and

School of Medicine, Tulane University

INTRODUCTION

"And Moses made a serpent of brass and set it upon the standard, and it came to pass that if a serpent had bitten any man, when he looked unto the serpent of brass, he lived." This quotation from Numbers 20:9 reflects the awareness of ancient and medieval physicians of the resistance of snakes to the venom of their own species as well as the venom of other snakes. On the assumption that the body of the snake contained substances which might neutralize the venoms and other toxic agents, extracts of snake flesh were commonplace in medical science during ancient and medieval times. This belief was so strong that such extracts were finally discarded from the British pharmacopoeia in the 17th century by a margin of only one vote. Far from being new knowledge, therefore, the concepts concerning the resistance of snakes to venoms are ancient and intertwined with legend, literature, history, religion and the use of the snake as the symbol of the medical profession.

REACTIONS TO VENOM

The resistance of snakes to inoculations of reptilian venom or the bites of venomous reptiles is so widely recognized (Swanson, 1946), that much of the scientific literature since 1861 has been devoted to establishing that the resistance is not absolute. The pioneering work of Mitchell (1861) was followed by a number of studies utilizing the venom of crotalids. Unfortunately, the results of these studies were mixed (Keegan and Andrews, 1942; Nicholl et al., 1933; Noguchi, 1904; Philpot and Smith, 1950). The varying dosages of venom, the species envenomated as well as the source and purity of the venoms undoubtedly contributed to the results of these studies. Regardless of these factors, however, the dosage of venom required to kill a snake was considerable (Keegan and Andrews, 1942), requiring between 0.7 to 2.0 mg/gm body weight or the equivalent of approximately 75 gm of dried crotalid venom for the average adult man. Similar reports exist for vipers (Boquet, 1945; Phisalix, 1927), elapines (Kellaway and LeMessurier, 1936) and the gila monster, Heloderma suspectum (Tyler, 1946).

From these studies it is evident that resistance of reptiles to homologous or heterologous venoms is not absolute, but the dosage required to produce death in the homologous species is usually very great. For example, the tiger snake, Notechis scutatus, has been reported to be 108,000 times more resistant to its own venom than is the guinea pig, Cavia porcellus (Kellaway and LeMessurier, 1936).

NEUTRALIZATION OF VENOM

The fresh serum of venomous reptiles contains a toxic factor which is inactivated when heated for 15 minutes at 56 C, and a neutralizing factor which is destroyed at temperatures of 70 C to 75 C (Boquet, 1945; Peterson and Koivastik, 1942; Philsalix, 1927; Tyler, 1946). The neutralizing factor is associated with the globulin fraction of the serum in both snakes and the gila monster (Boquet, 1945) and was believed to be highly specific for the homologous venom and the venom of closely related species. However, a recent study by Ovadia and Kochva (1977) reported that while sera from representatives of the families Elapidae, Viperidae, Crotalidae and Colubrida all neutralized the venom of Vipera palestinae, these same sera, including that of the homologous species, failed to neutralize the venom of the elapid, Walterinnesia aegyptia.

The non-venomous snakes, Elaphe quadrivirgata and Lampropeltis getulus, have sera which will neutralize the hemorrhagic and lethal effects of crotalid venoms (Philpot, 1954; Philpot and Smith, 1950; Rosenfield and Glass, 1940). The serum of L. getulus has an unexpectedly high potency of neutralization as compared to commercial antivenins. Mortality in mice, Mus musculus, injected with 2.5 LD_{50} of Crotalus adamanteus venom was 100%, but when the mice were passively immunized with 0.4 cc/kg of kingsnake serum, there was a 47% survival rate. This compares to a survival rate of only 27% when mice were give 0.8 cc/kg of a commercial crotalid antivenin preparation (Philpot and Smith, 1950). Inasmuch as the antivenin preparation contained 8 gm of protein/100 ml and the kingsnake serum preparation 5 gm or less of protein, the specific activity of the snake serum in neutralization of the lethal effects of venom was more than twice that of the commercial antivenin preparation. Mice inoculated with the snake serum immediately following the inoculation of the venom were protected as well as those mice which received venom mixed with the serum prior to inoculation. Similar results were obtained when mice were administered venom from Agkistrodon piscivorus.

The detoxified serum of C. adamanteus has been found to have a neutralization capacity equal to that of kingsnake serum in protecting mice from the hemorrhagic and lethal effects of rattlesnake or A. piscivorus venoms (Philpot and Deutsch, 1956) and to be superior to commercial crotalid antivenin preparations (Straight et al., 1976). In addition, the detoxified serum of the habu, Trimersesurus flavoviridis, was found to be 2 to 3 times more potent than antiserum from horses hyperimmunized with habu venom (Omori-Satoh et al., 1972).

MECHANISM OF NEUTRALIZATION

Enzymes were the first clearly recognized components of snake venoms and considerable effort was devoted to correlate venom action with enzymic function (Didisshem and Lewis, 1956: Friederich and Tu, 1971; Iwanaqa et al., 1976; Szabo and Gennaro, 1978). However, current research has elucidated that the highly toxic components of venom, in particular the neurotoxins and membrane active toxins, are polypeptides (Zeller, 1977). While highly active polypeptides dominate the action of hydrophiid venoms, they appear to play a lesser role in crotalid venom action as compared with enzyme components (Tu et al., 1966). Enzymes are involved in many levels of venom action (Kocholaty et al., 1971; Murata et al., 1963), such as by serving as spreading factors or by producing very active agents (bradykinin, lysolecithin) in the tissues of envenomated animals. Several instances are known which indicate that some enzymes may potentiate the action of other enzymes, hence the analysis of a single enzyme may not reveal its complete biofunction in venom action (Zeller, 1977).

A correlation between the neutralization of the proteolytic enzymes of venom and the neutralization of the toxicity of the venom has been established for a number of species (Ohsaka, 1960; Ovadia et al., 1976; Peterson and Koivastik, 1942; Philpot and Deutsch, 1956). While the venom of C. adamanteus is considered more toxic to man than the venom of A. piscivorus, its proteolytic enzymes in the natural state are weaker (Philpot and Deutsch, 1956). This paradox can be explained by the fact that biocarbonate ion in human serum has an activating effect on the venom proteases of C. adamanteus (Philpot, 1959; Philpot and Deutsch, 1956). These proteases, however, are inhibited by serum from L. getulus and C. adamanteus.

Ovadia (1978) established a relationship between the proteolytic activity of V. palaestinae venom and the hemorrhagic effect of the venom. This same relationship, however, was not found with T. flavoviridis venom (Takahasi and Ohsaka, 1970a,b) in which the proteolytic and hemorrhagic principles are separate.

Kellaway and LeMessuricr (1936) described the vasodepressive action of N. scutatus venom on experimental animals. The responsible principle was subsequently identified as bradykinin (Guest et al., 1947; Hamberg and Rocha e Silva, 1957), which was released from mammalian serum by the action of trypsin and snake venom. Deutsch and Diniz (1955) described the liberation of bradykinin by the action of 15 different crotalid venoms and that all venoms digested fibrinogen far more rapidly than fibrin. Factors present in the sera of snakes belonging to the families Crotalidae and Colubridae are known to block the release of bradykinin (Philpot et al., 1978a).

The release of bradykinin could account for many of the symptoms produced by crotalid venoms. Although it has been postulated that venom protease is responsible for bradykinin liberation, there are convincing arguements which link esterase activity to the bradykinin formation (Hamberg and Rocha e Silva, 1957; Henriques and Evseeva, 1969). Philpot et al. (1978a) proposed a simplified mechanism for crotalid venoms leading to hemorrhage and death. In this mechanism, the proteases and hyaluronidase play important roles. The proteases liberate bradykinin and destroy fibrinogen. Bradykinin causes bronchial constriction, vasodilation and hypotension. Hyaluronidase, which is present in the venom of the crotalids, depolymerizes the mucopolysaccharide which holds the vascular cells together, thereby making the capillary bed permeable and leading to hemorrhage. If the fibrinogen is degraded to amino acids and peptides, the result will be delayed clotting. The observed antivenin action of the sera of reptiles then best is explained by the presence of an antiprotease which prevents bradykinin liberation and fibrinogenolysis.

An interesting observation is the inhibition of the proteolytic activity and lethal effects of venom from species of Viperidae and Crotalidae by the albulmin fraction of the egg of the bushmaster, Lachesis muta (Philpot et al., 1978b). Unpublished studies by the authors have demonstrated that this property is present in the egg of a wide variety of venomous and non-venomous snakes.

The biochemical nature of the protease inhibitor factor in the serum of snakes is elusive and there are contradictory reports in the literature (Bonnet and Guttman, 1971; Boquet, 1945; Clark and Voris, 1969). However, electrophoretic studies have demonstrated that the inhibitory activity is due not to albumin or some small molecule bound to albumin, but rather to a separate antigenic protein with a molecular weight of 50,000 to 100,000 (Omori-Satoh et al., 1972; Ovadia et al., 1977; Philpot et al., 1978a; Straight et al., 1976). This protein is resistant to the action of trypsin and strong acid, but is destroyed by pronase (Philpot et al., 1978a,b). While it has been characterized as an antibody (Bonnet et al., 1971), experimental studies have not supported this position (Juratsch and Russell, 1971). In addition, the finding of the inhibitor in the eggs of venomous and non-venomous snakes shows very clearly that it is present from hatching and that it is not the result of active stimulation (Philpot et al., 1978b).

SIGNIFICANCE

If the term protease is considered in its broadest sense, e.g., bradykinin liberation or thrombin and fibrinolysin activity, then the toxic action of crotalid venom is closely related to the protease content of the venom. Neutralization of these enzymes closely parallels the neutralization of toxicity of the venom. Protease inhibition by snake serum or by snake eggs is analogous to trypsin inhibition by mammalian serum or avian eggs, both mechanisms protecting the animal against autodigestion by its own proteolytic enzymes.

The study of the process of venom neutralization by snake serum has several implications to human medicine (Maeno and Mitsuhashi, 1961; Ouyana and Huang, 1977; Ovadia et al., 1977; Takahashi et al., 1974). Of interest is the identification of proteolytic enzymes in venom which are associated with the inflammatory process and which are not neutralized by the serum of most mammals. In addition, the discovery of inhibitors of fibrinolysin, thrombin and bradykinin suggest the possible use of snake serum derivatives in the treatment of hemorrhagic conditions related to tissue destruction and shock. And, finally, the crude serum and its purified derivative from certain snake species compares very favorably to the action of equine derived antivenin and is considerably less toxic than the equine antivenin.

REFERENCES

Bonnet, D.E., and Guttman, S.I., 1971, Inhibition of moccasin (Agkistrodon piscivorus) venom proteolytic activity by the serum of the Florida king snake, Toxicon, 9:417-425.

Boquet, P., 1945, Sur les Prorietes Anbvenemeuses du Serum de Vipera Aspis, Ann. Inst. Pasteur, 71:340-343.

Clark, W.C., and Voris, H.K., 1969, Venom neutralization by rattlesnake albumin, Science, 164:1402-1404.

Deutsch, H.F., and Diniz, C.R., 1955, Some proteolytic activities of snake venom, J.Biol. Chem., 216: 17-26.

Didisshem, P., and Lewis, J.H., 1956, Fibrinolytic and coagulant activities of certain venoms and proteases, Proc. Soc. Exp. Biol. Med., 93:10-13.

Friederich, C., and Tu, A.T., 1971, Role of metals in snake venoms of hemorrhagic, esterase and proteolytic activities, Biochem. Pharmacol., 20:1549-1556.

Guest, M.M., Murphy, B.C., Bodyer, S.R., Ware, A.G., and Seegers, W.H., 1947, Physiological effects of a plasma protein: Blood pressure, leucocyte concentration, smooth and cardiac muscle activities, Amer. J. Physiol., 150:397-405.

Hamberg, V., and Rocha e Silva, M., 1957, On the release of bradykinins by trypsin and snake venoms, Arch. Int. Pharmacol. Dyn. Gand., 110:222-238.

Henriques, O.B., and Evseeva, L., 1969, Proteolytic esterase and kinin-releasing activities of some Soviet snake venoms, Toxicon, 6:205-209.

Iwanaqa, S., Oshima, G., and Suzuki, T., 1976, Proteinases from the venom of Agkistrodon halys biomhoffi, Methods Enzymol., 45:459-468.

Juratsch, C.E., and Russell, F.E., 1971, Immunological studies on snakes injected with Crotalis venom, Southwestern Herpetol. Soc., 6:1-4.

Keegan, H.L., and Andrews, T.F., 1942, Effects of crotalid venom on North American snakes, Copeia, 1942: 251-254.

Kellaway, C.H., and LeMessurier, D.H., 1936, The vasodepressant action of the venom of the Australian copperhead, Australian J. Exp. Biol. Med. Sci., 14:57-76.

Kocholaty, W.F., Ledford, E.B., Daly, J.G., and Billings, T.A., 1971, Toxicity and some enzymatic properties and activities in the venoms of Crotalidae, Elapidae and Viperidae, Toxicon, 9:131-137.

Maeno, H., and Mitsuhashi, S., 1961, Studies of Hb proteinase of habu venom with special reference to substrate specificity and inhibitory effect of serum, J. Biochem. (Tokyo), 51:330-336.

Mitchell, E.W., 1861, Researches on the venom of the rattlesnake with an investigation of the anatomy and physiology of the organs concerned, Smithsonian Contributions to Knowledge, 12 Article, 6:145.

Murata, Y., Satake, M., and Suzuke, T., 1963, Studies on snake venom, XII Distribution of proteinase activities among Japanese and Formosan snake venoms, J. Biochem. (Tokyo), 53:431-437.

Nicoll, A.A., Douglas, V., and Peck, L., 1933, On the immunity of rattlesnakes to their venom, Copeia, 1933:211.

Noguchi, H., 1904, The action of snake venom upon cold-blooded animals, Carnegie Institute Washington Publ., 12;1-16.

Ohsaka, A., 1960, Proteolytic activities of habu snake venom and their separation from lethal toxicity, Jap. J. Med. Sci. Biol., 13:33-41.

Omori-Satoh, T., Sadahiro, S., Ohsaka, A., and Murata, R., 1972, Purification and characterization of an antihemorrhagic factor in the serum of Trimeresurus flavoviridis, a crotalid, Biochem. Biophysica Acta, 285:414-426.

Ouyana, C., and Huang, T., 1977, The properties of the purified fibrinolytic principle from Agkistrodon acutis snake venom, Toxicon, 15:161-167.

Ovadia, M., 1978, Isolation and characterization of three hemorrhagic factors from the venom of the Vipera palestinae, Toxicon, 16:469-487.

Ovadia, M., and Kochva, E., 1977, Neutralization of Viperidae and Elapidae snake venoms by sera of different animals, Toxicon, 15:541-547.

Ovadia, M., Kochva, E., and Moav, B., 1977, The neutraliztion mechanism of Vipera palaestinae neurotoxin by a purified factor from homologous serum, Biochem. Biophysica Acta, 491:370-386.

Ovadia, M., Moav, B., and Kochva, E., 1976, Factors in blood serum of Vipera palaestinae neutralizing toxic fractions of its venom, Animal Plant Microbial Toxins, 1:137-141.

Peterson, H., and Koivastik, T., 1942, Toxicity of serum of adder (Vipera berus berus) and its antitoxic properties with reference to homologous and heterologous snake venoms, Z. Immunatsforsch. Exp. Therap., 102:324-331.

Philpot, V.B., 1954, Neutralization of snake venom in vitro by serum from the non-venomous Japanese snake, Elaphe quadrivirgata, Herpetologica, 10:158-160.

Philpot, V.B., 1959, Activation of venom proteases and reversal of chelating effects by sodium bicarbonate, Proc. Soc. Exp. Biol. Med., 101:79-80.

Philpot, V.B., and Deutsch, H.F., 1956, Inhibition and activation of venom proteases, Biochem. Biophysica Acta, 21:524-530.

Philpot, V.B., and Smith, R.G., 1950, Neutralization of pit viper venom by king snake serum, Proc. Soc. Exp. Biol. Med., 74:521-523.

Philpot, V.B., Ezekiel, E., Laseter, Y., Yaeger, R.G., and Stjernholm, R.L., 1978a, Neutralization of crotalid venoms by fractions of snake sera, Toxicon, 16:603-609.

Philpot, V.B., Young, P., Ezekiel, E., and Stjernholm, R.L., 1978b, Antivenom activity of proteins from snake eggs, Fed. Proc., 37:673.

Phisalix, M., 1927, Independence of antirabitic and antivenomous properties of blood of adder of genus Coluber, Bull. Soc. Pathol. Exot., 20:986-988.

Rosenfeld, S., and Glass, S., 1940, The inhibitory effect of snake blood upon the hemorrhagic action of viper venoms in mice, Amer. J. Med. Sci., 199:482-486.

Straight, R., Glenn, J.L., and Snyder, C.C., 1976, Antivenom activity of rattlesnake blood plasma, Nature, 261:259-260.

Swanson, P.L., 1946, Effects of snake venoms on snakes, Copeia, 1946:242.

Szabo, P.L., and Gennaro, J.F., 1978, Tissue necrosis and protease content in snake venoms, Toxicon, 16 (Suppl. 1):397-413.

Takahashi, T., and Ohsaka, A., 1970a, Purification and characterization of a proteinase in the venom of Trimeresurus flavoviridis: Complete separation of the enzyme from hemorrhagic activity, Biochem. Biophysica Acta, 207:293-307.

Takahashi, T., and Ohsaka, A., 1970b, Purification and some properties of two hemorrhagic principles (HR2 and HR2b) in the venom of Trimeresurus flavoviridis: Complete separation of the principle from the proteolytic activity, Biochem. Biophysica Acta, 207:65-75.

Takahashi, T., Iwanaga, S., and Suzuki, T., 1974, Snake venom proteinase inhibitors: I. Isolation of two inhibitors of kallikrein, trypsin, plasma and II. Chymotrypsin from the venom of Russell's viper (Vipera russelli), J. Biochem., 76:709-719.

Tu, A.T., Chua, A., and James, G.P., 1966, Proteolytic enzyme activities in a variety of snake venoms, Toxicol. Appl. Pharmacol., 8:218-223.

Tyler, A., 1946, On natural auto antibodies as evidenced by antivenin in serum and liver extract of gila monster, Proc. Nat. Acad. Sci., 32:195.

Zeller, E.A., 1977, Snake venom action: Are enzymes involved in it?, Experimentia, 33:143-284.

EUTHANASIA, NECROPSY TECHNIQUE AND COMPARATIVE HISTOLOGY OF REPTILES

Fredric L. Frye

School of Veterinary Medicine

University of California

EUTHANASIA

There are occasions when a captive reptile must be euthanized. Safety for the operator, humane dispatch of the animal, and salvage of the specimen for pathologic examination and/or museum preservation are all valid considerations which may determine which method of euthanasia is selected; often the size of the animal dictates the choice.

Venomous species can be euthanized by saturating their airspace with chloroform, diethylether, methoxyflurane, halothane or other volatile anesthetic agent. All of these agents pose potential health hazards to humans and should be used in properly closed containers in a well-ventilated area. Diethylether is highly flammable and requires additional caution when used. The length of time required to induce loss of consciousness varies with the species, body size, state of nutrition, ambient temperature, partial pressure of the anesthetic agent, etc., but usually requires only a brief exposure. Some reptiles can survive prolonged periods of hypoxia or even anoxia. Large crocodilians are particularly difficult to euthanize with volatile anesthetic agents, therefore, intracoelomic injection of a concentrated barbiturate solution or commercially-prepared euthanasia agent also may be employed.

For relatively small animals, a brief exposure to subfreezing temperature in a freezer compartment is a humane and highly effective method for inducing an unconscious state, followed by decapitation or other procedure which causes immediate death. If histopathologic studies are to be performed, it is essential that no actual freezing of the tissues occur because the formation of intracellular ice crystals and their subsequent thawing will destroy the value of such tissues for microscopic study.

With most methods, the reptilian heart will continue to contract for some time after the animal is clinically dead and the circulating blood, therefore, is readily available for gathering and study. Generally, sufficient blood will remain within the ventricle to allow adequate sampling.

NECROPSY TECHNIQUES

In order to facilitate data retrieval, each submitted animal should receive an accession number. Once the specimen has been euthanized or is already dead, a routine and standardized necropsy examination and gathering of samples for microbiological and histopathologic processing should be executed. The sequential procedure described here is of personal preferecne and it may be varied to suit the individual. The major point is that some standardized technique should be developed and adhered to so that oversights may be avoided. Jacobson (1978) described a most useful protocol by which specimens can be systematically prosected. In addition to physical observations, this protocol also allows for the inclusion of data pertaining to capture and/or captivity, i.e., husbandry practices, exposure to environmental conditions and abstracts of clinical diseases and medications administered.

Since many of the organisms affecting reptiles also are pathogenic for man, certain precautions should be employed to protect the operator from contamination and possible infection: 1) a separate necropsy area should be assigned for this specific purpose; 2) rubber gloves and protective post-mortem examination clothing including a protective respiratory mask and an eye shield or goggles should be worn; and, 3) rubber boots which can be immersed in disinfectant foot baths which lead into and out of the necropsy area should be worn to help protect resident animals and personnel from contamination.

Equipment

Special equipment will vary with the nature of the collection and physical facility as well as overall operating budget, but should include a variety of scalpel handles and blades, scissors, tissue forceps, mechanical bone or cast-cutting saw, drills for piercing chelonian shells, etc. Sterile instruments should be available for gathering uncomtaminated microbiological specimens. Some of the disposable hospital dressing packs which are employed in human hospitals are ideal for this purpose and are inexpensive.

Appropriate microbiological specimen containers and related equipment needed for the gathering of laboratory material for culture are essential. A Bunsen burner or alcohol lamp for flaming loops and blades used in gathering uncontaminated specimens for culture should be provided. A variety of containers filled with tissue fixatives should be provided. Ten percent buffered formalin solution is generally satisfactory for routine histologic techniques; absolute methanol and ethanol, Bouin's, Carney's, Kolmer's, Zenker's or Zenker-Formalin are useful fixatives essential for fixation of some tissues desired for special studies.

Tissue destined for electon microscopic processing must be fixed in appropriate media. Generally, such tissues are cut into blocks of not more than 1 mm square and fixed in freshly prepared cold 3% glutaraldehyde solution. Often, entire organs will require perfusion prior to selection and blocking of smaller specimens. After sufficient primary fixation, these small blocks may be transferred to osmium tetroxide or other agents. Because many of these tissue fixatives are highly toxic to the skin, respiratory and other mucosal surfaces, adequate ventilation and protective gloves must be provided and employed.

Photographic equipment with appropriate light sources is very useful to document findings. If the work volume and budget permit, a foot-activated tape recorder will help minimize oversight in transcribing the findings of the necropsy examination.

Reference texts relating to the specific anatomy of the species commonly examined should be readily available. Ashley (1955), Chiasson (1962), Goin and Goin (1971), McCauley (1956), Oldham et al. (1970, 1975), Porter (1972) and Weichert (1951) are some of the reference materials most often used for gross anatomy. In addition, the multivolume works edited by Gans and Parsons (1970) are immensely helpful in the identification and interpretation of many organs and tissues.

Blood collection

If possible, a whole blood specimen should be obtained for microbiological and/or hematological analysis. Direct cardiocentesis is a convenient method for drawing the specimen which is then used to inoculate appropriate culture media and make blood films on glass microscopic slides or cover slips.

Preliminary procedures

Whenever practicable, the specimen should be dissected upon a paraffin wax block or similar non-absorbing substance. After opening the coelomic cavity, the dependent body parts may be pinned securely to the surface thus placing them out of the way of the operator.

The integument or shell should be inspected for evidence of trauma (fight wounds, thermal burns, etc.), cutaneous or subcutaneous masses, changes in pigmentation and parasites.

Most non-chelonian specimens are placed in dorsal recumbency and, if necessary, are positioned with bolsters or blocks to help maintain this position. A ventral midline incision is made from the mandibular symphyseal region to the cloacal vent or beyond. Ideally, the skin should be reflected away from the ventral midline so that the subcutaneous tissues may be inspected.

In hard-shelled chelonians, the plastron is separated from the carapace by severing the bridges joining these structures on each side of the body between the fore and hindlegs. Depending upon the size of the animal, these bridges may be cut with a cast-cutting saw or shears. Using a long, thin-bladed boning knife, the plastron is then separated completely by severing any muscular attachments.

Respiratory system

After examining the upper respiratory system including the external nares and oral cavity, transect the upper jaw rostral to the eyes, exposing the nasal and vomeronasal areas. If the skulls of rare specimens are to be preserved for osteologic and/or museum study, this step may have to

be omitted; in such cases, nasal swabs, curettage specimens
or washings may be examined microscopically. The trachea
and mainstem bronchi are incised along their full length.
In smaller specimens, straight or curved iris scissors
and fine pattern, Brown-Adson-type thumb forceps are useful
for this operation. The lungs are explored. In snakes,
the left lung is vestigial or absent entirely. Chelonians
and crocodiles possess paired lungs. In most of the
chelonians, crocodilians and many lizards, the caudal
portions of the lungs may be represented by thin, sac-like
structures and will quickly collapse once the system has
been entered. Particular attention should be paid to the
presence of parasites, exudate, pneumonic areas, cysts,
hemorrhage, foreign bodies and neoplasms. With small
reptiles, a dissecting microscope should aid in identifying
lesions. Areas of pigmentation are common and normal in
the respiratory tissues of chelonians and some lizards.

Cardiovascular system

If radiographs have revealed evidence of pathologic
mineralization of the great vessels, remove portions of
the affected segments for histopathology. Arteriosclerosis
is a common finding in captive reptiles (Frye, 1981).

The heart is found anteriorally in all reptiles and
is enclosed in a fibrous pericardial sac. Inspect this
structure for the presence of foreign substances. A small
amount of clear fluid is normal. With the exception of
the crocodilians, all reptiles have a single large
ventricle; the crocodilians have a complete interventricular septum dividing the right and left sides. Two well
developed atria are present in all reptilian hearts and
all reptiles have both right and left aortic arches. A
single pulmonary vein is present in snakes and most
lizards. In crocodilians and most other reptiles, the
sinus venosus is a large triangular-shaped structure which
receives six seperate veins: the two superior (or anterior)
vena cavae; the post cava; the two hepatic veins; and,
the coronary vein (Chiasson, 1962; Weichert, 1951).

Endocrine system

The pituitary gland is located on the floor of the
cranial vault within the sella turcica of the sphenoid
bone. The paired optic nerves serve as a landmark, with
the pituitary lying on the midline and posterior to these
two large cranial nerves. The pituitary ranges in color
from white to light pink or gray and usually is spherical
to slightly elongated (Saint Girons, 1970).

The adrenal glands are paired in reptiles and, depending upon the order, may be elongated thin structures in snakes and most lizards or more compact and flattened in the chelonian and crocodilian species (Gabe, 1970). They usually can be located caudo-medial to the gonads within the mesorchium of the male or the mesovarium of the female. In chelonians, they lie against the kidneys; in crocodilians, they are retrocoelomic. The adrenals usually are yellow-orange or darkly pigmented and are well supplied by a vascular network originating and terminating in the abdominal aorta and vena cava, respectively. The cortical tissue usually is much lighter than the darker, red-brown medullary portions, but distinct zones may be lacking.

The thyroid and parathyroid glands are located anterior and dorsal to the heart base and its great vessels, near the bifurcation of the trachea (in those species which possess paired lungs and dual mainstem bronchi). The thyroid is single in some lizards; in others, it may be bilobed or paired among different members of the same family (Lynn, 1970). It usually is pink. The parathyroids usually are seen as one or two pairs of pale cream to white nodules. In most lizards, the cranial pair lies adjacent to the bifurcation of the common carotid artery. In most snakes, the parathyroids are represented as two pairs of glands; the caudal pair usually is located between and often medial to the anterior and posterior thymic lobes; the cranial pair is adjacent to and often intimately associated with the common carotid artery. In the crocodilians, there may be either one or two pairs anterior to the heart base and very near the common carotid artery. Chelonians possess two pairs; the anterior pair is within the thymus while the posterior pair usually is near the aortic arches and ultimobranchial body (Clark, 1970; Miller and Lagios, 1970).

The pancreas may be almost spherical, finger-shaped or triangular in snakes and some chelonia, or more flattened and elongated in most lizards, crocodilians and chelonians. It is located very near the duodenum and gall bladder in snakes and some lizards and usually is in close proximity to the spleen in most reptiles. In some chelonians, it is separated from the spleen entirely. The pancreas of most lizards possesses three limbs running along the bile duct towards the gall bladder; the third also runs along the small intestine as a thin strand which approaches the spleen (Miller and Lagios, 1970). In snakes, the pancreas usually is in contact with the proximal duodenum. In some chelonians, the pancreas is in direct contact with the spleen; in others, it is confined to the duodenal attachments along the mesentery. It is pale orange or pink in most reptiles.

The gonads are paired in reptiles and can be found partially attached to the mesorchium in males and the mesovarium in females. In the sexually active reptile, the ovaries are yellow to white, grape-like, irregular structures. The irregular surfaces are due to the presence of developing follicles. In snakes, the right ovary usually is anterior to the left. The ovarian pedicle is diffuse and poorly delineated in most reptiles. In most species, the paired testes are elongated, rounded and white to cream in color. The oviducts empty into the cloaca. The ducti deferentia may join the ureters and enter the cloaca together or may enter separately. Male chelonians and crocodilians have a single erectile penis (more papilla-like in the crocodilia). Snakes and lizards possess paired erectile intromittant organs called hemipenes. The tuatara, Sphenodon punctatus, lacks an intromittant organ.

Urinary system

In most reptiles, the urinary system consists of paired, well-lobulated kidneys whose ureters empty directly into the urodeum portion of the cloaca or, if present, a urinary bladder. In snakes and some particularly elongated species of lizards, excluding Ophiosaurus, the kidneys are situated with the right kidney anterior to the left and are located dorsally and medially, adjacent to the spinal column. In most lizards and chelonians, a thin membranous urinary bladder exists as a temporary reservoir for renal wastes. Urinary calculi are common in the terrestrial chelonians and some lizards which eat artifical diets or which have restricted access to water.

Digestive system

The digestive system of reptiles consists of a mouth, buccal cavity, esophagus, stomach, small intestine, large intestine, saccular cecum (in some species), and colon which empties into the proctodeum portion of the cloaca. There are also the accessory digestive components, namely the liver, gall bladder and exocrine pancreatic tissue.

Except in chelonians, the oral cavity with its teeth is lined by a mucous epithelium. The esophagus usually is folded longitudinally and ends at the cardiac sphincter. The stomach may be divided into cardiac, fundic and pyloric regions which are grossly distinct or may be more subtle in its divisions. At the caudal end of the stomach is the pyloric sphincter. The cardiac and pyloric sphincters are firm, pale-colored, muscular valves which aid in confining the ingesta within the various segments of the upper and mid digestive tract.

The gall bladder may be located some distance away from the liver in snakes and some lizards. It is connected to the liver by a long cystic duct and empties into the doudenum via the bile duct which may be of variable length.

The exocrine secretions of the pancreas empty into the duodenum via a short pancreatic duct. Some reptiles possess more than a single duct leading from the pancreas.

The liver of some species of reptiles may be heavily pigmented. This pigmentation is of no clinicopathological significance.

Particular attention should be paid to looking for parasites, especially ochetostomid trematodes which are common inhabitants of the buccal cavities and anterior pharyngeal areas of snakes whose diets include fish and amphibians. These flukes also may be found within the respiratory system. Gastrointestinal nematodes, acanthocephalans, cestodes and trematodes also may observed within the lumens of the esophagus, stomach, small and large intestine. The biliary passages and gall bladder should be incised and inspected for the presence of helminths, calculi and neoplasms.

Reticulo-endothelial system

The reticulo-endothelial system of most reptiles consists of the thymus gland, spleen, bone marrow, lymphoid aggregates or nodules scattered along the alimentary and respiratory tracts and Kupffer cells within the hepatic sinusoids. In addition, lymphoid nodules are found within the wall of the urinary bladder, vascular system and within the bone marrow. A cloacal structure similar in function to the avian bursa of Fabricius has been described in the snapping turtle, Chelydra serpentina (Borysenko and Cooper, 1972), and in the alligator, Alligator mississippiens (Good et al., 1966; McCauley, 1956). The thymus and spleen probably represent the major sites of immunocompetence in reptiles.

The reptilian thymus usually is composed of paired lobes of pale tissue located in the cervical region adjacent to the major blood vessels and nerves. Usually, these pairs of thymic lobes are separated from each other and the number and shape of the lobes vary within and between each order. The tuatara and most lizards possess two paired non-lobulated lobes, a cephalic and a caudal thymus, lying lateral to the pharyngeal wall on each side. The caudal pair usually reaches the level of the carotid arch posteriorally. Both lobes lie ventral to the internal carotid artery and medial to the internal jugular veins and vagus nerves (Bockman, 1970).

In snakes, the unlobulated pair of thymic lobes are located immediately cranial to the heart base, adjacent to the great vessels. Chelonians usually have distinctly lobulated thymic lobes and a third pair is common in some species within the order. The crocodilians have a thymus which is more elongated and fusiform and which extends cranially from the heart base and great vessels along the cervical region almost to the level of the head; it is bounded by the common carotid artery, jugular vein and vagus nerve on each side (Bockman, 1970).

The spleen is usually spherical or triangular in shape and is located near the stomach and/or pancreas. It is dark pink to deep red in color. Most reptiles have a specialized "lymph heart" lying within the pelvic canal. Lymph flows within a large, thin-walled subvertebral vessel which extends from the pelvic area cranially and drains into the cardinal veins, thence into the heart.

Central nervous system

The central nervous system of reptiles consists of the brain; forebrain, olfactory bulbs and associated tracts, cerebral hemispheres; diencephalon; midbrain, optic lobes and cerebral peduncles; hindbrain, cerebellum and medulla oblongata (continuous with the spinal cord); spinal cord; and, the special sense organs which consist of the lateral eyes, parietal eye (in those species which possess one), ears, sensory portions of the tongue, Jacobson's or vomeronasal organ and the maxillary (or facial) and labial pits in the Crotalidae and Boidae, respectively. The only reptiles which have functional, externally visible ears with auditory canals opening to the integumentary surface are the crocodilians and lizards. Middle and inner ear structures are present in the tuatara and snakes, although they may be much reduced in some families within an order.

The major organs within the central nervous system that are removed routinely during a post-mortem examination are the brain and lateral eyes. It is impractical to ever attempt to remove the brain in small reptiles; instead, the entire head is removed, fixed thoroughly and then decalcified for step-sectioning. The final result will be of higher quality than if the brain is extracted separately. Furthermore, step-sectioning will allow the worker to study individual organs in situ, with their natural relationships to other structures undisturbed.

In larger animals, the brain may be removed after the cranium has been opened and the meninges have been incised and reflected. Often the most simple method is to saw the head in its sagittal plane; this will afford direct access to the contents of the cranial vault while preserving almost all of the structures in their natural locations. Moreover, this method allows the fixative to more easily penetrate the soft tissues prior to dissection.

The lateral eyes may be removed and placed in an appropriate fixative which will preserve them for sectioning. Kolmer's solution is particularly useful for occular tissues.

Except in larger reptiles and for special circumstances, it is not practical to remove the entire spinal cord from the cadaver. Removal of short segments may be accomplished after the dorsal laminae have been removed. Smaller animals may be skinned and, after adequate fixation, portions of their axial skeletons are placed in a decalcifying solution prior to gross sectioning and histologic processing.

The smaller and more delicate special sense organs usually are studied by examining stained histologic sections of selected regions.

COMPARATIVE HISTOLOGY

A comparison with normal reference tissue is essential in order to appreciate the anatomic and morphological alterations observed in abnormal tissues. Isolated papers describing the histologic and ultrastructural features of individual organs and tissues have been published, but unified reference sources are rare (Frye, 1981). In this section, the histologic appearance of the major organ systems and tissues are illustrated. The scope of this chapter does not permit an in-depth treatment of the entire order with familial differences exhibited in each organ or tissue, but rather an overview with which the generalist may compare gross features.

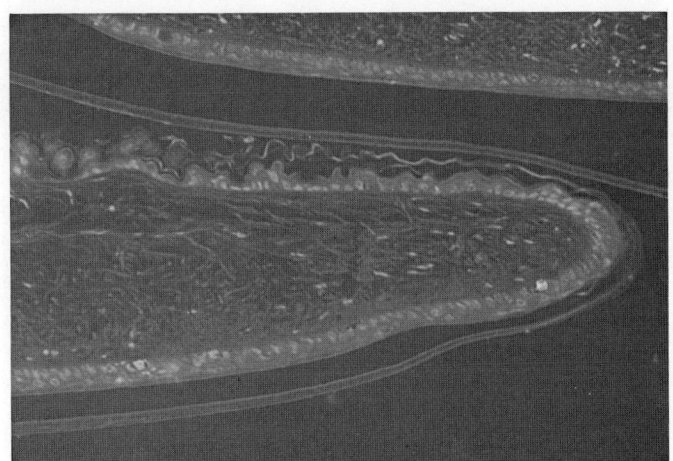

Fig. 28.1. Integument of a typical snake, Lampropeltis getulus californiae. Note dark-staining basal layer (b.l.), stratum malpighii (s.m.), stratum granulosum (s.g.), stratum lucidum (s.l.), and stratum corneum (s.c.). The keratinized layer is shed periodically. Note melanin pigment (m.p.). X40

Unless otherwise specified, the tissues illustrated have been stained with hematoxylin and eosin by routine histologic techniques.

Integument

The integumentary system of all living reptiles (other than a few turtles) consists of a covering of well developed epidermal scales. The skin of snakes and lizards is formed by foldings of both epidermis and outer dermis, while that of the chelonians and crocodilians is formed as large flat keratinous shields (Porter, 1972). In snakes and most lizards, the outer epidermal layer is shed periodically in a more or less intact fashion.

Figures 28.1 and 28.2 illustrate the skin of a snake and semi-aquatic turtle, respectively. The plates of most chelonians consist of trabecular bone overlaid by a dense keratin mantle. The intertrabecular spaces may be partially filled by bone marrow. The soft-shelled turtles possess smooth, pliant, leathery shells and have relatively scaleless skin covering their extremities. The integument of the tuatara is similar to that of the lizards, although the dermal plates located on the dorsal and dorsolateral

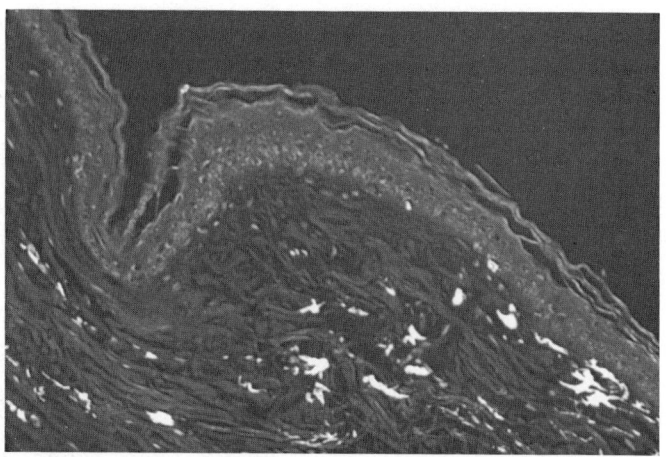

Fig. 28.2. Skin from the foreleg of a semi-aquatic turtle
Clemmys marmorata. Note the similarity to tha
of the snake. X40

surfaces of these animals, being composed of bone inbedded
in the dermis, more closely resemble those in the crocodilians.

Digestive system

The buccal cavity of reptiles is similar in its lining
to that observed in the higher vertebrates, although some
marked differences exist. In some terrestrial chelonians
and marine turtles, dense, horny, keratinous surfaces cover
much of the anterior or cranial digestive tract, including
much of the esophagus. In chelonians in general, teeth
in a dental arcade have been replaced by a horny beak.
Well developed cornified papillae cover much of the surface
of the posterior pharynx and esophagus, a feature characteristic of the sea turtles. In other species within the
testudines, the palatine and pharyngeal surfaces may be
lined with only lightly keratinized squamous epithelium.
To a large extent, this reflects the nature of the animal's
diet. In those chelonians which ingest scabrous items,
the anterior tract will be found to be more heavily keratinized than that of chelonians which eat softer diets.
The buccal cavity of those reptiles possessing teeth are
lined by non-keratinized squamous epithelium and typical
gingivae in the regions surrounding the teeth.

The tongue is covered with stratified squamous epithelium and is heavily muscled. In many lizards and

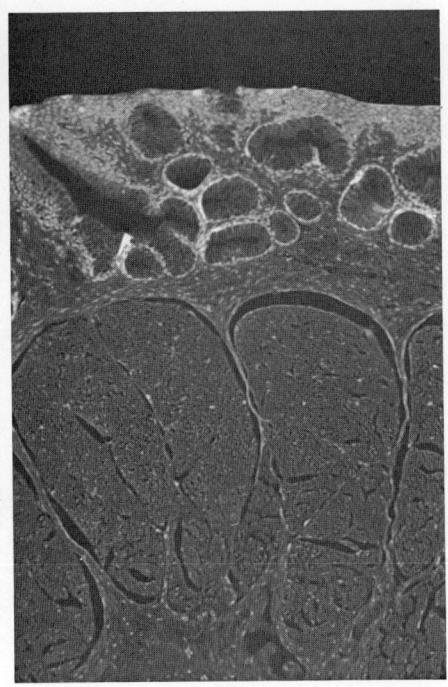

Fig. 28.3 Tongue of a desert tortoise, <u>Gopherus agassizi</u>. Note the population of mucus-secreting glands whose ducts open onto the lingual squamous epithelial surface. Basal cells of epithelium (b.c.), stratified squamous epithelium (s.s.), lamina propria (l.p.), skeletal muscle (s.m.) and mucus acini (m.a.). X60

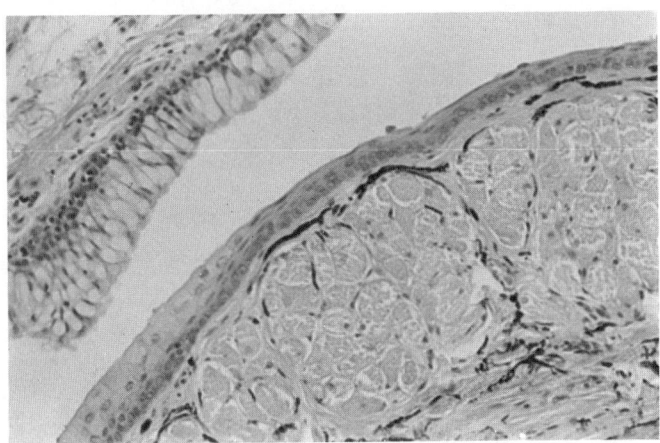

Fig. 28.4. Tongue (T.) and lingual sheath (L.S.) of a small python, <u>Liasis childreni</u>. Note the glandular acini (g.a.) and mucinous lobules within the lingual sheath whose secretions are carried to the surface and furnish lubrication for the epithelial surfaces. X60

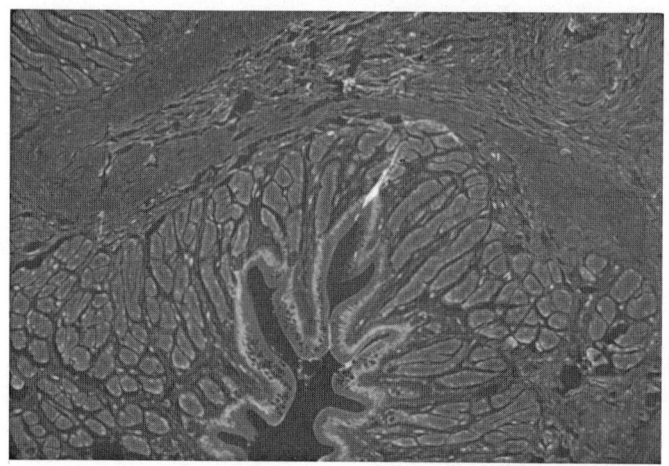

Fig. 28.5. Stomach (gastric fundus) of a boa constrictor, Boa constrictor imperator. Note gastric pits (g.p.), fundic glands (f.g.), chief cells (c.c.), parietal cells (p.c.), lamina propria (l.p.), muscularis mucosa (m.m.) and the circular muscle layer (c.m.). X40

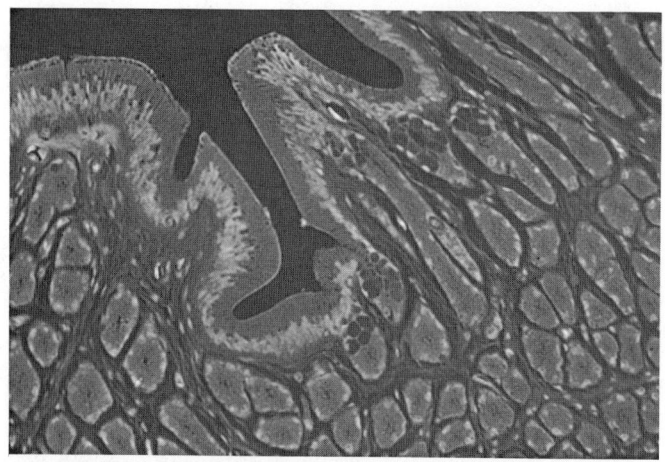

Fig. 28.6. Same snake as in Fig. 28.5. X80

chelonians, mucus glands are located subjacent to the basal layer of the lingual epithelium and are partially surrounded by skeletal muscle fibers (Fig. 28.3). These glands are absent in the tongues of snakes whose lingual epithelium is lubricated and moistened by secretions originating in the mucous epithelial lining of the lingual sheath (Fig. 28.4).

Except as noted above, the esophagus is morphologically similar to that seen in higher vertebrates. The stratified squamous epithelium rests upon rugose folds. Subjacent to the basement membrane are the fibrocollagenous connective tissue lamina propria, muscularis mucosae, loose areolar tissue and circular and longitudinal muscle layers. Mucus glands are numerous and their secretory products are carried to the luminal surface by short epithelium lined ducts. Small lymphoid aggregates are located just beneath the basement membrane. The outermost layer of the esophagus consists of a thin adventitia, as in other vertebrates, i.e., a serosal membrane is lacking.

The stomach is similar to that in higher vertebrates. The cranial or cardiac gastric mucosa exhibits a transition from the squamous epithelium of the terminal esophagus to a columnar epithelium as the fundic portion of the stomach is reached. In most reptiles, the fundic stomach comprises the largest portion of the glandular organ. The tall columnar epithelium lining the fundic portion contains numerous mucus-secreting goblet cells located at the asices of the gastric pits (Figs. 28.5 and 28.6). These pits and the microvilli at the tips of the gastric folds can be demonstrated easily when the section is stained with Alcian-PAS. Gastric glands usually are well demarcated by mucus neck cells (Fig. 29.7). The gastric glands are composed of polyhedral to plump cuboidal cells with pale blue-gray cytoplasm and other, smaller cells with distinctly eosinophilic cytoplasm. The first are the chief, or zymogenic, cells. Their nuclei may be either basal or apical in location. The second smaller and eosinophilic cells are the parietal cells whose nuclei tend to be mostly centrally located.

The caudal, or pyloric, portion of the glandular stomach terminates at the pyloric sphincter and exhibits an abrupt transition from the rich glandular mucosa of the fundus to an epithelium characterized by deeper gastric pits, and pyloric glands lined by a single type of cell whose cytoplasm is a uniform pink color when stained with hematoxylin and eosin. The lamina propria contains smooth muscle fibers originating in the muscularis mucosae, and

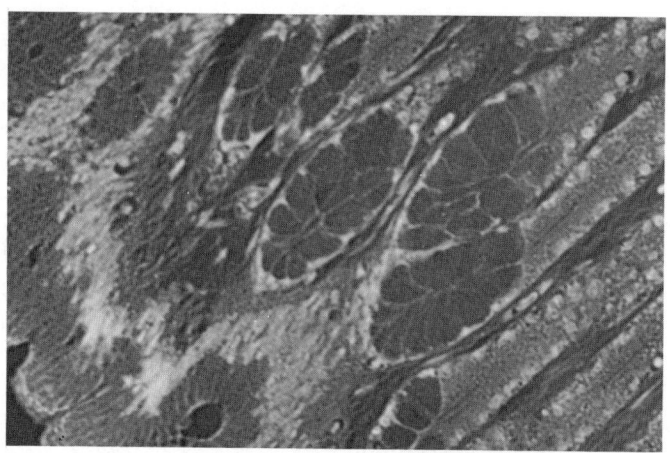

Fig. 28.7. Stomach: gastric fundus of the boa constrictor in Fig. 28.5, higher magnification. Simple columnar mucus epithelium (s.c.), gastric pits (g.p.), fundic glands (f.g.), chief cells (c.c.) and parietal cells (p.c.). X210

an occasional lymphatic aggregate or nodule. The number and distribution of these nodules is variable. As one descends the length of the stomach, the number of mucin-secreting goblet cells increases.

The small intestine usually is much shorter than that found in many mammals of the same size and whose diet is similar to that of reptiles. The duodenum commences at the caudal end of the pyloric sphincter and exhibits a marked change from the gastric pyloric mucosa. The duodenal mucosa is carried on elongated villi composed of an inner core or lamina propria containing connective tissue, smooth muscle fibers, lymphatics and small blood vessels. In the deeper layers of the mucosa are crypts (glands) of Lieberkuhn, above the muscularis mucosae (Fig. 28.8). These deep crypts tend to have very narrow lumens when compared to two adjacent intestinal villi. The luminal surfaces are covered by a simple columnar epithelium whose cells have distinctly basal nuclei. Goblet cells become more numerous as the mucosa descends caudally. Duodenal (Brunner's) glands are lacking. The muscularis mucosae and muscularis externa are well developed. Within the submucosa are randomly distributed lymphatic nodules containing populations of small, dark-staining lymphocytes and occasional paler-staining large macro-

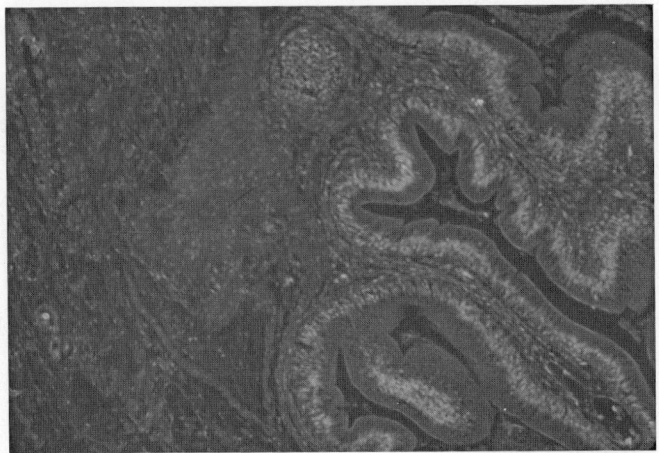

Fig. 28.8. Duodenum of a ratsnake, Elaphe guttata guttata. The lumen is lined by a simple columnar epithelium (s.c.) carried upon intestinal villi (v.) forming crypts of Lieberkuhn (c.L.). A supporting lamina propria (l.p.), lymphoid nodules (ly.), circular (c.m.) and longitudinal (l.m.) smooth muscle are present as in higher vertebrates. X60

phages. The outer surface of the intestine is covered by a serosal membrane as in higher vertebrates. Adipose tissue also is seen, particularly near the mesenteric attachments. Branches of the mesenteric arteries penetrate the gut wall at these mesenteric junctions and give rise to numerous arterioles and capillaries.

The large intestine also is lined by a simple columnar epithelium containing abundant mucin-producing goblet cells, particularly within the crypts formed by adjacent villi and folds. Lymphatic nodules appear more frequently than in the small intestine and may extend almost all the way out to the lumenal surface in some sections. There usually is less smooth muscle within the lamina propria of the large intestine than previously noted in the small bowel. In those herbivorous species with a cecum-like sacculated extension of the large intestine, the wall tends to be thinned and the mucosa is often heavily populated by goblet cells.

The large bowel empties into the proctodeum portion of the cloaca whose folded mucosa is lined by a simple

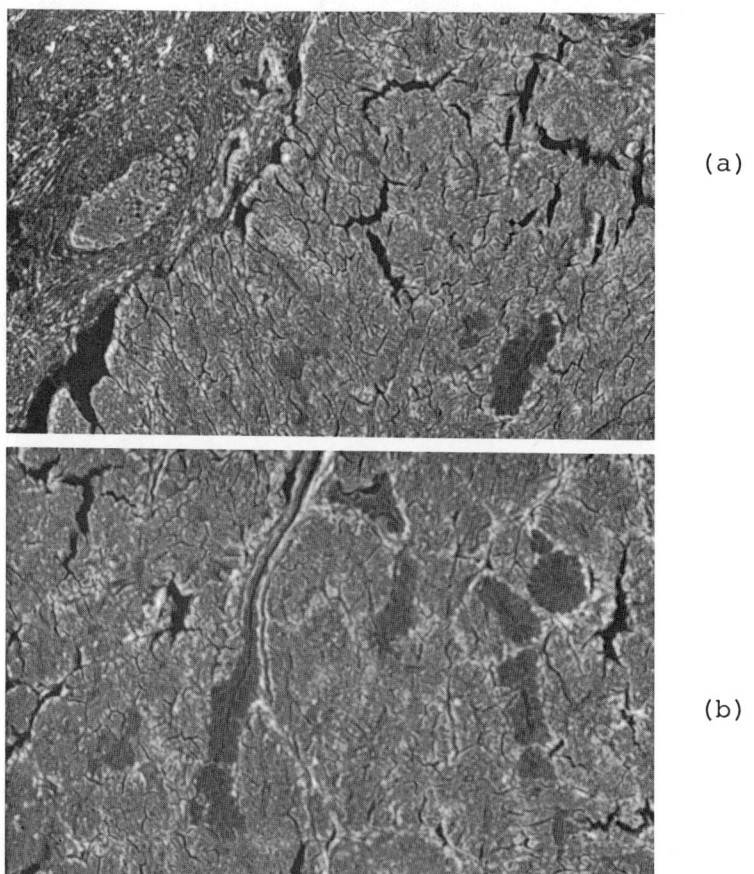

Fig. 28.9a,b. Modified venom producing salivary gland of a rattlesnake, Crotalus enyo. Note the well developed mixed glandular parenchyma consisting of lobules producing both venom and non-toxic salivary components. Ducts (d.) lined by high cuboidal to columnar epithelium course through the lobules. Myoepithelial cells (m.e.) and bundles of muscle fibers (m.) surrounding the glandula acini and lobules, respectively, aid in expelling the venom at the moment of purposeful envenomation. X60

cuboidal to low columnar epithelium, again, well supplied with goblet cells. The terminal cloaca may be lined by a non-cornified squamous epithelium in some species; otherwise, it is lined by a mucosa similar to that of the terminal colon, but with few, if any, villi; rather, the mucosa tends to be carried on loose folds arranged longitudinally.

The salivary glands are well developed lobular-alveolar structures in most reptiles. Typically, they are mixed mucoserous in their secretory output. Their acini are lined by cuboidal glandular epithelial cells whose basally located nuclei and abundant finely granular cytoplasm stain pale lavender to pink with hematoxylin and eosin, depending upon the nature of the secretory product. The serous acini which are lined by smaller cells tend to be darker staining than the paler and somewhat larger mucus secreting cells. The interacinar connective tissue septa may or may not be abundant, depending upon the species and the amount of smooth or skeletal muscle fibers within and investing the glands.

In poisonous snakes, some of the salivary glandular tissue is modified to secrete highly complex venoms containing enzymatic and neurotoxic substances. These products are carried to the fangs via excretory ducts originating within the glandular parenchyma (Fig. 28.9a and b). In the venomous Helodermatidae, the venom is produced within eight modified salivary glands located in the mandibular soft tissue and rather than being carried to the fangs (which do not contain hollow cavities or venom canals), merely seeps into wounds made by the teeth as the animal chews its prey or victim. In at least some of the Crotalidae, the venom glands are partially invested by a mantle of skeletal muscle which continues down as septa dividing the parenchyma into lobules. Myoepithelial-like cells are seen at the periphery of the acini and partially surrounding the smaller lobules. Accesory glands (Duvenoy's) may or may not be present.

As compared to higher vertebrates, the reptilian liver is less distinctly organized into lobules. The classical hepatic lobule can, nevertheless, be observed in the liver tissue of some species. Portal areas contain branches of the hepatic artery, portal vein and bile duct(s), respectively, and are supported by interlobular connective tissue. The central vein, when present, is located at the hub of the lobule with cords of polyhedral to cuboidal hepatocytes separated by endothelium-lined hepatic sinusoids radiating outward (Fig. 28.10). Small

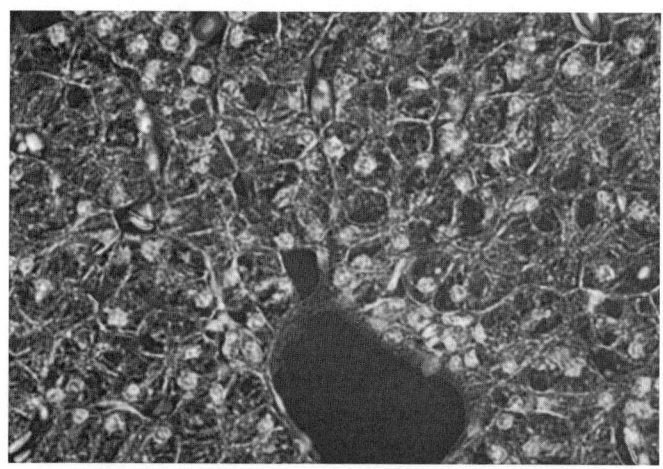

Fig. 28.10. Liver of an Iguana iguana. In this section, the hepatic parenchyma is arranged in a typical lobular fashion. Many reptiles have livers which are less distinctively organized into lobules. A central vein (c.v.) is surrounded by radiating cords of hepatocytes (h.c.), hepatic sinusoids (s.), small, flat, dark-staining Kupffer cells (K.c) and packets of pigment carried within randomly scattered chromatophores. Portal areas supporting branches of the hepatic artery (h.a.), branches of the portal vein (p.v.) and bile ducts (b.d.) are surrounded by interlobular connective tissue (c.t.). X120

dark-staining Kupffer cells are situated within the sinusoids and tend to be more flattened or spindle-shaped. In those reptiles with less distinctly organized liver morphology, the hepatocytes are arranged in branching cords, usually two cells wide. Between these branching cords are vascular spaces lined by endothelium and containing the above-mentioned Kupffer cells. Bile canaliculi tend to run within fine connective tissue septa-like interdigitations supporting the hepatic cords. Multiple branches of the bile ducts are commonly observed within the same high power field in some sections.

One feature of the reptilian liver is the large amount of melanin pigment distributed throughout the parenchyma. This material usually is confined in dense packets without particular anatomic pattern (Fig. 28.11).

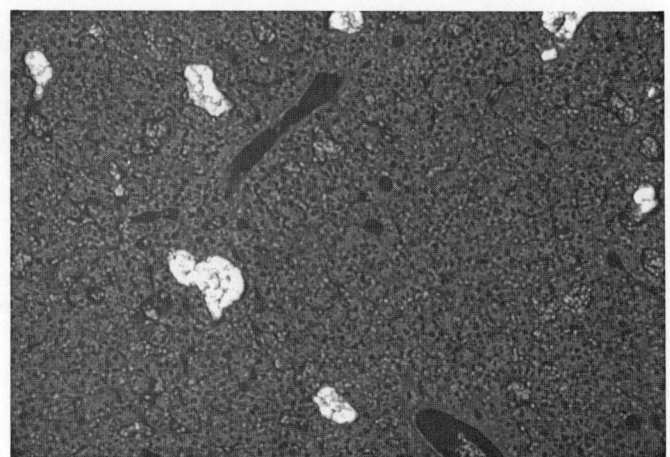

Fig. 28.11. Liver of a gopher tortoise, Gopherus agassizi. Note the aggregates of melanin pigment. This is a normal finding in these animals. X26

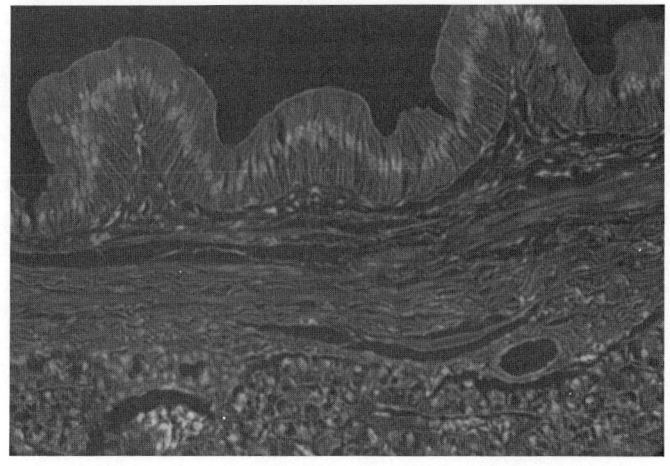

Fig. 28.12. Gall bladder of the same tortoise. Note the simple columnar epithelium (s.c), lamina propria (l.p.), basement membrane (b.m.), fibromuscular tunic (f.t.) and perimuscular connective tissue (c.t.) and stroma (s.). X40

The gall bladder may or may not be contigous with the hepatic tissue. It is lined by a simple or psuedostratified columnar epithelium. Subjacent to the thin lamina propria is a fine smooth muscle tunic and a few mucin secreting glands or goblet cells. These may be lacking in some reptiles (Fig. 28.12).

Pancreas

The reptilian pancreas, like that of the higher vertbrates, secretes both exocrine and endocrine secretory products. While similar in gross form and secretory function, the reptilian pancreas is morphologically different than that observed in mammals.

The exocrine parenchyma of the reptilian pancreas consists of branching tubules rather than the typical acini and lobules seen in mammals. However, the histolog is still recognizable as pancreatic tissue to the microscopist. Eosinophilic zymogen granules are located in the apical portions of the darker-staining exocrine cells whose nuclei occupy a basal position. A prominent nucleolus usually is present. These cells usually lie with their bases adjacent to a capillary surface (Miller and Lagios, 1970) (Fig. 28.13).

The endocrine or islet tissue may not be clearly distinguished from the exocrine portion. The islet tissue of some snakes, especially members within the Colubridae, is restricted to the splenic pole of the pancreas where semi-confluent giant islets are associated with first-order exocrine ducts (Miller and Lagios, 1970). A dual distribution of islets is observed in the chelonians (Titlbach, 1966). Isolated islet cells are intercalated within the pancreatic ductal epithelium together with larger masses of islet tissue, lacking separate basement membranes isolating them from exocrine tubules. In crocodilians, the distribution is similar with the islets separated from the exocrine cells; the beta cells are located more centrally and a population of alpha cells is found peripherally.

The pancreatic excretory ducts are lined by pale-staining, low columnar cells with basal nuclei. These ducts usually have thick walls and may be surrounded by dense fibrocollagenous connective tissue (Fig. 28.14).

Thyroid

The reptilian thyroid is morphologically similar to that seen in other vertebrates. Numerous follicular acini

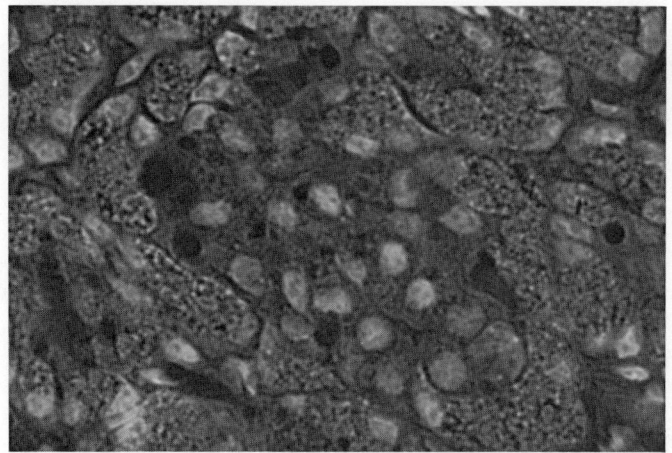

Fig. 28.13. Pancreas of a bullsnake, Pituophis melanoleucus catenifer. Note the discrete paler staining islets of Langerhans (i.L.) within the surrounding exocrine parenchyma which consists of branching tubules of cells (ex.). A branch of the pancreatic artery (a.) and vein (v.) also are illustrated. X40

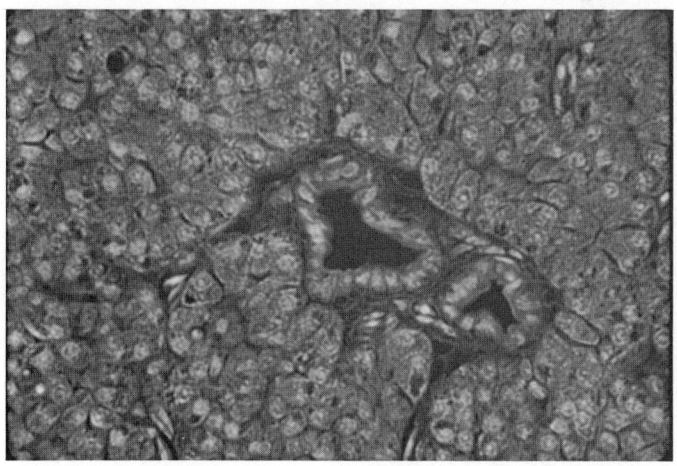

Fig. 28.14. Intralobular pancreatic duct from a python, Python sebae. Duct (d.) is lined by a low columnar epithelium (c.e.). Tubular acini (a.), vein (v.) and interlobular connective tissue (c.t.) are shown. X80

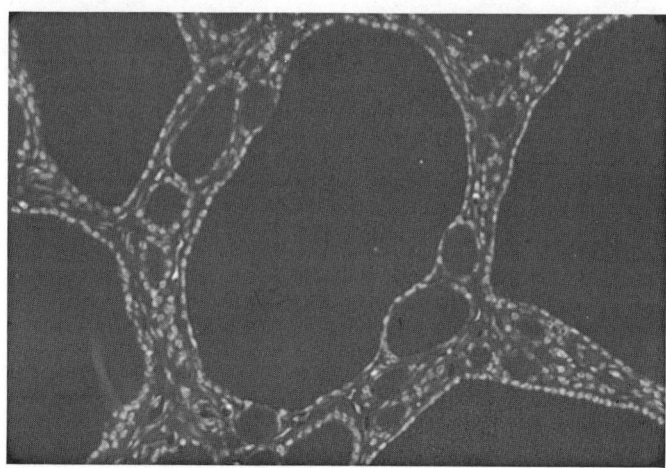

Fig. 28.15. Thyroid of a turtle, Chrysemys scripta elegans. The follicles (f.) are lined by a single layer of cuboidal to nearly squamous glandular epithelium (e.c.). The colloid (c.) contained within the follicles may exhibit irregular vacuolization (v.). X160

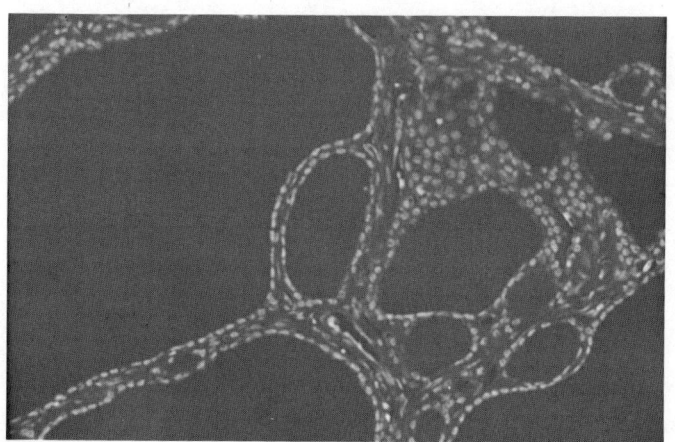

Fig. 28.16. Thyroid. This section was from a desert tortoise, Gopherus agassizi. Note the increased number of parafollicular or C-cells (p.f.). X160

are lined by a single layer of low cuboidal epithelial cells with more centrally located nuclei. The lumens of these follicles are filled with pink-staining, usually homogenous colloid (Fig. 28.15). Metabolic alteration may affect changes in the height of the epithelial cells lining the follicles and the quality of the enclosed colloid. Most reptiles, particularly those originating from temperate life zones, will exhibit cyclical changes in the follicular cell morphology. These are related to seasonal or climatic changes. The gland becomes more inactive during hibernation or periodic torpidity. The usually cuboidal shape of the acinar epithelium becomes either more columnar or flattens markedly and becomes squamous. Parafollicular cells are present within the interfollicular connective tissue stroma (Fig. 28.16).

Parathyroid

Reptiles possess one or two pairs of parathyroid glands. Unlike those observed in mammals, in most species of reptiles examined, the parathyroid has been found to consist of a single cell type which corresponds to the chief cell in the mammalian organ. In contrast to this finding, at least two species of lizards, Tiliqua occipitalis and Trachydosaurus rugosus have been shown to have three distinguishable cell types (Rogers, 1963). As noted earlier, the glands are located adjacent to the great vessels and/or heart base. In chelonians they may be imbedded within the thymus.

Generally, the cells of the parathyroid are arranged in cords or fascicles but, occasionally, follicle-like acini may be found. The chief-like cells typically are epithelial in form and contain round or ovoid nuclei and finely granular cytoplasm (Fig. 28.17).

Adrenal

Of interest to the histologist is the fact that the darker staining cells of the adrenal gland which are responsible for the secretion of adrenocorticosteroids, are situated in the more central or medullary portion of the gland, and the typical medullary portion (in the mammalian sense), i.e. chromaffin tissue, is located peripherally and tends to stain more lightly with hematoxylin and eosin. In most reptiles, the two major cell types are not distinctly separated into discrete zones (Fig. 28.18). In chelonians the interrenal tissue is composed of radially arranged cells with clusters of chromaffin cells distributed irregularly. In other reptiles, the

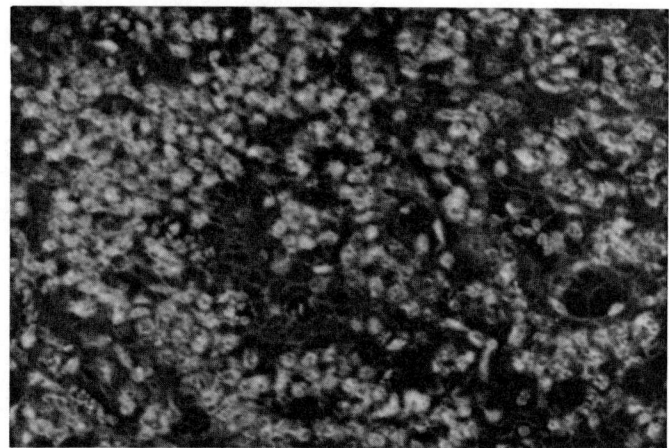

Fig. 28.17. Parathyroid of a desert tortoise, Gopherus agassizi. Most reptiles possess parathyroid glands with a single cell type. These are the chief cells (c.c.) which are arranged in cords. Capillaries (c.), veins (v.) and connective tissue comprise the balance of the gland. In at least two species of lizards, the parathyroid consists of at least three distinct cell types. X60

cells are arranged radially in cords, each one appearing to be two cells thick and with a capillary carried within a thin connective tissue stromal support in the middle. The entire gland is enveloped in a thin capsule which, in some species, expands to become interfascicular septa. Histologic sections frequently reveal isolated nerve cells along with an occasional dendritic melanocyte.

Pituitary

Two morphologically distinct portions of the pituitary are recognized in reptiles: the neurohypophysis and the adenohypophysis. The median eminence and neural lobe, pars nervosa, constitute the neurohypophysis. The intermediate lobe, pars intermedia, distal lobe, pars distalis and the pars tuberalis constitute the adenohypophysis (Saint Girons, 1970).

The histology of the pituitary glands of the different orders of reptiles has been described (Saint Girons, 1970) and, for the sake of brevity, will only be abstracted here.

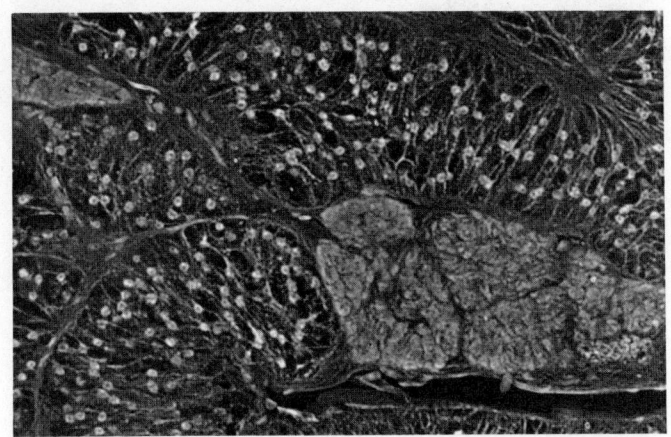

Fig. 28.18. Adrenal gland of a desert tortoise, Gopherus agassizi. Note the two distinct cellular types. The darker-staining "medullarly" cells (m.c.) secrete adrenal corticosteroid hormonal substances. The lighter-staining chromaffin cells (ch.) secrete neurosecretory products. The cells comprising these populations are arranged in branching cords which are separated from each other by thin connective tissue septa bearing vascular elements. X160

In transverse section the median eminence, from dorsal to ventral surfaces, is characterized by 1) a layer of ependymal cells, 2) a layer composed mainly of pituicytes, but containing a number of horizontal neurosecretory fibers, 3) a thicker layer than 1 or 2, formed mostly by straight or vertical neurosecretory fibers as well as by extensions from the basal poles of the glial cells. Above this is a mass containing connective tissue and a rich network of capillaries. The location of the median eminence varies with the order of reptile and may be much reduced in some.

The neural lobe in the tuatara, lizards, chelonians and the crocodilians is penetrated deeply by the infundibular recess, where extensive lateral hollow lobules are formed. In snakes the neural lobe is solid and incompletely divided into lobules by connective tissue septa (Saint Girons, 1970).

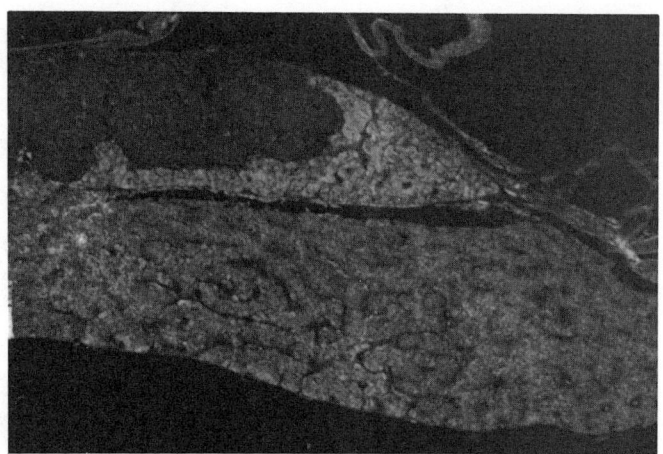

Fig. 28.19. Pituitary gland of a python, <u>Liasis childreni</u>. Note the pars distalis (p.d.) bottom, pars intermedia (p.i.), mid-field, and the pars tuberalis (p.t.), uppermost. X26

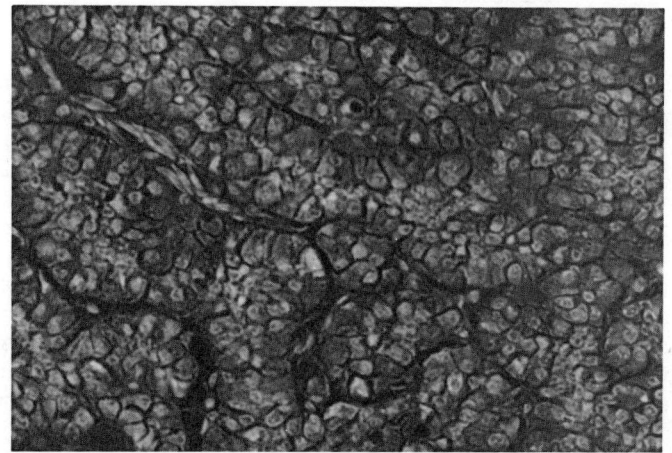

Fig. 28.20. Pituitary, pars distalis, same section as Fig. 28.19. Higher magnification illustrates cellular detail. Acidiphilic cells (a.c.), chromophobic cells (c.h.) and basophilic cells (b.c.). Sinusoids (s.) course through the glandular parenchyma. X160

Except in snakes, the pars nervosa resembles the structure of the median eminence. In snakes the ependymal cells are present only at the cranial extremity of the neural lobe, which is composed mainly of clustered neurosecretory fibers and an occassional pituicyte (Saint Girons, 1970).

The more highly developed and cellular distal lobe contains regular and moderately thick cords of chromophilic (i.e., erythrophilic and cyanophilic) secretory cells at their periphery and chromophobic cells nearer their centers. Vascular sinuses and fine connective tissue septa supporting capillaries separate these cords of cells (Figs. 28.19 and 28.20). Additionally, other morphologically distinct secretory cells may be found in some sections. The gland is covered by a thin connective tissue mantle, and numerous small blood vessels supply the organ, penetrating it from its base.

The pars tuberalis varies morphologically between the major orders of reptiles. In the chelonia it is continuous with the anterior part of the pars distalis and is composed of numerous small chromophobic cells and lesser numbers of large ovoid cells filled with large PAS-positive cytoplasmic granules. In the crocodilians the pars tuberalis consists of small groups of cells forming follicle-like structures along the ventral surface of the infundibular recess, especially in the region of the median eminence (Saint Girons, 1970). The pars tuberalis is vestigial or lacking in snakes and lizards.

Ultimobranchial bodies

These small gland-like structures are located near the thymus and/or parathyroid glands and are embryological derivatives of the pharyngeal pouches. Their number is variable, but usually there are two. They are enveloped in a fine connective tissue capsule and consist of delicate cords of small secretory epithelial cells whose function remains obscure. They have exhibited seasonal variations in secretory activity corresponding to those of the thyroid and, in fact, will respond to TSH administration in the same way as the thyroid (Lynn, 1970). In silver-stained histologic sections, nerves were observed entering the ultimobranchial bodies and thymuses of turtles. Cytologically, the cells of the ultimobranchial bodies resemble the chief-like cells of the parathyroid gland and stain rather darkly with hematoxylin and eosin (Figs. 28.21 and 28.22).

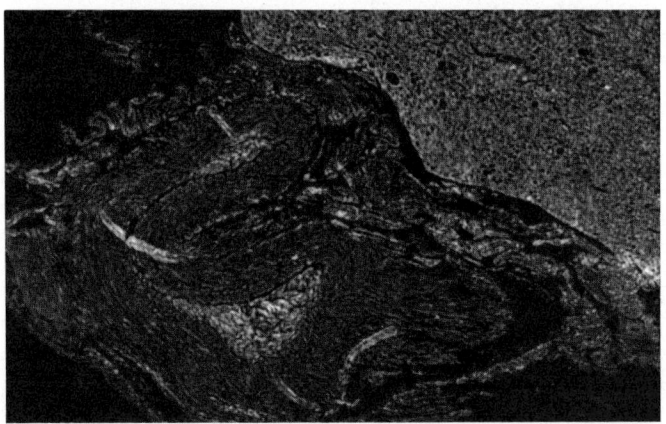

Fig. 28.21. Ultimobranchial body (u.b.) of a Boa constrictor. Note the close relationship with the common carotid artery (c.a.). X13

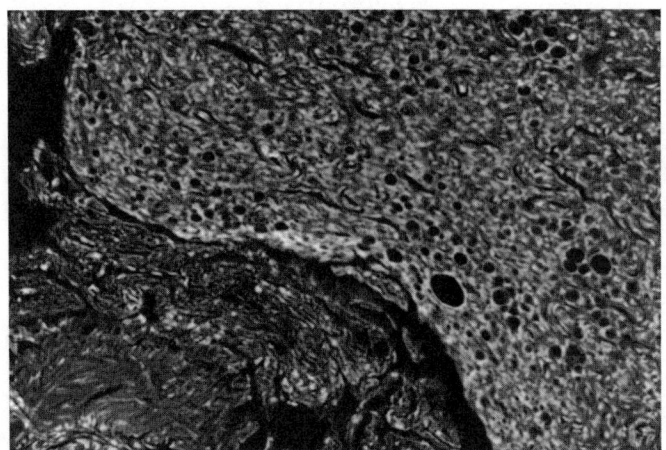

Fig. 28.22. Ultimobranchial body. This is a higher magnification of the same section shown in Fig. 28.21. Note the secretory nature of the epithelial cells (e.c.) which often contain clear vacuoles (v.). X160

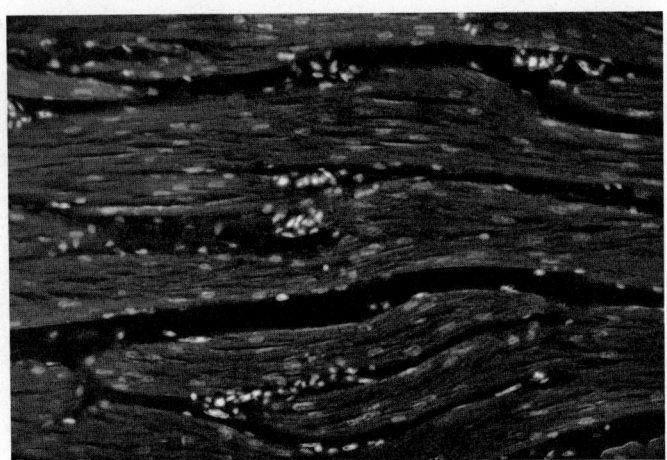

Fig. 28.23. Myocardium of a common iguana, Iguana iguana. Myocardial cell (m.c.), nucleus (n.), intermysial connective cell nuclei (c.t.). X160

Circulatory system

The myocardium of reptiles is similar to that seen in other vertebrates, although the wall of the solitary ventricle appears relatively thicker. This distinction is less apparent in the hearts of crocodilians which possess an interventricular septum dividing the ventricle. Freshly fixed myocardial fibers clearly exhibit cross striations when they are sectioned longitudinally (Fig. 28.23). These striations correspond to the A, I, H and Z bands seen in skeletal myofibers. Intercalated discs may be seen oriented transversely across the long axis of some fibers. These discs are bounded on both sides by the Z bands. The myocardial fiber nuclei are numerous and are located in the interior, usually axial portion of the fibers, and are oval to elongated in shape.

Arteries tend to be thick-walled, mostly due to their heavy muscular and elastic fiber tunics. Veins are thin-walled. Lymphatics, like those in other vertebrates, are characteristically very thin-walled and consist of endothelial cells whose cell processes are arranged into a tube. Conduction nerve fibers and capillaries may be seen coursing through the intermysial connective tissue.

Adipose tissue may be seen on the anterior epicardial surfaces of the hearts of obese individuals, but this is not a feature of the majority of reptilian hearts.

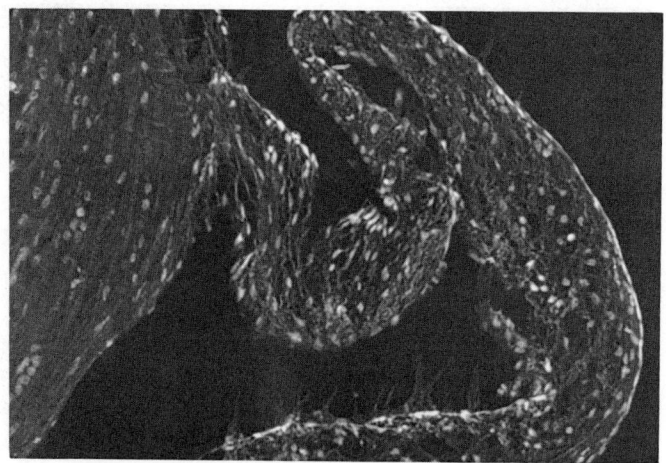

Fig. 28.24. Atrioventricular valve leaflet from an _Iguana iguana_. This structure is similar to the valves of higher vertebrates and is essentially avascular and receives its nutrition and gas exchange by direct diffusion from the surrounding blood. X160

The relatively avascular atrioventricular valvular cusps or leaflets are similar to those found in other vertebrate hearts. They are composed of loosely arranged, occasionally stellate or multipolar, irregular cells within a stroma of delicate collagen fibers, and homogenous ground substance. The free or lumenal surfaces of the valve leaflets are covered with a thin endothelium (Fig. 28.24).

Spleen

The spleen of most reptiles is spherical or triangularly elongated and is histologically similar to splenic tissue from other vertebrates. It consists of red pulp populated by splenic cords and endothelium lined sinusoids containing erythrocytes and occasional leukocytes, and a white pulp containing numerous lymphoid nodules and germinal centers. These centers usually are found to surround a splenic arteriole and are characterized by a collar or sheath of germinal small lymphocytes with rather large, densely-staining nuclei. Occasional histiocyte-like macrophages may be found within the centers of these lymphoid aggregates. Smooth muscle trabeculae may be seen partially dividing the parenchyma in some species. A dense connective tissue capsule surrounds the organ and

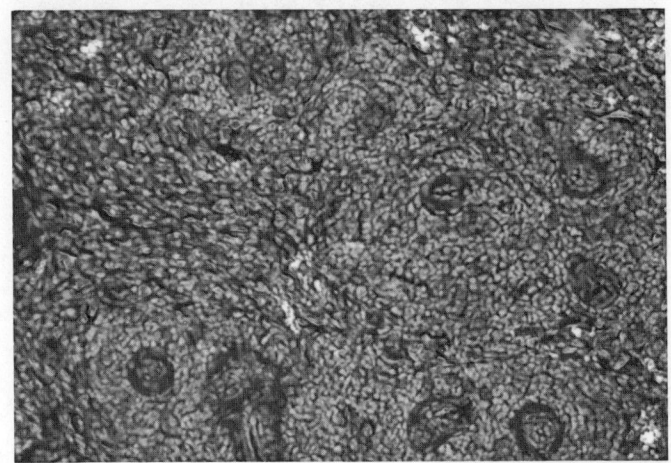

Fig. 28.25. Spleen from an Iguana iguana. Note the sheathed arterioles (s.a.) with their cuffs of small lymphocytes (ly.) and macrophages (m.), trabeculae (t.) and germinal center (g.c.). X60

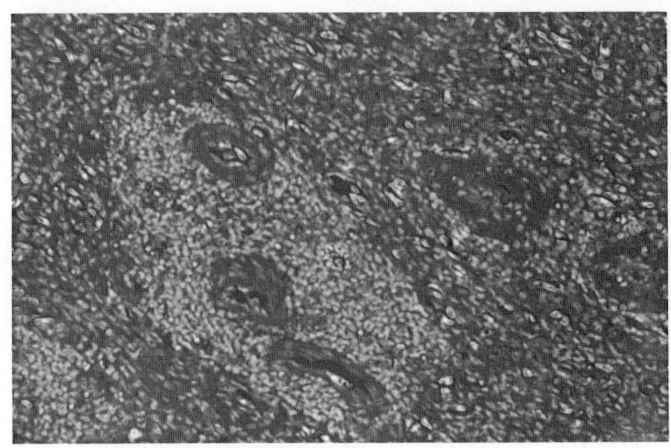

Fig. 28.26. Spleen, same section as in Fig. 28.25. X160

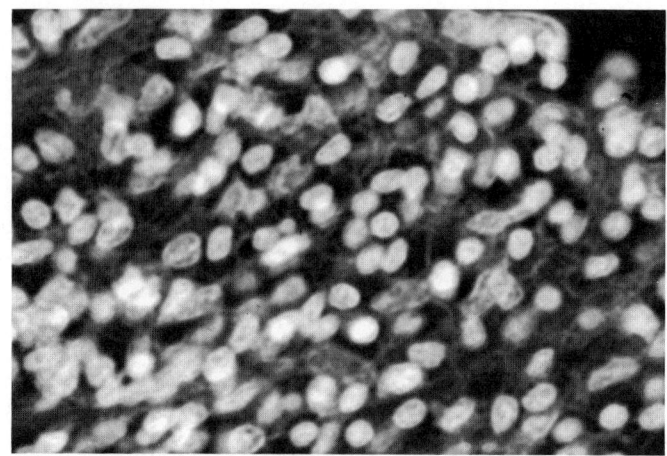

Fig. 28.27. Thymus of a <u>Boa</u> <u>constrictor</u>. This organ in snakes, lizards, crocodilians and tuatara lacks the lobulation observed in the chelonian thymus. Most of the tissue is composed of small densely-staining lymphocytes (ly.) bearing large nuclei. Large myoid cells with prominent single or multiple nuclei form loosely arranged fibers throughout the thymic parenchyma. Epthelioid cells (e.p.) are characterized by their pale-staining nuclei and tonofilaments, seen under high magnification. X210

may contribute extensions or septa which further divide the parenchyma. This is a feature most often observed in members of Boidae whose spleens usually are distinctly lobular in longitudinal section. One or more branches of the splenic arborization from the gastrosplenic or hepatosplenic artery penetrate the organ at the hilus. One or more splenic veins exit at the same site (Figs. 28.25 and 28.26).

<u>Thymus</u>

Thymic tissues contained within a variable number of lobulated or non-lobulated glands or nodules are found in reptiles. In snakes, lizards, crocodilians and tuatara, the thymus is unlobulated. Only in the thymus of the testudines are distinct lobules found. As noted previously, the thymic tissue is located in the cervical region and may be contigous with the parathyroid glands and adjacent to the ultimobranchial bodies and great vessels.

Histologically, the organ is populated by small, round lymphoid thymocytes characterized by their high nucleus to cytoplasm ratio, nuclear membrane indentation and densely clumped nuclear chromatin (Fig. 28.27). These cells are arranged in zones; those cells situated within the cortex are more closely packed than those within the medulla. The demarcation of cortical and medullary regions is not as clear in mature or aging animals as the thymus undergoes atrophic involution. The thymus may involute reversibly during nutritional stress or torpidity. Epithelial cells often exhibiting fine tonofilaments or desmosomes may be seen in some sections under high magnification. The epitheaial cells are characterized by their pale-staining nuclei and prominent nucleoli. Large oval myoid cells with single or multiple central nuclei are scattered throughout the thymic parenchyma. These cells, when sectioned longitudinally and appropriately stained, may exhibit cross banding with A, I, H, M and Z bands or lines. These myoid fibers are loosely arranged throughout and lend support to the tissues. Granulocytes, particularly heterophils, are seen frequently within the medulla. Thymic cysts are found occasionally. When present, these cysts are composed of epithelioid cells forming circular entities within whose lumens may be found pink-staining proteinaceous material.

Respiratory system

The trachea is similar to that present in higher vertebrates. Well developed hyaline cartilaginous tracheal rings support the tubular structure. These rings are joined at their dorsal edges by thin strands of tracheal muscle. The lumen is lined by ciliated columnar epithelium containing numerous mucus-secreting goblet cells (Figs. 28.28 and 28.29). Depending upon the species, mucinous and serous acini may be more or less well represented and tend to be more commonly observed in the caudal portions of the trachea and mainstem bronchi. Small lymphoid cell aggregations also may be scattered subjacent to the tracheal mucosa.

In the chelonians the trachea bifurcates into two mainstem bronchi at a more proximal or cranial location than in other reptiles. The bronchi retain the histologic features of the trachea to a level of the larger bronchioles at which point the cartilaginous rings are lost. The bronchiolar and respiratory epithelium flattens from a columnar or cuboidal shape to one which is more low cuboidal or even squamous as the airway cross-sectional diameter diminishes and where active gas transport and exchange occurs.

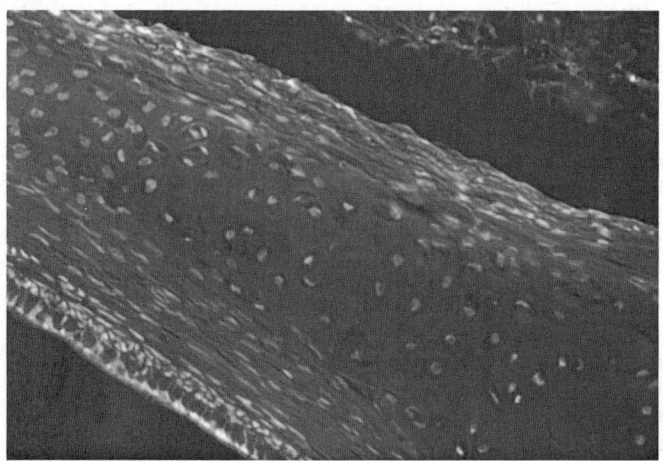

Fig. 28.28. Trachea from a sub-adult desert tortoise, Gopherus agassizi. Note the tracheal cartilage (t.c.), fibrous connective tissue (c.t.) and pseudostratified ciliated columnar epithelium (c.e.) lining the lumenal surface. X160

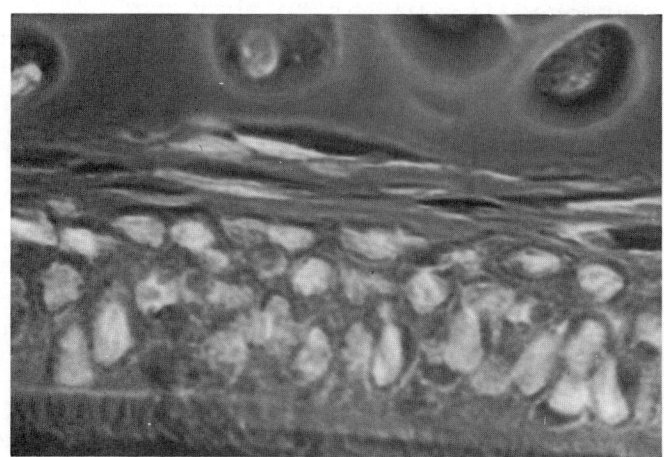

Fig. 28.29. Trachea, same as in Fig. 28.28, higher magnification illustrating the ciliated epithelium and stereocilia. X430

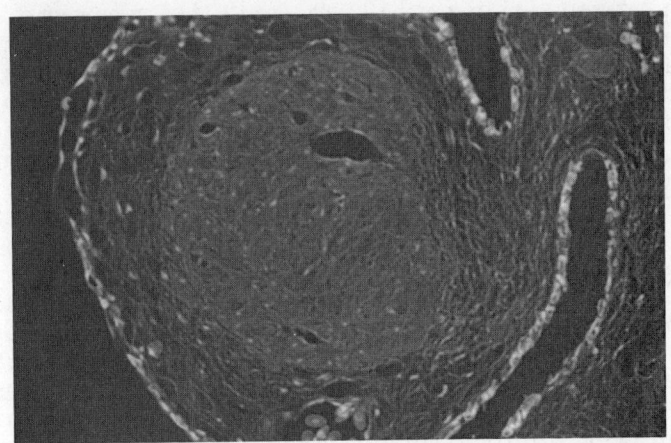

Fig. 28.30. Lung from a green sea turtle, Chelonia mydas mydas. Note the abundant smooth muscle (s.m.) supporting the respiratory epithelial surfaces. X60

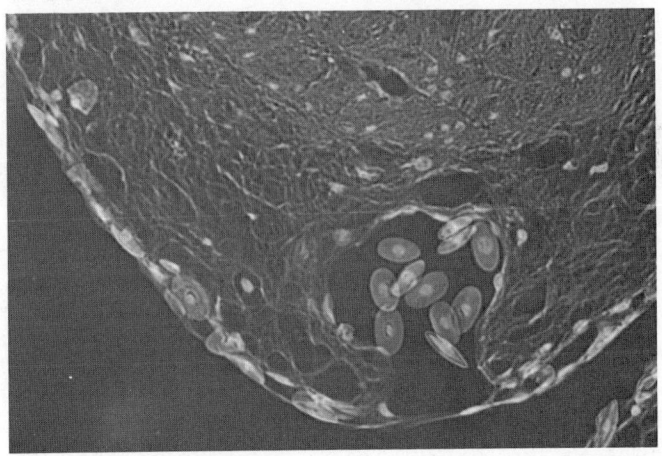

Fig. 28.31. Lung, same section as in Fig. 28.30. Note the rich capillary vasculature (cap.) and its intimate relationship to the respiratory gas exchange surface (ep.), endothelial cell nucleus (end.) and lumen of an air saccule (l.). X430

Most reptiles possess a far more simplified pulmonary gas exchange bed than that found in mammals. Similar to the avian organ, the reptilian lung is composed of a series of reticulated, open-end sacs. The air sac septa are lined by thin alveolar-like epithelial cells on both sides with thin-walled capillaries coursing between the two gas exchange surfaces (Figs. 28.30 and 28.31). One feature of the reptilian lung that is outstanding is the ample amount of smooth muscle included within the suporting architecture. Pulmonary arterioles and venules course throughout the more basilar portions of the lung. Occasional lymphoid cell nodules or aggregates may be seen, but their distribution in any single individual is variable. They are most common at the junctions of bronchioles and smaller bronchi. In those reptiles possessing lungs with a preponderance of air sacs, these thin-walled cul-de-sacs are lined by a very thin squamous to low cuboidal epithelium lying upon a fine basement membrane. In these lungs, the smooth muscle is rare or may be entirely lacking.

Excretory system

The kidneys of reptiles are variably uricotelic, with considerable differences between groups and species. The major nitrogenous excretory by-products of protein metabolism and catabolism are uric acid and its salts rather than urine composed of urea, per se.

Reptiles are unable to concentrate urine of greater osmolarity than that of their blood plasma. There are extrarenal concentrating mechanisms in many species. Numerous reptiles have salt-secreting glands near the eyes and nasal structures or beneath the tongue and lingual sheath (particularly in some sea snakes). These extrarenal salt-secreting organs actively release sodium, potassium and chloride ion products, thus conserving water. Minute quantities of allantoin, varying amounts of urea and ammonium ion or free ammonia also are excreted by the kidneys.

The typical glomeruli, proximal and distal convoluted tubules, are present, but an interposed loop of Henle is lacking (Figs. 28.32 and 28.33). This structure is of major evolutionary importance for water reabsorption in higher vertebrates which are capable of excreting a concentrated urine.

The reptilian nephron consists of the glomerulus (glomerular or Bowman's membrane with its parietal and visceral surfaces, and glomerular tuft composed of coiled

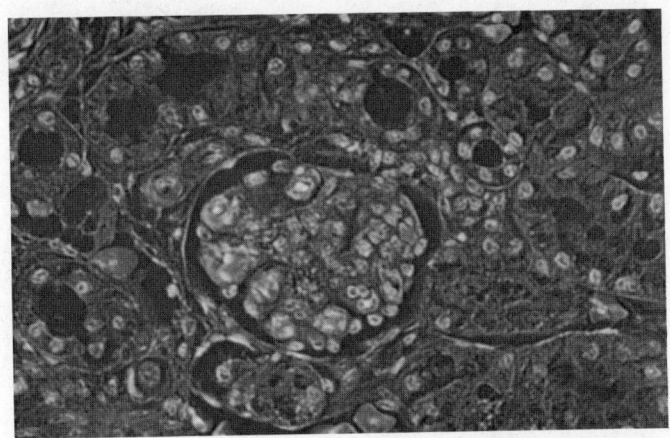

Fig. 28.32. Kidney of a kingsnake, Lampropeltis calligaster rhombomaculata. Note the glomerulus (g.), glomerular afferent arteriole (g.a.), glomerular tuft (g.t.), Bowman's membrane (B.m.), glomerular space (g.s.), proximal (p.t.) and distal (d.t.) tubules and interstitial connective tissue (c.t.). X160

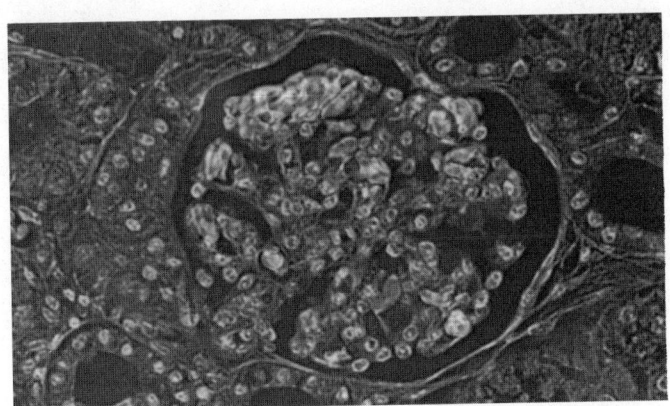

Fig. 28.33. Same section of kidney as in Fig. 28.32, higher magnification. X360

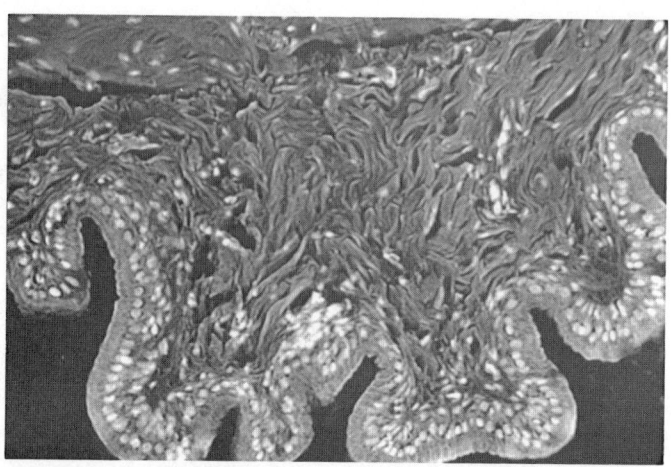

Fig. 28.34. Urinary bladder of a desert tortoise, Gopherus agassizi. A transitional epithelium (ep.) covers the easily distensible connective tissue wall which invests numerous smooth muscle fibers (s.m.). X60

capillary vasculature); a rather short neck piece, first and second portions of the proximal convoluted tubule; the distal convoluted tubule; and, collecting tubules which drain into the calyses thence into a ureter-like mesonephric duct. In some reptiles, the mesonephric duct empties into a true urinary bladder (Fig. 28.34). The bladder empties into the cloaca. In others, the excretory wastes empty into the urodeum of the cloaca and are passed through the cloacal vault.

Histologically, the glomeruli are found within the cortical portions of the renal tissues. The finely coiled or folded, anastomosing capillaries receive blood from the afferent arteriole and are surrounded by the endothelial cells and an occasional connective tissue cell. Bowman's membrane is composed of an outer, or parietal epithelium, and an inner, or visceral, epithelium. The space between the glomerular capillary tuft and the visceral surface of Bowman's membrane is the glomerular or uriniferous space. Plasma ultrafiltrate enters this space and is drained by a uriniferous tubule of the most proximal portion of the proximal convoluted tubule. This tubule has a relatively small lumen and is lined by cuboidal epithelium. High-power magnification will reveal a brush border to these cells. The cells of the distal convoluted

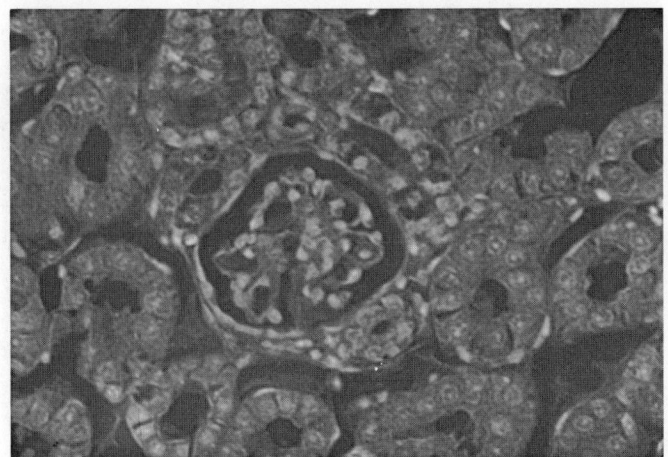

Fig. 28.35. Sexual segment granules (s.s.g.) contained within renal tublue epithelial cells within the sexual segment of the kidney of a male rattlesnake, Crotalus atrox. Note the cellular hypertrophy. X220

tubule are similar to those lining the proximal tubules, but the distal tubules tend to have larger lumens and lack a brush border. Both cell types tend to stain more intensively with hematoxylin and eosin than the larger, cuboidal cells lining the wide-lumen collecting tubules.

A juxtaglomerular apparatus may be found in some sections of reptilian kidney and consists of small cuboidal basophilic epithelial-like cells adjacent to the afferent arteriole.

Some male snakes and lizards exhibit a sexual segment granulation of the renal epithelial cells lining the distal convoluted tubules (Fig. 28.35). Cells lining a segment of the preterminal distal tubule become hypertrophied and markedly columnar in shape. They are observed to contain numerous eosinophilic intracytoplasmic granules. Beyond this hypertrophied segment usually is a normal length of tubule which empties into the collecting tubules. This hypertrophy tends to be seasonally cyclic, with regression in some species coinciding with peak testicular activity. In other species, the cyclical nature of the sexual segment is far less pronounced.

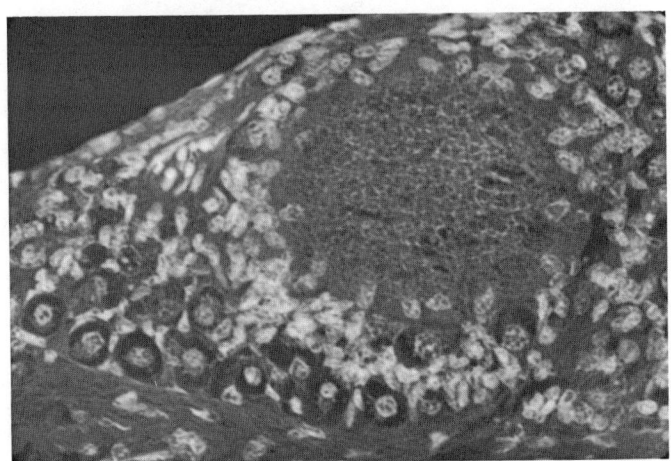

Fig. 28.36. Ovary from a Texas tortoise, Gopherus berlandieri. The developing follicle contains an early maturing oocyte (o.). Vacuolated primary follicles (p.f.) are seen partially surrounding the follicle. X210

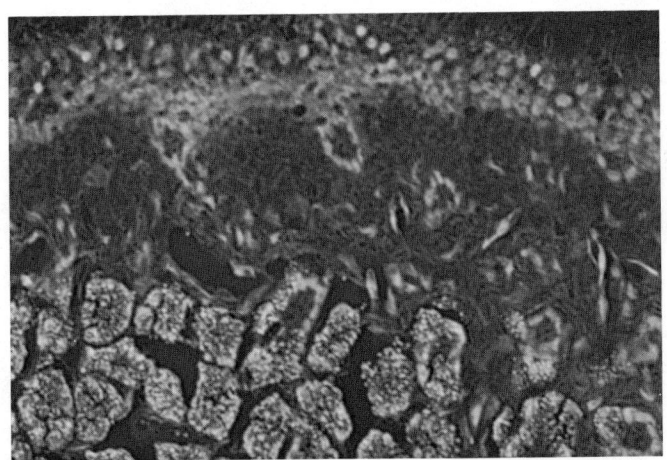

Fig. 28.37. Shell gland portion of the oviduct from a gravid desert tortoise, Gopherus agassizi. Numerous glandular lobules (lob.) are seen subjacent to the lumenal epithelium within the wall of the organ. The oviductal lumen is lined by a low columnar epithelium which contains occasional goblet cells. X60

Reproductive system

Paired ovaries or testes are found in female and male reptiles, repectively. True intersexual animals have been reported a number of times and there are populations of hermaphroditic snakes. A number of all female parthenogenic lizard species have been described.

Depending upon the phase of the ovulatory cycle, the ovary in the mature female reptile contains successively maturing follicles surrounding oocytes (Fig. 28.36) and/or corpora lutea; it is amply supported by a dense connective tissue stroma through which numerous small blood vessels and lymphatics pass. The oviduct is lined by a ciliated columnar epithelium containing occasional mucin-secreting goblet cells. In oviparous female reptiles, the oviduct becomes modified at its caudal end prior to emptying into the cloaca. Numerous submucosal lobular-alveolar glands containing acini lined with small, highly eosinophilic cuboidal epithelial cells can be seen microscopically (Fig. 28.37). These glands lie subjacent to the basement membrane of the oviductal epithelium and contribute the substances of which the calcareous or leathery egg shell is composed. This material is secreted and deposited as the eggs move down the oviduct.

The testes consist of numerous seminiferous tubules separated from each other by interstitial connective tissue. Each tubule is lined by a well defined basement membrane, upon which rests heavily staining primary spermatogonia and an occasional large, polyhedral Sertoli cell which usually is more pale-staining. More mature primary and secondary spermatocytes and finally spermatids and tailed spermatozoa are seen nearer the center of the tubules (Fig. 28.38). Small, eosinophilic cellular remnants of successively maturing germinal cells may be observed scattered among the spermatids and tailed spermatozoa. The interstitial connective tissue invests numerous small blood vessels and nests of interstitial cells of Leydig.

The spermatozoa are transported from the seminiferous tubules through a much coiled epididymis (Fig. 28.39). The tubular epididymis is lined by a ciliated columnar epithelium arranged in a single layer lying upon a well defined basement membrane. The nuclei of the ciliated columnar cells are in a sub-basal or central position. Their sterocilia are quite long, often occupying up to 25% of the lumninal diameter. The tubules are supported by a fine connective tissue stroma containing a few smooth

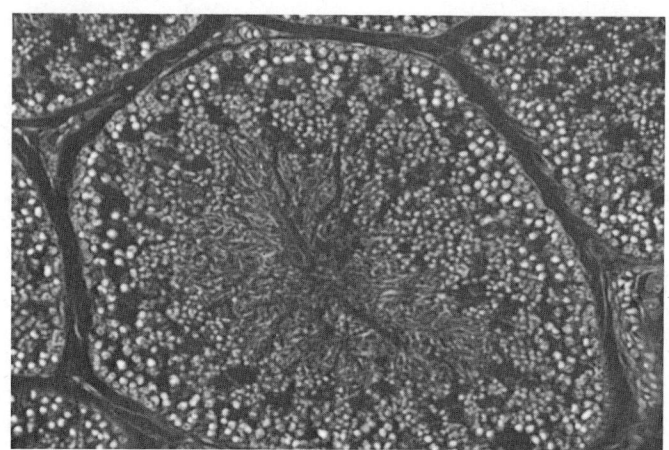

Fig. 28.38. Testis from a sexually mature and active collared lizard, Crotaphytus collaris collaris. Note the seminiferous tubules (s.t.), primary spermatogonia (p.s.), primary spermatocytes (I°.s.), secondary spermatocytes (II°.s.), spermatids (spt.), maturing tailed spermatozoa (m.s.), Sertoli cells (S.c.), basement membrane (b.m.) and interstitial cells (i.c.) lying within the intertubular connective tissue stroma (c.t.). X260

muscle fibers. From the epididymis, the spermatozoa are transported to the cloaca either directly or via the ureter through the thicker and more muscular walled ductuli deferentia, also lined by a strongly stereociliated columnar epithelium.

Central nervous system

The brains of reptiles are far less complex than those of the higher vertebrates. The cerebral and cerebellar cortices lack the sulci and gyri which give a much folded appearance to most mammalian brains. Granular, pyramidal, Purkinge, ependymal and various glial cells are, nonetheless, present (Fig. 28.40). The cerebellum contains a cortical molecular layer surrounding a more densely populated granular layer with Purkinge and glial cells imbedded within the neurophil. Within the cerebrum, large pyramidal nerve cells and their dendrites may be seen surrounded by abundant neuropil and glial cells. Small blood vessels are numerous and penetrate the nervous

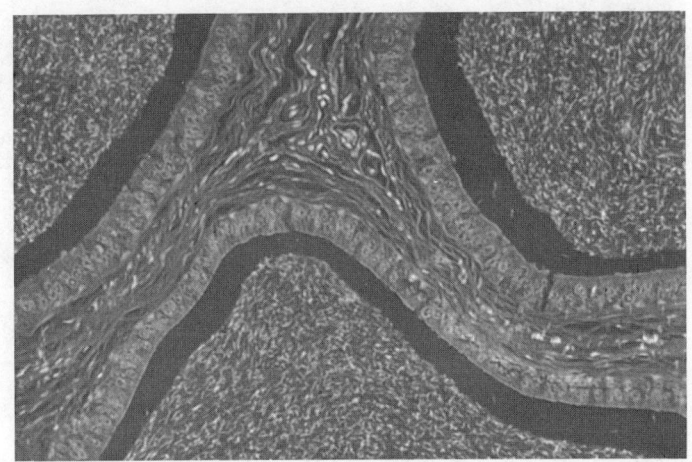

Fig. 28.39. Epididymis of a spotted ratsnake, <u>Spilotes pullatus</u>. A myriad number of spermatozoa (sp.) are contained within the lumen of the coiled tubular organ. The structure is lined by a ciliated columnar epithelium (c.e.) bearing stereocilia (st.). Numerous smooth muscle fibers (s.m.) course within the connective tissue stroma suporting the tubular epididymis as it forms numerous U-bends. The epithelium is carried on a thin basement membrane (b.m.). X60

tissue in several planes. The cranial nerve ganglia may appear far more complex in celluarity than one would expect in animals with such simple brains.

Lateral eyes

The ocular apparatus differs from one group of reptiles to another. Generally, the eyes of snakes and some lizards contain a tertiary spectacle which covers the outermost ocular tissue of the cornea (Peters, 1964). In most lizards, the substantia propria of the cornea is relatively thin, but its acellular Bowman's membrane is thick and is covered by a relatively thin bulbar conjunctiva. Between the substantia propria and the inner mesothelium is a thin, non-cellular Decemet's membrane (Underwood, 1970) (Fig. 28.41). Bowman's membrane is lacking in snakes, chelonians and crocodilians. Decemet's membrane is thin in snakes and testudines and may be lacking in some lizards, excluding some geckos.

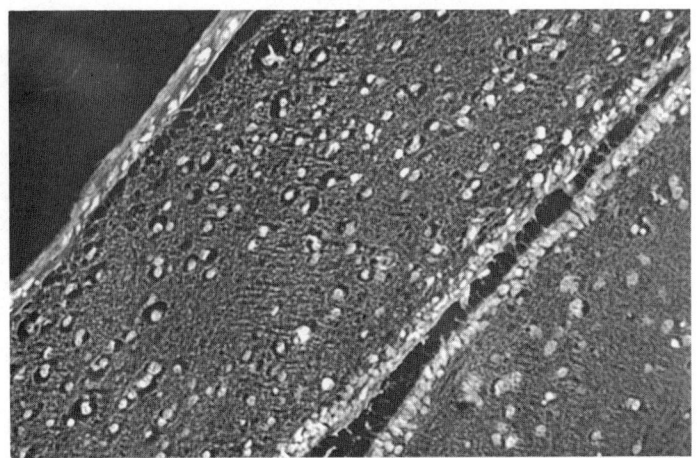

Fig. 28.40. Brain of <u>Uta stansburiana</u>; mid-coronal cross-section. Nerve cell nuclei (n.c.), glial cells (g.), ependymal cells (ep.) and neurophil (n.). X120

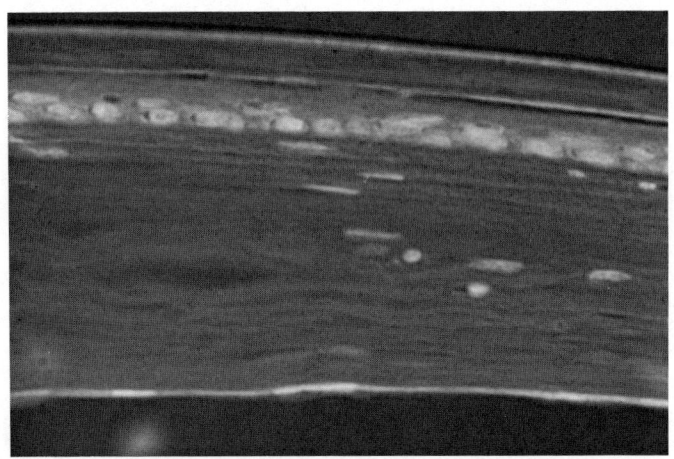

Fig. 28.41. Cornea of <u>Naja</u> sp. Note the spectacle shield (s.s.), anterior epithelium composed of squamous cells (s.c.), substantia propria (s.p.), Decemet's membrane (D.m.), and, posterior epithelium (p.e.). Note that Bowman's membrane is lacking in snakes, crocodilians and chelonians, although present in the cornea of some lizards. X220

The sclera is supported by curved scleral ossicles in lizards, snakes, some chelonians and the tuatara; these are lacking in the crocodilians. The conjunctival space is drained by the lacrimal duct via a single canaliculus.

The ciliary body is a circular structure lying within the globe, internal to the ring of scleral ossicles. It is covered with a double epithelium, the pars ciliaris retinae, which is contiuous with the two layers of the retina. Radially arranged fibers arising from the ciliary body attach to the crystalline lens. The lens is composed of spiral fibers arranged around its axis. In mid cross-section, these fibers appear to be radially oriented columns (Underwood, 1970). The lens is covered with a thin epithelium whose nuclei are distinctly flattened. This membranous surface is thickest at the equator of the lens where it attaches to the ciliary body. Some nocturnal lizards have lost the ciliary muscle and the amphisbaenids have lost the ciliary body. The ciliary bodies of the crocodilians and chelonians are much folded, forming ciliary processes whose tips may touch the lens capsule in the latter.

The iris is a continuation of the ciliary body and the double-layered pars ciliaris retinae which becomes the pares inrdiaca retinae. The outermost layre is more heavily pigmented than the inner. The mesodermal stroma of the iris consists of blood vessels, pigment cells and smooth muscle fibers. It is thickest at the pupil. The iris of the chelonian eye is similar to that in the lizards.

The retina of most diurnal lizards is composed of single and double cone cell layers. The sensory retina consists of the pigment epithelium, the visual cell layer and the nervous layers. The retina itself is avascular. The conus papillaris arises from the head of the optic nerve and tapers to a point that juct fails to touch the posterior surface of the lens. The conus is highly vascular and usually is heavily pigmented. It contains neuroglia and its blood supply enters via the optic nerve (Underwood, 1970). The conus is lacking in adult chelonians and crodilians. Some snakes retain it into adulthood; in others, it atrophies during embryonic development. It is most highly developed in some of the large-eyed lizards (Underwood, 1970).

The retinal histology of reptiles has been elegantly described (Underwood, 1970). The pigmented epithelium consists of a single layer of cells. Between the pigment

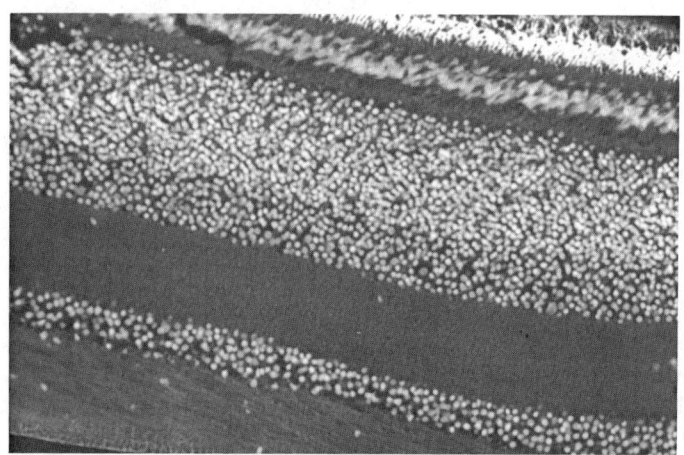

Fig. 28.42. Retina of an Iguana iguana. From the top down, the layers are as follows: inner limiting membrane (ilm.), ganglion cell layer (glc.), inner molecular layer (iml.), inner nuclear layer (inl.), outer molecular layer (oml.), outer nuclear layer (onl.), outer limiting membrane (olm.), and pigment epithelium (pe.). This section was taken temporal to the fovea centralis. X26

epithelium and the choroid is Bruch's membrane, consisting of elastic lamina. The visual cell layer consists of cone cells held together by a zone of terminal bars linking visual cells and neuroglia, the outer limiting membrane. The nuclei of the visual cells lie in the outer nuclear layer. The foot pieces of the visual cells synapse with the bipolar and horizontal cells and form the outer plexiform layer. The inner nuclear layer contains the nuclei of four cell types; the middle layer consists of the nuclei of bipolar cells which synapse with visual cells and ganglion cells, respectively; innermost, within the nuclear layer, are the nuclei of amacrine cells that synapse with the ganglion cells; the inner plexiform layer contains synapses between the bipolar and amacrine cells and ganglion cells. Neuroglia pass radially through the full thickness of the retina (Underwood, 1970) (Fig. 28.42).

Some snakes have retinas in which rods only, or rods in association with cones, form a duplex layer. The visual cells of snakes lack the oil droplets characteristic of cone cells in the lizard retina. The tuatara possesses a retina in which single and double cones bearing colorless oil droplets are present. The retina of the chelonian eye contains single or double cones similar to those of lizards, although rods have been described in some species (Walls, 1942). Crocodilians have retinas with single and double cones and single rods, but the rods predominate (Underwood, 1970).

In those non-crocodilian species of reptiles with moveable eyelids, the upper lid contains smooth muscle fibers. In addition, the lower lid contains a cartilaginous plate imbedded within the palpebral fascia. This is the tarsus which supports the lower lid as it slides over the cornea. In the crocodilians, the upper eyelid contains a bony tarsus and is mobile; the lower lid, being less mobile, lacks a tarsus of any kind.

The eyelids are covered on their outer surfaces by integument similar to and continuous with the rest of the animal's epidermis. The inner surface is covered by a conjunctival mucosa which extends inward from the mucocutaneous junction and covers the sclera. Some reptiles have a nictitating membrane extending between the fornices formed by the conjunctival mucosa. In some lizards, the nictitating membrane contains three vertical crescents of cartilage (Underwood, 1970). In the crocodilians, a single cartilaginous plate is present within the nictitating membrane.

Parietal eye

A parietal, or so-called "third", eye is found in the tuatara and in several lizard species, particularly in members of the Iguanidae. This extra-ocular photoreceptor is connected to the pineal body via a discrete parietal nerve at the base of the eye. This nerve passes through the parietal foramen in the cup-shaped depression in which the eye resides within the parietal bone. A thin epithelial scale covers an unpigmented cellular cornea several cell layers thick. An epithelial lens is present and is composed of a single layer of tall columnar cells in which the nuclei are oriented toward the center of the eye (Figs. 28.43 and 28.44). Beneath the cellular lens is a space containing clear fluid and an occasional macrophage-like leukocyte. The ventral, or basal segment, of the eye is lined by a pigmented, retina-like layer of photoreceptor cells and ganglion cells. The floor of the parietal eye is covered by a connective tissue capsule which is penetrated by an artery, vein and nerve serving the structure (Eakin, 1973; Gundy, 1976).

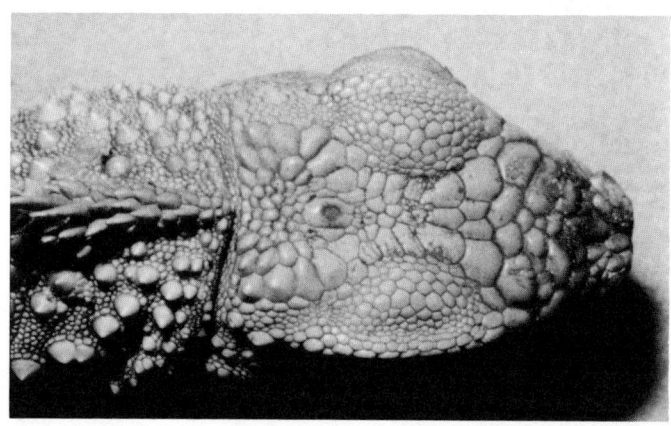

Fig. 28.43. Parietal eye from an Iguana iguana, in situ.

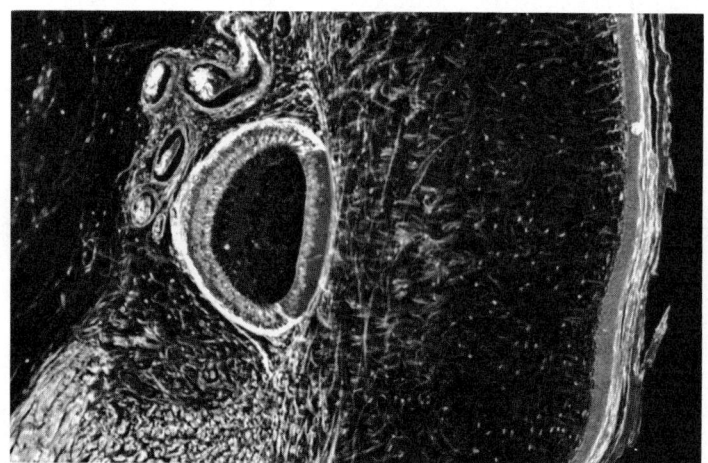

Fig. 28.44. Photomicrograph of a histological section from the same eye as in Fig. 28.43. Unpigmented scale (sc.) covers the dorsal surface; cellular cornea (c.); epithelial lens (l.); ocular fluid (fl.); and, retina (r.). X26

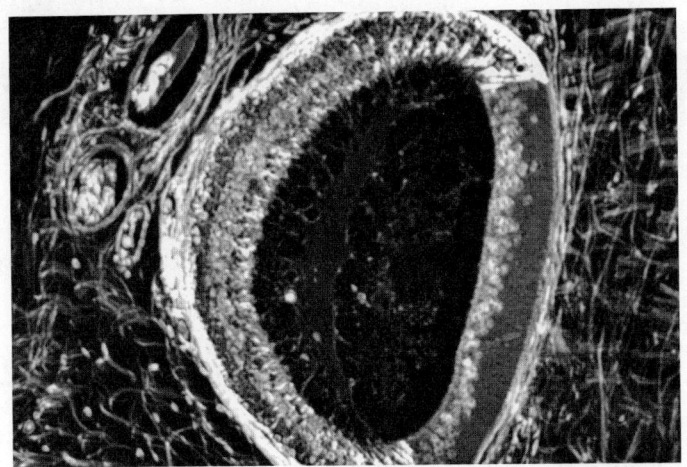

Fig. 28.45. Jacobson's or vomeronasal organ from an Iguana iguana. Note the ciliated columnar epithelium and numerous mucin-secreting goblet cells. Special stains have revealed delicate nerve endings penetrating between adjacent ciliated cells and extending out to the lumenal surface. X220

Jacobson's organ

Most highly developed in snakes and some lizards, this specialized oflactory epithelial structure is located dorsal to the anterior lingual sheath in snakes, or tongue in some lizards, i.e., on the underside of the buccal surface of the vomerine roof. This tissue consists of a highly ciliated columnar epithelium, similar to that of the upper respiratory surfaces, but it lacks basal cells. A rich network of nerve fibers penetrates along the basement membrane which invests numerous pigmented dendritic cells and small capillary vessels (Fig. 28.45). Special staining techniques applied to thin histologic sections have demonstrated delicate dendritic nerve endings passing between adjacent ciliated columnar cells and emerging on the lumenal surface of the organ (Frye, 1981).

REFERENCES

Ashley, L.M., 1955, "Laboratory anatomy of the turtle," Wm.C. Brown Co., Dubuque.

Bockman, D.G., 1970, The thymus, in: "Biology of the Reptilia," vol. 3, C. Gans and T.S. Parsons, eds., Academic Press, New York.

Borysenko, M., and Cooper, E.L., 1972, A histological stud of lymphoid tissue in the snapping turtle, Chelydra serpentina, J. Morphol., 138:487-497.

Chiasson, R.B., 1962, "Laboratory anatomy of the alligator," Wm.C. Brown Co., Dubuque.

Clark, N., 1970, The parathyroid, in: "Biology of the Reptilia, Vol. 3, C. Gans and T.S. Parsons, eds., Academic Press, New York.

Dolensek, E.P., 1971, Necropsy techniques in reptiles, J. Amer. Vet. Med. Ass., 159:1616-1617.

Eakin, R.M., 1973, "The third eye," Univ. California Press, Berkeley.

Frye, F.L., 1981, "Biomedical and surgical aspects of captive reptile husbandry," V.M. Publ. Co., Edwardsville.

Gabe, M., 1970, The adrenal, in: "Biology of the Reptilia," Vol. 3, C. Gans and T.S. Parsons, eds., Academic Press, New York.

Goin, C.J., and Goin, O.B., 1971, "Introduction to herpetology," 2nd ed., Freeman, San Francisco.

Good, R.A., Finstad, J., Pollara, R., and Gabrielsen, A., 1966, Morphologic studies on the evolution of the lymphoid tissues among lower vertebrates, in: "Phylogeny of immunity," R.T. Smith, P.A. Meischer and R.A. Good, eds., Univ. Florida Press, Gainsville.

Gundy, G.C., 1976, Parietal-pineal morphology in lizards and its physiological implications, Anat. Rec., 185:419-431.

Jacobson, E.R., 1978, Reptile necropsy protocol, J. Zoo Animal Med., 9:7-13.

Lynn, W.G., 1970, The thyroid, in: "Biology of the Reptilia," Vol. 3, C. Gans and T.S. Parsons, eds., Academic Press, New York.

McCauley, W.J., 1956, The gross anatomy of the lymphatic system of Alligator mississippiensis, Amer. J. Anat., 99:189-209.

Miller, M.M., and Lagios, M.D., 1970, The parathyroid, in: "Biology of the Reptilia," Vol. 3., C. Gans and T.S. Parsons, eds., Academic Press, New York.

Oldham, J.C., and Smith, H.M., 1975, "Laboratory anatomy of the iguana," Wm.C. Brown Co., Dubuque.

Oldham, J.C., Smith, H.M., and Miller, S.A., 1970, "A laboratory perspectus of snake anatomy," Stipes Publ. Co., Champaign.

Peters, R., 1964, "Dictionary of herpetology," Hafner Publ. Co., New York.

Porter, R., 1972, "Herpetology," W.B. Saunders, Philadelphia.
Rogers, D.C., 1963, A cytological and cytochemical study on the "epithelial body" on the carotid artery of the lizards, Trachydosaurus rugosus and Tiliqua occipitalis, Quart. J. Microscop. Sci., 104:197-205.
Saint Girons, H., 1970, The pituitary, in: "Biology of the Reptilia," Vol. 3, C. Gans and T.S. Parsons, eds., Academic Press, New York.
Schwartz-Karsten, H., 1933, Uber entwicklung und bau der brille bei ophidiern and lacertiliern und der anatomie ihrer travenwege, Morphol. J., 72:499-540.
Titlbach, M., 1966, Licht-und elektonenmikroskopische untersuchungen der lanerhanschen inseln von schildkroten (Testudo graeca), Z. Zellforsch. Mikrosk. Anat., 70:21-35.
Underwood, G., 1970, The eye, in: "Biology of the Reptilia," Vol. 3, C. Gans and T.S. Parsons, eds, Academic Press, New York.
Walls, G.L., 1942, The vertebrate eye and its adaptive radiation, Bull. Cranbrook Inst. Sci., 19:1-795.
Weichert, G.K., 1951, "Anatomy of the chordates," McGraw-Hill Book Co., Ltd., New York.

CONTRIBUTORS

Marilyn P. Anderson, D.V.M., Ph.D.
Department of Pathology
School of Medicine
University of California-San Diego
LaJolla, CA, 92037, U.S.A.

Roger E. Brannian, D.V.M.
Kansas City Zoological Park
Swope Park
5605 E. 63rd St.
Kansas City, MO, 64130, U.S.A.

Daniel R. Brooks, Ph.D.
Department of Zoology
University of British Columbia
6270 University Blvd.
Vancouver, BC, V6T 1W5, Canada

David G. Brownstein, D.V.M.
Section of Comparative Medicine
School of Medicine
Yale University
375 Congress Ave.
New Haven, CT, 06510, U.S.A.

Harold W. Casey, D.V.M., Ph.D.
Department of Veterinary Pathology
Armed Forces Institute of Pathology
Washington, DC, 20306, U.S.A.

John E. Cooper, D.T.V.M., M.R.C.V.S., F.I. Biol.
Comparative Pathology
Royal College of Surgeons of England
35-43 Lincoln's Inn Fields
London, WC2A 3PN, England

Gerald E. Cosgrove, M.D.
Department of Pathology
Zoological Society of San Diego
P.O. Box 551
San Diego, CA, 92112, U.S.A.

C. Bruce Cropp, M.S.
Bureau of Laboratories
Vector-borne Diseases Division
Center for Disease Control
United States Public Health Service
P.O. Box 2087
Ft. Collins, CO, 80522, U.S.A.

Dennis E. Deakins, M.D., Ph.D.
Physician/Surgeon
Grove, OK, 74344, U.S.A.

Werner Frank, Prof. Dr. rer. nat.
Department of Parasitology
Univerity of Hohenheim
Stuttgart, Federal Republic of Germany

Fredric L. Frye, D.V.M.
741 Plum Lane
Davis, CA, 95616, U.S.A.

Diane M. Hoff, B.S.
6705 NW Evelyn
Kansas City, MO, 64151, U.S.A

Gerald L. Hoff, Ph.D.
Division of Communicable Disease Control
Kansas City Health Department
1423 E. Linwood Blvd.
Kansas City, MO, 64109, U.S.A.

Elliott R. Jacobson, D.V.M., Ph.D.
Division of Laboratory Animal and Wildlife Medicine
College of Veterinary Medicine
University of Florida
Gainsville, FL, 32610, U.S.A.

George V. Kollias, Jr., D.V.M.
Department of Special Clinical Sciences
College of Veterinary Medicine
University of Florida
Gainsville, FL, 32610, U.S.A.

CONTRIBUTORS

Samuel V. Machotka, II, D.V.M.
Pathology Department
Hazelton Laboratories, Inc.
9200 Leesburg Turnpike
Vienna, VA, 22180, U.S.A.

Robert G. McKinnell, Ph.D.
Department of Genetics and Cell Biology
University of Minnesota
250 Biological Sciences Center
St. Paul, MN, 55108, U.S.A.

George Migaki, D.V.M.
Registry of Comparative Pathology
Armed Forces Institute of Pathology
Washington, DC, 20306, U.S.A.

Akira Oya, M.D.
Department of Virology and Rickettsiology
National Institute of Health
10-35 Kamiosaki 2-chome
Shinagawa-Ku
Tokyo, Japan

Van B. Philpot, Jr., M.D.
Department of Biochemistry
Tulane School of Medicine
Tulane University
1430 Tulane Ave.
New Orleans, LA, 70100, U.S.A.

Robert E. Schmidt, D.V.M., Ph.D.
Comparative Pathology Branch
U.S. Air Force School of Aerospace Medicine
Brooks Air Force Base, TX, 78235, U.S.A.

J. Teague Self, Ph.D.
Department of Zoology
University of Oklahoma
Norman, OK, 73019, U.S.A.

Kennedy F. Shortridge, Ph.D.
Department of Microbiology
University of Hong Kong
Pathology Building
Queen Mary Hospital Compound
Hong Kong

Emmett B. Shotts, Jr., Ph.D.
Department of Medical Microbiology
College of Veterinary Medicine
University of Georgia
Athens, GA, 30602, U.S.A.

Kurt P. Snipes, M.S.
Department of Veterinary Microbiology
School of Veterinary Medicine
University of California
Davis, CA, 95616, U.S.A.

John F.A. Sprent, Ph.D., D.Sc., F.R.C.V.S., F.A.A.
Department of Parasitology
Univerity of Queensland
St. Lucia
Queensland, 4067, Australia

Rune L. Stjernholm, Ph.D.
Department of Biochemistry
Tulane School of Medicine
Tulane University
1430 Tulane Ave.
New Orleans, LA, 70100, U.S.A.

Sam R. Telford, Jr., Ph.D.
Parasitology
Florida State Museum
University of Florida
Gainsville, FL, 32610, U.S.A.

Franklin H. White, Ph.D.
Department of Preventive Medicine
College of Veterinary Medicine
University of Florida
Gainsville, FL, 32610, U.S.A.

INDEX

Ablepharus boutonni
  arboviruses, 120
Absidia, 183
Acanthamoeba, 322-323
Acanthophis antarctieus
  neoplasia, 539, 560, 562
Acanthorhabdias, 214
Acanthotaenia, 248
Acenthixalus spinosus
  protozoans, 364
Acris gryllus
  protozoans, 281, 296,
      302, 361
Acrochordus javanicus
  neoplasia, 536, 568
Actinomyces bovis, 196
Actinomyces israelii, 196
Adenocarcinoma
  of frogs, 581-597
Aedes aegypti
  arboviruses, 109-110
  rhabdoviruses, 152
Aedes albopicta
  protozoans, 429
Aedes albopictus
  arboviruses, 110
Aedes atlanticus
  arboviruses, 110
Aedes canadensis
  arboviruses, 110
Aedes sierrensii
  protozoans, 433
Aedes sollicitans
  arboviruses, 110
Aedes stephensi
  protozoans, 433
Aedes sticticus
  arboviruses, 110

Aedes togoi
  arboviruses, 110
  protozoans, 429, 433
Aedes triseriatus
  arboviruses, 110
Aedes trivittatus
  arboviruses, 110
Aedes vexans
  arboviruses, 110
Aegyptianella, 475-476, 478
Aeromonas
  control, 53
  diagnosis, 53
  distribution, 50-51
  etiology, 49-50
  pathology, 51-53
Aeromonas hydrophila
  stomatitis, 38
Agama
  filiariasis, 498
  protozoans, 330
Agama agama
  pirhemocytonosis, 485
  protozoans, 387
Agama caucasica
  protozoans, 432
Agama nupta fusca
  protozoans, 468, 470-471
Agama sanguinolenta
  protozoans, 386, 388
Agama stellio
  protozoans, 386-389
Agama tuberculata
  protozoans, 416-417
Aging
  criteria of, 625
  maximums, 626

Agkistrodon contortrix
  pentastomiasis, 206
Agkistrodon halys
  neoplasia, 540
Agkistrodon piscivorus
  arboviruses, 119
  helminths, 236
  hyperplastic pancreatic
      regeneration, 629
  neoplasia, 540, 555-556,
      561-563, 566, 568
  pentastomiasis, 206
  protozoans, 486-487
  venom components, 696
  venom neutralization,
      695
Alaria americana, 255
Alexeiefella, 283
Alligator mississippiensis
  age, 626
  amyloidosis, 627
  arboviruses, 122
  bacteria, 26, 52, 85
  fungi, 185, 188, 192,
      197
  glomerulosclerosis, 628
  helminths, 233-234
  immunity, 73, 668, 710
  neoplasia, 532, 548
  nutritional deficiency,
      650
  pentastomiasis, 206
  protozoans, 430
Almpiwar virus, 120
Alofia, 206
Alsophis cathigerus pepei
  helminths, 236
Amblyomma dissimile
  protozoans, 429-433
Amblyomma flavomaculatum
  Q fever, 102
Amblyomma latum
  Q fever, 102
Amblyomma nitidum
  protozoans, 409
Amblyomma nuttali
  Q fever, 101-102
Ambystoma jeffersonianum
  protozoans, 276, 296-
      297, 361

Ambystoma maculatum
  protozoans, 276, 282, 285,
      296-297
Ambystoma mexicanum
  immunity, 680
  protozoans, 276, 278, 282,
      285, 296, 302, 308,
      361, 365
Ambystoma opacum
  protozoans, 276, 285, 294,
      297, 361
Ambystoma tigrinum
  fungi, 170
  protozoans, 278, 282, 285,
      296-297, 302, 360
Ameiva ameiva
  arboviruses, 120
  protozoans, 275, 332, 445-
      496
  rhabdoviruses, 152
Ameiva festiva
  protozoans, 332
Ameiva leptophrys
  protozoans, 332
Ameiva quadrilineata
  protozoans, 332
Amphibolurus barbatus
  filiariasis, 496
  fungi, 185, 197
Amphisbaena alba
  protozoans, 409
Amphiuma
  protozoans, 296
Amplicaecum, 241
Amyloidosis, 626-628
Anaplasma, 478
Aneides lugubris
  protozoans, 293
Angusticaecum holopterum,
      221, 227, 229, 230,
      242
Anolis
  protozoans, 386, 400, 407
Anolis auratus
  protozoans, 445, 455-457
Anolis carolinensis
  arboviruses, 120
  bacteria, 6, 40, 62
  fungi, 194
  herpesviruses, 160

Anolis carolinensis (continued)
  neoplasia, 533, 550
  protozoans, 275, 428, 431, 433, 444, 455, 458, 461, 463
Anolis cybotes
  protozoans, 419-420
Anolis equestris
  bacteria, 60-63
Anolis limifrons
  protozoans, 448, 456-457, 462-463
Anolis lionatus
  protozoans, 445, 448
Anolis poecilopus
  protozoans, 395, 445
Anopheles
  arboviruses, 109
Anopheles albimanus
  protozoans, 433
Anopheles quadrimaculatus
  arboviruses, 110
  rhabdoviruses, 152
Anopheles stephensi
  protozoans, 429
Aponoma halla
  Q fever, 101
Arboviruses
  diagnosis, 128-140
  etiology, 108-128
  hosts, 118-123
  vectors, 110-111
Arizona
  classification, 71-72
  diagnosis, 75-76
  distribution, 70-71
  pathogenesis and pathology, 72-75
  treatment, 76-77
Arizona elegans
  neoplasia, 537, 560
Armigeres subalbatus
  arboviruses, 110
Armillifer, 206
Arthritis, 61-63
Ascaris, 219
Ascorbic acid deficiency, 643-644
Aspergillosis, 185-188

Aspergillus amstelodami, 187, 191
Aspergillus fumigatus, 185
Aspidites
  helminths, 237
Atelopus varius
  protozoans, 421, 480
Atheris albolabus
  neoplasia, 540, 568
Atractaspis leucomeles
  protozoans, 326
Aufwuchs, 362-365
Austramphilina, 250
Austrelaps superba
  protozoans, 329

Balantidium, 360, 363
Bartonella, 478
Basidiobolus ranarum, 184
Basiliscus
  arboviruses, 110
  protozoans, 275
Basiliscus basiliscus
  protozoans, 332
Basiliscus plumifrons
  neoplasia, 533, 552
  protozoans, 332
Basiliscus vittatus
  bacteria, 60
Batrachotaenia, 248
B-cells, 662
Beauchampia, 249
Beauveriosis, 192-193
Beauveria bassiana, 192-193, 198
Befilaria, 489-490
Bertariella, 478-480
Besnoitia, 325-333
Betramia, 350
Biotin deficiency, 643
Bitis arietans
  fungi, 186
  helminths, 240
  neoplasia, 540, 557, 560, 569
  protozoans, 342
Bitis atrox
  neoplasia, 540
Bitis gabonica
  neoplasia, 540, 555, 557

Bitis lachesis
  protozoans, 344
Bitis nasicornis
  helminths, 215
  neoplasia, 540, 559-561, 563
Boa constrictor
  filiariasis, 487, 491, 496-498
  fungi, 194, 196
  helminths, 256
  histology of, 716, 718, 732, 736
  hypovitaminosis, 645, 647
  neoplasia, 568
  protozoans, 281, 295, 321, 324-325, 396, 424, 426, 428, 431, 433
  starvation, 637
Boidae
  age of, 626
Bombina bombina
  protozoans, 302
Bombina variegata
  protozoans, 302
Bone marrow, 663
Boodon lineatus
  protozoans, 480
Bothridium, 248
Bothriocephalus, 248
Bothrops alternata
  arboviruses, 119
  protozoans, 403-404
Bothrops atrox
  neoplasia, 558
  paramyxoviruses, 38
Bothrops moojeni
  protozoans, 424
Bothrops pradoi
  bacteria, 93
Bradykinin, 696
Brevimulticaecum, 222, 230, 235
Brygoofilaria, 489-490
Bufo
  bacteria, 74, 86
  humidity tolerance, 618
  Q fever, 102

Bufo (continued)
  protozoans, 302
Bufo alvarius
  fungi, 170
Bufo americanus
  bacteria, 60, 62
  herpesviruses, 160
  protozoans, 278, 285, 296-297, 302-303, 360-361
Bufo blombergi
  fungi, 170, 175-178
Bufo bufo
  fungi, 170
  immunity in, 679-680
  protozoans, 278, 281-283, 285, 291, 296-297, 302-303, 308, 349, 350, 360-361
Bufo houstonensis
  fungi, 173-174, 179
Bufo japonicus
  arboviruses, 113
Bufo lentiginosus
  protozoans, 350
Bufo marinus
  bacteria, 86
  fungi, 170, 172
  immunity in, 97, 677-678
  protozoans, 303, 330
Bufo melanostictus
  fungi, 170
  protozoans, 291, 294, 303
Bufo regularis
  protozoans, 303, 305
Bufo terrestris
  protozoans, 296-297
Bufo valliceps
  protozoans, 304
Bufo vulgaris
  protozoans, 350
Bunamide, 256
Bungarus fasciatus
  arboviruses, 119
  herpesviruses, 160
Bunyamwera virus, 121
Butantinella, 206

Cage paralysis, 651
Caimans
  hypovitaminosis, 648-650

Caimans (continued)
 pentastomiasis, 206
Caiman crocodylus
 herpesviruses, 160
Caiman sclerops
 fungi, 188-189
 immunity in, 668
Calopistes maculatus
 neoplasia, 534, 554-555
Calotes mystaceus
 fungi, 197
Calotes nemoricola
 protozoans, 282
Calotes versicolor
 arboviruses, 120
 filiariasis, 496
 immunity in, 665, 675,
  680-682
 protozoans, 291, 341,
  478, 483
Candidiasis, 189-190
Candida albicans, 190
Candida tropicalis, 190
Cardianema, 488-490
Cardiovascular system
 histology of, 733-734
 necropsy of, 707
Caretta caretta
 fungi, 189
 helminths, 241
 protozoans, 478
Caryospora, 338-339, 345
Catadiscus, 252
Causus rhombeatus
 protozoans, 288
Central nervous system
 histology of, 746-753
 necropsy of, 711-712
Cepedea, 300-301, 303
Cepedietta, 361, 363
Cephalobaena, 206
Cephaloclamys, 248
Cephalosporiosis, 188-189
Ceramodactylus doriae
 protozoans, 386
Cercomonas, 287
Chaco virus, 120, 150-156
Chalcides ocellatus
 protozoans, 326
Chalcides tridactylus
 protozoans, 352

Chamaeleo bitaeniatus
 fungi, 190
Chamaeleo brevicornis
 protozoans, 405-406
Chamaeleo dilepis
 fungi, 194
 neoplasia, 533, 548
Chamaeleo fisheri
 protozoans, 326, 331, 474
Chamaeleo jacksonii
 fungi, 184-185
 protozoans, 345
Chamaeleo lateralis
 protozoans, 405, 485
Chamaeleo oustaleti
 filiariasis, 492
 protozoans, 485
Chamaeleo pardalis
 filiariasis, 492
 protozoans, 485
Chamaeleo verrucosus
 filiariasis, 492
Chamaeleo vulgaris
 protozoans, 386
Chamaeleo zeylanicus
 protozoans, 291
Charleville virus, 115, 120
Chelodina longicollis
 helminths, 242
Chelonia mydas
 fungi, 189, 192-193
 helminths, 241
 herpesviruses, 161-164
 histology of, 739
 immunity in, 667
 neoplasia, 521, 528-530,
  543, 545-547
 protozoans, 313, 343-344,
  360, 476, 479
Chelydra serpentina
 arboviruses, 121
 bacteria, 95, 97
 fungi, 191
 immunity in, 666, 710
 protozoans, 309, 407, 473
Chilomstix, 279-280
Chinemys reevesi
 arboviruses, 114
Chironius
 bacteria, 84

Chitra indica
  protozoans, 467
Chondropython viridis
  helminths, 237
Chromomycosis
  classification, 170-171
  diagnosis, 176-179
  distribution, 169-170
  immunity to, 179-180
  pathogenesis and pathology, 172-176
  transmission, 171-172
Chrysemys concinna
  protozoans, 433, 469
Chrysemys marginata
  protozoans, 364
Chrysemys nelsoni
  bacteria, 85
Chrysemys ornata
  fungi, 189
Chrysemys picta
  arboviruses, 121
  bacteria, 60, 85, 97
  herpesviruses, 160-161, 163
  immunity in, 667, 672
  neoplasia, 530, 542-543
  protozoans, 308, 402, 407, 468, 472
Chrysemys scripta
  arboviruses, 121
  bacteria, 60, 74, 85, 93
  herpesviruses, 160
  histology of, 726
  hypovitaminosis, 642
  neoplasia, 530, 543
  protozoans, 303, 472-473
Chrysops callidus
  vector, protozoa, 468
Chrysosporiosis, 193
Chrysosporium keratinophilum, 193
Ciliophora, 359-365
Cingula, 480
Citrobacter, 62
Cladosporiosis, 171, 196
Cladosporium carrionii, 171
Claudius angustatus
  protozoans, 307-309

Clelia clelia
  filiariasis, 491
Clemmys
  neoplasia, 530, 547
  protozoans, 285
Clemmys caspica
  arboviruses, 121
Clemmys guttata
  arboviruses, 121
  protozoans, 407
Clemmys insculpta
  arboviruses, 121
Clemmys marmorata
  herpesviruses, 160-161, 163
  histology of, 714
Clinostomum, 256
Cnemidophorus
  arboviruses, 120
  protozoans, 275
Cnemidophorus lemniscatus
  protozoans, 332
Colpoda, 363
Colubridae
  age of, 626
Coluber
  protozoans, 294-295
Coluber carbonaria
  protozoans, 352
Coluber constrictor
  arboviruses, 118
  immunity in, 670
Coluber gemonensis
  protozoans, 316, 319, 352
Coluber hippocrepis
  protozoans, 321
Coluber karelini
  protozoans, 388
Coluber rhodorhachis
  protozoans, 388
Coluber viridiflavus
  protozoans, 330, 336
Complement
  amphibian immunity, 676
  reptilian immunity, 671-672
Congenital transmission
  protozoans, 424
Conispiculum, 489-490
Conophis vittatus
  filiariasis, 491
Constrictor constrictor
  bacteria, 40

Constrictor constrictor
        (continued)
    neoplasia, 536, 559,
        561-564
Contracaecum, 230
Cordylus cataphractus
    filiariasis, 491
Cordylus polyzonus
    neoplasia, 533, 549
Cordylus vittifer
    protozoans, 457, 485
Corytophanes, 407
Cotylaspis, 249
Coxiella burneti, 101-104
Coxiellosis (see Q fever)
Crepidobothrium, 248
Crocodilians
    immunity in, 668
Crocodilurus lacertinus
    fungi, 190
Crocodylus
    neoplasia, 532, 548
Crocodylus acutus
    fungi, 185, 187
    neoplasia, 532, 547
Crocodylus crocodilus
    fungi, 194
Crocodylus moreleti
    fungi, 185
Crocodylus niloticus
    fungi, 185, 194
    protozoans, 396
Crocodylus porosus
    neoplasia, 532, 547-548
    protozoans, 313
Crotalus adamanteus
    hyperplastic pancreatic
        regeneration, 629
    venom components, 696
    venom neutralization,
        695
Crotalus atrox
    arboviruses, 119
    bacteria, 60, 75
    histology of, 743
    neoplasia, 540, 564
    protozoans, 293
Crotalus basiliscus
    filiariasis, 491
Crotalus cerastes
    protozoans, 344

Crotalus confluens
    protozoans, 342
Crotalus durissus
    neoplasia, 396, 424, 428,
        433
Crotalus enyo
    histology of, 720
Crotalus horridus
    neoplasia, 521-522, 541,
        556, 558-559, 561-
        564
    protozoans, 345
Crotalus mitchelli
    bacteria, 39
    neoplasia, 541, 558
Crotalus ruber
    neoplasia, 541, 564-565
Crotalus triseriatus
    bacteria, 60
Crotalus viridis
    neoplasia, 541, 555
    Q fever, 102
    protozoans, 294, 344
Crotaphytus collaris
    histology of, 746
    protozoans, 461
Cryptosporidium, 346-347
Crysticercus fasciolaris, 527
Ctenosaura acanthura
    amyloidosis, 627
    bacteria, 72
    protozoans, 309, 361
Cubirea, 206
Culex dolosus
    vector, protozoa, 403, 422
Culex fatigans
    vector, rhabdoviruses, 152
Culex hayashii
    vector, arboviruses, 110,
        113
Culex infantulus
    vector, arboviruses, 111-
        112, 114
Culex pipiens
    vector, arboviruses, 111
    vector, protozoa, 404,
        421-422, 429, 433,
        451-452, 468
Culex quinquefasciatus
    vector, protozoa, 433

Culex resturans
  vector, arboviruses, 111
Culex salinanius
  vector, arboviruses, 111
Culex tarsalis
  vector, arboviruses, 109,
    111
  vector, protozoa, 423,
    429, 433
Culex territans
  vector, arboviruses, 111
  vector, protozoa, 403
Culex tritaeniorhynchus
  vector, arboviruses, 111-
    113
Culesita
  vector, arboviruses, 109
Culesita melanura
  vector, arboviruses, 111
Culesita minnesotae
  vector, arboviruses, 111
Culesita morsita
  vector, arboviruses, 111
Cuora amboinensis
  protozoans, 285-286
C-virus, 522, 527
Cyclagras gigas
  paramyxoviruses, 134
  protozoans, 433
Cyclospora, 338, 344
Cyclura cornuta
  neoplasia, 533, 553
Cyclura ricordi
  neoplasia, 533, 549
Cynops pyrrhogaster
  protozoans, 308
Cyrtodactylus scaber
  protozoans, 432
Cystoisospora, 338
Cytamoeba, 474, 477, 480-
    482

Dactylosoma, 473-475
Deblockotaenia, 248
Dehydration (see water
    deprivation)
Deirochelys reticularia
  bacteria, 39
Demansia psammophis
  protozoans, 344

Dendrelaphis punctulatus
  protozoans, 339
Dendroaspis angusticeps
  bacteria, 41, 84
Dendroaspis jamesoni
  bacteria, 41
  trauma, 609
Dendroaspis polylepis
  bacteria, 41
Dermatophilosis, 196-197
Dermatophilus congolensis,
    196-197
Dermocystidium, 347-348
Dermomycoides, 347
Dermosporidium, 347
Desmognathus fuscus
  protozoans, 276, 278, 285,
    6294, 361
Dicercomonas, 284, 287
Diesingia, 206
Digestive system
  histology of, 714-724
  necropsy of, 709-710
Diochetos, 248
Diplodiscus, 252
Diplodocus, 553
Diploglossus fasciatus
  protozoans, 462
Diplorchis, 249
Dipsosaurus dorsalis
  bacteria, 40
  immunity in, 73, 668-669,
    673
Dispholidus typus
  neoplasia, 537, 555-556
Distomum constrictum
  and neoplasia, 528, 543
Dorisiella, 339
Draco maculatus
  protozoans, 449
Drowning, 619-620
Drymarchon corais
  fungi, 185
  pentastomiasis, 206
  protozoans, 295, 423, 428,
    431, 491, 496
Drymobius bifossatus
  protozoans, 308
Dujardianascaris, 221, 230,
    235
Duthiersia, 248

INDEX

Echis carinatus
  bacteria, 84
  protozoans, 388
Edwardsiella tarda
  classification, 86-87
  diagnosis, 87-88
  distribution, 84-86
Egernia cunninghami
  immunity in, 673, 669
Eggs
  bacterial penetration, 72
Eimeria, 338, 340, 343-345
Elaphe
  filiariasis, 498
  helminths, 213
  protozoans, 295
Elaphe guttata
  arboviruses, 119
  histology of, 719
  neoplasia, 527, 537,
    556, 565-566
Elaphe obsoleta
  arboviruses, 119
  herpesviruses, 160
  immunity in, 670
  neoplasia, 537, 555,
    557, 563, 566-568
Elaphe quadrivirgata
  venom neutralization,
    695
Elaphe rufodorsata
  arboviruses, 116, 119
Elaphe schrenckii
  arboviruses, 119
Elaphe subocularis
  bacteria, 40
Elaphe vulpina
  immunity in, 670
Elapidae
  age of, 626
Electrocution, 610-611
Elenia, 206
Embadomonas, 281
Emyda vittata
  protozoans, 402
Emydoidea blandingi
  bacteria, 95
  protozoans, 407
Emys orbicularis
  bacteria, 93, 95

Emys orbicularis (continued)
  helminths, 242
  neoplasia, 530, 547
  protozoans, 276-279, 285,
    352
Encephalitis viruses, 109,
    116-122
Encylometra bolognensis, 354
Endocrine system, reptiles
  histology of, 724-732
  necropsy of, 707-709
Entamoeba
  classification, 306-312
  diagnosis, 317-320
  pathogenesis and pathol-
    ogy, 312-317
  treatment, 320-321
Enteromonas, 280
Entomelas, 214
Environment
  in neoplasia, 525-526
Enzymes
  in venoms, 695-698
Eperythrozoon, 458, 478
Epicrates cenchris
  bacteria, 38
  fungi, 194
  protozoans, 396, 403
Epidermophyton, 197
Epistylis, 364
Eremias oliveri
  protozoans, 326, 386
Erysipelothrix insidiosa, 187
Erythrolamprus bionus
  bacteria, 84
Eryx tataricus
  viruses, 527
Eublepharis macularis
  bacteria, 40
Eumeces fasciatus
  neoplasia, 534, 548
Eumeces inexpectatus
  protozoans, 481-482
Eumeces laticeps
  arboviruses, 120
Eunectes murinus
  fungi, 195-196
  neoplasia, 536, 556, 560,
    568
Eupolystoma, 249

Eurycea lucifuga
  protozoans, 361
Euspondylus brevifrontalis
  protozoans, 416-417
Euthanasia, 703-704
Eutrichomastix, 294

Fallisia, 434, 447-451
Fer-de-Lance virus, 133
Fibrocystis, 332
Fibrous osteodystrophy, 651-654
Filariasis
  classification, 488-489, 494
  diagnosis, 498
  distribution, 490-494
  pathogenesis and pathology, 495-498
  treatment and immunity, 498-499
Foleyella, 489-490
Fonsecaea pedrosoi, 171, 195
Frenkelia, 325, 334
Fungal infections
  in amphibians, 169-181
  in reptiles, 183-204
Fusarium oxysporum, 194

Gallinaceum, 458
Garnia, 447-448
Geckobiella texana
  vector, protozoa, 421, 429
Gedoelstascaris, 230, 235
Gehyra australis
  arboviruses, 115, 120
  protozoans, 294
Geimania, 365
Gekko gecko
  arboviruses, 120
  bacteria, 52, 60, 84
  herpesviruses, 160
  protozoans, 395, 422, 432
Gekko verticillatus
  protozoans, 428
Gekko vittatus
  protozoans, 294

Genetics
  in neoplasia, 525
Geochelone carbonaria
  neoplasia, 529-530
  protozoans, 286
Geochelone denticulata
  fungi, 189
Geochelone elegani
  protozoans, 286
Geochelone elephantopus
  fungi, 187, 191-192
  neoplasia, 529-530
  protozoans, 308
Geochelone emys
  neoplasia, 530, 543
Geochelone gigantea
  fungi, 184, 187, 191
  hyperthermia, 612
Geochelone nigrita
  fungi, 189
Geochelone sulcata
  protozoans, 308
Geochelone tritugu
  neoplasia, 547
Geomyda
  protozoans, 285
Geotrichosis, 190-191
Gerrhonotus multicarinatus
  protozoans, 462
Giardia, 284, 287-289
Gigliolella, 206
Glaucoma, 365
Glomerulosclerosis, 628-629
Glossina, 396-397, 403
Glossiphonia, 402
Glugea, 349, 352
Goezia holmesi, 222, 230, 235-236
Goiter, 654-657
Gonatodes albogularis
  protozoans, 395, 399, 448
Gonatodes taniae
  protozoans, 395
Gonyocephalus borneensis
  protozoans, 462-463
Gopherus agassizi
  bacteria, 25-34
  gout, 635
  histology of, 715, 723, 726, 728-729, 738, 742, 744

Gopherus agassizi tinued)
  hypovitaminosis, 641
  obesity, 658
  starvation, 638
Gopherus berlandieri
  arboviruses, 121
  histology of, 744
Gopherus polyphemus
  arboviruses, 120
  bacteria, 39-40
  hypovitaminosis, 646-647
Gout, 634-636
Grahamella, 478-480
Graptemys geographica
  protozoans, 407
Graptemys kohni
  bacteria, 70, 85
Grey patch disease, 161-165
Gymnodactylus caspius
  protozoans, 386, 388-389
Gyrodactylus, 249, 253

Haematoloechus, 252
Haementeria lutzei
  vector, protozoa, 403, 433
Haemocystidium, 467
Haemogregarines
  classification, 418-420
  diagnosis, 427-431
  distribution, 408-418
  immunity, 431-434
  pathogenesis and pathology, 424-427
  transmission, 421-424
Haemogregarina, 408, 418-433
Haemoparasites, reptiles, 385-517
Haemoproteiids
  classification, 467
  diagnosis, 472
  distribution, 465-467
  immunity, 472-473
  pathogenesis and pathology, 468-472
  transmission, 467-468
Haemoproteus, 466, 475, 493

Haldea valeriae
  arboviruses, 118
Haptophyra, 361, 363
Hartmannella, 322-323
Hastospiculum oncocercum, 488-490
Hegeriella, 300-304
Helicops modestus
  protozoans, 401
Heloderma horridum
  hypovitaminosis, 643
  protozoans, 295, 317
Heloderma suspectum
  age of, 626
  bacteria, 38, 73
  filiariasis, 490
  hypovitaminosis, 643
  immunity in, 666
  neoplasia, 533, 552-553
  protozoans, 281, 295
  venom, resistance to, 694
Hemidactylus
  protozoans, 276, 295
Hemidactylus brookii
  bacteria, 62
  protozoans, 386, 405, 471
Hemidactylus flavivirdis
  bacteria, 74
Hemidactylus frenatus
  arboviruses, 120
  protozoans, 404-405
Hemidactylus giganteus
  protozoans, 282
Hemidactylus mabuya
  protozoans, 341
Hemidactylus turcicus
  protozoans, 386
Hemolymph test, 104
Henneguya, 356
Hepatozoon, 409, 418-433
Herpes sarmini, 527
Herpesviruses, amphibians
  Lucke tumor virus, 582-593
Herpesviruses, reptiles
  classification, 161
  diagnosis, 164-165
  immunity, 165
  pathogenesis and pathology, 162-164
  transmission, 161-162

Herpetomonas, 274-277, 387
Heterodon
  helminths, 213
  protozoans, 294-295
Heterodon nasicus
  neoplasia, 537, 556
Heterodon platyrhinos
  arboviruses, 118
  bacteria, 93
  neoplasia, 522, 537, 560, 562
Heteronota binoei
  protozoans, 468
Hexamastix, 298, 294-295
Hexametra, 221, 230, 236
Hexametra angusticaecoides, 241
Hexametra boddaertii, 239-240
Hexametra hexametra, 241
Hexametra quadricornis, 239-240
Hexamita, 267-274, 280, 284-287
Hexamitus, 284
Hirstiella, 429
Histology, reptiles, 712-753
Hoarella, 338
Holbrookia texanus
  bacteria, 60
Homalopsis buccata
  neoplasia, 537, 557
Hormodendrum, 171, 195
Humidity, effects of, 618
Hyalomma aegyptium, 103, 105, 114
Hyalomma truncatum, 101
Hyaluronidase, 696-697
Hydraspis hilarii
  fungi, 186
Hydrosaurus amboinensis
  neoplasia, 533, 549
Hyla arborea
  protozoans, 302, 361
Hyla aurea
  protozoans, 358
Hyla caerulea
  fungi, 170

Hyla cinerea
  protozoans, 296, 302, 360
Hyla crucifer
  protozoans, 285, 296, 302, 360
Hyla suptentrionalis
  fungi, 170
Hyperplastic pancreatic regeneration, 629-631
Hyphomyces, 183
Hypoglycemia, 658
Hypotrichomonas, 295, 298
Hypovitaminosis, 640-650

Iguana iguana
  bacteria, 60
  fungi, 186, 193
  herpesviruses, 160-162
  histology of, 722, 733-735, 750, 752-753
  immunity in, 669
  neoplasia, 533, 548-549, 552-554
  protozoans, 276, 313, 321, 360, 420, 459, 461, 484, 487
Immune mechanisms
  amphibian
    cell-mediated, 679-680
    humoral, 676-679
    on metamorphosis, 680
    phagocytosis, 676
  reptilian
    cell-mediated, 674-676
    humoral, 664-674
    responses, 680-682
Immunoglobulins, 136-140, 665-671, 677-679
Integument, reptiles
  histology of, 713-714
  necropsy of, 706
Irradiation, 620-621
Isospora, 338, 340-342, 345
Ixodes nipponensis, 477, 482, 486
Ixodes persulcatus, 115
Ixodes ricinus, 115

Japalura polygonata
  filiariasis, 490

INDEX

Kachuga
  Q fever, 101
Kapsulotaenia, 248
Karotomorpha, 275, 278-279
Karyolysus, 416-431
Kentropyx calcaratus
  arboviruses, 120
  rhabdoviruses, 152
Klosiella, 324-325
Kidney, immunologic, 663
Kinixys belliana
  helminths, 242
Kinosternon leucostomum
  protozoans, 321
Kinosternon scorpioides
  protozoans, 283, 326, 331-332
Kinosternon subrubrum
  arboviruses, 122
Kiricephalus coarctatus, 205-206, 208
Klossiella, 418
Krefftascaris parenteri, 221, 242-243

Lacerta agilis
  arboviruses, 119
  bacteria, 93
  neoplasia, 526, 533, 551-552
  protozoans, 417, 428, 431
Lacerta dugesii
  protozoans, 333
Lacerta muralis
  bacteria, 73
  neoplasia, 534, 552
  protozoans, 323, 326, 354, 418-419, 433
Lacerta sicula
  neoplasia, 534, 552
  protozoans, 336
Lacerta strigata
  protozoans, 474
Lacerta tiliquerta
  protozoans, 336
Lacerta viridis
  arboviruses, 119
  fungi, 194
  neoplasia, 534, 551, 553

Lacerta viridis (continued)
  protozoans, 483
  viruses, 160-162
Lacerta vivipara
  protozoans, 417, 428, 431
Lachesis muta
  protozoans, 435
  venom, resistance to, 697
Laelaps echidninus, 422
Lainsonia, 418-428
Lamblia, 287
Lampropeltis
  helminths, 213
  protozoans, 288, 294-295
Lampropeltis calligaster
  histology of, 741
Lampropeltis doliata
  filiariasis, 491
Lampropeltis getulus
  arboviruses, 118
  bacteria, 84
  histology of, 713
  neoplasia, 538, 564-565, 568-569
  venom, neutralization of, 694
Lampropeltis triangulum
  fungi, 185
Lankesterella amania, 418, 474
Latastia longicauda
  protozoans, 386
Laticauda colubrina
  protozoans, 409
Leimadophis
  bacteria, 84
Leiololopisma metallica
  protozoans, 326
Leiperia, 206
Leishmaniasis
  classification, 386-387
  diagnosis, 390-391
  distribution, 387-389, 467-468, 493
  immunity to, 391
  pathogenesis and pathology, 390
  transmission, 389-390
Leptodactylus ocellatus
  fungi, 170
  protozoans, 303, 330

Leptodactylus pentadactylus
  fungi, 169-170
  protozoans, 478
Leptomonas, 274-275, 387
Leptospira
  classification, 93-97
  diagnosis, 96
  distribution, 93-94
  immunity, 96-97
  pathogenesis and pathology, 95
Leptotheca, 356
Levineia, 338
Liasis amethystinus
  helminths, 237
Liasis childreni
  histology of, 715, 730
Ligamifer, 206
Limax-amoebae, 321-322
Limnatis granulosa, 402
Lioheterodon modestus
  protozoans, 428, 433
Liopeltis vernalis
  lipoproteins, 137
Liophis jaegeri
  protozoans, 303
Lissemys punctata
  protozoans, 479
Lophotaspis, 249
Lucke tumor
  abundance, 585-588
  cloning, 597
  distribution
    geographic, 583-584
    seasonal, 584-585
  etiology, 588-592
  immunity to, 595-596
  pathogenesis and pathology, 593-594
  temperature relationship, 596-597
  transmission, 592-593
Lungworms
  classification, 214
  diagnosis, 214-215
  distribution, 213
  pathogenesis and pathology, 214
  treatment, 215-216
Lutzomyia stewarti, 451

Lutzomyia trinidadensis, 400, 404
Lutzomyia vexatrix, 451
Lycodon striatus
  Q fever, 101
Lygosoma himalayanum
  protozoans, 416-417
Lygosoma laterale
  protozoans, 461
Lyssemysia, 249

Mabuya carinata
  protozoans, 276
Mabuya mabouya
  protozoans, 460-462
Mabuya maculilabris
  filiariasis, 493
Mabuya striata
  filiariasis, 493
  protozoans, 404, 459
Mabuya quiquetaeniata
  filiariasis, 493
  protozoans, 405
Macdonaldius, 488-490
Madagascarophis colubrina
  protozoans, 428, 433
Madathamugadia, 489-490
Malaclemys terrapin
  arboviruses, 121
  bacteria, 85
Malacocherusus tornieri
  neoplasia, 528-530
Malaria
  diagnosis, 458-460
  distribution, 435-446
  etiology, 446-451
  immunity to, 461-463
  pathogenesis and pathology, 452-458
  transmission, 451-452
Mansonia perturbans, 109, 111
Marco virus, 120, 150-156
Martinezia, 309
Masticophis flagellum
  bacteria, 8
  neoplasia, 538, 559
  pentastomiasis, 206
Mauremys caspica
  bacteria, 85, 93
  protozoans, 286, 307

Mauremys leprosa
  protozoans, 475
Mayaro virus, 120
Megalodiscus, 252
Megastoma, 287
Melanochelys trijuga
  bacteria, 85
  neoplasia, 530, 542
Metabolic bone disease, 650-654
Metamorphosis
  and immune response, 680
Micrococcus, 72
Microspora, 348-355
Microsporidium, 349
Microsporum cookei, 197
Minerals, trace, 654-657
Monocercomonas, 279, 293-298
Monocercomonoides, 290
Morelia argus
  immunity in, 665-666
  protozoans, 326
Morelia spilotes
  fungi, 191
  helminths, 237
  protozoans, 321, 329, 334, 484
Mortierella, 183
Mucor, 183, 185, 199, 348
Multicaecum, 230, 235
Multicotyle, 249
Mycobacterium
  classification, 2-5
  diagnosis, 16-17
  pathogenesis and pathology, 5-6, 8-15, 609
  transmission, 7
  treatment, 17-19
Myxidium, 356
Myxobolus, 356, 358
Myxosporidians, 354-359
Myxosoma, 356

Naegleria, 322-324
Naja
  fungi, 196
  histology of, 748
  pentastomiasis, 209-210

Naja flava
  protozoans, 345
Naja melanoleuca
  neoplasia, 539, 555, 566
Naja naja
  arboviruses, 119
  bacteria, 74
  herpesviruses, 160, 162
  neoplasia, 539, 556-557, 560
Naja nigricollis
  neoplasia, 539, 556, 560
  protozoans, 476
Naja nivea
  neoplasia, 539, 568
Natrix
  protozoans, 281, 294-296, 330
Natrix natrix
  bacteria, 1, 73
  fungi, 188
  neoplasia, 538, 555, 569
  Q fever, 101
  protozoans, 293, 339, 352
Natrix stolata
  neoplasia, 538
Natrix viperinus
  protozoans, 339
Necropsy techniques, 704-712
Necturus
  protozoans, 361
Necturus maculosus
  immunity in, 677
Nematodes
  classification, 214, 221-222, 488-489
  diagnosis, 214-215, 232-243, 498
  distribution, 213, 220-221, 487-493
  immunity to, 498
  pathogenesis and pathology, 214, 228-232, 495-498
  transmission, 222-228, 494-495
  treatment, 215-216, 499
Neodiplorchis, 249
Neopolystoma, 249

Neoplasia
  in amphibians, 581-605
  classification of, 522-524
  in reptiles
    crocodilians, 532, 547-548
    lizards, 533-535, 548-555
    turtles, 528-547
    snakes, 536-541, 555-571
Neoseps reynoldsi
  protozoans, 294
Nerodia
  helminths, 213, 236
  pentastomiasis, 206
Nerodia erythrogaster
  arboviruses, 118
Nerodia rhombifera
  protozoans, 486
Nerodia sipedon
  arboviruses, 118
  bacteria, 72
  fungi, 190
  immunity in, 670
Newts
  protozoans, 281, 323, 360
Newt-pest (see Saprolegnia)
Ninia sebae
  protozoans, 344
Nosema, 349-350, 352
Non-specific inhibitors, 136-137
Notechis ater
  protozoans, 329
Notechis scutatus
  bacteria, 84
  venom
    components of, 696
    resistance to, 694
Notophthalmus viridescens
  protozoans, 356, 358
Nuttallia, 475-476
Nutritional disorders
  in reptiles, 633-660
Nycotherus, 360-361, 364
Nyctositum, 364
Nyctotheroides, 364

Obesity, 657-659
Octomastix, 284
Octomitus, 284, 289
Octosporella, 339
Oligodon arnensis
  bacteria, 74
Oncogenic viruses, 560, 563-566
Ondatra zibethica, 207
Oochoristica, 248
Oochoristica anolis, 253
Oochoristica bivitellobata, 253
Opalina, 299-305
Opercularia, 364
Opheodrys aestivus
  arboviruses, 118
Opheodrys vernalis
  protozoans, 344
Ophidascaris, 221, 223-224, 229-230, 233, 236-241
Ophis meremmii
  protozoans, 303
Ophisaurus apodus
  immunity in, 666
  protozoans, 276, 321
Ophisaurus attenuatus
  arboviruses, 120
Ophionyssus natricis, 51
Ophiophagus hannah
  Q fever, 101
Ophiotaenia, 248
Ophiovalipora, 248
Orneoascaris, 221, 230, 241-243
Ornithodos talaje, 495
Ortleppascaris, 230, 235
Osteodystrophia fibrosa cystica, 651
Osteogenesis imperfecta, 651
Osteomalacia, 651
Oswaldofilaria, 488-490
Ozobranchus branchiatus
  and neoplasia, 528, 543
Ozobranchus shipleyi, 422

Pachydactylus capensis
  protozoans, 478
Paecilomyces fumoso-roseus, 191, 198

Pancerina, 248
Paraheterotyphlum, 220, 230, 235-236
Parapolystoma, 249
Parasites
 in neoplasia, 527-528
Pasteurella
 classification, 25, 27
 diagnosis, 32
 distribution, 27
 immunity to, 34
 pathogenesis and pathology, 29-31
 transmission, 28
 treatment, 32
Pelobates fuscus
 protozoans, 302
Pelomedusa subrufa
 neoplasia, 531, 543
Pelusious subniger
 neoplasia, 529
Penicillium, 185, 189
Pentasomes
 diagnosis, 210-211
 distribution, 205-206
 pathogenesis and pathology, 208-210
 transmission, 207-208
Perkinsus, 348
Peromyscus maniculatus, 328, 335
Phagocytosis, 676
Phialophora, 171, 195
Philodryas nattereri
 protozoans, 404
Phlebotomus, 115
Phrynocephalus
 protozoans, 386
Phrynops hilari
 bacteria, 14
Phrynops geoffroanus
 neoplasia, 531, 542
Phrynosoma
 protozoans, 276, 282, 291, 294, 296, 461
Phrynosoma cornutum
 bacteria, 60
Phyrnosoma solare
 bacteria, 38, 73
 immunity in, 669

Phycomycosis, reptiles, 183-185
Phyllobates trinitatis
 fungi, 170
Phyllurus platurus
 protozoans, 485
Pipa
 protozoans, 357
Pirhemocyton, 458, 477-478, 482-487
Pitatuba, 488-490
Pituophis
 protozoans, 294-296
Pituophis catenifer
 protozoans, 291, 428, 431, 433
Pituophis melanoleucus
 arboviruses, 118
 bacteria, 70
 filiariasis, 490
 histology of, 725
 neoplasia, 538, 556, 558, 560, 564-565, 568
 protozoans, 281, 329, 335
Placobdella, 402-403, 420, 422
Plasmocytes, perihepatic, 663
Plasmodium, 434-465, 472, 475, 482, 485
Platyhelminths
 classification, 254-255
 distribution, 250-254
 pathogenesis and pathology, 256
 treatment, 256-257
Platysternon megacephalum
 protozoans, 309
Platyurus patyurus
 arboviruses, 120
Pleistophora, 349
Pleusios subniger
 neoplasia, 531
Plica umbra
 protozoans, 450
Plistophora (see Pleistophora)
Podacris sicula
 protozoans, 336
Podacris tiliquerta
 protozoans, 336

Polychrus marmoratus
    protozoans, 428
Polydelphis anoura, 219,
        221, 224, 230, 236
Polymastix, 279, 294
Polypeptides
    in venoms, 695-696
Polystoma, 249
Polystomoidella, 249
Polystomoides, 249
Porocephalus crotali, 205-
        208
Proteocephalus, 248, 252
Proteromonas, 275-277
Proteus vulgaris, 85
Protoopalina, 300-302, 306
Protozoa
    haemoparasitic, 385-473
    non-haemoparasitic, 259-
        384
Psammophis sehokari
    protozoans, 388
Pseudechis porphytiacus
    neoplasia, 539, 556,
        562-564
    protozoans, 347
Pseudoboa cloelia
    neoplasia, 539, 556
Pseudoboa nevwiedi
    bacteria, 84
Pseudomonas
    classification, 37
    diagnosis, 42-43
    distribution, 38-39, 194
    pathogenesis and pathol-
        ogy, 39-42
    treatment, 43-45
Pseudophryne bibronii
    protozoans, 302
Pseudopolystoma, 249
Pseudothamugadia, 489-490
Pseudotriton
    protozoans, 282
Pternohyla fodiens
    fungi, 170
Ptyas korros
    arboviruses, 118
    Q fever, 101
Ptyas mucosus
    Q fever, 101

Python curtus
    helminths, 237
Python melanoleucus
    neoplasia, 568
Python molurus
    bacteria, 40
    filiariasis, 496
    helminths, 237
    neoplasia, 536-537, 555-557,
        560-561, 569
    protozoans, 337
    Q fever, 101, 103
Python regius
    bacteria, 40
    fungi, 201
    Q fever, 102
Python reticularis
    bacteria, 40
    filiariasis, 496
    fungi, 196
    helminths, 237
    neoplasia, 522, 537, 556,
        560, 566, 568
    protozoans, 329, 334-335,
        337, 340
Python sebae
    helminths, 237
    histology of, 725
    neoplasia, 537, 556, 568
    protozoans, 308, 310, 428,
        433
Pythonella, 339

Q fever
    diagnosis, 103-104
    etiology, 102
    pathogenesis and pathol-
        ogy, 103
    transmission, 102-103

Rachidelus brazili
    protozoans, 396, 403
Raillietiella bicaudata, 205-
        206, 208
Ramphiophis rostratus
    neoplasia, 539, 566
Rana
    helminths, 243
    humidity
        tolerance to, 618

Rana bufonis
  helminths, 213
Rana catesbeiana
  arboviruses, 122
  immunity in, 678
  protozoans, 281, 285,
    296, 303, 360
Rana clamitans
  arboviruses, 122
  neoplasia, 585
  protozoans, 281, 296,
    303, 360
Rana cyanophlyctis
  protozoans, 282, 294
Rana esculenta
  bacteria, 94
  protozoans, 284-285, 288,
    296, 302-303, 308,
    360-361
Rana fusca
  bacteria, 94
Rana japonica
  protozoans, 482
Rana nigromaculata
  arboviruses, 122
Rana palustris
  neoplasia, 584
  protozoans, 296, 302,
    360-361
Rana pipiens
  arboviruses, 122
  bacteria, 60-62, 93, 97
  fungi, 170
  herpesviruses, 160
  immunity in, 676-679
  neoplasia, 581-597
  protozoans, 276, 278,
    281-283, 285, 293,
    296-297, 302-303,
    330, 360-361
Rana pretiosa
  thermal stress, 613
Rana ridibunda
  arboviruses, 122
  bacteria, 74
  protozoans, 303
Rana rugosa
  protozoans, 474
Rana sylvatica
  helminths, 213

Rana sylvatica (continued)
  protozoans, 296, 302, 360-361
Rana temporaria
  bacteria, 6
  fungi, 170
  protozoans, 281, 283, 285,
    288, 294, 296, 302-
    303, 308, 324, 345,
    350, 356, 360
Rana terrestris
  protozoans, 303
Rana tigrina
  arboviruses, 120
  protozoans, 282
  Q fever, 102
Rana utricularia
  neoplasia, 584
Rattus fuscipes, 328, 334
Rattus norvegicus, 328, 335
Rattus triomanicus, 328, 337
Rattus rattus, 328
Red-leg, 51
Renal rickets, 651
Reproductive system
  histology of, 744-747
  necropsy of, 709
Respiratory system
  histology of, 737-740
  necropsy of, 706-707
Reticulo-endothelial system
  histology of, 734-737
  necropsy of, 710-711
Retortamonas, 279-280
Rhabdias, 213-216
Rhabdophis tigrina
  arboviruses, 118
Rhabdoviruses, 149-157
Rhacophorus
  fungi, 170
Rhinoclemys annulata
  bacteria, 85
Rhinoclemys punctularia
  protozoans, 286
Rhizopus, 183-185
Rhytidoides similis
  and neoplasia, 529
Rickettsia, 101-106, 473-487
Rous sarcoma virus, 527

Sarcocystis
  classification, 325-330
  hosts, 330-337, 340
  pathogenesis and pathology, 336-337
Salamandra
  protozoans, 276, 281-282, 291, 296
Salamandra atra
  protozoans, 344
Salamandra salamandra
  glomerulosclerosis, 629
Salmonella
  classification, 71-72
  diagnosis, 75-76
  distribution, 70-71
  pathogenesis and pathology, 72-75
  treatment, 76-77
Sambonia, 206
Saprolegnia, 609
Saurocytozoon, 434, 447-452
Sauromalus obesus
  bacteria, 38, 73
  immunity in, 668-669, 673
  protozoans, 295, 428
Sauromella, 478
Sauronyssus sauraram, 416-418, 421-424, 429
Sauroplasma, 476-478, 482
Saurositus, 489-490
Sceloporus
  protozoans, 276, 282, 291, 294, 407, 428, 431
Sceloporus clarkii
  protozoans, 309
Sceloporus ferrariperezi
  protozoans, 462
Sceloporus graciosus
  protozoans, 416-417
Sceloporus jarrovi
  protozoans, 416-417, 442
Sceloporus magister
  protozoans, 417
Sceloporus malachiticus
  protozoans, 332, 441
Sceloporus occidentalis
  protozoans, 326, 399, 417, 428, 433, 443-444, 451-452, 458

Sceloporus poinsetti
  bacteria, 60
  protozoans, 432
Sceloporus torquatus
  protozoans, 441
Sceloporus undulatus
  protozoans, 323, 428, 444, 453, 455, 458, 463
Sceloporus woodi
  protozoans, 458
Schellackia, 409, 418-428, 482
Schizobodo tarentolae, 276
Sebekia oxycephala, 52, 205-206, 208
Secondary nutritional hyperparathyroidism, 651
Semenoviella, 248
Sergentomyia, 115, 389, 396, 404
Serpentoplasma, 476, 479
Serratia
  classification, 60-61
  diagnosis, 63-64
  distribution, 59-60
  pathogenesis and pathology, 61-63
  transmission, 61
  treatment, 64-65
Shistosoma hematobium, 527
Shorttia, 214
Sicuophora, 364
Simondia, 467
Siredon mexicanum
  bacteria, 52
Sistrurus catenatus
  fungi, 185
  neoplasia, 541, 555
Solafilaria, 489-490
Sphenodon punctatus
  helminths, 220
  histology of, 709
  immunity in, 73, 666
  protozoans, 312-313, 349, 352, 354, 408
Sphyranura, 249
Spilotes pullatus
  histology of, 747
  neoplasia, 539, 558
  protozoans, 435
Spirocerca lupi, 527

Spirometra, 248
Spironucleus, 280, 287
Spirorchis, 253
Splendidofilaria, 488-490
Starvation, 637-640
Steatitis, 645-650
Sternotherus carinatus
    arboviruses, 121
Sternotherus niger
    neoplasia, 528, 530
Sternotherus odoratus
    bacteria, 62, 85
    fungi, 187
    neoplasia, 530, 546
Storeria dekayi
    bacteria, 62
    herpesviruses, 160
Storeria occipitomaculata
    arboviruses, 118
Stress
    in bacterial infections,
        28-34, 37, 45, 50,
        75
    in viral infections,
        125, 161-162, 165
Strongyloides, 215
Styphlodora, 256
Subtriquetra, 206
Sulcascaris, 220, 228, 230,
    241-242

Takydromus smaragdinus
    protozoans, 454
Takydromus tachydromoides
    arboviruses, 119
    protozoans, 419, 444,
        454, 458, 476-478,
        481-483, 485-486
Tantilla coronatum
    protozoans, 294
Tarentola annularis
    protozoans, 471
Tarentola gerrhonoti
    protozoans, 404
Tarentola mauritanica
    bacteria, 62
    protozoans, 276, 326,
        386, 404, 482
Tarentola sclepori
    protozoans, 404

T-cells, 662, 674-676
Tejidotaeinia, 248
Telorchis, 252
Telorchis elcolanii, 354
Tembusu virus, 136
Temperature
    effect on
        bacterial infection, 62
        fungal infection, 198-
            200
        immune response, 672-674,
            677, 681
        neoplasia, 596-597
        viral infection, 126
    hyperthermia, 611-615
    hypothermia, 615-617
Teratoscincus scincus
    filiariasis, 493
    protozoans, 388-390, 465-
        471
Terranova, 222, 230, 234-235
Terrapene carolina
    arboviruses, 121
    bacteria, 39-40, 85
    herpesviruses, 160
    irradiation, 621
    neoplasia, 531, 547
    protozoans, 285, 309
Terrapene ornata
    protozoans, 286
Testudo
    helminths, 242
    protozoans, 303, 330, 360
Testudo campanulata
    protozoans, 475
Testudo chilensis
    protozoans, 308
Testudo elegans
    protozoans, 281, 291
Testudo graeca
    bacteria, 73
    drowning, 620
    lipoproteins, 137
    protozoans, 308, 476
    Q fever, 101, 103
Testudo hermanni
    amyloidoisis, 626
    bacteria, 73
    protozoans, 531, 544

Testudo horsfieldi
  neoplasia, 531, 547
  protozoans, 286
  viruses, 527
Testudo ibera
  immunity in, 665, 667,
    674
Testudo marginata
  protozoans, 286
Testudo radiata
  fungi, 194, 196
Testudo rugosa
  immunity in, 675
Testudotaenia, 248
Tetrahymena, 363
Tetramastix, 279
Tetramitus, 279, 323
Tetratrichomonas, 298
Thamnodynastes pallidus
  protozoans, 435
Thamnophis
  arboviruses, 117
  bacteria, 75
  helminths, 213
  immunity in, 666
  pentastomiasis, 206
  protozoans, 281, 294,
    296, 309
  Q fever, 102
Thamnophis butleri
  bacteria, 62
Thamnophis elegans
  arboviruses, 118
  neoplasia, 539, 568
Thamnophis ordinoides
  immunity in, 670-671
Thamnophis proximus,
  thermal acclimatization,
    612
Thamnophis radix
  arboviruses, 119
  protozoans, 283
Thamnophis sauritus
  protozoans, 344
Thamnophis sirtalis
  arboviruses, 119
  bacteria, 95, 97
  fungi, 184, 190
  herpesviruses, 160
  neoplasia, 539, 556, 562-563, 568

Thamnophis sirtalis (continued)
  protozoans, 344
Thamugadia, 489-490
Thecadactylus rapicaudus
  protozoans, 400, 462, 463
Thiamine deficiency, 642-643
Thymus, immunologic, 663
Tiliqua
  hypovitaminosis, 643
Tiliqua gigas
  bacteria, 40
Tiliqua occipitalis
  histology of, 727
Tiliqua rugosa
  immunity in, 97, 672
Tiliqua scincoides
  bacteria, 84
  fungi, 197
Timbo virus, 120, 150-156
Toddia, 485-487
Tomodon dorsatus
  protozoans, 435, 439, 486
Toxoplasma, 325, 330-331
Toxorhynchites amboinensis,
    132
Trachydosaurus rugosus
  histology of, 727
  protozoans, 361
Transovarial transmission 72,
    125
Trauma, 607-610
Travassosacaris, 230, 236,
    239-240
Trepomonas, 280
Tricercomonas, 283
Trichoderma, 201
Trichodina, 361, 363
Trichomastix, 294
Trichomitus, 298
Trichomonas, 290-293, 295
Trichophyton, 197
Trichosporon, 194
Trigonomonas, 280
Trimersesurus flavoviridis
  venom neutralization, 695
Trimitus, 280
Trimophodon biscutatus
  filiariasis, 491, 496, 498
  protozoans, 476, 479

Trionyx
  starvation, 638
Trionyx ferox
  arboviruses, 121
  neoplasia, 531, 543
  protozoans, 433
Trionyx gangeticus
  protozoans, 309
Trionyx muticus
  protozoans, 364
Trionyx sinensis
  arboviruses, 121
Trionyx spinifer
  arboviruses, 121
  protozoans, 473
Tripteroides bambusa
  arboviruses, 111
Tritrichomonas, 299
Triturus
  protozoans, 276, 282
Triturus alpestris
  protozoans, 296, 303,
    360-361
Triturus cristatus
  protozoans, 285, 296,
    360-361
Triturus helveticus
  protozoans, 278, 302,
    361
Triturus torosus
  protozoans, 278, 285,
    296-297, 361
Triturus viridescens
  protozoans, 278, 283,
    285, 294, 296-
    297, 308, 361
Triturus vulgaris
  protozoans, 283, 302,
    349-350, 360-361
Tropidurus hispidus
  protozoans, 455-456
Tropidurus torquatus
  arboviruses, 120
  protozoans, 462
Trypanosoma
  classification, 391-395,
    401
  diagnosis, 406
  distribution, 395-400
  host specificity, 406-
    407

Trypanosoma (continued)
  pathogenesis and pathol-
    ogy, 402-406
Tunetella, 475-476
Tupinambis
  helminths, 220, 241
  hypovitaminosis, 643
  neoplasia, 522
Tupinambis nigropunctatus
  fungi, 186
  neoplasia, 534, 548, 552
Tupinambis rufescens
  neoplasia, 534, 548
Tupinambis teguixin
  bacteria, 60-63
  neoplasia, 534, 552
  protozoans, 420, 428, 432-
    433, 446
Tyzzeria, 339

Urinary system
  histology of, 740-743
  necropsy of, 709
Uromastix
  filiariasis, 498
  protozoans, 276
Uromastix acanthinurus
  neoplasia, 533, 549
Uromastix hardwickii
  bacteria, 74
  protozoans, 361
Urophagus, 284
Urosaurus ornatus
  bacteria, 60
Urotaenia, 111, 112
Uta stansburiana
  histology of, 748
  protozoans, 326, 416-417
Uukuniemi virus, 119

Vahlkampfia, 323
Varanus
  fungi, 197
  helminths, 220, 241
  hypovitaminosis, 643
  neoplasia, 535
  protozoans, 295
Varanus bengalensis
  neoplasia, 534, 549
  protozoans, 288
  neoplasia, 534, 549

Varanus dracoena
 neoplasia, 534, 553
Varanus gouldii
 protozoans, 326
Varanus griseus
 protozoans, 338
Varanus komodoensis
 neoplasia, 534, 548-549, 554
 protozoans, 312
Varanus niloticus
 neoplasia, 535, 549
 protozoans, 288, 303, 309
Varanus salvator
 lipoproteins, 137
 neoplasia, 535, 549-550
 protozoans, 318
Varanus varius
 protozoans, 326
Vasotrema, 252
Vatacrarus, 409
Venom
 and bacteria, 75
 and herpesviruses, 160, 162
 neutralization of, 694-697
 reactions to, 693-694
Vesicular stomatitis virus, 118-121
Vipera ammodytes
 bacteria, 73
Vipera berus
 neoplasia, 541
Vipera palestinae
 neoplasia, 541, 557
 venom neutralization, 694
Vipera russellii
 neoplasia, 522, 541, 563-564
 protozoans, 281, 291, 330
Vipera xanthina
 bacteria, 38
Viperidae
 age of, 626
Vitamin disorders, 640-650

Waddycephalus, 206
Walterinnesia aegyptia
 venom neutralization, 694

Water deprivation, 633-636
Wenyonella, 339
White muscle disease, 650

Xantusia
 protozoans, 276, 282, 291, 297, 361
Xenodon
 bacteria, 84
Xenodon merremi
 protozoans, 396
Xenodon neuwiedii
 protozoans, 396
Xenopus laevis
 bacteria, 6
 glomerulosclerosis, 628
 immunity in, 677-680
 protozoans, 288, 296, 302, 360
Xiphophorus
 neoplasia, 525

Zelleriella, 300-301, 303
Zoonosis, 180, 208, 211